LIVER BIOPSY INTERPRETATION

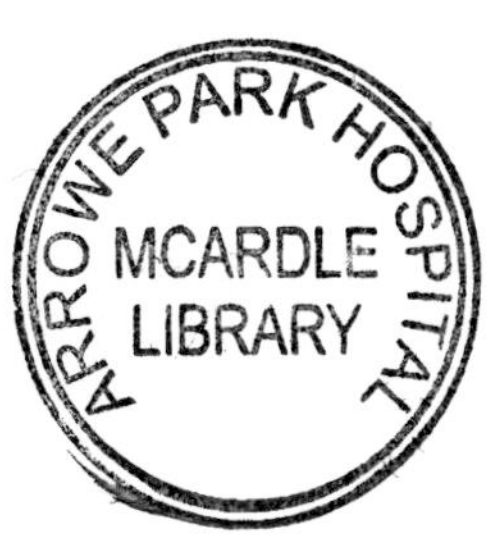

Commissioning Editor: Michael J. Houston
Project Development Manager: Sheila Black
Project Manager: Kathryn Mason
Production Assistant: Gemma Lawson
Senior Designer: Sarah Russell
Illustration Manager: Mick Ruddy
Illustrator: Deborah Maizels
Marketing Managers: Leontine Treur (UK), Ethel Cathers (US)

SEVENTH EDITION

LIVER BIOPSY INTERPRETATION

PETER J. SCHEUER
Professor Emeritus (Histopathology)
Royal Free & University College Medical School of University College London

JAY H. LEFKOWITCH
Professor of Clinical Pathology
College of Physicians & Surgeons of Columbia University
New York

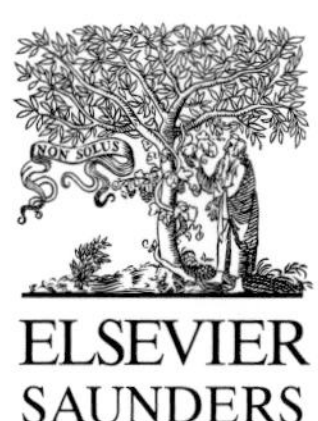

ELSEVIER
SAUNDERS

ELSEVIER
SAUNDERS

First edition 1968
Second edition 1973
Third edition 1980
Fourth edition 1988
Fifth edition 1994
Sixth edition 2000
Seventh edition 2005
Reprinted 2006

ISBN 1 4160 2621 5

British Library Cataloguing in Publication Data
A catalogue record for this book is available from the British Library

Library of Congress Cataloguing in Publication Data
A catalogue record for this book is available from the Library of Congress

Notice

Medical knowledge is constantly changing. Standard safety precautions must be followed, but as new research and clinical experience broaden our knowledge, changes in treatment and drug therapy may become necessary r appropriate. Readers are advised to check the most current product information provided by the manufactacturer or of each drug to be administered to verify the recommended dose, the method and duration of administration, and contraindications. It is the responsibility of the practitioner, relying on experience and knowledge of the patient, to determine dosages and the best treatment for each individual patient. Neither the Publisher nor the editors assume any liability for any injury and/or damage to persons or property arising from this publication.

The Publisher

Printed in China
C/02

The publisher's policy is to use **paper manufactured from sustainable forests**

Contents

Preface

For the first time since this book appeared in 1968 there is no foreword. Sheila Sherlock generously contributed a foreword to each of the first six editions. Sadly, she died in 2001. She was our teacher, friend and esteemed colleague and a great supporter of our efforts. We felt that it would not be appropriate or indeed possible to replace her and decided that the foreword should be omitted. We dedicate this edition to her memory. We also mourn the loss of Kamal Ishak, a great hepatopathologist who throughout his long career at the Armed Forces Institute of Pathology in Washington made important contributions to our knowledge of liver disease. The influence of Sheila Sherlock and Kamal Ishak remains with us, as does the teaching of Hans Popper.

Several changes mark the new edition. The most obvious is that virtually all black and white illustrations have now been replaced with figures in colour, leaving only naturally monochrome subjects such as silver impregnations and electron micrographs. Because of this and the need to illustrate a few more conditions, the seventh edition contains 141 new figures.

In spite of that, we have made strenuous efforts to keep the size of the book appropriate for its purpose. This emphasises once more our belief that a book used by pathologists at the bench should be reasonably concise and the information in it easily accessible. The pathologist or clinician faced with an immediate diagnostic problem should, we believe, be able to look up the relevant part of the book without spending a great deal of time. We have achieved this by rigorous editing of some chapters, by deleting figures which we considered no longer necessary and by keeping chapter bibliographies as short as possible. We apologise to those authors whose older papers have been omitted; no offence is intended and readers searching for old papers are advised to consult internet sources, larger textbooks or previous editions of this one. As before, we have provided lists of further general reading at the end of each chapter for those who want to explore a particular topic in greater depth.

Peter J. Scheuer
Jay H. Lefkowitch
2005

Acknowledgements

We are once more grateful to our colleagues, both pathologists and clinicians, who have maintained our knowledge of liver pathology by asking our opinion on liver biopsies. This book is particularly addressed to them.

The technical staff of the laboratories of the Royal Free Hospital, London and of the College of Physicians and Surgeons of Columbia University, New York provided us with excellent sections for photomicroscopy. For most of the new colour illustrations, this work was superbly done in London by Mr John Difford. Dr Kay Savage, Mr Paul Bates and Mr Francis Moll gave invaluable advice on digital photomicroscopy and on the subsequent editing of photographs for publication. Mr Neal Byron gave expert advice on laboratory techniques. In New York, histology manager Sunilda Valladares-Silva and her responsive technical team provided consistently high quality liver biopsy slides and special stains. Casey Schadie assisted with preparation of the manuscript. Several generous donors of slides and figures are acknowledged in the appropriate captions.

Our colleagues on both sides of the Atlantic helped us by critically evaluating parts of the new edition and by giving us the user's point of view. American colleagues helping in this way included Dr Elizabeth Brunt and Dr Neil Theise. In Europe, special thanks are due to Professor Paul Dhillon, Dr Alberto Quaglia, Professor Tania Roskams, Dr Richard Standish and Dr Claire Craig.

Finally, it has been a pleasure and a privilege to work with our publishers. Michael Houston, Sheila Black and Kathryn Mason of Elsevier supported our efforts throughout the planning and preparation of the seventh edition and contributed much to a book which we hope will help and please our readers.

GENERAL CONSIDERATIONS

Liver biopsy is one of many diagnostic tools used in the evaluation and management of patients with liver disease. Amidst a proliferation of radiological methods, gene tests and molecular studies, liver biopsy continues to play an important role because the concepts and classification of liver disease are rooted in morphology. Moreover, looking at a liver biopsy specimen under the microscope is a very direct way of visualising the morphologic changes that affect the liver in disease. The pathologist's *interpretation* (rather than mere enumeration) of these changes is used to answer important clinical questions such as disease causation and activity and the effects of therapy. A thorough and informed interpretation of liver biopsy findings therefore stands to have substantial impact on patient care. Questions of a more basic pathobiological nature can also be addressed by applying contemporary techniques of molecular and genomic medicine to liver biopsy material.

There are many reasons for liver biopsy[1] (Table 1.1), as will be apparent from the contents of this book. Establishing a tissue diagnosis of neoplastic disease, evaluation of jaundice of uncertain cause and assessment of pyrexia of unknown aetiology continue to be common diagnostic problems. Other issues have more recently gained emphasis, such as the grading and staging of chronic hepatitis,[2] which now occupies a sizeable portion of the pathologist's workload, especially for chronic viral hepatitis B and C. Formal scoring is often requested in these cases and several systems are available to choose from (these are discussed further in Ch. 9). In evaluating abnormal liver function tests in patients with negative serologic studies, liver biopsy is rarely normal.[3] In this regard, the importance of non-alcoholic fatty liver disease (NAFLD) (discussed in Ch. 7) as a major cause of abnormal serum aminotransferase levels[4] has grown with the widespread prevalence of obesity and diabetes, and liver biopsy is often obtained to investigate this possibility. The work-up of liver

Table 1.1 Reasons for liver biopsy

Evaluation of abnormal liver function tests
Investigation of pyrexia of unknown aetiology
Diagnosis of neoplasms
Evaluation of ascites and portal hypertension
Grading and staging of chronic hepatitis
Documentation of steatosis and its possible complications
Evaluation of liver dysfunction after liver, kidney and bone marrow transplantation
Investigation of jaundice of unclear aetiology
Monitoring effects of therapy

dysfunction following liver, kidney or bone marrow transplantation is also reliant on information from liver biopsies which must be reported promptly and with due consideration that the pathological changes in these patients may reflect more than one aetiologic factor.

TYPE AND ADEQUACY OF LIVER BIOPSY SPECIMEN

Several liver biopsy techniques and routes are now available for use (Table 1.2), each with inherent diagnostic advantages and disadvantages. Those with an interest in the history of liver biopsy, including the methods, risks, indications and contraindications will find this topic well covered in standard textbooks,[5] reviews[1] and editorials.[6,7] Liver biopsy is an invasive technique which requires a skilled operator and all possible safeguards to minimise the risk of complications. Precise guidelines vary from one centre to another.[8] Following the biopsy procedure, the needle track may be plugged with gelatine sponge (Fig. 1.1) or other materials[9] (Fig. 1.2)[10] to prevent bleeding.[11] The standard percutaneous suction needle biopsy popularised by Menghini[12] continues to be in active use, while biopsy samples obtained with thin needles under CT guidance and by the transjugular route are now seen more often. Whatever method is chosen, the operator should carefully consider whether the specimen obtained is likely to be adequate for the intended purpose. For example, a small needle specimen obtained with a small-bore needle guided by ultrasound or CT scan may be adequate for the diagnosis of hepatocellular carcinoma, but not necessarily suitable for the diagnosis and histological evaluation of chronic hepatitis.[13] With needles of the Menghini type, the biopsy core is aspirated and may fragment if the liver is cirrhotic. (This is discussed further in Ch. 10.) Cutting needles have been reported to produce better specimens,[14] but in patients with focal lesions, aspiration needles often sample both the lesion itself and the adjacent liver;[15] this is helpful in planning treatment.

Biopsy pathology differs from autopsy pathology in that there are pitfalls peculiar to small samples. A needle biopsy specimen of liver represents perhaps one fifty-thousandth of the whole organ and there is therefore an obvious possibility of sampling error. Some diseases of the liver are diffuse and involve every lobule, so that sampling error is unlikely; these can be diagnosed with confidence even in small specimens. A diagnosis of acute viral hepatitis can be established in a needle specimen only a few millimetres long whereas a specimen of similar size may not

Table 1.2 Liver biopsy techniques and routes

- Percutaneous
  - Suction (e.g. Menghini, Klatskin, Jamshidi needles)
  - Cutting (e.g. Vim-Silverman, Tru-cut needles)
  - Spring-loaded
- Transjugular
- Thin-needle with ultrasound/CT guidance
- Laparoscopic
- Operative wedge
- Fine-needle aspiration

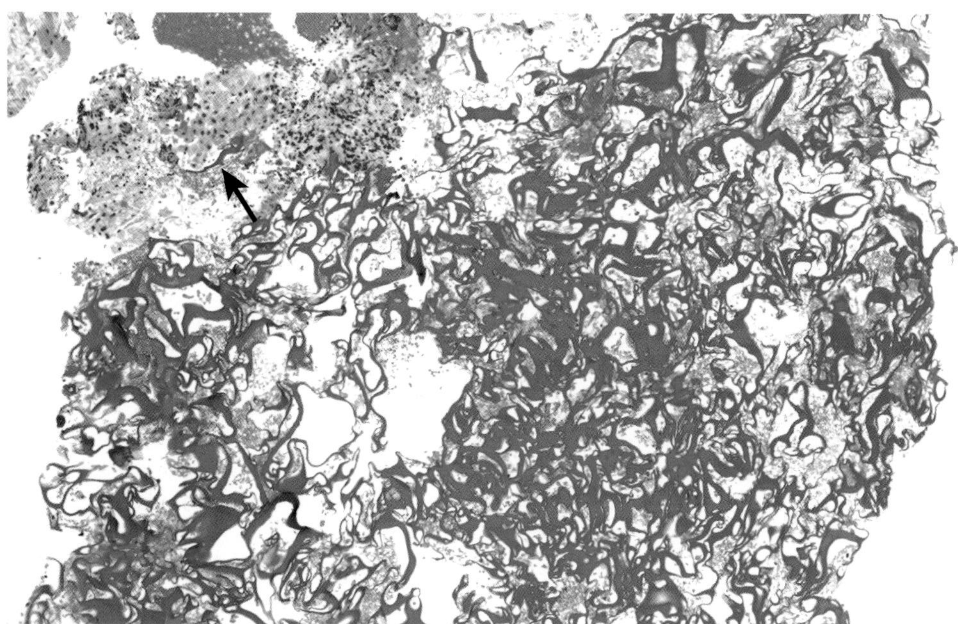

Figure 1.1 *Foreign material*. This is absorbable gelatine, which was used to plug a needle track. A small amount of liver tissue is seen at the point of the arrow. (Needle biopsy, H&E).

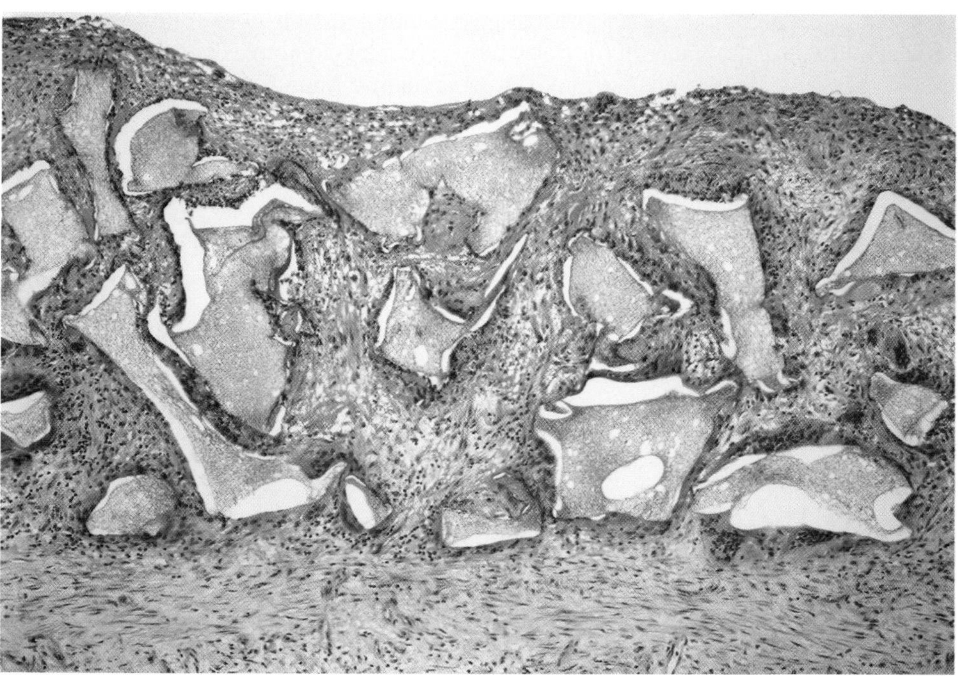

Figure 1.2 *Foreign material*. Material used to plug a needle track has here escaped and produced a peritoneal foreign-body giant cell reaction.[10] (H&E).

be adequate for the accurate diagnosis and evaluation of chronic liver disease,[16] for assessment of bile duct numbers or for the detection of focal lesions such as tumour deposits or granulomas. Focal or unevenly distributed lesions cannot be entirely excluded on the basis of their absence from an unguided needle biopsy specimen. When focal lesions are suspected, multiple biopsies may help to reduce sampling error.

Chronic hepatitis and cirrhosis present particular sampling problems. In some patients with hepatitis there is a zone of extensive necrosis immediately adjacent to the capsule, whereas the deeper parenchyma is less severely affected. A small specimen consisting of tissue from the subcapsular zone of the liver would then give a misleadingly pessimistic impression (Fig. 1.3). A related problem occurs in superficial wedge biopsies obtained surgically: the subcapsular zone often shows extensive fibrosis and accentuated nodularity in many forms of hepatitis and vascular disease and may result in the over-diagnosis of cirrhosis. The length of a biopsy core and the number of portal tracts present also have an impact on the accuracy of grading and staging chronic hepatitis.[16] In cirrhosis, the structure of a nodule is sometimes very similar to that of normal liver, so that a sample consisting almost entirely of the parenchyma from within a nodule may present serious diagnostic difficulties (Fig. 1.4). These are accentuated by the resistance of dense fibrous tissue; in a patient with cirrhosis an aspiration biopsy needle may glance off fibrous septa and selectively sample the softer nodular parenchyma. For this reason, some clinicians prefer to use cutting needles in patients with suspected cirrhosis.[17]

Abnormalities in a liver biopsy may represent changes remote from a pathological lesion rather than the lesion itself. In large bile duct obstruction, for example, the results of the obstruction are clearly seen in the biopsy sample whereas the cause of the obstruction is usually not visible. The biopsy may be taken from the vicinity of a focal liver lesion such as metastatic carcinoma and present one or more of a range of pathological features often puzzling to the interpreter[18] (Fig. 1.5). Similarly, disease elsewhere in the body may give rise to reactive changes in the liver; biopsy appearances are not normal, but at the same time do not indicate primary liver disease.

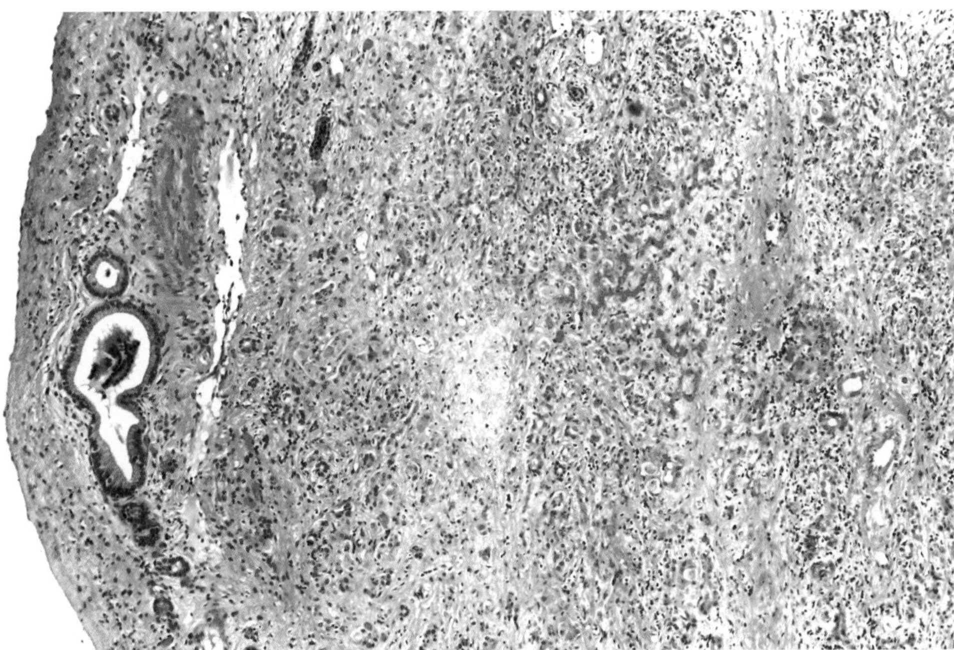

Figure 1.3 *Subcapsular necrosis*. There is a zone of multilobular necrosis immediately deep to the liver capsule (left) in this patient with chronic hepatitis. A small superficial sample would have presented problems of interpretation. (Needle biopsy, H&E).

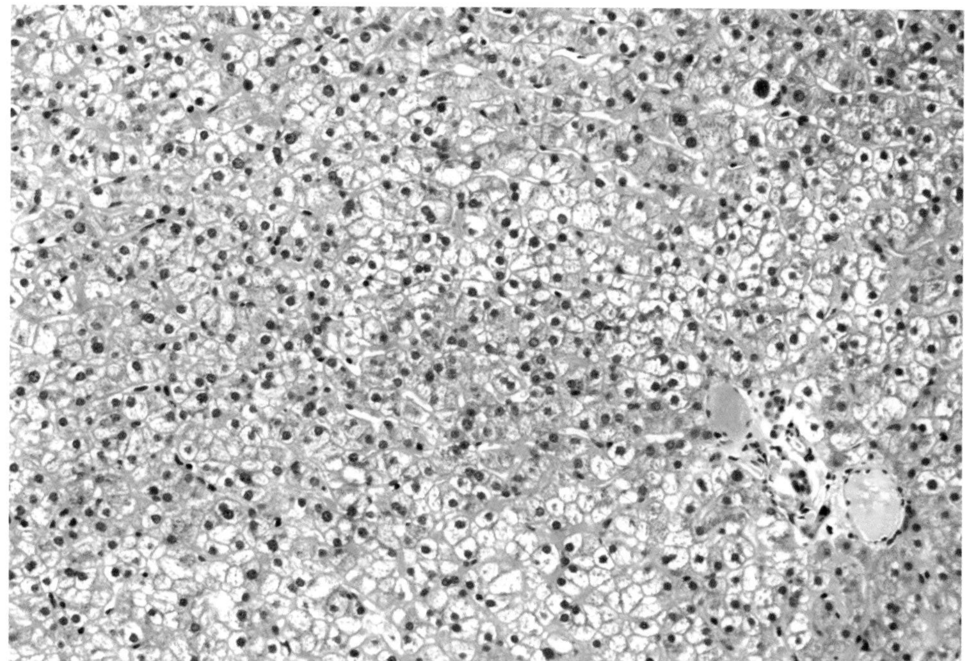

Figure 1.4 *Cirrhosis*. Appearances are nearly normal because the sample is from the centre of a nodule and does not include septa. A portal tract (at right, below centre) is small and poorly formed. (Needle biopsy, H&E).

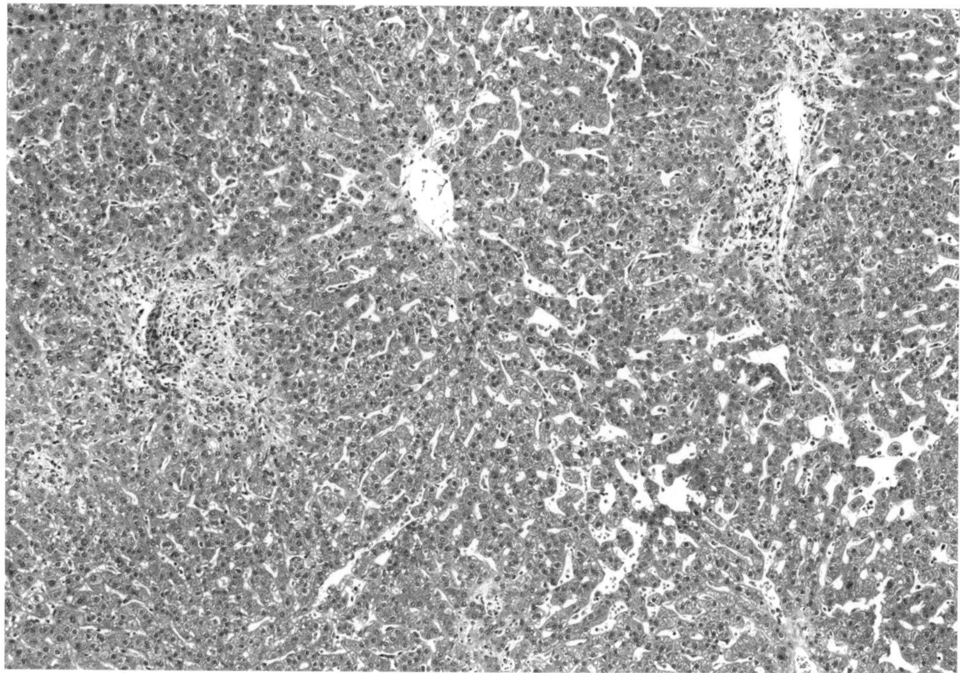

Figure 1.5 *Changes near metastatic tumour*. Portal changes like those of biliary obstruction are seen at left and top right, and there is sinusoidal dilatation in the perivenular area below right. (Needle biopsy, H&E).

Biopsies reveal lesions or diseases rarely seen at autopsy because of their relatively benign course, such as sarcoidosis. In other conditions, the evolution of a disease to an end stage means that the earlier and more characteristic pathological features are rarely seen at autopsy or even at liver transplantation. In such cases, liver biopsies provide valuable insights into the pathology of the disease.

Liver biopsy does not always provide a final or complete diagnosis. Sometimes it even fails to give helpful information. In most cases, however, an adequate and properly processed biopsy is an important item among the diagnostic tests to which the patient is subjected. The relatively limited range of morphological reactions of the liver to injury determines a need for full clinical, biochemical, immunological and imaging data to complement the biopsy findings. Pathologists need this information in order to avoid writing clinically unhelpful or even misleading reports, though they may prefer to read the slides before the clinical data to avoid bias.[19] Conversely, it is important that pathologists should produce clear and full reports on the biopsy findings for their clinical colleagues. Every report should attempt to answer one or more clinical questions, whether or not these are explicitly stated on the request form. The use of a standardised checklist has been advocated as a means of ensuring that no potentially useful information is omitted.[20] However, most pathologists currently write unstructured reports. These can be supplemented by a summary giving the essential message which the pathologist wants to convey.

THE SPECIMEN AT THE BEDSIDE AND IN THE LABORATORY

Before a liver biopsy is undertaken, the clinician may wish to discuss with the pathologist the need for any special treatment of the specimen such as freezing part of the specimen or taking tissue for electron microscopy.[19] Accurate assessment of the often subtle changes in a liver biopsy requires sections of high quality. The pathologist is usually aware of possible artefacts in liver biopsy material, as in any histological specimen. Artefacts should obviously be avoided whenever possible and recognised as such when they do occur. A biopsy of adequate size may be made undiagnosable by rough handling (Fig. 1.6), poor fixation, overheating, poor microtome technique and bad staining, all of which can obscure the criteria on which histological diagnoses are based. Poor fixation sometimes leads to potentially confusing liver-cell swelling, recognisable as artefact by its location away from the edges of the specimen (Fig. 1.7). False-positive staining for iron is evident when the staining is unrelated to particular cells or structures, or is in a different focal plane from the tissue.

This book is mainly about changes seen in conventionally-stained paraffin sections and cytological preparations. There are many other ways of looking at or investigating a tissue sample, some of them helpful in routine diagnosis. Several remain research tools for the time being but may become routine tests in the future. Immunocytochemical staining of tissue sections is particularly helpful for the detection of components of the hepatitis B virus (Figs 1.8,1.9), the hepatitis D virus (Fig. 6.16), cytomegalovirus and other infective agents. It is the most accurate way of diagnosing an α_1-antitrypsin deficiency morphologically. It is increasingly used as a research tool to study the expression and distribution of cytokeratins, cytokines, receptor molecules, matrix components, lymphocyte markers and other proteins. It is helpful in the diagnosis of neoplasms of doubtful histogenesis or differentiation

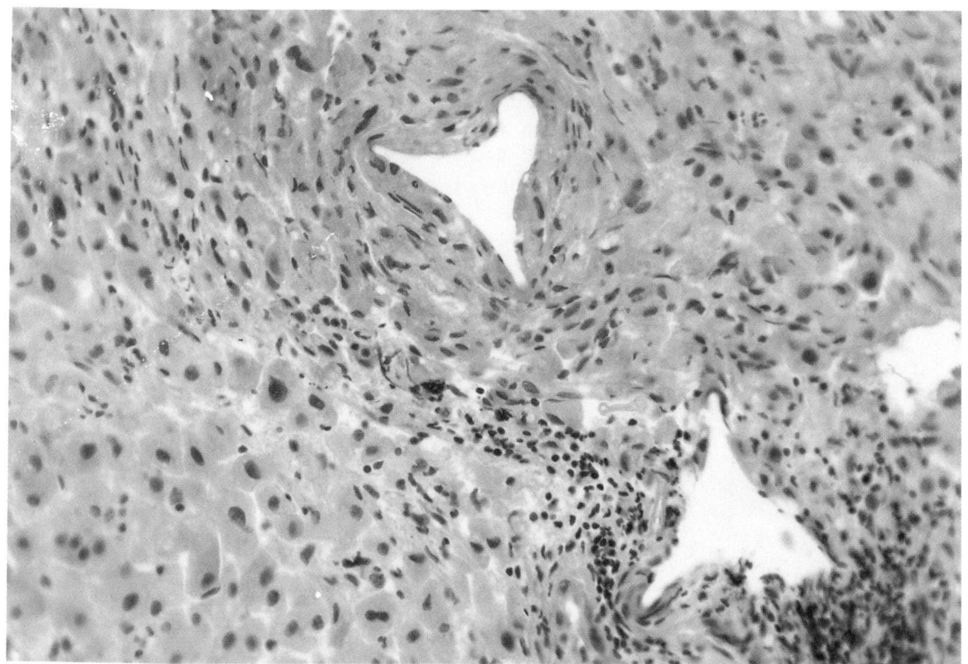

Figure 1.6 *Traumatic artefact*. The triangular spaces, which slightly resemble blood vessels, are artefacts caused by rough packing of the specimen between pieces of foam sponge (H&E).

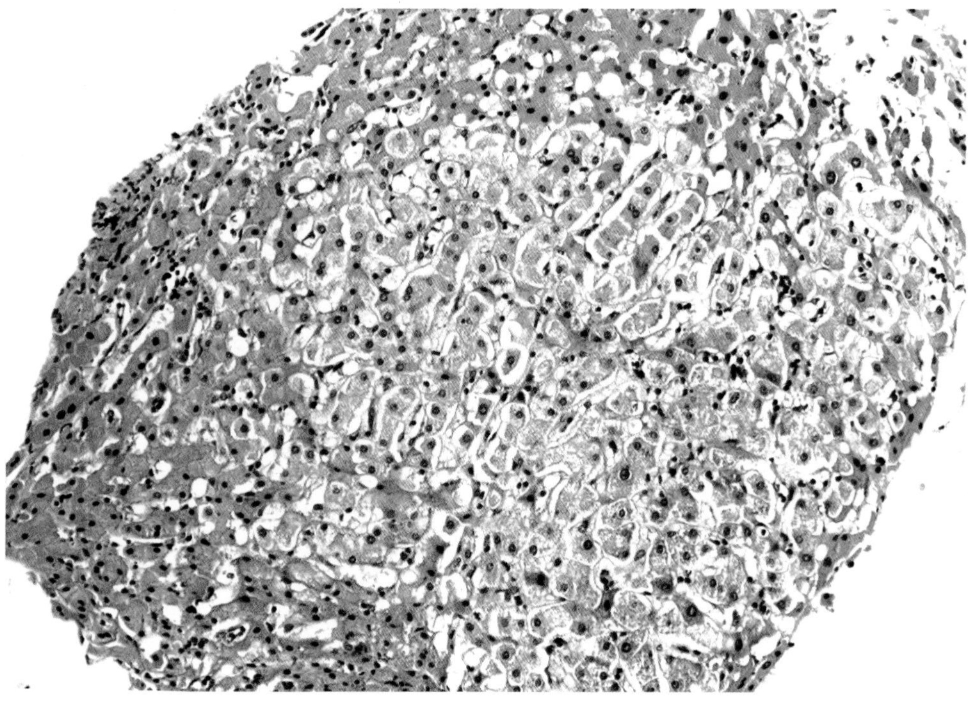

Figure 1.7 *Fixation artefact*. Hepatocytes in the central part of the specimen are swollen and pale-staining because of poor fixation. (Needle biopsy, H&E).

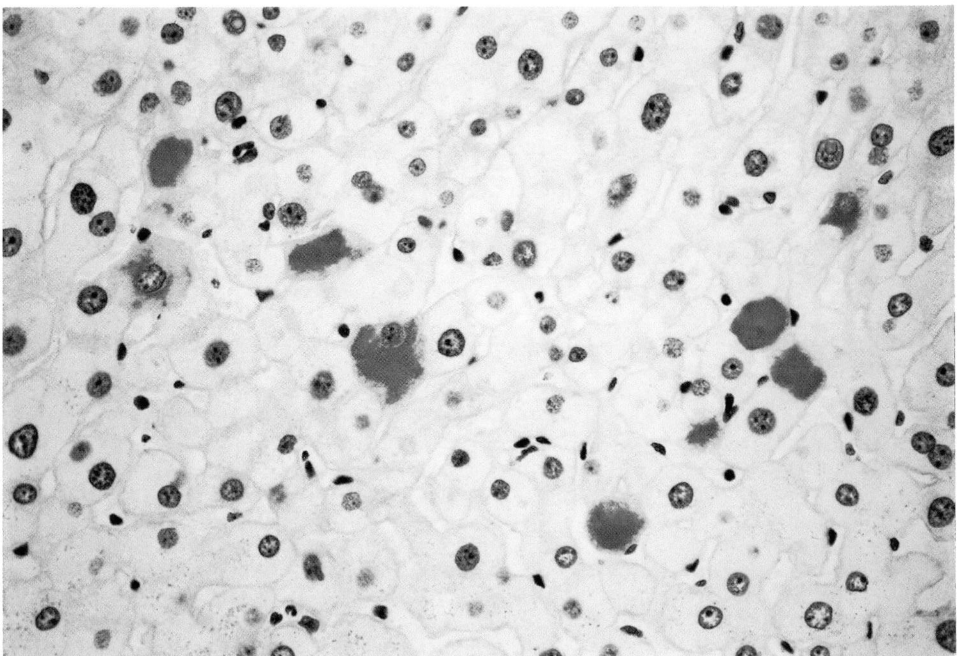

Figure 1.8 *Immunocytochemical demonstration of hepatitis B surface antigen (HBsAg).* Much of the cytoplasm is intensely stained in a minority of hepatocytes. These correspond to the ground-glass cells seen with other stains. (Needle biopsy, specific immunoperoxidase).

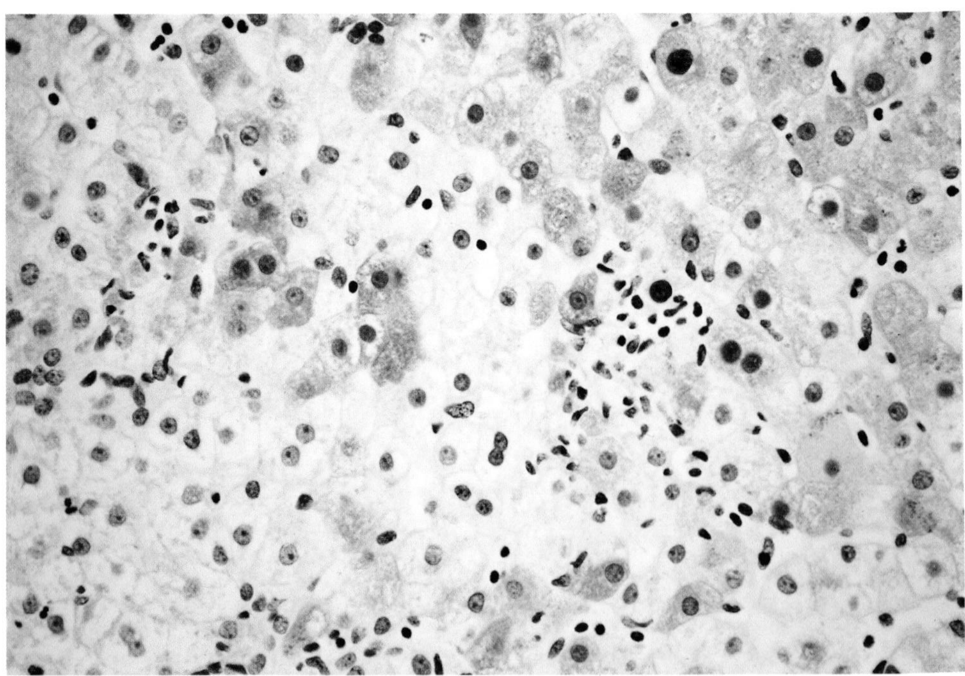

Figure 1.9 *Immunocytochemical demonstration of hepatitis B core antigen (HBcAg).* There is intense nuclear staining in several hepatocytes, as well as weaker cytoplasmic positivity. (Needle biopsy, specific immunoperoxidase).

and of hepatocellular carcinoma. Specific uses of immunocytochemistry are quoted in the appropriate chapters. Electron microscopy has a limited but well-defined place in liver pathology and is dealt with in the final chapter of this book.

In situ hybridisation has been applied to liver tissue for the identification or assessment of replication of hepatitis viruses and cytomegalovirus (Fig. 1.10). The polymerase chain reaction (PCR) can be applied to liver tissue[21,22] and provides more direct evidence of virus infection in the liver than serum PCR. DNA extracted from biopsy tissue has been used to test for the C282Y mutation of hereditary haemochromatosis[23,24] and for the PiZ mutation of α_1-antitrypsin.[25] Gene chip microarray analysis of liver tissue[26] holds the promise of making direct correlations between alterations defined in the genome and morphological changes.

Part of the biopsy specimen can be analysed for copper, iron or abnormally stored substances, and enzyme activities can be assayed by micromethods. In the case of copper and iron, these measurements can, if necessary, be made after paraffin embedding, as discussed in Chapter 14. Elution of Sirius red from sections provides an accurate method for the measurement of tissue collagen[27] and this stain is also used for image analysis of collagen.[28–30] *In situ* demonstration of enzymes can be achieved by immunocytochemical methods or by means of enzyme histochemistry and has provided convincing evidence of metabolic zonation in human liver.[31,32]

Well-established techniques of morphometry and image analysis have been applied to tissue sections to obtain data on relative volumes of tissue components in normal human liver[33,34] and in disease.[28–30,35,36] Three-dimensional reconstruction using a computer has helped in the understanding of disease processes and of the relationship between anatomical structures,[37–39] but is not yet a diagnostic tool for everyday use.

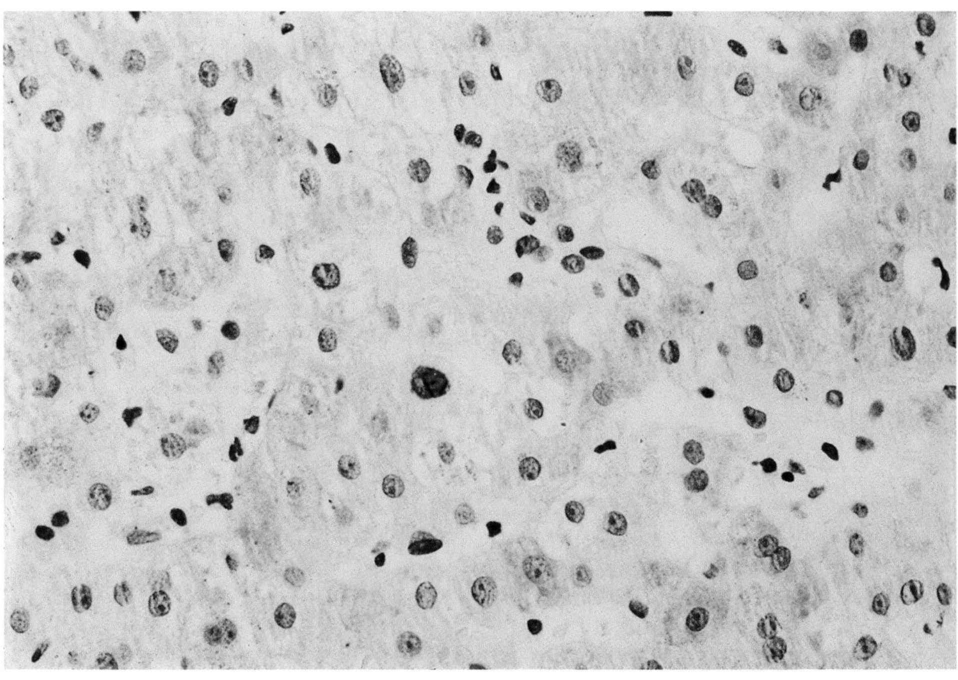

Figure 1.10 *In situ hybridization for cytomegalovirus DNA.* Positive staining of a hepatocyte nucleus (centre) indicates presence of viral DNA. (Fig. kindly provided by Dr Neil Theise, New York).

REFERENCES

1 Bravo AA, Sheth SG, Chopra S. Liver biopsy. *N Engl J Med* 2001; **344**: 495–500.
2 Brunt EM. Grading and staging the histopathological lesions of chronic hepatitis: the Knodell histology activity index and beyond. *Hepatology* 2000; **31**: 241–246.
3 Skelly MM, James PD, Ryder SD. Findings on liver biopsy to investigate abnormal liver function tests in the absence of diagnostic serology. *J Hepatol* 2001; **35**: 195–199.
4 Clark JM, Brancati FL, Diehl AM. Nonalcoholic fatty liver disease. *Gastroenterology* 2002; **122**: 1649–1657.
5 Sherlock S, Dooley J. Diseases of the Liver and Biliary System, 11th edn. Oxford: Blackwell Science, 2002: 37–46.
6 Bianchi L. Liver biopsy in elevated liver functions tests? An old question revisited. *J Hepatol* 2001; **35**: 290–294.
7 Demetris AJ, Ruppert K. Pathologist's perspective on liver needle biopsy size? *J Hepatol* 2003; **39**: 275–277.
8 Sue M, Caldwell SH, Dickson RC, et al. Variation between centers in technique and guidelines for liver biopsy. *Liver* 1996; **16**: 267–270.
9 Thompson NP, Scheuer PJ, Dick R, et al. Intraperitoneal Ivalon mimicking peritoneal malignancy after plugged percutaneous liver biopsy. *Gut* 1993; **34**: 16–35.
10 Mican JM, Di Bisceglie AM, Fong T-L, et al. Hepatic involvement in mastocytosis: clinicopathologic correlations in 41 cases. *Hepatology* 1995; **22**: 1163–1170.
11 Sawyer AM, McCormick PA, Tennyson GS, et al. A comparison of transjugular and plugged-percutaneous liver biopsy in patients with impaired coagulation. *J Hepatol* 1993; **17**: 81–85.
12 Menghini G. One-second needle biopsy of the liver. *Gastroenterology* 1958; **35**: 190–199.
13 Petz D, Klauck S, Röhl et al. Feasibility of histological grading and staging of chronic viral hepatitis using specimens obtained by thin-needle biopsy. *Virchows Arch* 2003; **442**: 238–244.
14 Sada PN, Ramakrishna B, Thomas CP, et al. Transjugular liver biopsy: a comparison of aspiration and Trucut techniques. *Liver* 1997; **17**: 257–259.
15 Van Leeuwen DJ. Liver biopsy. In: Tytgat GNJ, Mulder CJJ, eds. Procedures in Hepatogastroenterology, 2nd edn. Dordrecht: Kluwer, 1997: 193.
16 Colloredo G, Guido M, Sonzogni A, et al. Impact of liver biopsy size on histological evaluation of chronic viral hepatitis: the smaller the sample, the milder the disease. *J Hepatol* 2003; **39**: 239–244.
17 Colombo M, Ninno E Del, Francis R de, et al. Ultrasound-assisted percutaneous liver biopsy: superiority of the Tru-Cut over the Menghini needle for diagnosis of cirrhosis. *Gastroenterology* 1988; **95**: 487–489.
18 Gerber MA, Thung SN, Bodenheimer HC Jr. et al. Characteristic histologic triad in liver adjacent to metastatic neoplasm. *Liver* 1986; **6**: 85–88.
19 Desmet VJ. What more can we ask from the pathologist? *J Hepatol* 1996; **25 (Suppl 1)**: 25–29.
20 Foschini M, Sarti F, Dina RE, et al. Standardized reporting of histological diagnoses for non-neoplastic liver conditions in needle biopsies. *Virchows Arch* 1995; **426**: 593–596.
21 Lau GKK, Davis GL, Wu SPC, et al. Hepatic expression of hepatitis C virus RNA in chronic hepatitis C: a study by in situ reverse-transcription polymerase chain reaction. *Hepatology* 1996; **23**: 1318–1323.
22 O'Leary JJ, Chetty R, Graham AK, et al. In situ PCR: pathologist's dream or nightmare? *J Pathol* 1996; **178**: 11–20.
23 Aldersley MA, Howdle PD, Wyatt JI, et al. Haemochromatosis gene mutation in liver disease patients. *Lancet* 1997; **349**: 1025–1026.
24 Press RD, Flora K, Gross C, et al. Hepatic iron overload. Direct HFE (HLA-H) mutation analysis vs. quantitative iron assays for the diagnosis of hereditary hemochromatosis. *Am J Clin Pathol* 1998; **109**: 577–584.
25 Ortiz-Pallardó ME, Ko Y, Sachinidis A, et al. Detection of alpha-1-antitrypsin PiZ individuals by SSCP and DNA sequencing in formalin-fixed and paraffin-embedded tissue: a comparison with immunohistochemical analysis. *J Hepatol* 2000; **32**: 406–411.

26 Sreekumar R, Rosado B, Rasmussen D, et al. Hepatic gene expression in histologically progressive nonalcoholic steatohepatitis. *Hepatology* 2003; **38**: 244–251.
27 Jimenez W, Pares A, Caballeria J, et al. Measurement of fibrosis in needle liver biopsies: evaluation of a colorimetric method. *Hepatology* 1985; **5**: 815–818.
28 Chevallier M, Guerret S, Chossegros P, et al. A histological semiquantitative scoring system for evaluation of hepatic fibrosis in needle liver biopsy specimens: comparison with morphometric studies. *Hepatology* 1994; **20**: 349–355.
29 Pilette C, Rousselet MC, Bedossa P, et al. Histopathological evaluation of liver fibrosis: quantitative image analysis vs semi-quantitative scores. *J Hepatol* 1998; **28**: 439–446.
30 Masseroli M, Caballero T, O'Valle F, et al. Automatic quantification of liver fibrosis: design and validation of a new image analysis method: comparison with semi-quantitative indexes of fibrosis. *J Hepatol* 2000; **32**: 453–464.
31 Lamers WH, Hilberts A, Furt E, et al. Hepatic enzymic zonation: a reevaluation of the concept of the liver acinus. *Hepatology* 1989; **10**: 72–76.
32 Sokal EM, Trivedi P, Cheeseman P, et al. The application of quantitative cytochemistry to study the acinar distribution of enzymatic activities in human liver biopsy sections. *J Hepatol* 1989; **9**: 42–48.
33 Ranek L, Keiding N, Jensen ST. A morphometric study of normal human liver cell nuclei. *Acta Pathol Microbiol Scand A* 1976; **83**: 467–476.
34 Rohr HP, Lüthy J, Gudat F, et al. Stereology: a new supplement to the study of human liver biopsy specimens. In: Popper H, Schaffner F, eds. Progress in Liver Diseases, Vol. V, 1st edn. New York, NY: Grune & Stratton, 1976: 24.
35 Kage M, Shimamatu K, Nakashima E, et al. Long-term evolution of fibrosis from chronic hepatitis to cirrhosis in patients with hepatitis C: morphometric analysis of repeated biopsies. *Hepatology* 1997; **25**: 1028–1031.
36 Casali AM, Carbone G, Cavalli G. Intrahepatic bile duct loss in primary sclerosing cholangitis: a quantitative study. *Histopathology* 1998; **32**: 449–453.
37 Yamada S, Howe S, Scheuer PJ. Three-dimensional reconstruction of biliary pathways in primary biliary cirrhosis: a computer-assisted study. *J Pathol* 1987; **152**: 317–323.
38 Nagore N, Howe S, Boxer L, et al. Liver cell rosettes: structural differences in cholestasis and hepatitis. *Liver* 1989; **9**: 43–51.
39 Ludwig J, Ritman EL, LaRusso NF, et al. Anatomy of the human biliary system studied by quantitative computer-aided three-dimensional imaging techniques. *Hepatology* 1998; **27**: 893–899.

CHAPTER 2

LABORATORY TECHNIQUES

PROCESSING OF THE SPECIMEN

As soon as a needle biopsy specimen is obtained from the patient it should be expelled gently into fixative or onto a piece of glass, card or wood. Filter paper is less suitable because fibres tend to adhere to the tissue and may interfere with sectioning. The specimen must be treated with great care and excessive manipulation should be rigorously avoided; distortion of the specimen by rough handling at this stage may seriously interfere with accurate diagnosis, because diagnosis often depends on subtle criteria. At this stage, minute pieces can be put into an appropriate fixative for electron microscopy (Ch. 17), preferably by an operator experienced in this technique, and samples taken for chemical analysis or freezing. Frozen sections may be needed for demonstration of lipids. If porphyria is suspected, a very small amount of the unfixed tissue can be examined under ultraviolet light or with a suitable quartz halogen source, either whole or smeared onto a glass slide.

Tissue for paraffin embedding should be transferred to a fixative as soon as possible. When transit to the laboratory is likely to involve much movement, it is helpful to fill the container to the brim with fixative. Buffered formalin and formol saline are both suitable for routine fixation, which is accomplished after 3 h at room temperature or less at higher temperatures (Table 2.1). Operative wedge biopsies and larger specimens need longer fixation. Fixatives other than formalin are successfully

Table 2.1 Sample tissue schedules for liver biopsies

Agent	Manual	Routine overnight automatic	Routine overnight automatic (vacuum)[a]	Ultra-rapid automatic (vacuum)[a]
Buffered formalin	3 h	3 h	2 h	30 min
Formalin-ethanol-water (1:8:1)	overnight	–	–	–
70% ethanol	–	3 h	1 h	3 min
90% ethanol	–	3 h	1 h	2 min
100% ethanol	2 × 1 h	2 × 2 h	3 × 1 h	3 × 2 min
Xylene	3 × 1 h	3 × 1 h	4 × 1 h	4 × 5 min
Wax (60°C)	2 × 1 h	2 × 1 h	3 × 1 h	3 × 5 min
Total time	24 h	18 h	14 h	1 h 16 min

[a]All at 50°C except for wax step.

used in some centres; handbooks of laboratory technique should be consulted for optimum times and conditions for each fixative.

Minute fragments can be hand-processed more quickly than larger pieces and this also avoids undue shrinkage and hardening. Automated vacuum embedding allows the time of processing of needle specimens to be drastically reduced, as shown in the table; the ultra-rapid method by which a good section can be produced in about 2 h has become important because of the need for rapid decisions on treatment in patients who have undergone liver transplantation. Frozen sections, occasionally needed for a decision at surgery, can be cut by a standard method using a cryostat. They are sometimes adequate for diagnosis of obvious lesions such as neoplasms, but are unsuitable for recognition of subtle changes, and can even be dangerously misleading.

The exact number of sections routinely cut from a block varies widely from one laboratory to another. In the laboratory of one of the authors, at the Royal Free Hospital in London, ten or more consecutive sections 3–5 μm thick are cut from each block and alternate sections used for the staining procedures outlined in the next paragraphs. The remaining sections are stored. Step sections are used when discrete lesions such as granulomas or tumour deposits are suspected and for serial biopsies following liver transplantation. Large numbers of serial or near-serial sections rarely contribute to the diagnosis.

CHOICE OF STAINS

The stains routinely applied to liver biopsies vary according to local custom. The minimum advised is a haematoxylin and eosin (H&E) and a reliable method for connective tissue. The authors prefer a silver preparation for reticulin as the principal method for showing connective tissue for reasons discussed below, but trichrome stains also have important applications and can reveal changes not easily seen in a reticulin, such as the pericellular fibrosis of steatohepatitis. Routine staining for iron enables the biopsy to be used to screen for iron storage disease and the periodic acid-Schiff stain after diastase digestion (DPAS or PASD) provides a relatively crude, but practicable screening procedure for α_1-antitrypsin deficiency as well as showing activated macrophages and bile-duct basement membranes. Stains for copper-associated protein, elastic fibres and hepatitis B surface antigen are useful and arguably essential additions to the routine list. Some pathologists like to see two haematoxylin and eosin-stained sections, one from the beginning and the other from the end of a series of consecutive sections. Other methods are used as required for particular purposes. The extent to which 'special' stains form part of the routine set must be decided by each pathologist.

A **reticulin** preparation is important for accurate assessment of structural changes. Without it, thin layers of connective tissue and hence cirrhosis may be missed, as may foci of well-differentiated hepatocellular carcinoma in which the reticulin structure is often highly abnormal (see Fig. 11.12). Counterstaining is sometimes used, but is apt to distract rather than help, bearing in mind that the chief function of the reticulin preparation is to provide a sensitive low-power indicator of structural changes.

Stains for **collagen** such as Chromotrope-aniline blue (CAB) are important for the detection of new collagen formation, especially in alcoholic steatohepatitis and its imitators (see Ch. 7). Collagen staining is therefore advised for any biopsy showing substantial steatosis. It also helps to show blocked veins within scars; these are easily missed on haematoxylin and eosin. It is therefore wise to do a trichrome when vascular disease is suspected.

A stain for **elastic fibres** such as the orcein stain, Victoria blue or elastic-Van Gieson is also useful to identify blocked vessels. The stains often enable the pathologist to distinguish between recent collapse and old fibrosis, since only the latter is positive (see Ch. 6). Again, this distinction may be very difficult to make on H&E and even with the help of stains for collagen and reticulin. The orcein and Victoria blue also show copper-associated protein and hepatitis B surface material.

Staining for **iron** by Perls' or other similar method enables not only iron but also bile, lipofuscin and other pigments to be evaluated, as discussed in Chapter 3. Counterstaining should be light to avoid obscuring small amounts of pigment.

Staining of **glycogen** by means of the PAS method or Best's carmine demonstrates the extent of any liver-cell loss, and shows focal areas devoid of hepatocytes such as granulomas. **Glycoproteins** may be demonstrated by the PAS method after digestion with diastase to remove glycogen. This stain serves to accentuate hypertrophied macrophages, such as Kupffer cells filled with ceroid pigment after an acute hepatitis or episode of cholestasis. Alpha$_1$-antitrypsin bodies stain strongly, but the stain is not sufficiently sensitive to enable all examples of α_1-antitrypsin deficiency to be detected.

Staining for **copper** is mainly used in suspected Wilson's disease, although, as explained in Chapter 14, it is not always helpful and may even be negative. The rhodanine method is preferred because it is easy to distinguish the orange-red colour of copper from bile, a distinction which is occasionally difficult with rubeanic acid. In Wilson's disease, there is variable correlation between the presence of stainable copper and staining for **copper-associated protein**. In chronic cholestasis, however, the two usually correspond.

Other non-immunological methods useful on occasion include the Ziehl-Neelsen stain for **mycobacteria** and for the ova of *Schistosoma mansoni*. Specific staining for **bilirubin** is rarely necessary, but conjugated bilirubin stains a bright green colour by the van Gieson method (Fig. 4.3). **Amyloid** is stained by the usual techniques.

For **immunohistochemical staining**, standard techniques are applied. Among antibodies which are helpful in everyday practice are those against components of the hepatitis B virus, the delta agent, cytomegalovirus and α_1-antitrypsin. Neoplasms of doubtful histogenesis or differentiation are investigated by appropriate panels of antibodies, as in any other organ. In hepatocellular carcinoma, bile canaliculi between tumour cells may stain with a polyclonal anti-CEA, cross-reacting with a canalicular antigen. Assessment of bile duct loss may require staining of cytokeratins 7 and 19, characteristic of bile-duct rather than liver-cell cytoplasm and of the ductular reaction (see Ch. 4). The application of immunohistochemistry as well as of other modern techniques is discussed in more detail in Chapter 17.

Most of the staining methods mentioned above are used routinely in many laboratories, and can be found in the books listed under General Reading at the end of this chapter. A selection of methods is given below.

Silver impregnation for reticulin fibres (Gordon and Sweets)

1. Bring section to distilled water.
2. Treat with acidified potassium permanganate for 10 min; wash in distilled water.
3. Leave section in 1% oxalic acid until pale (about 1 min). Wash well in several changes of distilled water.
4. Mordant in 2.5% iron alum for 10 min. Wash in several changes of distilled water.
5. Treat with silver solution until section is transparent (about 10–15 s). Wash in several changes of distilled water.
6. Reduce in 10% formalin (4% aqueous solution of formaldehyde) for 30 s. Wash in tap water followed by distilled water.
7. Tone if desired in 0.2% gold chloride for 1 min. Rinse in distilled water.
8. Fix in 2.5% sodium thiosulphate for 5 min. Wash several times in tap water.
9. Transfer section to ethanol, clear and mount.

Reticulin appears black. The colour of the collagen varies according to whether step 7 is used; in untoned preparations it is yellow-brown.

Silver solution

To 5 ml of 10% aqueous silver nitrate, add strong ammonia (sp. gr. 0.88) drop by drop until the precipitate which forms is just dissolved. Add 5 ml of 3% sodium hydroxide. Add strong ammonia drop by drop until the resulting precipitate dissolves. The solution does not clear completely. Make up to 50 ml with distilled water. Scrupulously clean glassware should be used throughout.

Acidified potassium permanganate

To 95 ml of 0.5% potassium permanganate, add 5 ml of 3% sulphuric acid.

Chromotrope – aniline blue (CAB) method for collagen and Mallory bodies

(As used at Mount Sinai Hospital, New York; modified from Roque[1] and Churg & Prado[2])

1. Bring section to water
2. Stain nuclei by the Celestine blue-Lillie Mayer sequence or other method. Rinse in distilled water.
3. Immerse in 1% phosphomolybdic acid for 1–3 min. Rinse well in distilled water.
4. Stain with CAB solution for 8 min. Rinse well in distilled water. Blot.
5. Dehydrate quickly, clear and mount.

Collagen is stained blue. Mallory bodies stain blue or sometimes red. Giant mitochondria stain red.

CAB solution

1.5 g aniline blue is dissolved in 2.5 ml HCl and 200 ml distilled water with gentle heat. 6 g Chromotrope 2R is added. The pH should be 1.0.

Orcein stain for copper-associated protein, elastic fibres and hepatitis B surface material[3]

1. Bring section to water.
2. Treat with acidified potassium permanganate for 15 min.
3. Rinse in water and de-colorise in 2% oxalic acid.
4. Rinse in distilled water, then wash in tap water for 3 min.
5. Stain in commercial orcein solution for 30–60 min, at room temperature.
6. Rinse in water, then differentiate if necessary in 1% HCl in 70% ethanol.
7. Dehydrate, clear and mount.

Elastic fibres, copper-associated protein and hepatitis B surface material (HBsAg) stain brown. The method is less sensitive for HBsAg than immunohistochemical techniques. However, of the components listed, copper-associated protein is often the most difficult to stain reliably. Natural orceins seem to be more satisfactory than synthetic ones, but are difficult or impossible to obtain. In case of difficulty, doubling the concentration of orcein and the amount of HCl may help (Hans Popper, personal communication).

Acidified potassium permanganate

To 95 ml of 0.5% potassium permanganate, add 5 ml of 3% sulphuric acid.

Rhodanine stain for copper[4]

1. Bring section to distilled water.
2. Incubate in rhodanine working solution for 18 h at 37°C or 3 h at 56°C.
3. Rinse in several changes of distilled water and stain with Carazzi's haematoxylin for 1 min.
4. Rinse with distilled water and then quickly in borax solution. Rinse well in distilled water.
5. Dehydrate, clear and mount.

Copper deposits stain bright red. Bile stains green. Weakly positive stains tend to fade, but fading can be reduced by staining at the higher temperature and by using certain mounting media (e.g. Ralmount (Raymond A. Lamb), DPX or Diatex). Note the two alternative times and temperatures for the rhodanine working solutions. The staining time can be shortened further.[5]

Rhodanine stock solution

p-Dimethylaminobenzylidene rhodanine	0.2 g
Ethanol	100 ml

The working solution is prepared by diluting 3 ml of the well-shaken stock solution with 47 ml distilled water.

Borax solution

Disodium tetraborate	0.5 g
Distilled water	100 ml

Victoria blue method for copper-associated protein, elastic fibres and hepatitis B surface material[6]

1. Bring section to distilled water.
2. Treat with acidified potassium permanganate (see Gordon & Sweets' reticulin, above) for 5 min.
3. Treat with 4% aqueous sodium metabisulphite for 1 min.
4. Wash in running tap water.
5. Wash well with 70% ethanol.
6. Stain in Victoria blue solution in a Coplin jar for a minimum of 4 h, and preferably overnight.
7. Wash well with 70% ethanol. This is the differentiation step; ensure that the background of the section is clear.
8. Wash in running tap water for 1 min.
9. Stain with nuclear fast red solution for 5 min.
10. Wash in running water for 2 min.
11. Dehydrate, clear and mount.

Copper-associated protein, elastic fibres and hepatitis B surface material are stained blue on a pink background.

Victoria blue solution

Distilled water	200 ml
Dextrine	0.5 g
Victoria blue	2 g
Resorcinol	4 g

Slowly warm the mixture of the above until it boils. Gradually add 25 ml of boiling 29% ferric chloride solution and boil for a further 3 min. Cool and filter through fine paper. Dry the filtrate on the filter paper to complete dryness in a 56°C oven. Dissolve the filtrate in 400 ml 70% ethanol. Finally add 4 ml concentrated HCl and 6 g phenol. The solution is best left for 2 weeks before use.

Nuclear fast red

Dissolve 0.1 g nuclear fast red in 100 ml warmed 5% aluminium sulphate. Filter when cool.

REFERENCES

1 Roque AL. Chromotrope aniline blue method of staining Mallory bodies of Laennec's cirrhosis. *Lab Invest* 1953; **2**: 15–21.

2 Churg J, Prado A. A rapid Mallory trichrome stain (Chromotrope-aniline blue). *Arch Pathol* 1956; **62**: 505–506.

3 Shikata T, Uzawa T, Yoshiwara N, et al. Staining methods of Australia antigen in paraffin section – detection of cytoplasmic inclusion bodies. *Jpn J Exp Med* 1974; **44**: 25–36.

4 Lindquist RR. Studies on the pathogenesis of hepatolenticular degeneration. II. Cytochemical methods for the localization of copper. *Arch Pathol* 1969; **87**: 370–379.

5 Emanuele P, Goodman ZD. A simple and rapid stain for copper in liver tissue. *Ann Diagn Pathol* 1998; **2**: 125–126.

6 Tanaka K, Mori W, Suwa K. Victoria blue-nuclear fast red stain for HBs antigen detection in paraffin section. *Acta Pathol Jpn* 1981; **31**: 93–98.

GENERAL READING

Bancroft JD, Gamble M, eds. Theory and Practice of Histological Techniques, 5th edn. London: Churchill Livingstone, 2002.

Kiernan JA. Histological and Histochemical Methods: Theory and Practice, 3rd edn. Oxford: Butterworth-Heinemann, 1999.

Polak JM, van Noorden S. Introduction to Immunocytochemistry, 2nd edn. Microscopy Handbooks 37. Oxford: Bios Scientific Publishers, 1997.

Prophet EB, Mills B, Arrington JB, Sobin LH, eds. Laboratory Methods in Histotechnology. Washington, DC: American Registry of Pathology, 1992.

CHAPTER 3

THE NORMAL LIVER

STRUCTURES AND COMPONENTS

Functional units and nomenclature

Under the low power of the microscope, normal liver is seen to have a regular structure based on portal tracts and efferent veins. The smallest portal tracts contain portal venules, hepatic arterioles and small interlobular bile ducts. Blood from both venules and arterioles passes through the sinusoidal system to reach efferent hepatic venules. From these, the blood drains into successively larger veins to reach the inferior vena cava. Bile flows from the smallest ducts into larger ducts, to reach the small intestine by way of the common bile duct.

The functional relationship between these various structures has been the subject of much debate. The most widely used models are the classic lobule and Rappaport's acinus.[1] The lobule has an efferent venule at its centre and portal tracts at its periphery (Fig. 3.1). The acinus is based on a terminal portal tract, with blood passing from this, through successively less well-oxygenated parenchymal zones 1, 2 and 3, to efferent venules. It is worth emphasising that both lobules and acini are concepts rather than fixed anatomical structures. Several other models have been

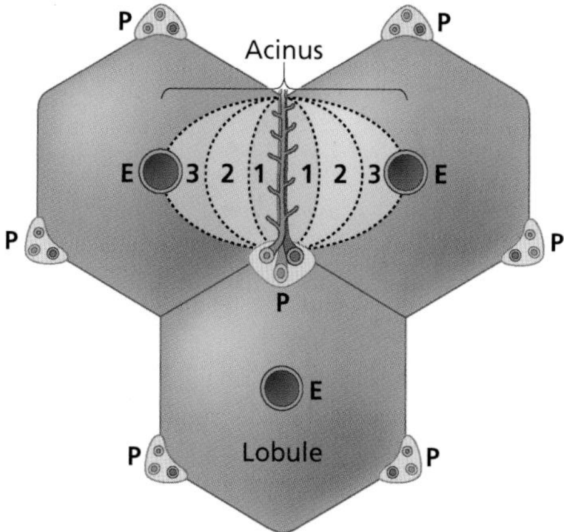

Figure 3.1 *Diagrammatic representation* of a simple acinus and its division into zones 1, 2 and 3, with three adjacent lobules for comparison. Portal tracts (P) contain bile ducts, arterioles and venules. E, efferent vein (central vein or terminal hepatic venule).

proposed, as well as modifications to the original lobular model.[2–4] From a pathologist's point of view, both lobular and acinar concepts have their merits in different situations. To give examples, the sinusoidal congestion of venous outflow obstruction is often more easily understood on the basis of the lobule, with maximum intensity at its centre. Bridging hepatic necrosis, however, is difficult to understand in terms of the lobule and has been explained as death of hepatocytes in acinar zones 3, the zones in which oxygen saturation is relatively low. In everyday practice it seems best to use words compatible with either model as far as possible. In this book we have therefore used the term *periportal* to describe the part of the parenchyma lying nearest to a small portal tract, and *perivenular* for the parenchyma near an efferent venule.

Portal tracts

Portal tracts of different size may be seen in biopsies (see Fig. 4.1). The smallest represent terminal tracts from which blood enters the parenchyma. Larger portal tracts contain vessels and ducts which convey blood and bile to and from the smaller tracts. Pathological processes do not necessarily affect large and small tracts to the same extent.

A typical small portal tract contains a bile duct, portal venule, hepatic arteriole and lymphatics, all embedded in connective tissue (Fig. 3.2). A few lymphocytes and mast cells may be seen even in normal subjects and nerve fibres can be demonstrated by appropriate staining. The exact contents are variable, however, depending in part

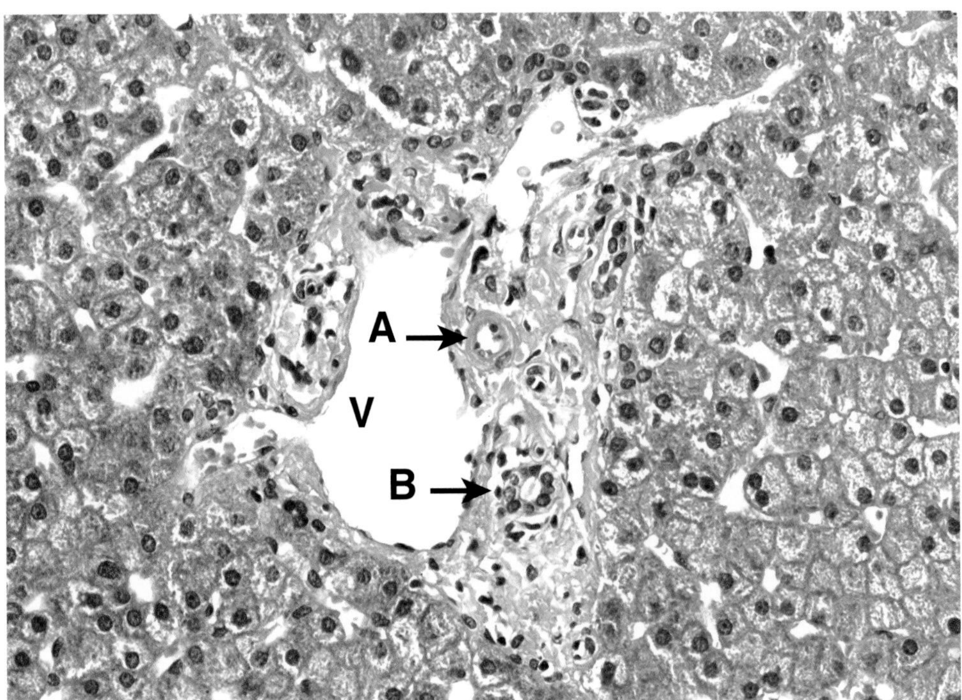

Figure 3.2 *Normal adult liver*. A small portal tract contains a portal venule (V), arteriole (A) and interlobular bile duct (B). (Needle biopsy, H&E).

on the angle of sectioning. In a study of 16 needle biopsies from normal subjects[5] 38, 9 and 7% of tracts did not contain a portal vein branch, hepatic arteriole or bile duct, respectively. Most, but by no means all, hepatic artery branches are accompanied by bile ducts. These observations have obvious implications for the histological diagnosis of bile duct or blood vessel loss. A confident diagnosis requires examination of several portal tracts.

Bile ducts

Near, or at the margins of the small portal tracts, the bile canaliculi, formed as spaces between adjacent hepatocytes, communicate with the canals of Hering.[6–8] These are lined partly by hepatocytes and partly by biliary epithelial cells. From the canals of Hering, bile drains into bile ductules lined entirely by biliary epithelium (see Fig. 5.1). Neither canals of Hering nor ductules are easily seen in normal liver, but they may become apparent in disease (Fig. 3.3). The exact location of the junction between the canals of Hering and bile ductules varies, the ductules sometimes having an intraparenchymal portion, seen in two-dimensional sections as apparently isolated ductules among hepatocytes. The canals of Hering and bile ductules have received much attention in recent years, because they are thought to be the site of a progenitor-cell compartment which becomes activated when a need for new hepatocytes and bile ducts cannot be adequately met otherwise.[8,9] Progenitor cells contain cytokeratins CK7 and CK19, and also stain with OV-6, an antibody used on frozen tissue to mark similar cells ('oval cells') in rodents.[10,11] The use of a combined

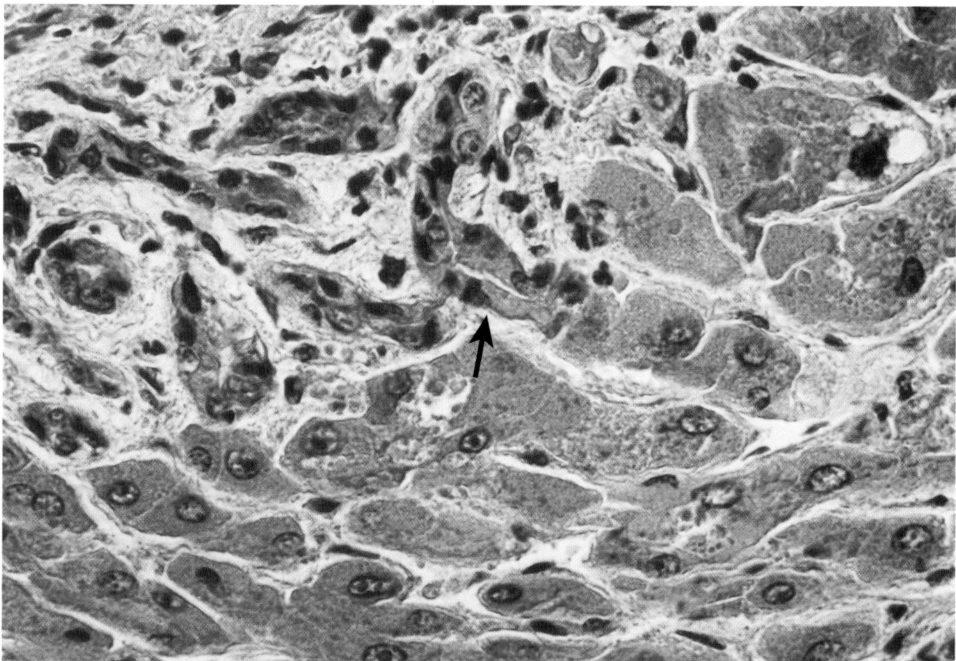

Figure 3.3 *Bile ductules and canals of Hering*. These are unusually prominent in this cirrhotic liver. A liver-cell plate is seen in continuity with a ductular structure (arrow). (Needle biopsy, H&E).

stain for CK7 and collagen has been proposed as an aid to the combined study of bile ducts, ductules, canals of Hering, progenitor cells and fibrosis.[12]

The interlobular ducts into which the ductules drain have an internal diameter of less than 100 μm and are more or less centrally located in the small portal tracts. They are lined by cuboidal or low columnar epithelium and have a basement membrane associated with diastase-PAS-positive material. Portal venules and hepatic arterioles usually lie close to these ducts but, as already noted, not all three structures are necessarily seen in a single plane of section. Positive identification of bile ducts in pathological states can be difficult, but is made easier by cytokeratin staining; ducts contain CK7 and CK19 in addition to CK8 and CK18, the latter two also found in hepatocytes.[13]

Bile drains from the interlobular ducts into septal bile ducts having an internal diameter of more than 100 μm. Septal ducts are lined by tall columnar epithelium, with basally located nuclei. These and larger ducts towards the hepatic hilum are sometimes associated with heterotopic exocrine pancreatic tissue.[14] Around the largest intrahepatic ducts there are peribiliary glands.[14]

Hepatic sinusoids, space of Disse and extracellular matrix

Hepatic sinusoids

The hepatic sinusoids are lined by specialised **endothelial cells**, which form an incomplete, porous barrier allowing easy exchange of materials between blood and hepatocytes. The endothelial cells are positive for CD4, CD13, CD14, CD16, Cdw32, CD36 and CD54 and thus have a different phenotype from capillary endothelium, portal venules and terminal hepatic venules; these stain for CD31 and CD34 and bind *Ulex europaeus* lectin.

Within the sinusoidal lumen lie the **Kupffer cells**, specialised hepatic macrophages. These have irregular processes, which may straddle the sinusoidal lumen. They are more numerous near portal tracts. Activated Kupffer cells, unlike endothelial cells, are diastase-PAS and muramidase positive. Phenotypically-distinct lymphocytes are found both within the sinusoidal lumens and in the portal tracts.[15] Lymphocytes in the lumens include pit cells having natural killer (NK) activity.[16]

Space of Disse

The space of Disse, lying between the sinusoidal endothelium and the hepatocytes, is not conspicuous in paraffin-embedded biopsies, but may be artefactually prominent in autopsy material. It contains components of the **extracellular matrix, nerves,**[17,18] and **hepatic stellate cells**.

Hepatic stellate cells are members of the myofibroblast family. There is international agreement that the term 'stellate cell' should be used rather than one of many synonyms in the literature[19] (see Glossary). Stellate cells are involved in fibrogenesis and in the control of sinusoidal blood flow.[20,21] They may also act as antigen-presenting cells. In childhood and adolescence stellate cells are positive for alpha smooth muscle actin, but thereafter become negative until activated under pathological conditions.[22] Both resting and activated stellate cells are positive for synaptophysin,[23] for vinculin after microwave pretreatment of paraffin sections[24] and for cellular retinol-binding protein-1 (CRBP-1).[25] Difficult to identify in normal liver in routine sections, stellate cells can be recognised in pathological conditions by their vacuolated cytoplasm and consequently scalloped nucleus (see Fig. 7.7). It is likely that the hepatic stellate cell is not the only cell type in the liver concerned with collagen synthesis.[26,27]

The **extracellular matrix** comprises many different components. Collagen types I and III predominate. Types IV, V, VI, VIII, XIV, XVIII and XIX are also present, together with proteoglycans and glycoproteins such as fibronectin and laminin.[28] Type III collagen is the main component of reticulin fibres in the space of Disse (Fig. 3.4), while type I is abundant in portal tracts and in the walls of efferent veins. Elastic fibres, abundant in portal tracts, are not demonstrable in sinusoidal walls in normal liver.[29]

Hepatocytes

The hepatocytes are arranged in plates separated by the sinusoidal labyrinth (Fig. 3.5). The layer of hepatocytes next to a small portal tract is known as the limiting plate. In adults, the hepatocyte plates are one cell thick, but in any one section a few plates will appear thicker because of tangential cutting. Widespread formation of twin-cell plates indicates hyperplasia, recent or current.

Hepatocytes are polygonal cells with well-defined cell borders. Each cell contains one or more nuclei. Most cells contain one nucleus; a few contain two in normal subjects. Nucleoli are often visible, mitotic figures rare. Most of the nuclei are diploid,[30] but smaller numbers of tetraploid and even larger nuclei are found, especially in older subjects.[31] Polyploidy and variation in nuclear size are therefore normal characteristics of adult human liver. A few nuclei may appear vacuolated because of glycogen accumulation, especially in children and adolescents.

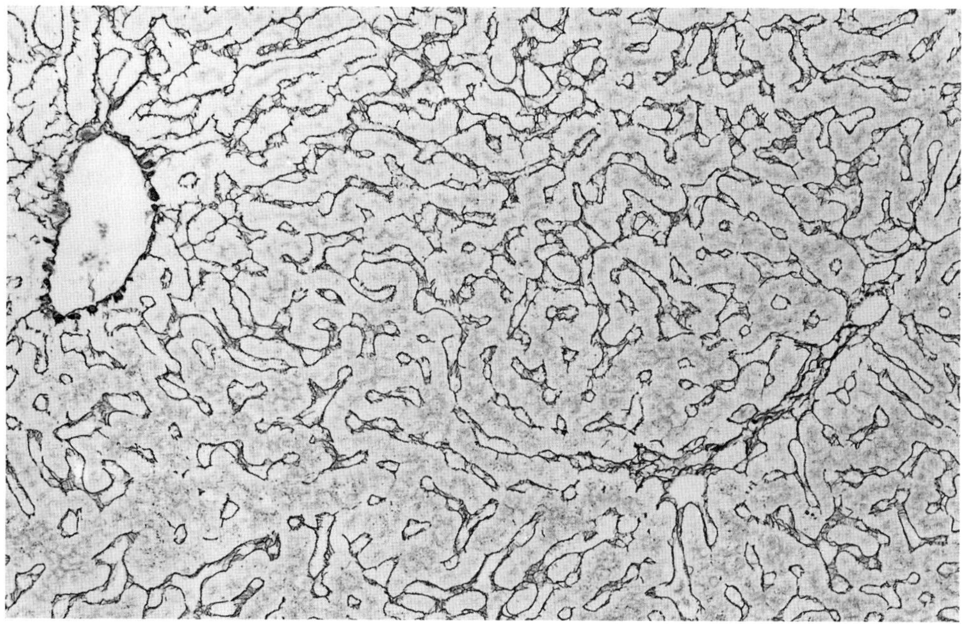

Figure 3.4 *Normal adult liver.* There is a regular reticulin network between the portal tract below right and the efferent hepatic venule to the left. (Needle biopsy, reticulin).

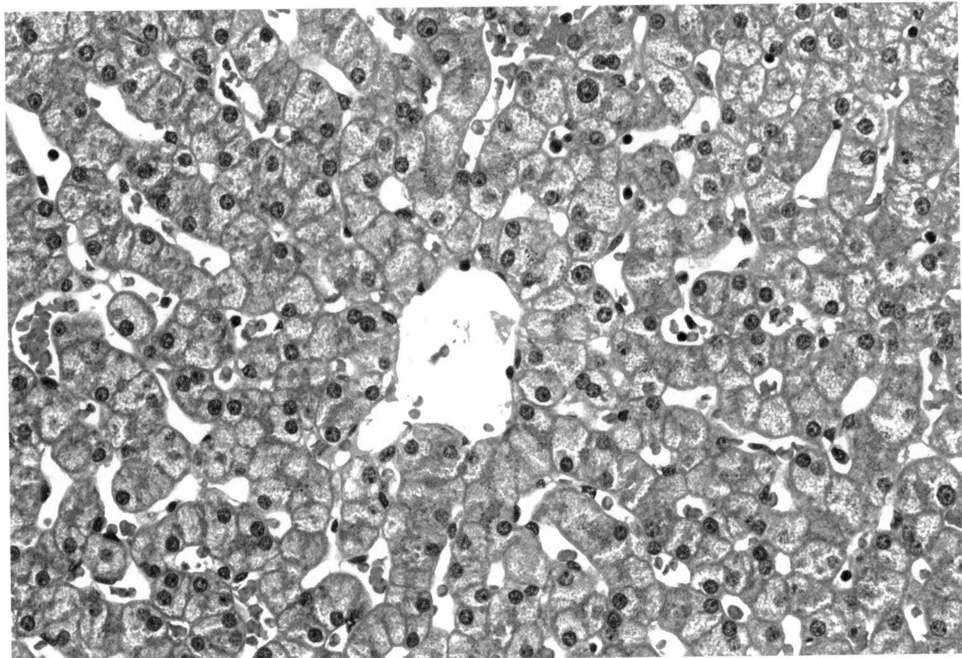

Figure 3.5 *Normal adult liver*. Hepatocyte plates, for the most part one cell thick, radiate out from the terminal venule in the centre. (Wedge biopsy, H&E).

Hepatocyte cytoplasm is normally rich in glycogen. In haematoxylin and eosin-stained sections the cytoplasm appears granular and often pale-staining centrally, where glycogen and endoplasmic reticulum predominate. A few fat vacuoles and occasional apoptosis may be seen in the absence of obvious disease. Many different proteins can be demonstrated in or on the hepatocytes, in keeping with the liver's many metabolic functions. These include secreted proteins such as albumin and cell surface proteins such as adhesion molecules.[32] Structural proteins include cytokeratins 8 and 18. Staining with the antibody Hep Par 1 is positive,[33] but this is not exclusive to hepatocytes.

Between the hepatocytes, their walls formed by two or three cells, are the bile canaliculi, already mentioned. They are usually too small to be readily seen by light microscopy in routine paraffin sections, but are occasionally visible as minute spaces at the biliary poles of the hepatocytes. Bile is rarely seen in normal subjects. The canalicular network can be demonstrated using a polyclonal antibody to CEA, which also reacts with a canalicular antigen (see Fig. 11.15).

Hepatocellular pigments (Table 3.1)

Within the hepatocytes, aggregated near the bile canaliculi and most abundant in perivenular areas, there are fine yellow-brown granules of lipofuscin pigment (Fig. 3.6). Lipofuscin is a normal constituent of adult liver, increasing in amount with age but also sometimes found in children. The granules represent lysosomes containing materials which cannot be further degraded. The amount of the pigment varies greatly in normal liver, making assessment of increase or decrease in disease subject

Table 3.1 Identification of hepatocellular pigments

	Haemosiderin	Lipofuscin	Dubin-Johnson pigment	Bile	Copper-associated protein
Distribution	Periportal	Perivenular	Perivenular, often also in Kupffer cells	Often perivenular; also in canaliculi and Kupffer cells	Periportal in chronic cholestasis
Intracellular site	Pericanalicular	Pericanalicular	Pericanalicular	Pericanalicular or diffuse	Variable
Granule size (approximate)	1 μm	1 μm	Often >1 μm	Variable	1 μm or less
Colour	Golden brown, refractile	Yellow-brown	Dark brown	Yellow, brown or green	Grey
Perls' stain for iron	+	–	–	–	–
Diastase-PAS stain	–	Variable	Variable	Variable	Often +
Long Ziehl-Neelsen stain	–	+	Often +	–	–
Orcein, Victoria blue stain	–	–	–	–	+

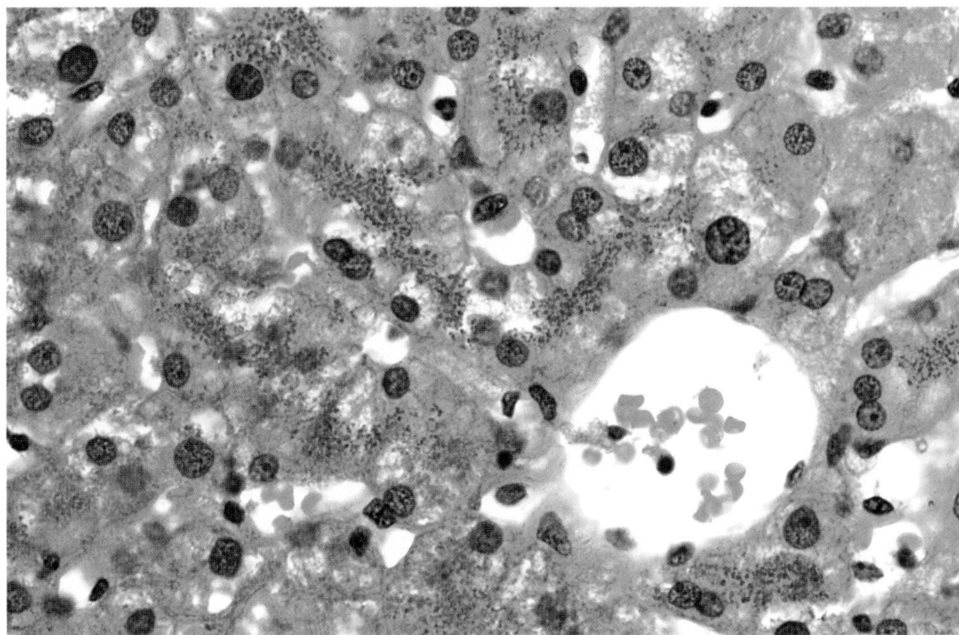

Figure 3.6 *Lipofuscin pigment.* In this normal liver from an adult there are prominent brown lipofuscin granules at the biliary poles of the hepatocytes. (Wedge biopsy, H&E).

to error in the absence of well-controlled morphometric data. Lipofuscin also varies in its staining properties according to its constituents and age. It is acid-fast, has reducing properties and stains variably with diastase-PAS. Perls' stain for iron is negative.

Large amounts of lipofuscin are difficult to distinguish from Dubin-Johnson pigment by light microscopy alone, but the latter is usually coarser and darker (see Fig. 13.19). Intracellular bile can be distinguished from lipofuscin by its bright green staining with van Gieson's method (see Fig. 4.3) and by the almost invariable presence of bile thrombi in canaliculi. An exception to this is liver following transplantation, in which diffuse intracellular bile is common in the absence of bile thrombi.

Normal liver is negative for stainable iron. All but very small amounts should be further investigated by appropriate biochemical and genetic methods. This is because it is important to identify patients with the common and treatable condition of hereditary haemochromatosis (Ch. 14).

Copper-associated protein is seen in high copper states as grey-brown intracytoplasmic granules, usually in a periportal location. It can be stained with orcein or Victoria blue.

NORMAL APPEARANCES IN CHILDHOOD

Haemopoiesis is active during the fetal period (Fig. 3.7) and continues until a few weeks after birth. Haemopoietic cells are present in portal tracts and sinusoids (Fig. 3.8). Hepatocyte plates are mainly two cells thick until the age of five or six, when the adult pattern of single cell plates is established. Hepatocytes and their

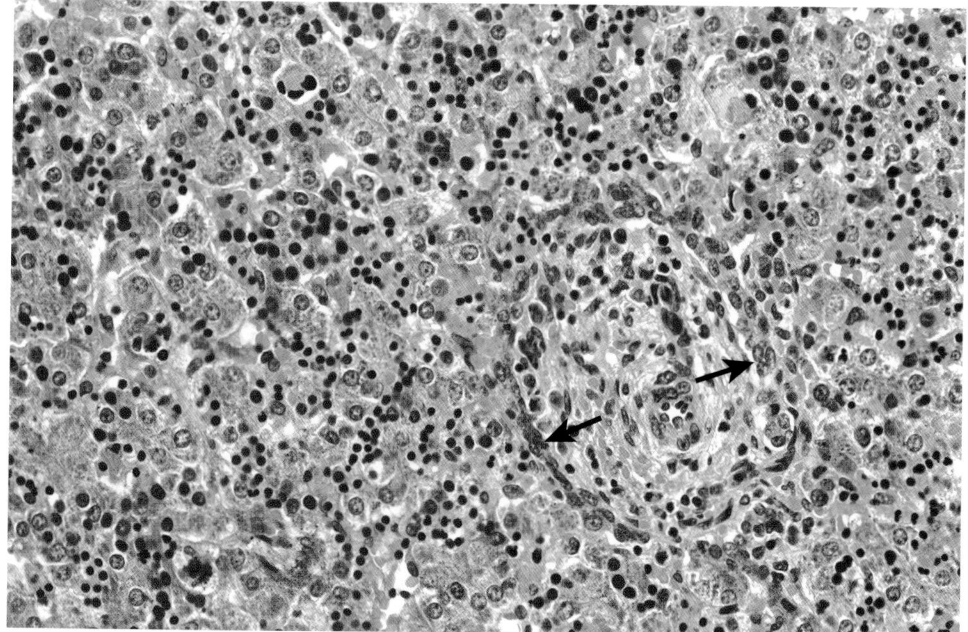

Figure 3.7 *Liver of fetus at 19 weeks' gestation*. Many haemopoietic cells are seen in sinusoids and in the immature portal tract. A ductal plate at the margin of the tract (arrows) indicates bile-duct formation. (Post-mortem liver, H&E).

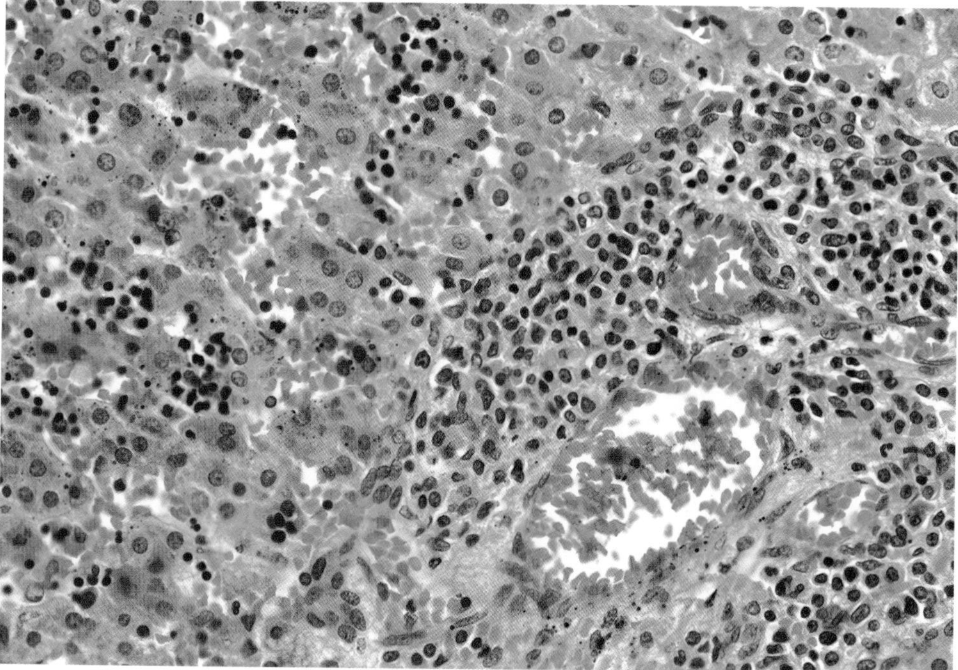

Figure 3.8 *Normal liver in a neonate*. Abundant haemopoietic cells are seen in the portal tract and in the sinusoids. (Post-mortem liver, H&E).

nuclei vary little in size. Glycogen vacuolation of nuclei is common in adolescents. Lipofuscin pigment is absent or scanty in the first two decades of life.

AGEING

The size of hepatocytes and their nuclei becomes more variable with increasing age (Fig. 3.9). This variation is due to greater numbers of polyploid cells,[31] with large nuclear and cell volumes. Lipofuscin pigment in hepatocytes is often abundant, especially around terminal hepatic venules (Fig. 3.6). Portal connective tissue becomes denser, and arteries may be thick-walled even in normotensive subjects. Pseudocapillarisation of the sinusoidal lining with loss of permeability may have important consequences for lipid metabolism and vascular disease.[34]

BIOPSY OF THE NORMAL LIVER

Percutaneous liver biopsies are necessarily taken though the liver capsule, which may be seen at one end of the core or as a separate piece. It sometimes contains vessels and bile ducts, but can be distinguished from a pathological septum by the density and maturity of the connective tissue. Deeper in the core, pathological septa

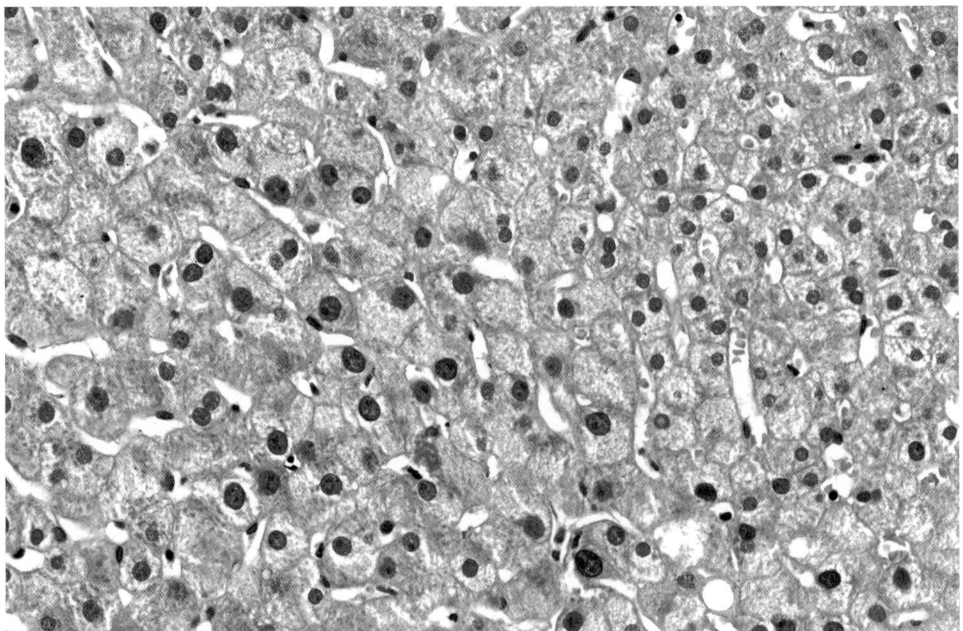

Figure 3.9 *Liver in an old person.* Hepatocyte nuclei vary considerably in size. (Needle biopsy, H&E).

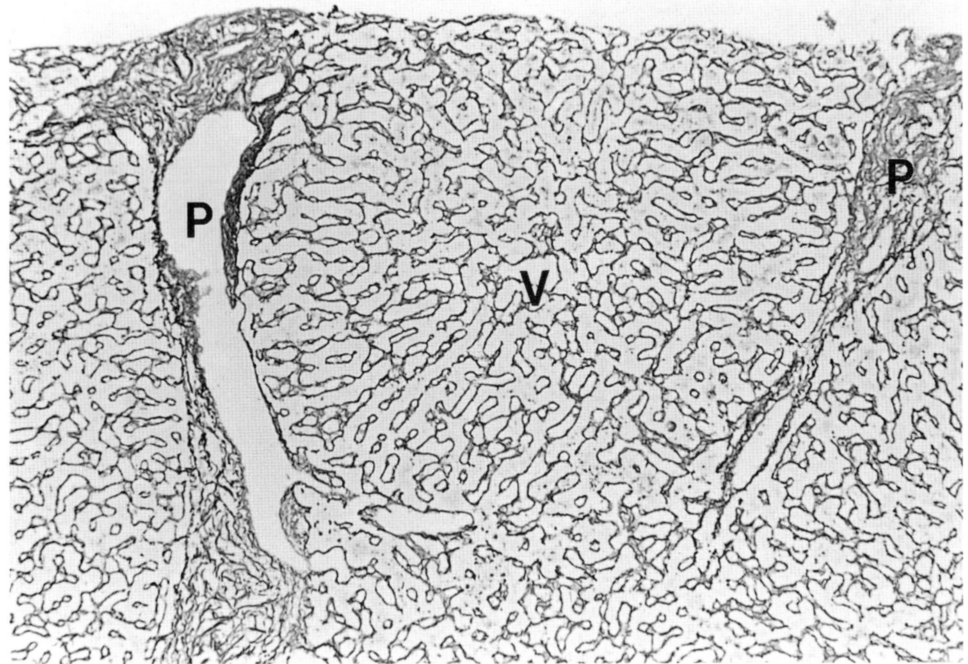

Figure 3.10 *Normal adult liver*. Two normal portal tracts (P), cut longitudinally, mimic septa. Between them is an efferent hepatic venule (V). (Needle biopsy, reticulin).

must also be distinguished from longitudinally-cut portal tracts (Fig. 3.10). The length and width of the liver core is often critical for diagnosis, as discussed under the heading of grading and staging in Chapter 9. Short pieces or slender cores taken with narrow needles may be inadequate for the diagnosis of unevenly-distributed, non-neoplastic lesions.

Other organs and tissues, especially skin, pleura and intercostal muscle, are sometimes included in the specimen. Close apposition to the liver core of fibrous tissue or of tumour does not necessarily reflect hepatic fibrosis or tumour within the liver.

Transjugular biopsy specimens may be small and fragmented, especially in patients with cirrhosis, but are usually adequate for histological diagnosis.

Surgical biopsies taken from the inferior margin of the liver are in the form of wedges covered on two aspects by capsule. The structure of the immediately subcapsular zone differs somewhat from the deeper tissue (Fig. 3.11), but there is good correlation between the volume fraction of non-parenchymal components in subcapsular and deeper zones.[35] Appearances mimicking cirrhosis do not usually extend for more than 2 mm into the liver, and confusion is unlikely except with very small samples.

In surgical biopsies taken some time after the beginning of an operation, neutrophil leucocytes accumulate under the capsule and in portal tracts, around terminal venules and focally within the parenchyma (Fig. 3.12). Here, there is focal loss of hepatocytes. Similar parenchymal changes have been reported after heavy sedation without full anaesthesia.[36] They are also found in patients infected with cytomegalovirus (Ch. 15).

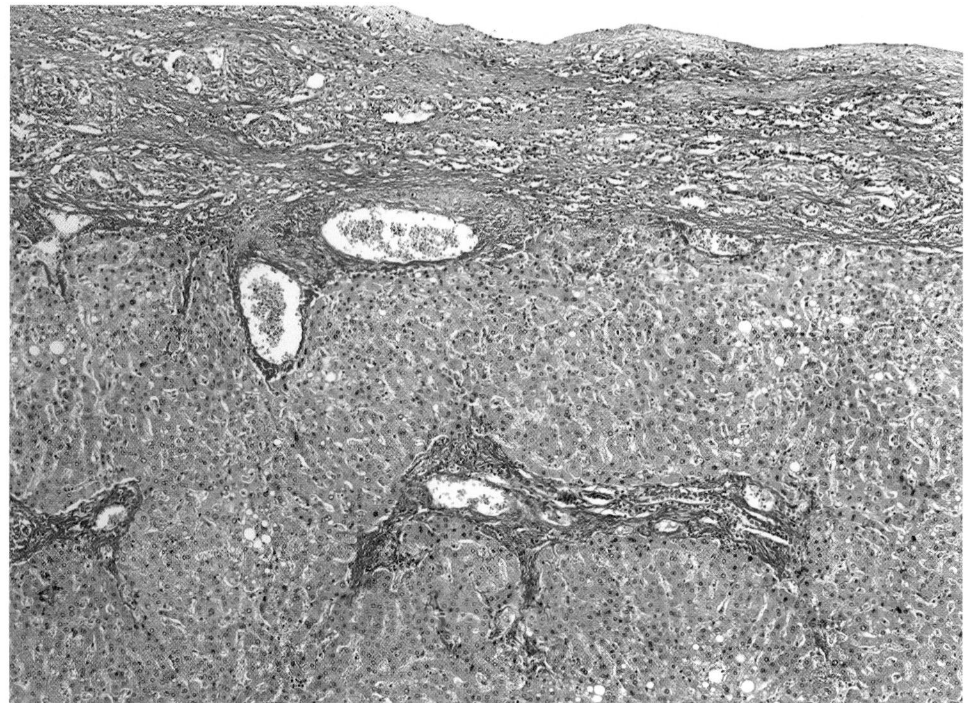

Figure 3.11 *Normal adult liver*. The capsule is thick and portal tracts are prominent. (Post-mortem liver, trichrome).

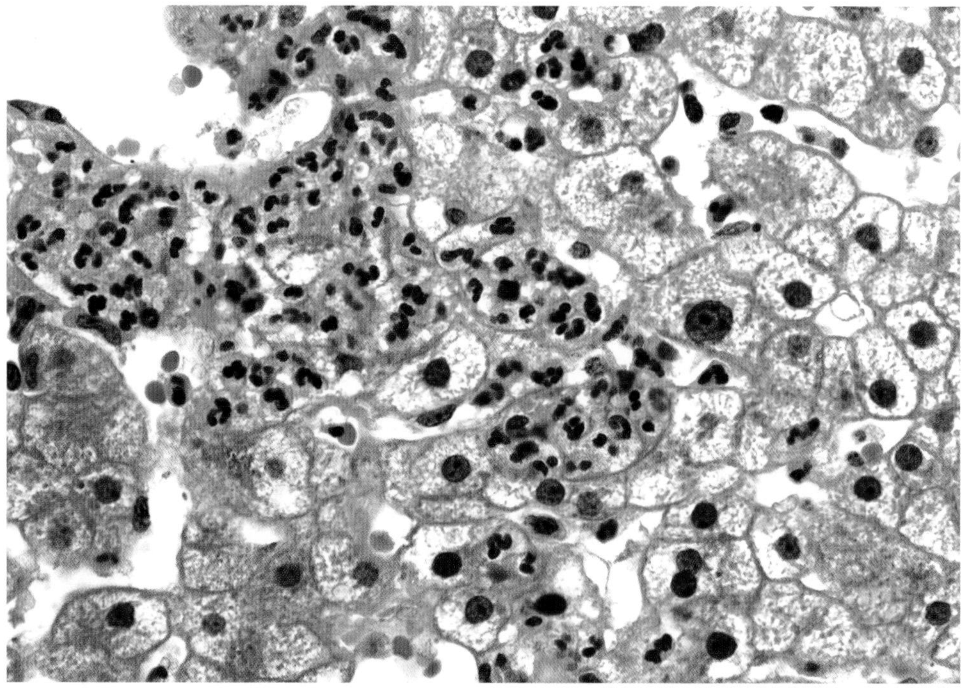

Figure 3.12 *Operative wedge biopsy*. Clumps of neutrophils mark sites of hepatocellular necrosis, resulting from the procedure. Part of an efferent venule is seen top left. (Wedge biopsy, H&E).

REFERENCES

1 Rappaport AM. The microcirculatory acinar concept of normal and pathological hepatic structure. *Beitr Pathol* 1976; **157**: 215–243.

2 Saxena R, Theise ND, Crawford JM, et al. Microanatomy of the human liver – exploring the hidden interfaces. Derivation of hepatocytes from bone marrow cells in mice after radiation-induced myeloablation. *Hepatology* 1999; **30**: 1339–1346.

3 MacSween RNM, Desmet VJ, Roskams T, et al. Developmental anatomy and normal structure. In: MacSween RNM, Burt AD, Portmann BC, et al., eds. Pathology of the Liver, 4th edn. London: Churchill Livingstone, 2002: 1.

4 Reuben A. Now you see it, now you don't. *Hepatology* 2003; **38**: 781–784.

5 Crawford AR, Lin X-Z, Crawford JM. The normal adult human liver biopsy: a quantitative reference standard. *Hepatology* 1998; **28**: 323–331.

6 Theise ND, Saxena R, Portmann BC, et al. The canals of Hering and hepatic stem cells in humans. *Hepatology* 1999; **30**: 1425–1433.

7 Saxena R, Theise N. Canals of Hering: recent insights and current knowledge. *Semin Liver Dis* 2004; **24**: 43–48.

8 Roskams TA, Theise ND, Balabaud C, et al. Nomenclature of the finer branches of the biliary tree: canals, ductules, and ductular reactions in human livers. *Hepatology* 2004; **39**: 1739–1745.

9 Roskams TA, Libbrecht L, Desmet VJ. Progenitor cells in diseased human liver. *Semin Liver Dis* 2003; **23**: 385–396.

10 Crosby H, Hubscher S, Fabris L, et al. Immunolocalization of putative human liver progenitor cells in livers from patients with end-stage primary biliary cirrhosis and sclerosing cholangitis using the monoclonal antibody OV-6. *Am J Pathol* 1998; **152**: 771–779.

11 Roskams T, De Vos R, van Eyken P, et al. Hepatic OV-6 expression in human liver disease and rat experiments: evidence for hepatic progenitor cells in man. *J Hepatol* 1998; **29**: 455–463.

12 Hytiroglou P, Tobias H, Saxena R, et al. The canals of Hering might represent a target of methotrexate hepatic toxicity. *Am J Clin Pathol* 2004; **121**: 324–329.

13 van Eyken P, Desmet VJ. Cytokeratins and the liver. *Liver* 1993; **13**: 113–122.

14 Terada T, Nakanuma Y, Kakita A. Pathologic observations of intrahepatic peribiliary glands in 1000 consecutive autopsy livers. Heterotopic pancreas in the liver. *Gastroenterology* 1990; **98**: 1333–1337.

15 Norris S, Collins C, Doherty DG, et al. Resident human hepatic lymphocytes are phenotypically different from circulating lymphocytes. *J Hepatol* 1998; **28**: 84–90.

16 Nakatani K, Kaneda K, Seki S, Nakajima Y. Pit cells as liver-associated natural killer cells: morphology and function. *Med Electron Microsc* 2004; **37**:29-36.

17 Tiniakos DG, Lee JA, Burt AD. Innervation of the liver: morphology and function. *Liver* 1996; **16**: 151–160.

18 Akiyoshi H, Gonda T, Terada T. A comparative histochemical and immunohistochemical study of aminergic, cholinergic and peptidergic innervation in rat, hamster, guineapig, dog and human livers. *Liver* 1998; **18**: 352–359.

19 International Consensus Group. Hepatic stellate cell nomenclature. *Hepatology* 1996; **23**: 193.

20 Pinzani M. Hepatic stellate (Ito) cells: expanding roles for a liver-specific pericyte. *J Hepatol* 1995; **22**: 700–706.

21 Rockey DC. Hepatic blood flow regulation by stellate cells in normal and injured liver. *Semin Liver Dis* 2001; **21**: 337–349.

22 Schmitt-Graff A, Kruger S, Bochard F, et al. Modulation of alpha smooth muscle actin and desmin expression in perisinusoidal cells of normal and diseased human livers. *Am J Pathol* 1991; **138**: 1233–1242.

23 Cassiman D, van Pelt J , De Vos R, et al. Synaptophysin: A novel marker for human and rat hepatic stellate cells. *Am J Pathol* 1999; **155**: 1831–1839.

24 Kawai S, Enzan H, Hayashi Y, et al. Vinculin: a novel marker for quiescent and activated hepatic stellate cells in human and rat livers. *Virchows Arch* 2003; **443**: 78–86.

25 Lepreux S, Bioulac-Sage P, Gabbiani G, et al. Cellular retinol-binding protein-1

expression in normal and fibrotic/cirrhotic human liver: different patterns of expression in hepatic stellate cells and (myo)fibroblast subpopulations. *J Hepatol* 2004; **40**: 774–780.

26 Cassiman D, Roskams T. Beauty is in the eye of the beholder: emerging concepts and pitfalls in hepatic stellate cell research. *J Hepatol* 2002; **37**: 527–535.

27 Ramadori G, Saile B. Mesenchymal cells in the liver – one cell type or two? *Liver* 2002; **22**: 283–294.

28 Schuppan D, Ruehl M, Somasundaram R, et al. Matrix as a modulator of hepatic fibrogenesis. *Semin Liver Dis* 2001; **21**: 351–372.

29 Porto LC, Chevallier M, Peyrol S, et al. Elastin in human, baboon, and mouse liver: an immunohistochemical and immunoelectron microscopic study. *Anat Rec* 1990; **228**: 392–404.

30 Deprez C, Vangansbeke D, Fastrez R, et al. Nuclear DNA content, proliferation index, and nuclear size determination in normal and cirrhotic liver, and in benign and malignant primary and metastatic hepatic tumors. *Am J Clin Pathol* 1993; **99**: 558–565.

31 Kudryatsev BN, Kudryatseva MV, Sakuta GA, et al. Human hepatocyte polyploidization kinetics in the course of life cycle. *Virchows Arch B Cell Pathol* 1993; **64**: 387–393.

32 Hinchliffe SA, Woods S, Gray S, et al. Cellular distribution of androgen receptors in the liver. *J Clin Pathol* 1996; **49**: 418–420.

33 Wennerberg AE, Nalesnik MA, Coleman WB. Hepatocyte paraffin 1: a monoclonal antibody that reacts with hepatocytes and can be used for differential diagnosis of hepatic tumors. *Am J Pathol* 1993; **143**: 1050–1054.

34 Le Couteur DG, Fraser R, Cogger VC, et al. Hepatic pseudocapillarisation and atherosclerosis in ageing. *Lancet* 2002; **359**: 1612–1615.

35 Ryoo JW, Buschmann RJ. Comparison of intralobular non-parenchyma, subcapsular non-parenchyma, and liver capsule thickness. *J Clin Pathol* 1989; **42**: 740–744.

36 McDonald GS, Courtney MG. Operation-associated neutrophils in a percutaneous liver biopsy: effect of prior transjugular procedure. *Histopathology* 1986; **10**: 217–222.

GENERAL READING

Crawford AR, Lin X-Z, Crawford JM. The normal adult human liver biopsy: a quantitative reference standard. *Hepatology* 1998; **28**: 323–331.

Geerts A. History, heterogeneity, developmental biology, and functions of quiescent hepatic stellate cells. *Semin Liver Dis* 2001; **21**: 311–335.

Kita H, Mackay IR, Van De WJ, et al. The lymphoid liver: considerations on pathways to autoimmune injury. *Gastroenterology* 2001; **120**: 1485–1501.

MacSween RNM, Desmet VJ, Roskams T, et al. Developmental anatomy and normal structure. In: MacSween RNM, Burt AD, Portmann BC et al., eds. Pathology of the Liver, 4th edn. London: Churchill Livingstone, 2002: 1.

Reuben A. Now you see it, now you don't. *Hepatology* 2003; **38**: 781–784.

Roskams TA, Libbrecht L, Desmet VJ. Progenitor cells in diseased human liver. *Semin Liver Dis* 2003; **23**: 385–396.

Roskams TA, Theise ND, Balabaud C, et al. Nomenclature of the finer branches of the biliary tree: canals, ductules, and ductular reactions in human livers. *Hepatology* 2004; **39**: 1739–1745.

Schuppan D, Ruehl M, Somasundaram R, et al. Matrix as a modulator of hepatic fibrogenesis. *Semin Liver Dis* 2001; **21**: 351–372.

Strain AJ, Crosby HA, Nijja S, et al. Human liver-derived stem cells. *Semin Liver Dis* 2003; **23**: 373–384.

CHAPTER 4 ASSESSMENT AND DIFFERENTIAL DIAGNOSIS OF PATHOLOGICAL FEATURES

INITIAL EXAMINATION AND REPORTING

Naked-eye examination and description of biopsy specimens

While these are of limited diagnostic value, they reduce the possibility of specimen identification error. The pathologist should make sure that the whole specimen has been adequately sectioned by comparing the size of the sectioned and stained tissue with the measurement recorded on macroscopic examination. Naked-eye examination also helps in the selection of suitable areas for electron microscopy. Needle biopsy specimens from cirrhotic liver are often irregular in calibre or obviously nodular, with brown or green nodules separated by grey or white fibrous tissue. The specimen may easily break into smaller pieces on handling or processing. Specimens with metastatic tumour or primary hepatocellular carcinoma also often fragment. The normal liver, however, gives rise to cylinders of even colour and thickness, which do not fragment easily. Cholestasis imparts a green colour, while fatty liver is pale brown or yellow and may float in the fixative. In cholesterol ester storage disease and Wolman's disease, the specimen is bright orange; this should warn the pathologist of the need to keep some tissue for frozen sectioning and electron microscopy. A black or very dark brown colour is characteristic of the Dubin-Johnson syndrome. Metastatic tumour, like fibrous tissue, is often white. Congested liver is deep red in colour. The clinician should record if the specimen was difficult to obtain from the patient and whether the liver felt hard when the needle was inserted, as in many cases of cirrhosis, or very hard as in congenital hepatic fibrosis.

Routine microscopy

Routine microscopy of liver biopsies should include systematic assessment of overall structure, portal tracts and their contents, terminal hepatic venules, hepatocytes and sinusoidal cells. Some pathologists use a proforma or checklist in order to avoid omitting relevant data.[1]

The following sections are intended to help in the evaluation of pathological changes. Most of the information is also found in other parts of the book, under individual diseases. There is inevitably some repetition, because many of the listed features are found in combination. The final part of the chapter contains guidance on the differential diagnosis of acute cholestasis and of individual pathological findings.

Structural changes, collapse and fibrosis

Minor structural changes are difficult to assess in sections stained with haematoxylin and eosin (H&E) and may indeed be missed altogether. Examination of a connective tissue preparation is therefore often important. Normal liver tissue shows a hierarchy of ramifying portal tracts of varied sizes, which are present in needle and wedge biopsy samples (Fig. 4.1). The subdivisions of these portal tracts parallel the hierarchy of hepatic artery and portal vein branches and bile ducts as they distribute throughout the liver and can thereby be roughly subdivided into segmental, area, conducting (septal) and terminal portal tract units (compare with Fig. 5.1). For detection of the most minor abnormalities an uncounterstained silver impregnation for reticulin is generally best, although pericellular fibrosis is most easily detected in sections stained for collagen.

Using these methods, an impression may be gained that although portal tracts and terminal venules are normally related to each other, the portal tracts are enlarged and perhaps even linked by fibrous septa. This is consistent with mild chronic viral hepatitis or with one of the conditions in which portal changes typically predominate; these include biliary tract disease, haemochromatosis, congenital hepatic fibrosis and schistosomiasis. If however, the reticulin framework of the parenchyma is distorted, lesions characterised by lobular damage should be considered. These include acute and chronic hepatitis as well as forms of biliary

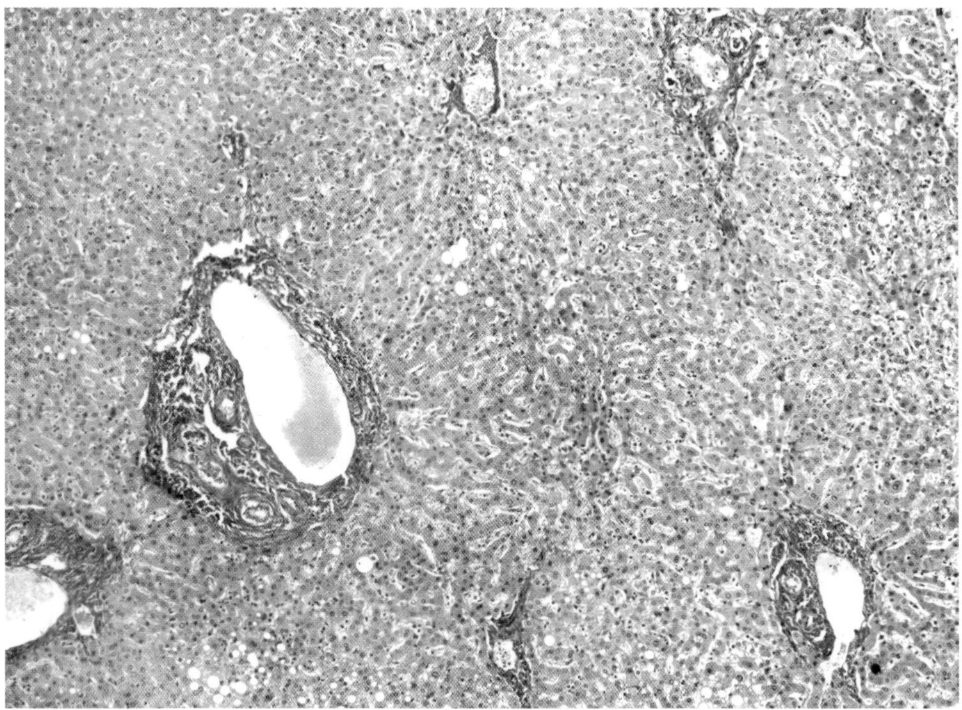

Figure 4.1 *Portal tract size variations.* Biopsies contain portal tracts ranging in size from larger conducting tracts (at left) to the small terminal tracts (right top and bottom) from which blood enters the parenchyma. (Wedge biopsy, CAB).

disease in which there is also hepatocellular damage, notably primary biliary cirrhosis. Venous congestion leads to regular condensation of perivenular reticulin.

Recent collapse and fibrosis are sometimes difficult to distinguish even with the help of good collagen stains. A stain for elastic tissue can help to resolve this problem because the presence of elastic fibres outside the portal tracts is an indication of long standing disease. Collagen stains are helpful for the recognition of blocked veins, for example in necrotic areas, alcoholic liver disease, venous outflow obstruction and epithelioid haemangioendothelioma. Collagen staining is important for the detection of pericellular fibrosis, as already indicated, and should therefore be used whenever there is substantial steatosis or a suspicion of steatohepatitis.

The histological diagnosis of cirrhosis is fully discussed in Chapter 10. Once cirrhosis has developed, the pattern of fibrosis is one of the features that may help to determine its cause. In primary or secondary biliary cirrhosis, for example, fibrosis expanding and linking the portal tracts is a more important early factor in pathogenesis than hepatocellular regeneration; this is reflected in the morphological picture of broad perilobular septa surrounding irregularly-shaped islands of parenchyma (as in Fig. 5.11). In hereditary haemochromatosis and chronic venous outflow obstruction, the impression is also of fibrosis rather than regeneration as the principal pathogenetic factor. In these diseases with a long pre-cirrhotic phase of fibrosis, transected parenchymal peninsulas may be mistaken for true regenerative nodules. This is particularly common just deep to the liver capsule. Isolated subcapsular nodules in an otherwise not nodular biopsy should therefore be interpreted with caution.

Hepatocellular damage

Death of individual hepatocytes or small groups of these cells is loosely called *focal* necrosis, although the mechanism may in fact be apoptosis. The distinction cannot always be made easily by routine microscopy unless apoptotic bodies are seen. Focal necrosis is associated with accumulation of inflammatory cells of various types, including macrophages. *Spotty* necrosis is used for the same lesion in the context of acute hepatitis. Focal necrosis is a common finding which does not in itself indicate primary disease of the liver, because it is often part of a non-specific reaction to disease elsewhere in the body. While degenerating hepatocytes or cell fragments are sometimes seen within the focal inflammatory infiltrate, the inflammatory reaction is usually more obvious than the necrosis, and the latter is assumed to have taken place because of a gap in a liver-cell plate (liver-cell 'drop-out').

Confluent necrosis

Confluent necrosis (see Fig. 8.4) refers to substantial areas of liver-cell death. The commonest cause of this type of necrosis in biopsy material is hepatitis, either viral or drug-related, in which case the necrosis is accompanied by an inflammatory reaction. Confluent necrosis with little or no inflammation is seen in hypoperfusion of the hepatic parenchyma, as in shock or left ventricular failure and in heat-stroke (see Fig. 12.2). Paracetamol (acetaminophen) poisoning produces a similar lesion. In all the above examples the necrosis is typically perivenular but it may, if severe and extensive, form bridges linking vascular structures (see below). Some poisons, including ferrous sulphate, typically cause periportal (zone 1) necrosis. Haphazardly distributed areas of necrosis are found in disseminated herpes virus infections (e.g. herpes simplex, varicella) (see Fig. 15.4) and in mycobacterial diseases. Tumour necrosis may be so extensive that no recognisable tumour tissue is present in the section; in such cases the reticulin pattern may help to establish a diagnosis.

Bridging necrosis

Bridging necrosis describes the location rather than the type of necrosis. It usually results from extensive necrosis of confluent type. The term has been used for necrosis linking any of the vascular structures, but it is now more often restricted to the linking of terminal hepatic venules (centrilobular veins) to portal tracts (Fig. 4.2). A possible explanation of this type of bridging is that it represents necrosis of acinar zones 3, which touch both the veins and the larger portal tracts (as in Fig. 3.1). Linking of portal tracts to each other is common in conditions in which portal tracts are widened, for example by chronic hepatitis or biliary tract disease; this is partly because the chance of obtaining a longitudinal section of a widened portal tract is greater than for one of normal width. Linking of perivenular areas to each other is found in some examples of parenchymal hypoperfusion and venous outflow obstruction.

Bridging of terminal hepatic venules to portal tracts is a fairly common feature of acute hepatitis of viral type, when the bridges contain few or no elastic fibres. It is also seen in exacerbations of chronic hepatitis. Old bridges contain elastic fibres as

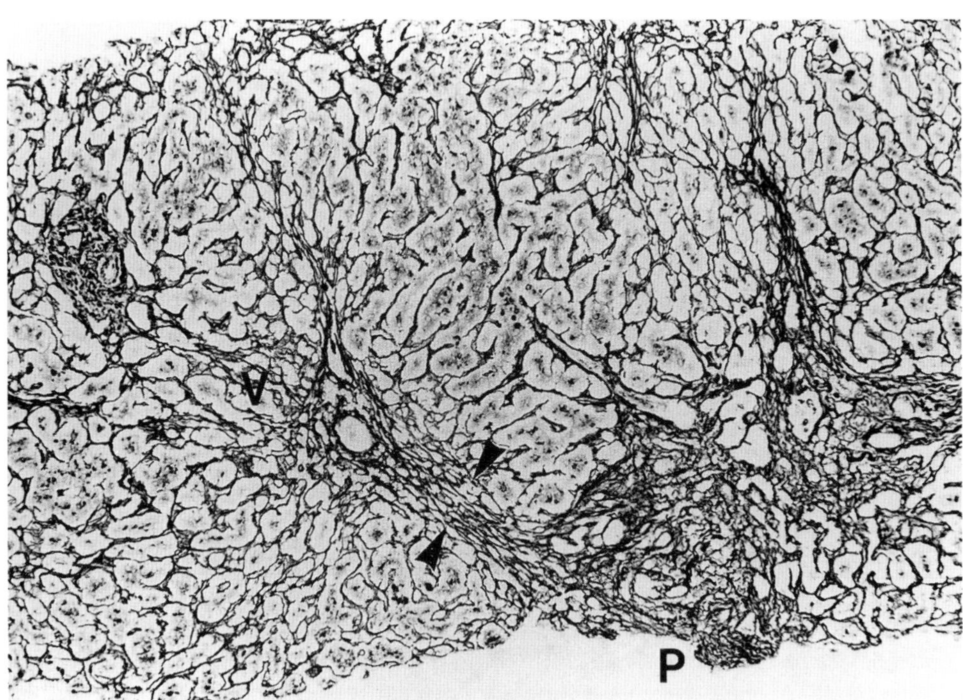

Figure 4.2 *Acute hepatitis with bridging necrosis.* Collapsed reticulin here gives a false impression of chronic liver disease. A bridge or passive septum (arrowheads) links an expanded portal tract (P) with a terminal hepatic venule (V). (Needle biopsy, reticulin).

well as collagen fibres. Such bridging fibrosis is an important component both of the more severe examples of chronic viral hepatitis and of steatohepatitis. Contraction of collagen-rich bridges may produce rapid and severe distortion of the normal hepatic microstructure, with correspondingly rapid progression to cirrhosis.

Panlobular and multilobular necrosis

Panlobular (panacinar) and multilobular (multiacinar) necrosis are terms used to describe confluent necrosis involving entire single lobules or several adjacent lobules respectively. They are further discussed in the chapter on acute viral hepatitis.

Interface hepatitis (piecemeal necrosis)

Interface hepatitis (piecemeal necrosis) (see Figs 9.3 and 9.4), is a process of inflammation and erosion of the hepatic parenchyma at its junction with portal tracts or fibrous septa. The term interface hepatitis was introduced because the death of hepatocytes probably involves apoptosis rather than, or as well as necrosis[2–5] and because it takes place at the parenchymal-connective tissue interface. It is common in chronic viral hepatitis but is also found in other conditions (see Table 9.2). The inflammatory infiltrate is composed mainly of lymphocytes, with or without recognisable plasma cells, and is accompanied by fibrosis of the affected areas with new formation of collagens and other extracellular matrix components.[6] The process is sometimes referred to as classical or lymphocytic piecemeal necrosis in order to distinguish it from biliary, ductular and fibrotic piecemeal necrosis, processes found in chronic biliary tract disease and described in the section on primary biliary cirrhosis in Chapter 5.

Cholestasis

In morphological terms, cholestasis is the presence of visible bile in tissue sections. It is also known as bilirubinostasis because the main component seen by light microscopy is bilirubin. Bile is rarely seen in normal liver and then only in minute amounts; cholestasis should therefore be regarded as pathological. The location of the bile varies. The commonest is in dilated bile canaliculi between hepatocytes. This canalicular form of cholestasis, sometimes called acute cholestasis, may be accompanied by bile accumulation in the cytoplasm of hepatocytes and Kupffer cells. Canalicular cholestasis is typically perivenular. In contrast, in patients with chronic biliary tract disease, bile may accumulate in periportal hepatocytes. This is also known as cholate stasis because abnormal bile salts are thought to contribute to its pathogenesis.

In large bile-duct obstruction in adults, bile is not usually visible under the microscope within canals of Hering, bile ductules or bile ducts even though the biliary tree may be dilated. The commonest cause of ductular cholestasis is sepsis. Dense bile is also visible in ducts in different forms of ductal plate malformation and in extrahepatic biliary atresia. In transplanted livers it may result from inadequate graft function, but sepsis should always be considered as an alternative possibility.

Canalicular cholestasis

Canalicular cholestasis takes the form of bile plugs (bile thrombi) in dilated canaliculi (see Fig. 5.2). There is often brown or yellow pigment in nearby hepatocytes and Kupffer cells, but the distinction of this pigment from others such as lipofuscin and ceroid is not a serious practical problem; this is because the presence of bile in the canaliculi makes the diagnosis of cholestasis obvious. In general, cholestasis should only be diagnosed with great caution in the absence of bile plugs in canaliculi, although cytoplasmic liver-cell bilirubinostasis without canalicular bile is quite common after liver transplantation. The perivenular location of canalicular cholestasis is partly an artefact of paraffin embedding, but also reflects real functional differences between the various parts of the lobule.

The colour of bile under the microscope varies according to pigment concentration and the degree of oxidation. It may be dark brown, green or yellow, and is occasionally so pale as to make detection difficult at first glance. The van Gieson stain, which stains bilirubin green, may then be helpful (Fig. 4.3). Pale counterstaining, as commonly used in Perls' method for iron, also makes bile easier to see. Specific histochemical methods for bilirubin are rarely necessary in ordinary diagnostic work.

When acute cholestasis is prolonged, the relationship of hepatocytes to each other may undergo focal change. Instead of the normal arrangement of two or three hepatocytes around a small bile canaliculus, the number of cells is increased and the lumen of the canaliculus considerably enlarged. The new structures are called cholestatic rosettes (Fig. 4.4). The lumens of the rosettes are part of the biliary tree, but the bile may be lost during processing. Even apparently empty rosettes should therefore be regarded as an indication of cholestasis. Other hepatocellular changes in

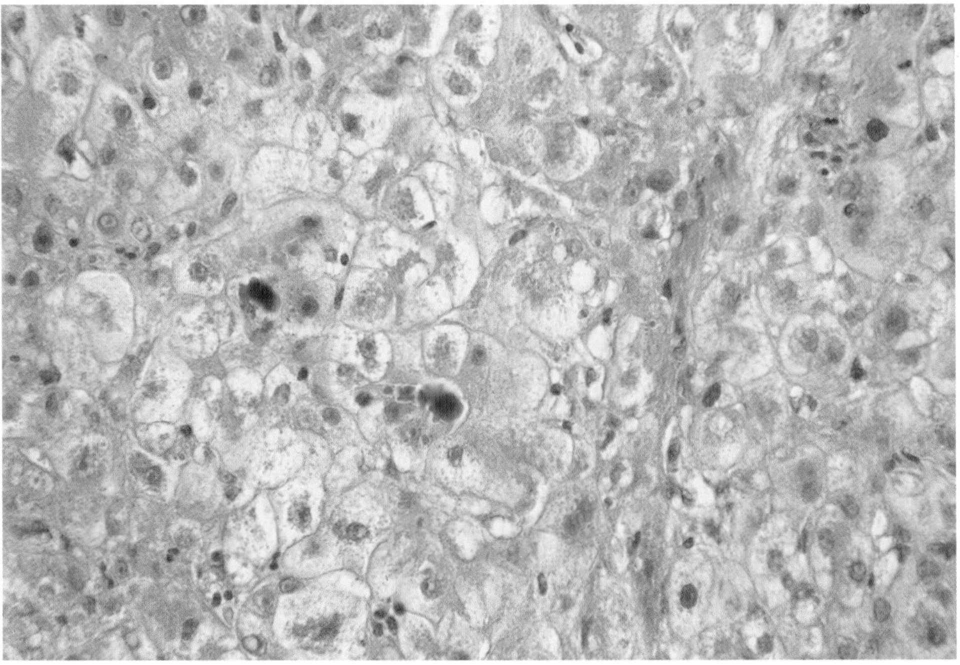

Figure 4.3 *Cholestasis.* Bile thrombi in dilated canaliculi are stained bright green. The red material is collagen. (Needle biopsy, haematoxylin & van Gieson).

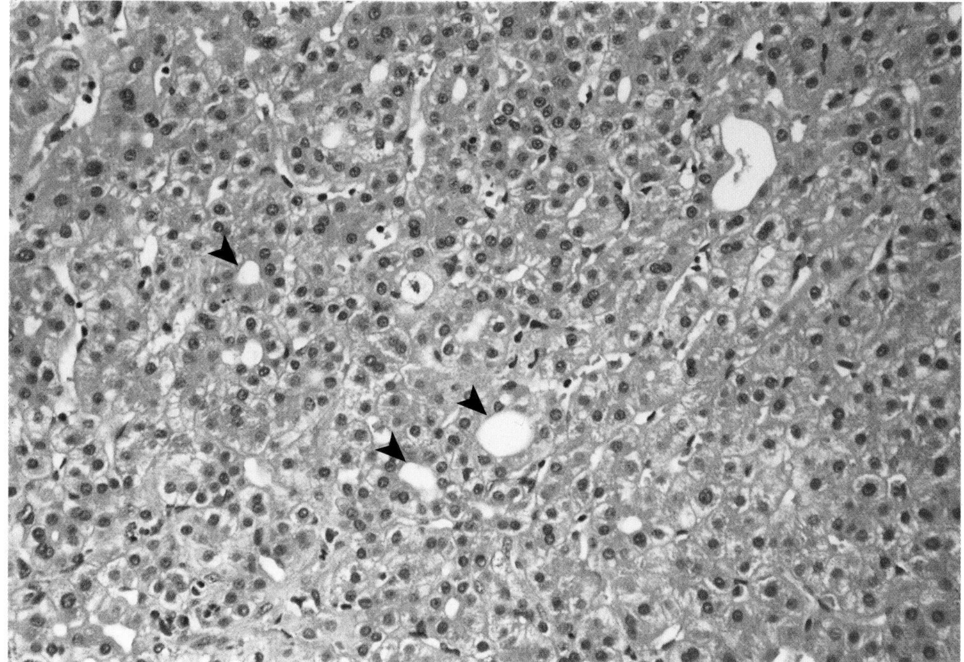

Figure 4.4 *Cholestasis.* Several liver-cell rosettes, glandular formations around prominent lumens, are marked by arrowheads. (Wedge biopsy, H&E).

cholestasis are described in Chapter 5, in the section on large bile-duct obstruction. Very occasionally prolonged canalicular cholestasis is associated with the accumulation of copper and copper-associated protein, but this is much more characteristic of the chronic periportal form of cholestasis, discussed below.

Canalicular cholestasis in perivenular areas is mainly seen in the conditions listed in Tables 4.1 and 4.2. Cholestasis of less regular distribution is common in chronic liver diseases with severe hepatocellular dysfunction or with associated sepsis.

Chronic cholestasis

Chronic cholestasis (cholate stasis, pseudoxanthomatous change, precholestasis; see Fig. 5.10) is seen in chronic liver diseases, especially those involving the biliary tree, and is the result of interference with bile flow at the level of the portal tracts. Bile (i.e. bilirubinostasis) may or may not be obvious, and the lesion is more easily recognised by hepatocellular swelling and pallor, and by the accumulation of copper and copper-associated protein in the affected cells. Mallory bodies may also be present. In some instances these are associated with an infiltrate of neutrophils, in which case the distinction from steatohepatitis must be made on the overall appearances and clinical context. The connective tissue adjacent to an area of chronic cholestasis is often oedematous. It may show a ductular reaction containing proliferated ductule-like structures which have the cytokeratin profile of bile ducts.[7] They express cytokeratins 7 and 19 which are not normally demonstrable in hepatocytes. Because the ductular reaction is often associated with disruption of the limiting plates of hepatocytes around the portal tracts, it has given rise to the concept of ductular

Table 4.1 Common causes of canalicular cholestasis

Obstruction to major bile ducts
Acute hepatitis
Cholestatic drug jaundice
Sepsis
Cholestatic syndromes (see Table 5.1)

Table 4.2 Main causes of bland intrahepatic cholestasis

Drugs (e.g. contraceptive steroids)
Sepsis
Benign recurrent intrahepatic cholestasis
Cholestasis of pregnancy
Post-transplant bile flow impairment or rejection
Lymphomas

piecemeal necrosis.[8] Chronic cholestasis, unlike acute canalicular cholestasis, is not necessarily associated with clinical jaundice or a high level of serum bilirubin, but the serum alkaline phosphatase level is characteristically raised.

DIFFERENTIAL DIAGNOSIS OF INDIVIDUAL FINDINGS

Acute cholestasis

Modern imaging methods have greatly reduced the need for liver biopsy in acutely jaundiced patients. Biopsy is nevertheless still helpful in some instances when the cause of a presumed intrahepatic jaundice is in doubt, when there is a need to distinguish between acute and chronic liver disease and when other investigations give equivocal results. Liver transplantation has led to a striking increase in liver biopsies for evaluation of the cause of jaundice. The pathologist may also need to assess surgical biopsy specimens from jaundiced patients. Accurate histological diagnosis is important because correct treatment may depend upon it and a wrong answer can lead to dangerous mismanagement. It has to be admitted, however, that the pathologist cannot always give a clear answer to the questions put by the clinician.

In essence, the pathologist faced with a liver biopsy from an acutely jaundiced patient is asked to decide between the options in Table 4.3. The last two items are discussed in detail in the relevant chapters, and it is only necessary here to note that it is sometimes difficult to distinguish between chronic hepatitis and severe acute hepatitis with bridging necrosis. This clinically important distinction is made more easily with the help of a stain for elastic fibres. The main problem lies in the differentiation of the first four possibilities, bile-duct obstruction, acute hepatitis and various other forms of intrahepatic cholestasis, including that due to sepsis. These

Table 4.3 Decisions in the acutely jaundiced patient

Are the patient's major bile ducts obstructed?
Has the patient got an acute viral or drug-related hepatitis?
Is there evidence for a diagnosis of sepsis?
Does the patient have one of the intrahepatic conditions listed in Table 4.2?
Does the patient have steatohepatitis?
Does the patient have chronic liver disease with an acute exacerbation rather than acute liver disease?

can usually be distinguished by careful and methodical examination of abnormalities in the lobules and in the portal tracts (Fig. 4.5).

Lobular changes

Obstruction to large bile ducts within or outside the liver leads to morphological cholestasis in perivenular areas. Bile canaliculi are dilated and contain bile thrombi (canalicular cholestasis). There is a variable degree of liver-cell swelling, inflammatory cell infiltration and Kupffer-cell hypertrophy in the cholestatic areas, but elsewhere the parenchyma appears substantially normal. The inflammatory infiltration is usually modest or even absent and liver-cell plates remain for the most part intact. A few apoptotic bodies and liver-cell mitoses may be seen, reflecting increased liver-cell turnover. Bile infarcts sometimes develop in the elderly, in whom duct obstruction is a very important cause of acute jaundice; there is sometimes more liver-cell damage than in the young.

By contrast, in acute hepatitis there is usually disruption of cell plates and widespread swelling, shrinking and loss of hepatocytes, usually most striking in perivenular areas but often widely distributed. In some forms of viral hepatitis, especially hepatitis A, there is sometimes substantial necrosis and lymphoplasmacytic infiltration of the periportal parenchyma. Cholestasis may be seen in acute hepatitis, again commonly in hepatitis A, but canalicular dilatation is slight and hepatocellular changes are not confined to areas of cholestasis. In patients on immunosuppressive therapy, for example after liver transplantation, the inflammatory infiltrate of an acute viral hepatitis may be relatively inconspicuous.

In other forms of intrahepatic cholestasis such as drug-induced cholestasis, benign recurrent cholestasis and cholestasis of pregnancy, the changes within the lobules are much the same as in bile-duct obstruction, except that bile infarcts are unusual and, if present, small. Canaliculi are less dilated than in bile-duct obstruction, except in liver-cell rosettes, which often form in intrahepatic cholestases and which are described and illustrated above. There may be striking liver-cell swelling and multinucleation. Inflammatory infiltration is variable; in most forms of intrahepatic cholestasis inflammation and liver-cell damage are absent or slight, but in a minority of cases of idiosyncratic drug cholestasis they are sufficient to justify a label of cholestatic hepatitis.

Portal changes

Examination of portal tracts (Fig. 4.6) provides further discrimination, particularly between bile-duct obstruction and the other conditions. In bile-duct obstruction the

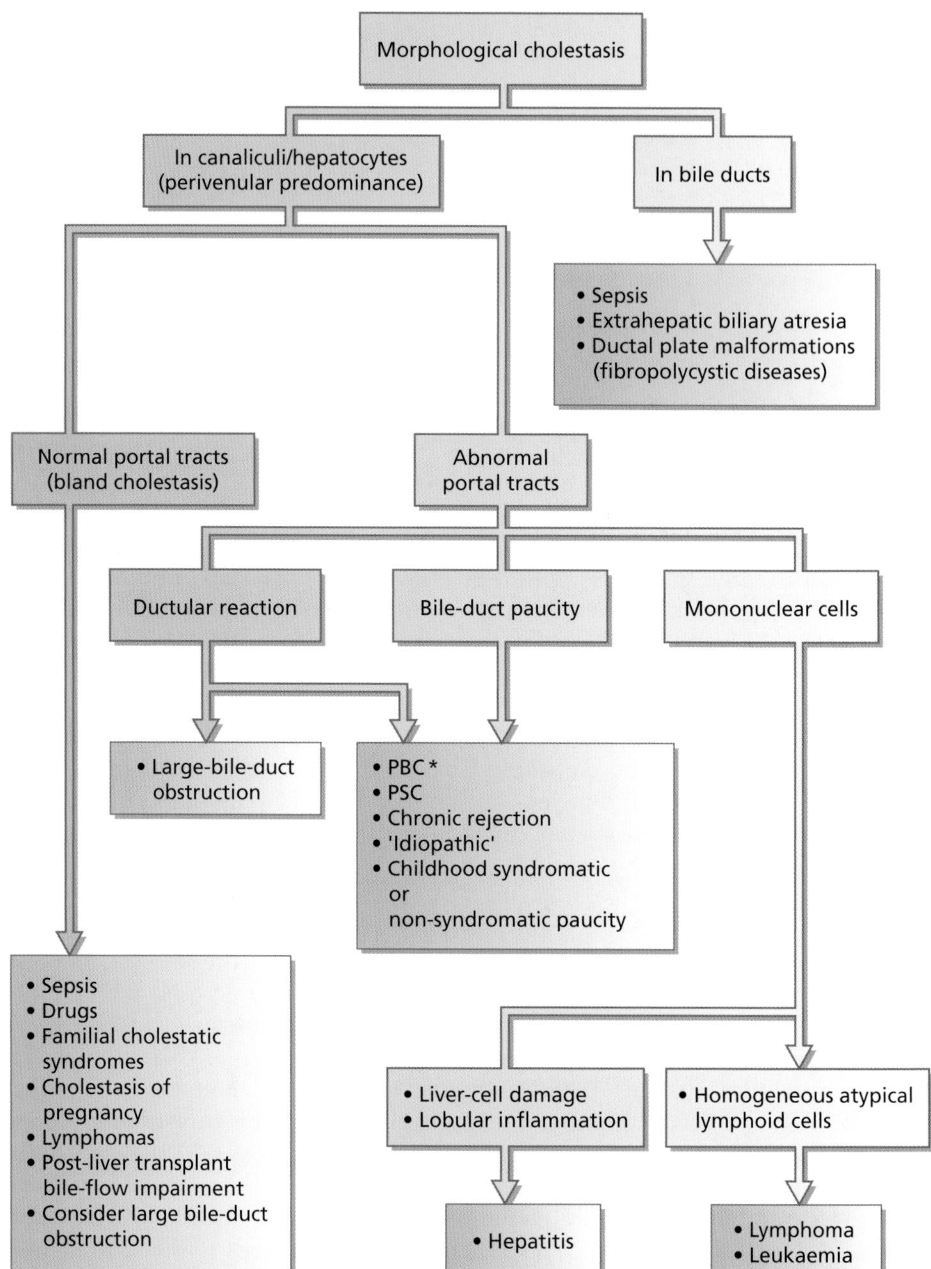

Figure 4.5 *Algorithmic approach to morphological cholestasis.* Once the site of cholestasis is identified pathologically, careful assessment of portal tracts and lobular changes allows the major differential diagnosis to be established.
*In PBC, morphological cholestasis is usually only apparent in later, advanced disease.

portal tracts are typically expanded and oedematous, with a pale watery appearance to the connective tissue. There is an increased number of bile-duct profiles at the margins of the tracts, most of these ducts lying roughly parallel to the portal-parenchymal interface (see section on the ductular reaction, below). An associated inflammatory infiltrate includes neutrophils. Not all portal tracts are equally affected. Bile extravasates may be seen. The margins of the portal tracts are usually

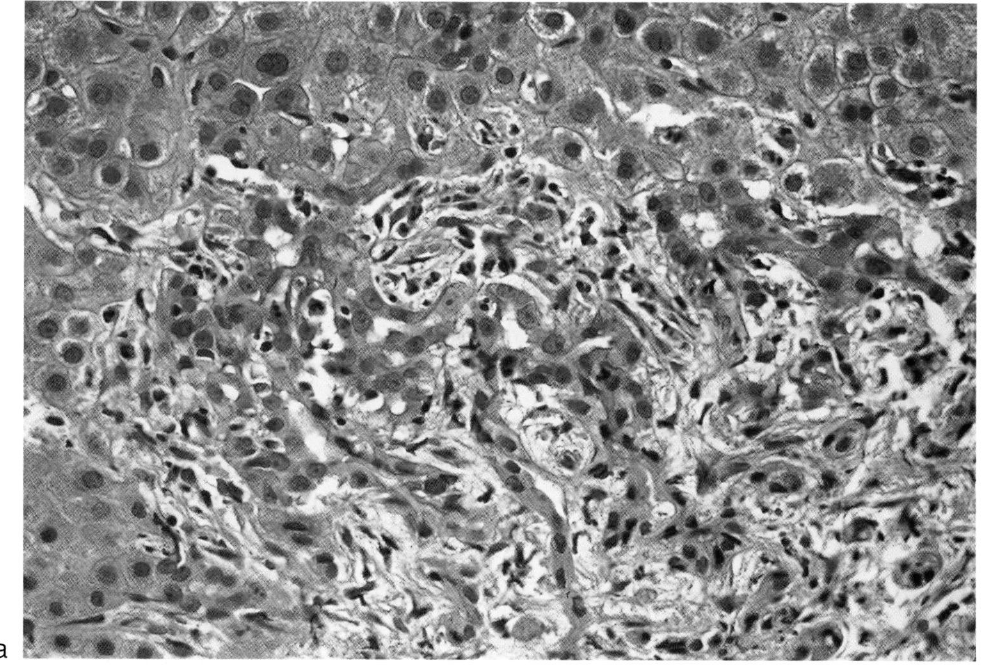

a

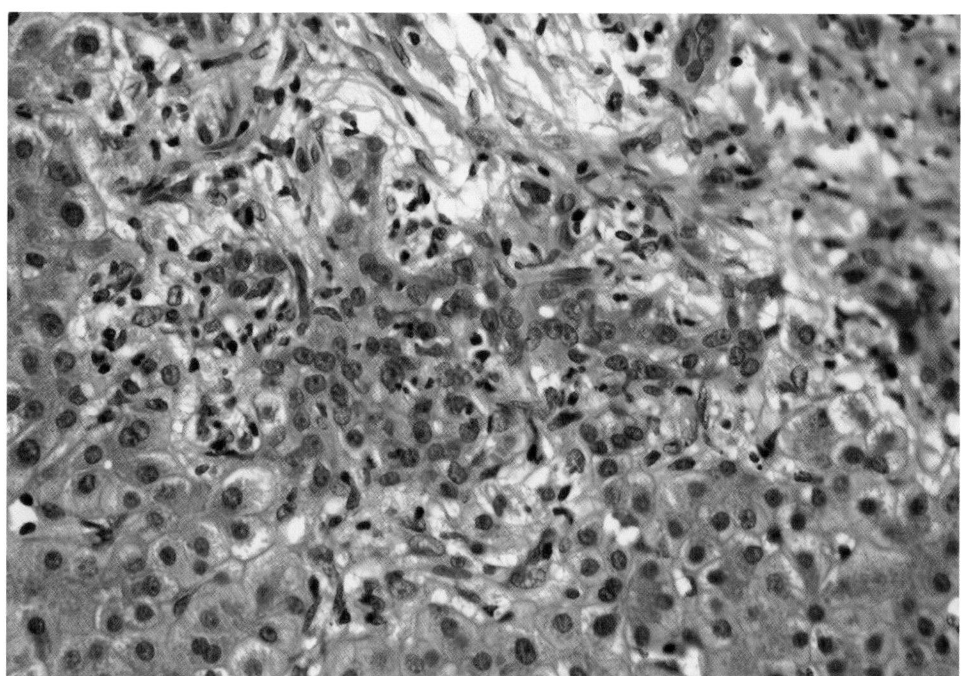

b

Figure 4.6 *The ductular reaction in different diseases.* (a) Ductular structures at edge of portal tract in bile-duct obstruction. (b) Tangle of ductules in primary biliary cirrhosis. *Continued*

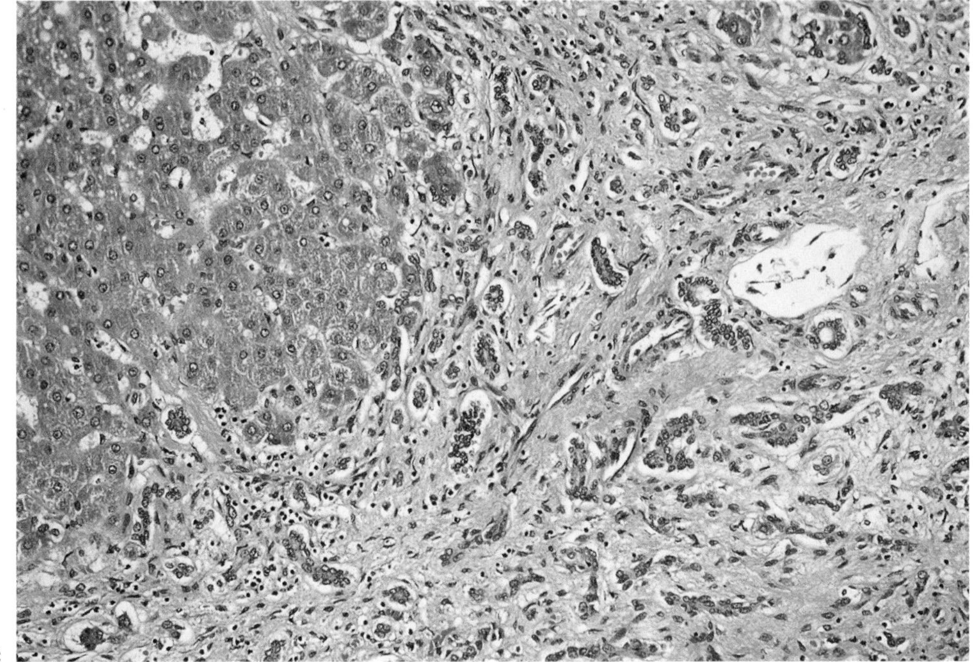

c

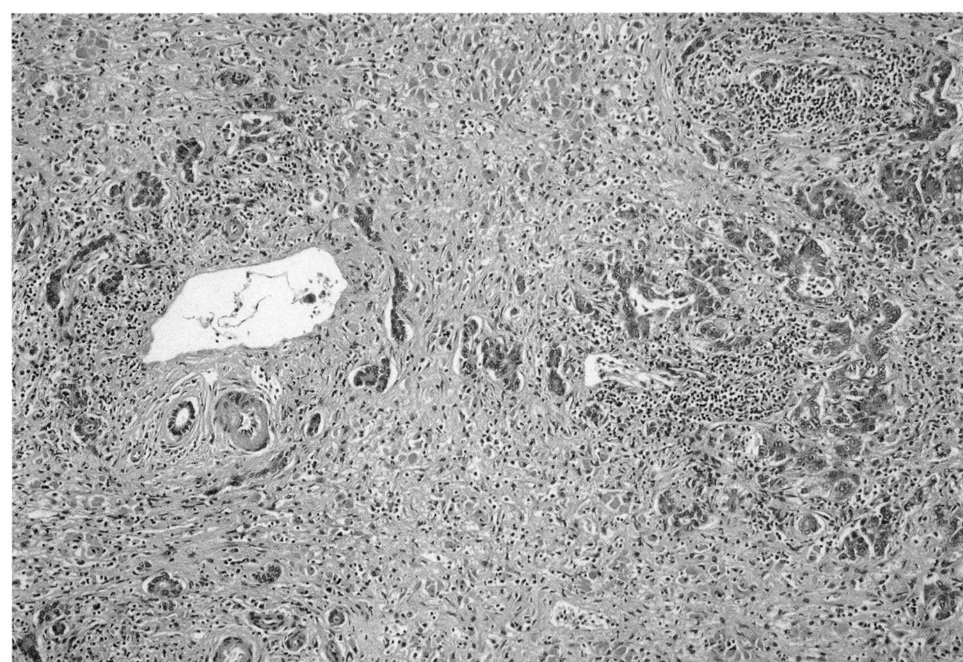

d

Figure 4.6, cont'd *The ductular reaction in different diseases.* (c) Non-biliary cirrhosis: ductular structures near the edge of the nodule and within the fibrotic portal tract. (d) Multilobular necrosis: the duct-like structures probably reflect progenitor-cell activity in the absence of adequate hepatocellular regeneration. (H&E).

irregular, leading to possible confusion with interface hepatitis. The latter is accompanied by a lymphocytic infiltrate, rather than neutrophils, and the cholestasis, portal oedema and duct proliferation of duct obstruction are absent.

Paradoxically, the portal bile ducts are not always strikingly dilated when major ducts are obstructed, although the main duct system is seen to be dilated on cholangiography. When small ducts or canals of Hering are dilated, filled with bile and infiltrated or surrounded by neutrophils, sepsis rather than bile-duct obstruction should be suspected as the cause of the patient's jaundice (see Fig. 15.11).

In acute hepatitis the portal infiltrate is mainly composed of lymphocytes although a few other cells are commonly seen. Ductular reaction is not usually conspicuous but ducts may be damaged (see Fig. 6.7). In the less common examples of acute hepatitis in which the portal reaction mimics that of duct obstruction, the parenchymal changes of hepatitis make the diagnosis clear.

The ductular reaction

The ductular structures which develop as a prominent feature in a variety of biliary and other conditions may arise from periportal progenitor cells, canals of Hering or other sources (see Ch. 5) and are typically associated with neutrophil infiltrates and stromal oedema with variable degrees of fibrosis, collectively referred to as the *ductular reaction*. The ductular reaction can be viewed as a stereotypical periportal response to injury,[9] which is exemplified by acute biliary obstruction, but which also occurs in several other pathological settings.

Certain features help in interpreting the diagnostic significance of the ductular reaction. In acute biliary obstruction, the ductular structures are arranged in parallel to the portal-parenchymal interface, associated with the portal oedema and scattered neutrophils previously mentioned (Fig. 4.6a). In chronic biliary tract diseases such as primary biliary cirrhosis, the ductular profiles may lie at an angle to the interface or form convoluted tangles (Fig. 4.6b). Hepatocellular diseases may also act as a stimulus for the ductular reaction. In a minority of patients with acute hepatitis with much cholestasis, as seen for example in hepatitis A, a ductular reaction may accompany portal infiltrates of lymphocytes and plasma cells.[10] The picture can mimic that of biliary obstruction, and the distinction requires careful consideration of the lobular changes. Ductular reaction is virtually always associated with neutrophils, so that the presence of these cells is not in itself evidence of bile-duct obstruction. Ductular reaction also is seen in some examples of non-biliary cirrhosis in which the ductular structures are not necessarily limited to the margins of portal tracts or the septal-parenchymal interface, but extend to greater distances into the fibrous tissue (Fig. 4.6c). However, extensive ductular reaction accompanied by other features of chronic cholestasis suggests cirrhosis of biliary origin.

In panlobular necrosis, seen for example in patients with fulminant or subacute viral hepatitis or in severe hepatotoxicity, extensive loss of hepatocytes is often associated with an exuberant ductular reaction extending from periportal regions further inward toward the centres of lobules (Fig. 4.6d). Finally, it should be noted that a ductular reaction of varying degree may develop in chronic hepatitis, including chronic hepatitis B and C.[11,12] It may be unusually prominent in fibrosing cholestatic hepatitis which develops in a minority of patients with recurrence of hepatitis B or C after liver transplantation (see Fig. 16.16). In any situation in which the relative diagnostic importance of the ductular reaction must be established, immunostains for cytokeratin 7 or 19 are useful for highlighting the ductular structures (see Figs 5.24 and 5.25).

Bile duct loss

Loss of interlobular bile ducts is a key feature of several diseases in childhood and adult life. These are sometimes referred to as **vanishing bile duct syndromes**. The principal causes in children are syndromatic and asyndromatic paucity of intrahepatic bile ducts, α_1-antitrypsin deficiency and early-onset sclerosing cholangitis. Some uncommon familial cholestatic syndromes and Langerhans cell histiocytosis should also be considered. In adults (see Table 5.3), the commonest causes are primary biliary cirrhosis, primary sclerosing cholangitis, graft-versus-host disease and chronic liver graft rejection.

In assessing duct loss, it is important to bear in mind that not every small portal tract is seen to contain a bile duct in the plane of section. In a study of normal human liver biopsies,[13] 7% of sectioned portal tracts did not contain a bile duct. For confident assessment of duct numbers a biopsy must therefore contain several portal tracts. Loss of ducts is accompanied in many, but not all cases, by the features of chronic cholestasis outlined above. This depends on the extent of duct loss, the underlying aetiology and the degree of fibrosis. A significant ductular reaction develops in some conditions of bile duct loss (primary biliary cirrhosis, primary sclerosing cholangitis) but not others (Alagille's syndrome in children, chronic liver graft rejection).

Copper-associated protein

Granules of the copper-associated protein metallothionein can be stained by several methods, including orcein and Victoria blue. They are usually positive with PAS after diastase digestion. Their most common location is in periportal hepatocytes or, in cirrhotic livers, in hepatocytes at the periphery of nodules. This reflects inability of the hepatocytes to excrete copper efficiently. Some granules can be seen in cirrhosis of any cause, but large amounts should lead to a suspicion of chronic biliary tract disease or intrahepatic cholestasis.[14] Copper itself is usually demonstrable in the same location, and there may be other features of chronic cholestasis such as ductular proliferation, neutrophils, intercellular fibrosis and oedema. A few granules of copper-associated protein are sometimes seen deeper within the lobules in prolonged acute cholestasis.

Copper-associated protein also accumulates in Wilson's disease, as discussed in Chapter 14. As a rule neither the protein nor copper itself is demonstrable by staining in the early stages of the disease. When cirrhosis develops in Wilson's disease some nodules may be rich in copper-associated protein and copper (although one may be demonstrable without the other), while others are negative. The copper and the protein are usually diffusely distributed throughout a nodule, in contrast to their location in chronic cholestasis.

Hepatocyte swelling

Normal hepatocytes are polygonal in shape, with abundant pale-staining granular cytoplasm rich in glycogen. Moderate swelling is sometimes due to adaptive hyperplasia of the smooth endoplasmic reticulum in response to drugs (see Fig. 8.1). More severe swelling with rounding of the cell outlines, or hepatocellular ballooning, is a feature of cell damage. It may accompany canalicular cholestasis (see Fig. 5.2) but is most characteristically found in various forms of hepatitis (see Fig. 6.2). This is recognised by disruption of the liver-cell plates and by accompanying inflammatory-cell infiltration. Perivenular liver-cell ballooning associated with inflammation and a pericellular network of 'chicken-wire' fibrosis is characteristic of steatohepatitis due to various causes[15] (see Fig. 7.12). Following liver transplantation, ballooned hepatocytes can result from perfusion injury, hypoperfusion or hepatitis (see Fig. 16.2). In microvesicular steatosis, the cytoplasm of hepatocytes is expanded by minute fat droplets which are sometimes too small to resolve by routine microscopy. The frequent presence of larger fat vacuoles and the clinical context should help to make the diagnosis.

Apoptosis

An occasional apoptotic body may be seen in normal liver. In cholestasis from any cause, and in donor livers shortly after transplantation, there is often an increase in the number of apoptotic bodies as well as in mitotic figures in hepatocytes. Abundant apoptotic bodies (acidophil bodies) are found in acute hepatitis from any cause. They were first described by Councilman in yellow fever, so that the term Councilman body should strictly speaking be confined to that disease.

Inflammatory-cell infiltration

Neutrophils

Neutrophils are most numerous in portal tracts in large bile-duct obstruction, and in any condition in which there is an extensive ductular reaction (see above). In ascending cholangitis they are found in the lumens and walls of bile ducts. In intra- or extrahepatic sepsis there may be neutrophils around ducts and bile within their lumens. Neutrophils are also seen in the sinusoids. A few neutrophils in a predominantly lymphocytic-plasmacytic portal infiltrate are common in acute hepatitis from any cause, but predominance of neutrophils suggests possible drug-related liver injury.

Diffuse infiltration of the parenchyma by neutrophils is unusual. It may represent a classical acute inflammatory response to extensive tissue destruction from any cause. Localised infiltrates are found in steatohepatitis, especially when alcohol-related. However, a mainly lymphocytic infiltrate does not exclude the diagnosis if other features are present. Focal accumulations of neutrophils (microabscesses) are a feature of cytomegalovirus infection and of perfusion injury in liver grafts. They are also seen in many other complications of liver transplantation, though usually in smaller numbers than in cytomegalovirus infection.[16] Clusters of neutrophils may be found within sinusoids in any wedge biopsies taken in the course of surgery (as seen in Fig. 3.12) and should not then be taken as indicating specific hepatic pathology.

Eosinophils

Portal infiltrates in many different liver diseases include occasional eosinophils, and their presence does not necessarily imply drug hypersensitivity or toxicity. Portal tracts often show a few eosinophils accompanying lymphocytes and plasma cells in chronic viral hepatitis. They are common in primary biliary cirrhosis and are occasionally abundant.[17] After liver transplantation they are one of the manifestations of cellular rejection.[18] An infiltrate with very prominent eosinophils suggests drug toxicity, systemic conditions with eosinophilia, parasitic disease or eosinophilic gastroenteritis.[19] Focal accumulations of eosinophils are seen in the parenchyma within some granulomas, notably those due to parasites.

Plasma cells

Portal and lobular plasma cell infiltrates are often striking in autoimmune hepatitis, but they may also be seen in acute or chronic viral hepatitis. They are sometimes abundant in hepatitis A. Plasma cells form an important part of the portal infiltrates of primary biliary cirrhosis.

Lymphoid follicles

Portal follicles are common and large in many patients with hepatitis C.[20] In this condition they may have easily identifiable germinal centres. Similar follicles are found in primary biliary cirrhosis and autoimmune hepatitis. Less prominent follicles without germinal centres, sometimes referred to as lymphoid aggregates, may be seen in hepatitis B, hepatitis C and other chronic liver diseases.

REFERENCES

1 Foschini M, Sarti F, Dina RE, et al. Standardized reporting of histological diagnoses for non-neoplastic liver conditions in needle biopsies. *Virchows Arch* 1995; **426**: 593–596.

2 Yoon J-H, Gores GJ. Death receptor-mediated apoptosis and the liver. *J Hepatol* 2002; **37**: 400–410.

3 Patel T, Gores GJ. Apoptosis and hepatobiliary disease. *Hepatology* 1995; **21**: 1725–1741.

4 Kerr JFR, Searle J, Halliday WJ, et al. The nature of piecemeal necrosis in chronic active hepatitis. *Lancet* 1979; **ii**: 827–828.

5 Hiramatsu N, Hayashi N, Katayama K, et al. Immunohistochemical detection of Fas antigen in liver tissue of patients with chronic hepatitis C. *Hepatology* 1994; **19**: 1354–1359.

6 Takahara T, Nakayama Y, Itoh H, et al. Extracellular matrix formation in piecemeal necrosis: immuno-electron microscopic study. *Liver* 1992; **12**: 368–380.

7 Roskams T, Desmet V. Ductular reaction and its diagnostic significance. *Sem Diagn Pathol* 1998; **15**: 259–269.

8 Portmann B, Popper H, Neuberger J, et al. Sequential and diagnostic features in primary biliary cirrhosis based on serial histologic study in 209 patients. *Gastroenterology* 1985; **88**: 1777–1790.

9 Roskams T. Progenitor cell involvement in cirrhotic human liver diseases: from controversy to consensus. *J Hepatol* 2003; **39**: 431–434.
10 Teixeira MR Jr., Weller IVD, Murray AM et al. The pathology of hepatitis A in man. *Liver* 1982; **2**: 53–60.
11 Fotiadu A, Tzioufa V, Vrettou E, et al. Progenitor cell activation in chronic viral hepatitis. *Liver Int* 2004; **24**: 268–274.
12 Eleazar JA, Memeo L, Jhang JS, et al. Progenitor cell expansion: an important source of hepatocyte regeneration in chronic hepatitis. *J Hepatol* 2004; **41**: 983–991.
13 Crawford AR, Lin X-Z, Crawford JM. The normal adult human liver biopsy: a quantitative reference standard. *Hepatology* 1998; **28**: 323–331.
14 Guarascio P, Yentis F, Cevikbas U, et al. Value of copper-associated protein in diagnostic assessment of liver biopsy. *J Clin Pathol* 1983; **36**: 18–23.
15 Gramlich T, Kleiner DE, McCullough AJ, et al. Pathologic features associated with fibrosis in nonalcoholic fatty liver disease. *Hum Pathol* 2004; **35**: 196–199.
16 Lamps LW, Pinson CW, Raiford DS, et al. The significance of microabscesses in liver transplant biopsies: a clinicopathological study. *Hepatology* 1998; **28**: 1532–1537.
17 Terasaki S, Nakanuma Y, Yamazaki M, et al. Eosinophilic infiltration of the liver in primary biliary cirrhosis: a morphological study. *Hepatology* 1993; **17**: 206–212.
18 Datta Gupta S, Hudson M, Burroughs AK, et al. Grading of cellular rejection after orthotopic liver transplantation. *Hepatology* 1995; **21**: 46–57.
19 Schoonbroodt D, Horsmans Y, Laka A, et al. Eosinophilic gastroenteritis presenting with colitis and cholangitis. *Dig Dis Sci* 1995; **40**: 308–314.
20 Scheuer PJ, Ashrafzadeh P, Sherlock S, et al. The pathology of hepatitis C. *Hepatology* 1992; **15**: 567–571.

GENERAL READING

Ludwig J, Batts K. Practical Liver Biopsy Interpretation: Diagnostic Algorithms, 2nd edn. Chicago: ASCP Press, 1998.
Roskams T, Desmet VJ. Ductular reaction and its diagnostic significance. *Semin Diagn Pathol* 1998; **15**: 259–269.

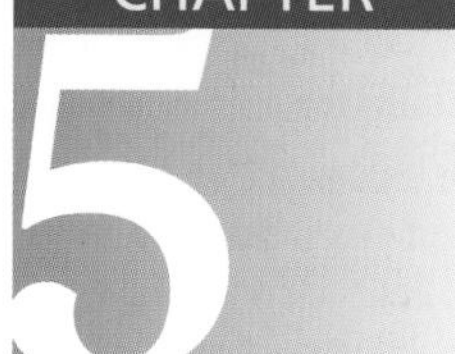

BILIARY DISEASE

INTRODUCTION

There are many sites along the biliary tree where bile flow may be interrupted, from the bile canaliculi and smallest intrahepatic ducts to the large bile ducts and duodenum (Fig. 5.1). Damage or obstruction at these various sites may result in visible bile in histological sections (cholestasis), altered bile duct morphology, changes within the portal tracts and periportal parenchyma, or combinations of these. Diseases of the larger ducts must be distinguished from diffuse intrahepatic diseases

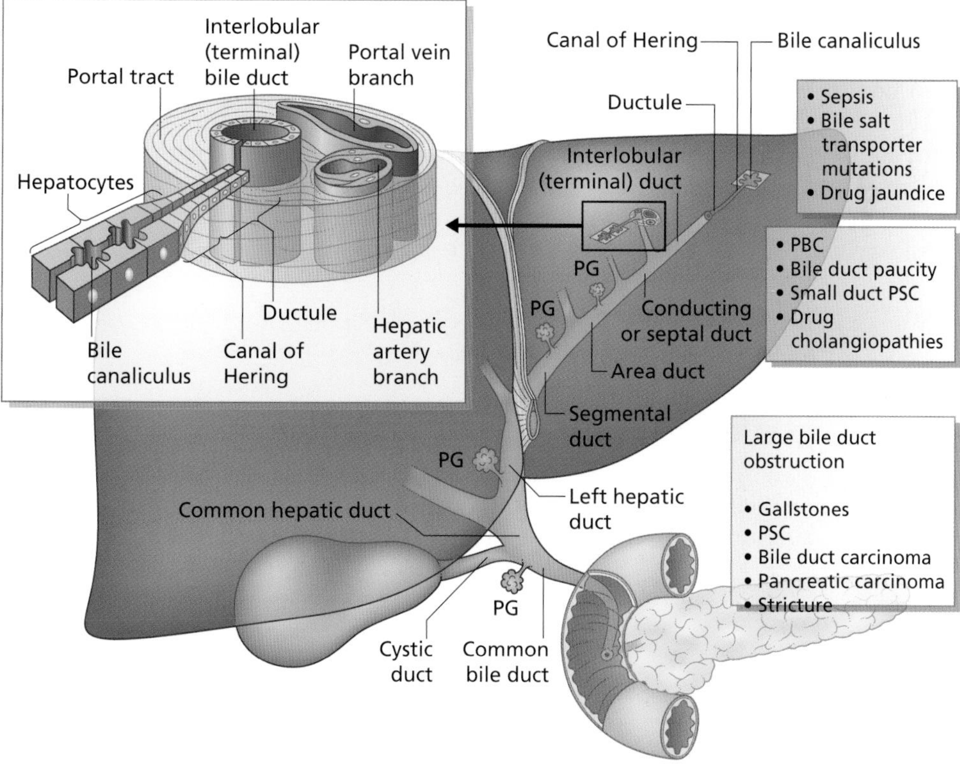

Figure 5.1 *The biliary tree*. The ramifying structures of the biliary system are shown schematically. The large, segmental and area ducts have peribiliary glands (PG). The finer branches are shown in an enlargement at upper left. Boxes at right show examples of biliary disease at the specific levels affected.

because of different clinical management and liver biopsy is often helpful in this respect. However, diseases of large bile ducts outside and within the liver share pathological features and may be amenable to similar forms of treatment; for this reason, the term 'extrahepatic biliary obstruction' is not used in this chapter. Carcinoma of the main hepatic ducts, for example, may be situated wholly within the liver, yet lead to the changes of large-duct obstruction. This chapter discusses these changes as well as the pathology of primary biliary cirrhosis and primary sclerosing cholangitis, the diagnostic problem of overlap with autoimmune hepatitis and several bile duct paucity disorders.

CHOLESTASIS

The term *cholestasis* in clinical and pathological usage refers to impairment of bile flow. Under the microscope, cholestasis (sometimes called **bilirubinostasis**) is defined as the presence of bile pigment within bile canaliculi, hepatocytes and other sites. It is the morphologic correlate of clinical jaundice. Cholestasis is an important finding in large bile-duct obstruction or in extensive intrahepatic bile duct disease, but may also accompany the parenchymal damage in certain types of hepatitis. Pure (bland) cholestasis as an isolated lesion requires consideration of several possible aetiologies (Table 5.1), which may not be distinguishable by light microscopy alone. For example, in neonatal and childhood jaundice, cholestasis may result from mutations in bile salt transport proteins on the canalicular membrane[1] or from mitochondriopathies[2] (discussed further in Chapter 13). In adults, drug hepatotoxicity, circulating endotoxin in septicaemia[3] and cytokine release from extrahepatic lymphoma[4] are further examples of functional disorders of bile secretory physiology that may lead to intrahepatic cholestasis (see Ch. 4). The pathologist's first priority when cholestasis is present, nevertheless, is careful examination of the portal tracts for possible changes of mechanical large bile-duct obstruction, which are described below.

LARGE BILE-DUCT OBSTRUCTION

Biopsies from patients with large bile-duct obstruction are much less often seen than formerly, because of improved imaging methods. However, the pathologist needs to

Table 5.1 Causes of intrahepatic cholestasis

Septicaemia
Drug hepatotoxicity
Bile salt transporter mutations (e.g. Byler disease)
Extrahepatic lymphoma
Mitochondriopathies (e.g. Navajo neurohepatopathy)
Early large bile-duct obstruction

be able to recognise the characteristic changes, especially following liver transplantation. From the first weeks of obstruction, there is cholestasis in perivenular areas; that is to say, bile is visible under the microscope in the form of bile thrombi (bile plugs) in canaliculi and as yellow-brown pigment in hepatocytes and Kupffer cells (Fig. 5.2). The presence of canalicular bile thrombi distinguishes cholestasis from other pigmentations (see Table 4.1). Kupffer cells in cholestatic areas are enlarged and pigmented, containing both bile and diastase-resistant PAS-positive material. In recovering obstruction the Kupffer-cell changes persist while bile thrombi become smaller and less numerous. Finally, as in residual acute hepatitis, a few diastase-PAS-positive Kupffer cells may provide the only histological evidence of a recent episode of jaundice.

At first, the hepatocytes in areas of cholestasis show little change, but with time they often become swollen. Their nuclei increase in size and number and a few apoptotic bodies and mitoses may be seen, indicating increased cell turnover. Individual hepatocytes or small groups of cells undergo *feathery degeneration*, characterised by rarefied and reticular cytoplasm (Fig. 5.3). The lesion is focal and the affected cells are typically surrounded by more or less normal hepatocytes. Feathery degeneration may be difficult to distinguish from the ballooning degeneration of hepatitis (see Fig. 6.2) or following liver transplantation, but in ballooning the cytoplasm is often granular rather than feathery and the lesion is more widespread in the lobule.

In a minority of patients with obstructed ducts **bile infarcts** form (Fig. 5.4). These are substantial areas of hepatocellular degeneration or death containing pale or bile-stained hepatocytes or discrete rounded cells difficult to distinguish from macrophages. There are variable amounts of bile and fibrin, the latter often abundant. Reticulin fibres become progressively more difficult to demonstrate. Bile

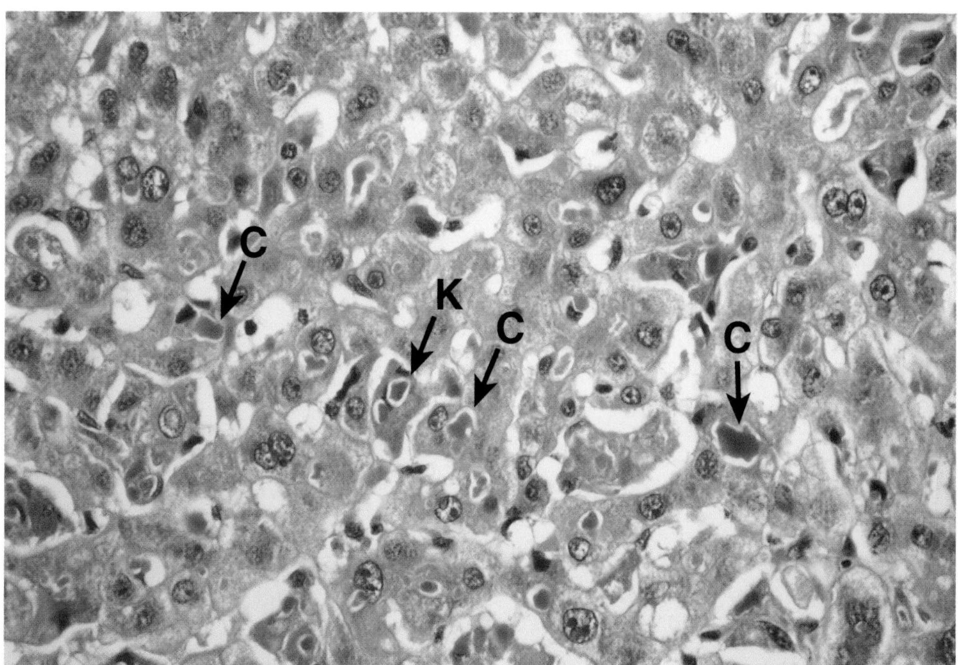

Figure 5.2 *Cholestasis*. Bile is seen in the form of bile thrombi (bile plugs) in dilated canaliculi (C), as well as in Kupffer cells (K). (Needle biopsy, H&E).

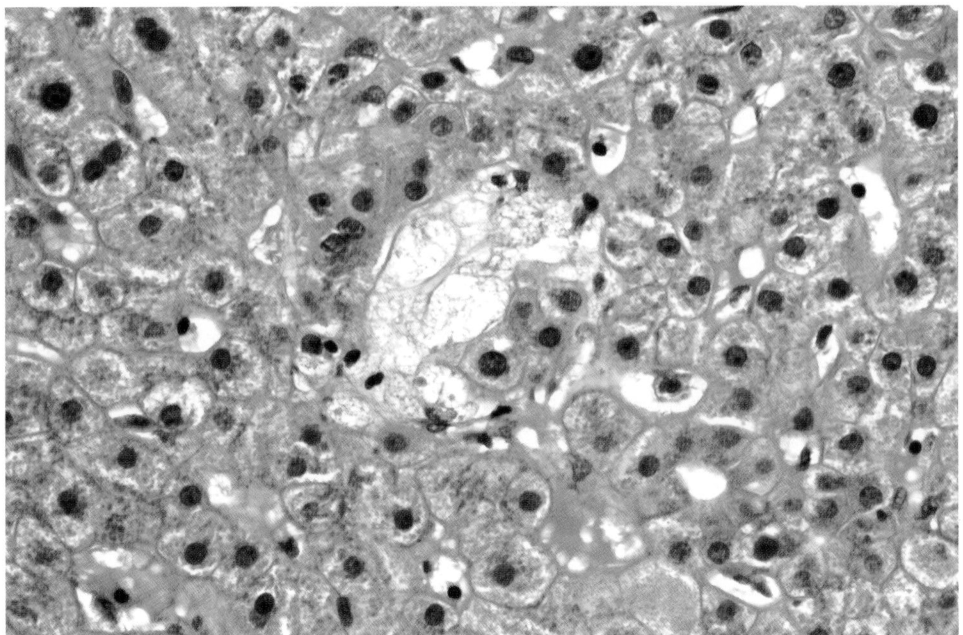

Figure 5.3 *Cholestasis.* Small groups of swollen hepatocytes at centre have undergone feathery degeneration. Adjacent hepatocytes appear normal. (Wedge biopsy, H&E).

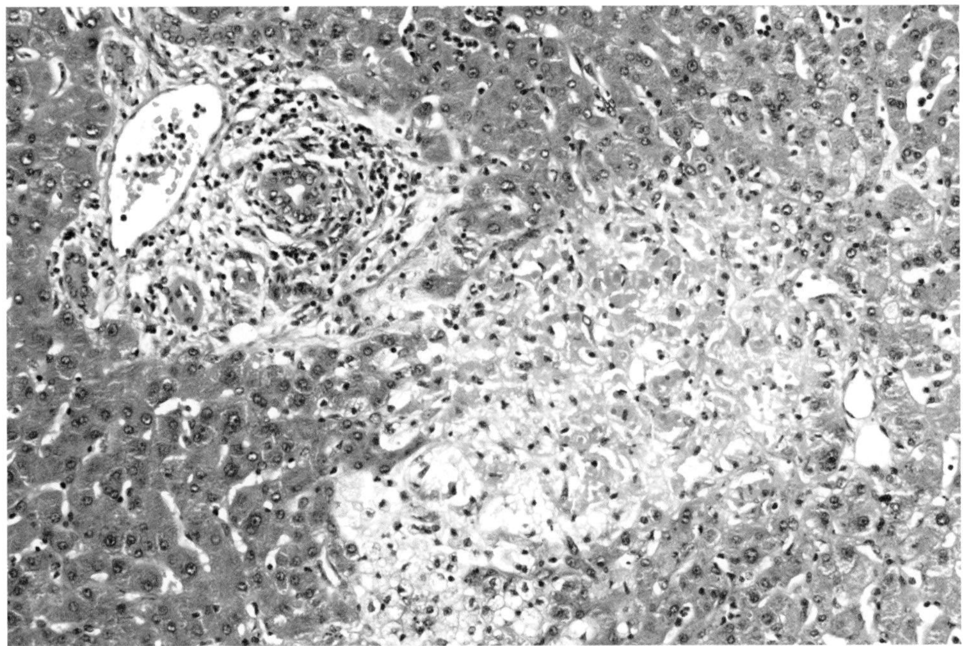

Figure 5.4 *Large bile-duct obstruction with bile infarct.* A bile infarct is seen at the centre of the field near the portal tract. Hepatocyte nuclei are pyknotic within the infarct. Some of the pink strands represent fibrin. (Wedge biopsy, H&E).

eventually leaches out of the infarct to leave a barely pigmented and scarcely stained lesion containing the ghosts of hepatocytes. Small bile infarcts may be found in severe cholestasis from any cause; larger infarcts such as the one shown in Fig. 5.4, especially if adjacent to a portal tract, are highly suggestive of bile-duct obstruction. However, because such infarcts are only seen in a minority of patients with obstructed ducts, the diagnosis must usually be established by other criteria.

As a result of these various forms of hepatocellular damage in biliary obstruction and indeed in cholestasis generally, a certain amount of inflammatory infiltration of the parenchyma is commonly seen after a period of some weeks. This infiltration is usually mild and restricted to the cholestatic areas, unlike the inflammation of an acute hepatitis. When cholestasis resulting from duct obstruction is prolonged, especially in older patients, inflammation and liver-cell damage are occasionally severe enough to raise the alternative possibility of an acute hepatitis. It is then helpful to note that in bile-duct obstruction the liver-cell plates remain for the most part intact, whereas in hepatitis they become irregular as a result of cell loss, swelling and regeneration. Central-portal (zone 3) bridging necrosis is not a feature of biliary obstruction.

Within a few days or weeks of the onset of duct obstruction a characteristic triad of portal changes develops,[5] consisting of portal oedema and swelling (Fig. 5.5), infiltration by inflammatory cells and increased numbers of bile-duct profiles at the margins of the portal tracts (Figs 5.6, 5.7). These marginal bile-duct structures are the most consistent finding in the portal tracts and are rarely absent.[5] They may originate

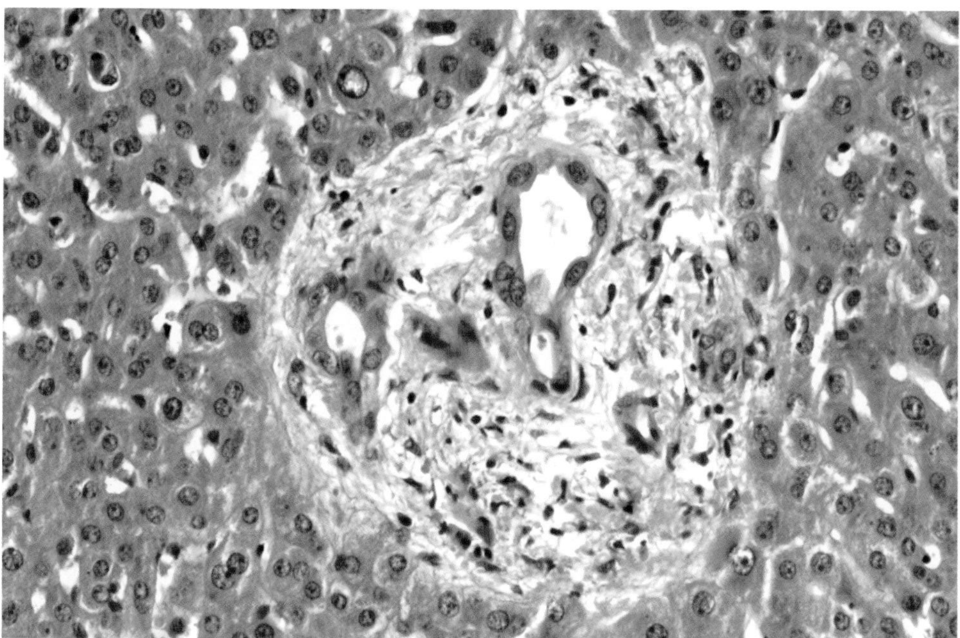

Figure 5.5 *Large bile-duct obstruction*. The connective tissue of a small portal tract is oedematous. There is little inflammation in this example. (Wedge biopsy, H&E).

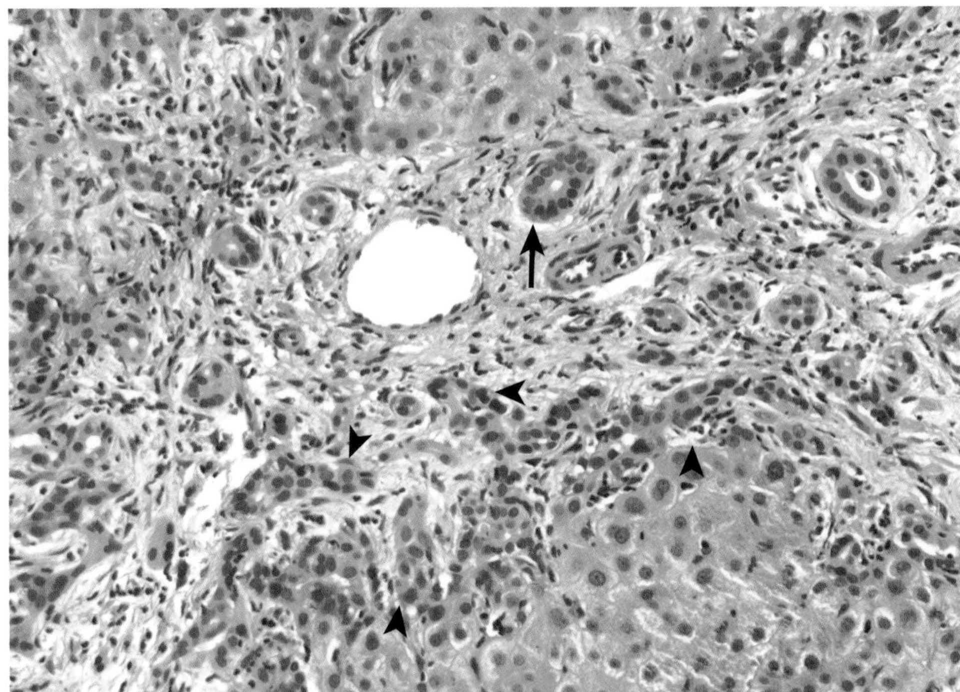

Figure 5.6 *Large bile-duct obstruction.* A prominent ductular reaction (arrowheads) is present at the edge of an inflamed and oedematous portal tract. The original interlobular duct is marked by an arrow. (Needle biopsy, H&E).

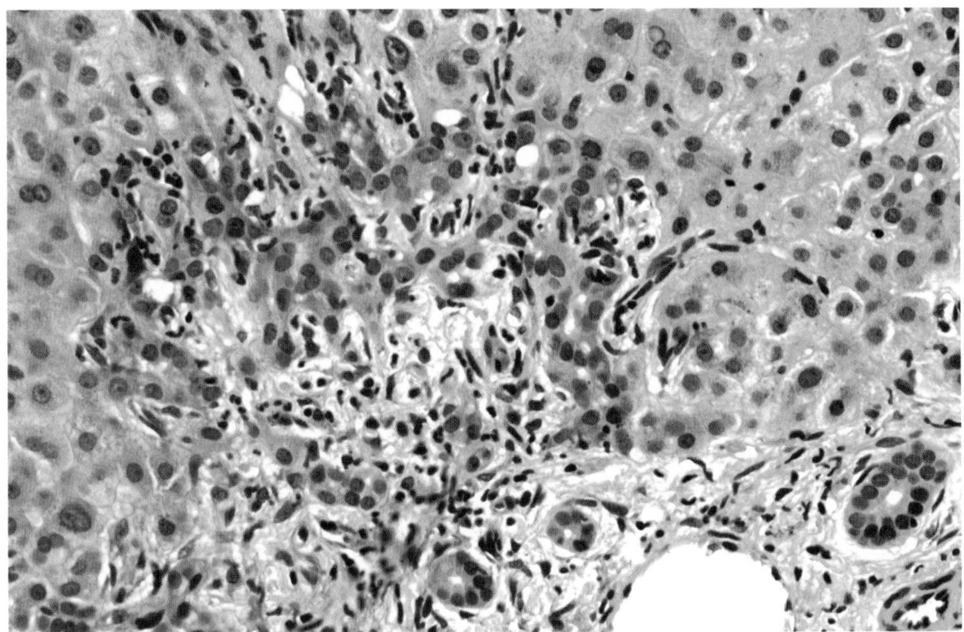

Figure 5.7 *Ductular reaction in large bile-duct obstruction.* The upper left-hand portion of Figure 5.6 is shown at higher magnification. The irregular ductular structures at the edge of the portal tract show compressed, narrow lumens and an associated neutrophil infiltrate. (Needle biopsy, H&E).

from canals of Hering, periportal stem cells or other sources[6] and are an early response to the increased portal tract pressure due to obstruction, circulating mediators[7] and expression of developmental proteins such as Notch receptors and Jagged proteins.[8] The term *ductular reaction* refers to these proliferated bile ductules accompanied by inflammation and stromal changes at the edges of the portal tracts.[9] Usage of 'ductular reaction' is now preferable to 'bile ductular proliferation' or 'typical' and 'atypical' bile ductules which embody considerable imprecision.[6] The ductular structures may be of normal calibre or dilated, but are often flattened with small or imperceptible lumens (Fig. 5.7) and variations in nuclear size, staining and location. These structures can be highlighted by immunostaining for cytokeratin 7 or 19 (see Figs 5.24, 5.25). Surprisingly, bile is not usually seen within dilated ducts or ductules in uncomplicated obstruction; when it is present, sepsis should be suspected. The differentiation of the ductular reaction of biliary obstruction from that of chronic liver disease has already been discussed in Chapter 4.

Within the oedematous, swollen portal tracts, especially around proliferated bile ducts, an inflammatory infiltrate develops, mediated by the complex interactions of cytokines and cellular adhesion molecules (some produced by biliary epithelium itself[10]) and proinflammatory agents such as endotoxin.[3] Neutrophils are prominent but there may be other cells including lymphocytes and eosinophils. The presence of a few eosinophils is therefore not in itself sufficient evidence for a diagnosis of drug jaundice. As a result of the proliferative and inflammatory changes of bile-duct obstruction, the outlines of the portal tracts become irregular and the limiting plates of hepatocytes are disrupted to a variable extent. This disruption should be distinguished from interface hepatitis in which the infiltrate is predominantly composed of lymphocytes and plasma cells and in which the acute inflammatory changes of bile-duct obstruction are not seen.

In a few patients with bile-duct obstruction the portal changes are inconspicuous (Fig. 5.5) or even absent. Biliary obstruction should therefore be considered in the differential diagnosis of canalicular cholestasis without portal reaction (so-called pure or bland cholestasis). Conversely, portal changes resembling those of duct obstruction are occasionally found in severe acute hepatitis, when the parenchymal alterations make the diagnosis clear. Sometimes, similar portal changes are seen without cholestasis near space-occupying lesions such as metastases,[11] usually together with sinusoidal dilatation. Portal inflammation without cholestasis is also found in patients with disease affecting one or other part of the biliary tree but without current obstruction of the segment biopsied. It is seen in chronic pancreatitis[12] and in patients with acute cholecystitis or choledocholithiasis.[13] Biopsies showing only an increased number of well-differentiated bile ductules at the portal interface, unaccompanied by inflammation or stromal changes, have been noted in patients with idiopathic **isolated ductular hyperplasia (IDH)**[14] (Fig. 5.8). These patients have longstanding abnormalities in serum alanine aminotransferase and/or gamma glutamyl transferase, no proven biliary tract disease and an apparently good prognosis (although the cause of this reactive lesion is uncertain).

In a few instances of biliary obstruction, bile escapes from a duct into the connective tissue of a portal tract, giving rise to a *bile extravasate*. This leads to a phagocytic reaction, with or without foreign-body giant cells (Fig. 5.9). Bile extravasates, like large bile infarcts, are almost diagnostic of obstruction, but are only seen in a minority of patients. If the extravasate extends beyond the confines of a portal tract into the adjacent parenchyma, the appearances at the periphery of the lesion are very like those of a bile infarct.

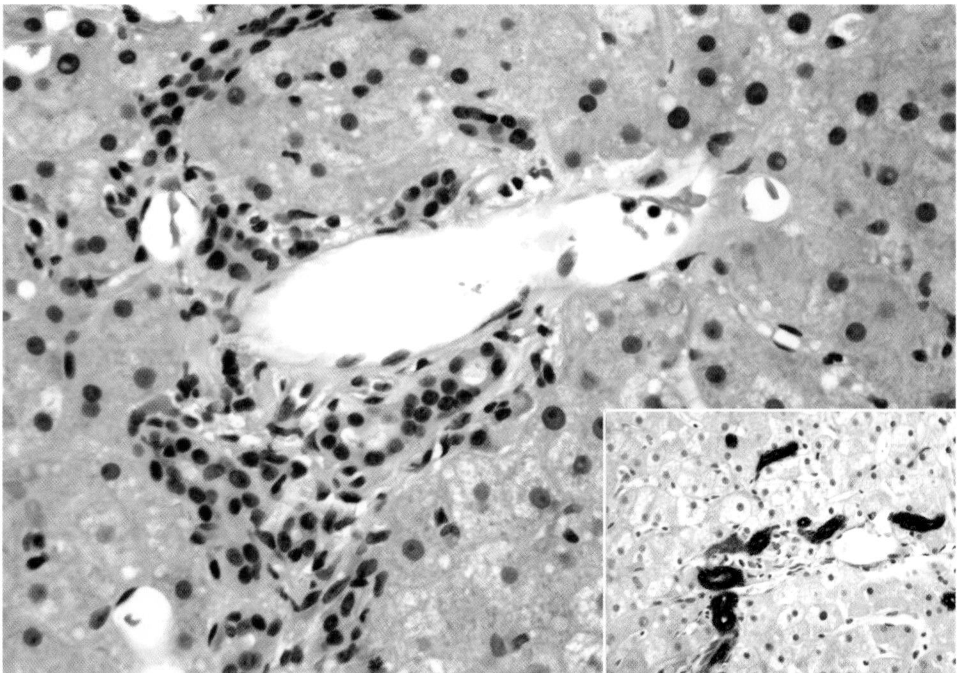

Figure 5.8 *Isolated ductular hyperplasia.* Well-differentiated hyperplastic bile ductules are present in this biopsy from a patient with persistent liver function test abnormalities unrelated to viral hepatitis or demonstrable biliary disease. The absence of oedema and inflammation help distinguish this lesion from large bile-duct obstruction. (Needle biopsy, H&E). *Inset*: Immunostain for cytokeratin 7 on a deeper level highlights the bile ductules. Needle biopsy, specific immunoperoxidase. (Case kindly provided by Drs Bernard Traub and John B. Herrington, III, Sleepy Hollow, New York).

Chronic bile-duct obstruction and biliary cirrhosis

When bile-duct obstruction persists, the acute inflammatory reaction in the portal tracts is followed by increasing fibrosis. Production of fibrogenic cytokines by bile duct epithelium contributes to this process.[15] Eventually the tracts are linked by broad fibrous septa. There is a variable degree of acute and chronic inflammatory infiltration, the chronic element less striking than in primary biliary cirrhosis. In some patients, the lesion appears to progress more by cholangitis than by obstruction and cholestasis is therefore not always prominent or even present.

Interference with normal secretion of bile leads to several changes in hepatocytes adjacent to portal tracts and fibrous septa. The cells become swollen and separated by fibrous tissue, inflammatory cells and ductular structures (neocholangioles) derived from hepatocytes or bipotential stem cells.[16–18] Their cytoplasm is rarefied and may contain visible bile pigment, Mallory bodies, copper and copper-associated protein (Fig. 5.10). The latter is seen in the form of fine brown granules staining variably with diastase-PAS and strongly with orcein or Victoria blue. The combination of all these changes is known as **chronic cholestasis** or **cholate stasis** (**pseudoxanthomatous change, precholestasis**) on the basis that some of the alterations probably result from the accumulation of toxic bile salts. Canalicular cholestasis is sometimes seen between the affected hepatocytes. The hepatocellular changes, ductular reaction and associated fibrosis in the periportal or

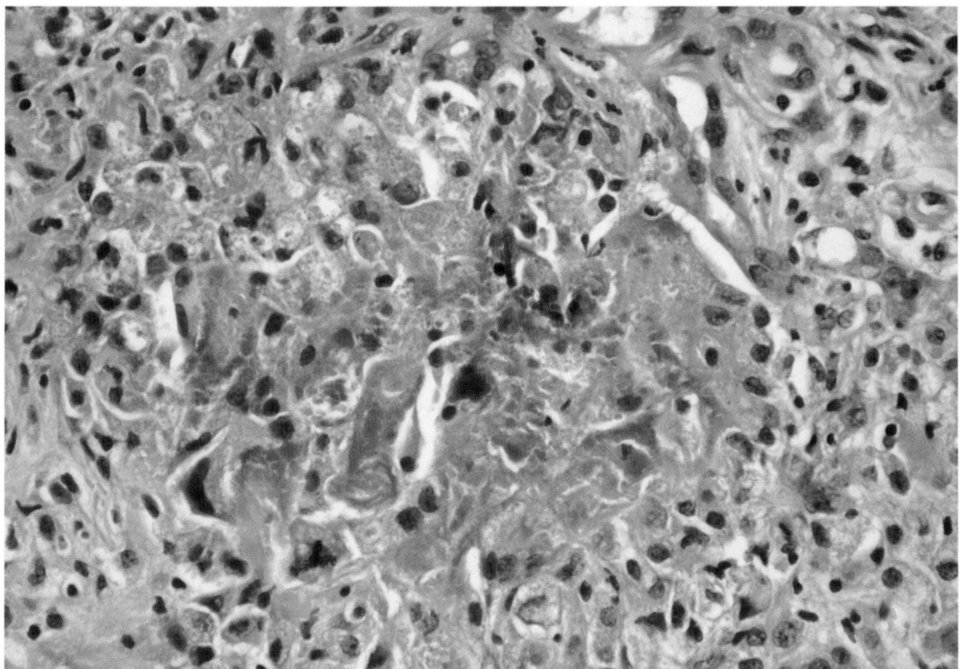

Figure 5.9 *Large bile-duct obstruction.* Bile extravasate. Bile has escaped from a duct and has evoked a phagocytic reaction. (Needle biopsy, H&E).

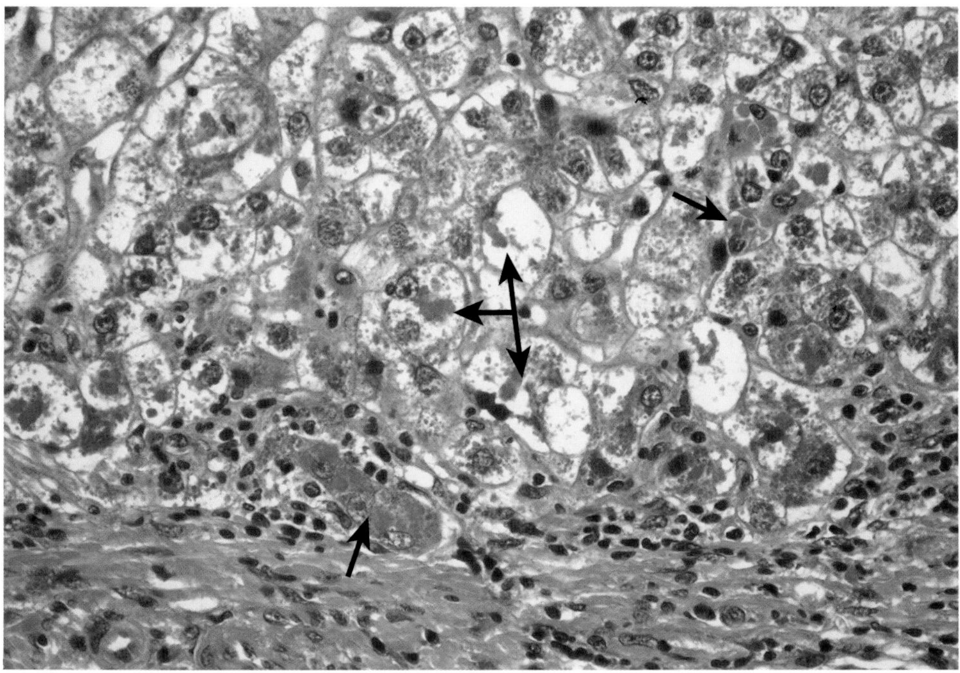

Figure 5.10 *Chronic cholestasis.* Hepatocytes near a portal tract (below) are swollen and pale-staining. Many contain Mallory bodies (lower arrow and triple arrow). Bile thrombi are also seen (top arrow). (Wedge biopsy, H&E).

periseptal region in effect produce an irregular interface with the parenchyma which has in the past been linked with the term 'piecemeal necrosis'.[19] However, distinction from the interface hepatitis of chronic hepatitis (see Ch. 10) is usually apparent from the aforementioned features.

The fibrous septa, which eventually form in chronic biliary tract disease, surround and outline groups of classical hepatic lobules, leaving the normal vascular relationships essentially intact. Islands of parenchyma with characteristic protruding studs resemble the pieces of a jigsaw puzzle or land-masses on a map (Fig. 5.11). Spherical nodules are sparse at first, in spite of evidence of liver-cell hyperplasia in the form of thickened liver-cell plates, seen particularly in patients with associated portal hypertension.[20] An occasional rounded parenchymal island may merely represent a tangential section of a complex parenchymal mass such as the one shown in Fig. 5.11, rather than a true regeneration nodule of cirrhosis. This is especially common just deep to the liver capsule. A histological diagnosis of cirrhosis should therefore be made with caution, because at a fibrotic, pre-cirrhotic stage, considerable resolution can occasionally result if an obstruction is relieved.[21] Eventually, true *secondary biliary cirrhosis* develops, its biliary origin still evident from nodule shape and the regular, broad fibrous septa composed of loose collagen bundles with parallel arrangement (Figs 5.11 and 5.12). A zone of oedema containing a ductular reaction is often diagnostically helpful and may be striking even at low magnification (Fig. 5.11). Thus, many different structural characteristics make it possible to diagnose chronic biliary tract disease even in the absence of cholestasis. Finally, however, an end-stage cirrhosis forms, no longer necessarily recognisable as biliary in origin.

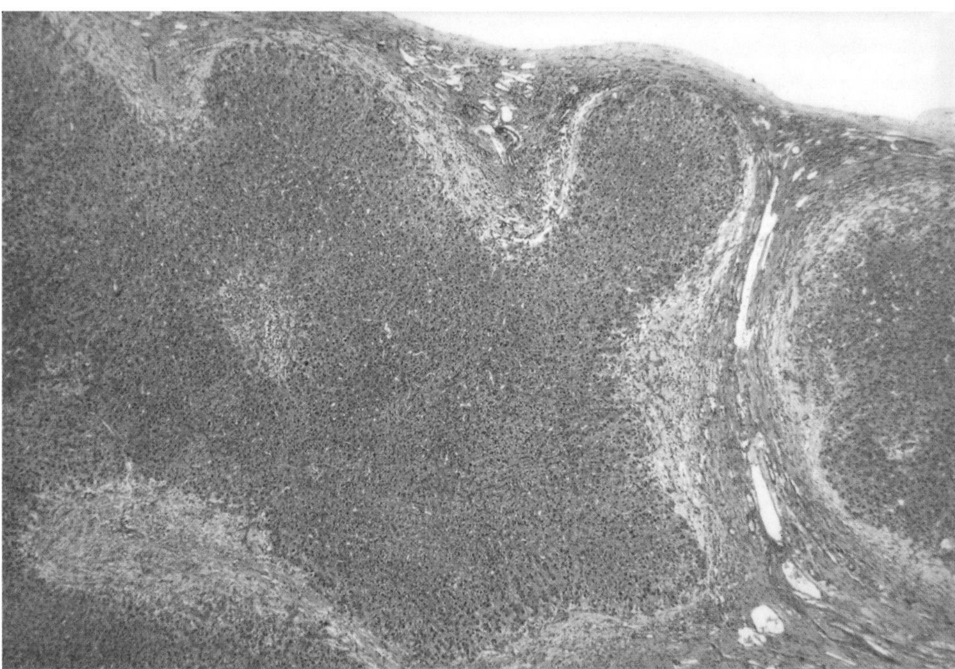

Figure 5.11 *Secondary biliary cirrhosis.* Irregular nodules resemble pieces of a jigsaw puzzle. Note the narrow zone of oedema and ductular reaction at the nodule margin. (Wedge biopsy, H&E).

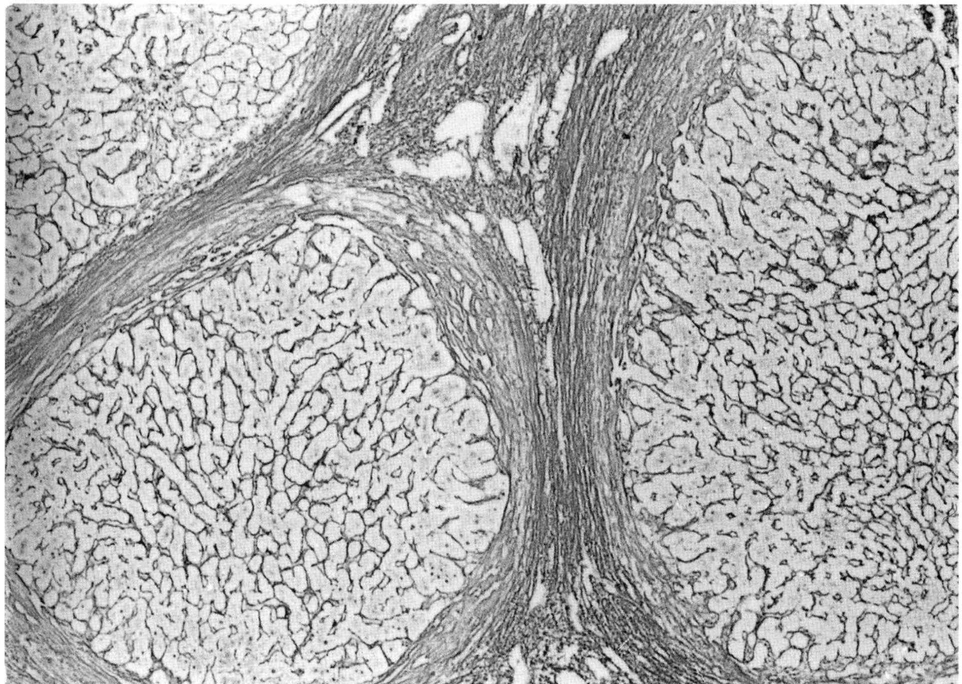

Figure 5.12 *Secondary biliary cirrhosis.* Nodules are surrounded by loose bundles of parallel collagen fibres showing little compression. (Wedge biopsy, reticulin).

CHOLANGITIS: INFECTION OF THE BILIARY TREE

In biliary obstruction, the inflammatory infiltrate around bile ducts in small portal tracts typically includes neutrophils. There is therefore cholangitis in a strictly histological sense, but this does not imply that there must be bacterial infection of the biliary tree or clinical ascending cholangitis. In the latter, neutrophils are more numerous and are found not only around ducts but also in their walls and lumens[22] (Fig. 5.13). Paradoxically, interlobular bile ducts are most affected and larger ducts may appear histologically normal. The wall of a small duct may rupture, leading to abscess formation in the portal tract. Neutrophils are seen in the sinusoids and abscesses may form in the lobules. Associated lesions include fibrin thrombi in portal vein branches, pyelophlebitis and various degrees of parenchymal necrosis,[23] the latter probably related to hypoperfusion of the parenchyma. Cholestasis is more often absent than present. Causes of ascending cholangitis include cholecystitis and choledocholithiasis, strictures including those due to primary sclerosing cholangitis, intrahepatic biliary stones,[24] pancreatitis, neoplasia of the biliary tree and Caroli's disease. In patients with AIDS, cholangitis is frequently associated with infection by *Cryptosporidium*, CMV or species of microsporidia.[25,26]

If cholangitis persists or recurs over a period of years, secondary biliary cirrhosis may develop. The histological features are then as described above in the section on bile-duct obstruction.

Septicaemia and other forms of sepsis are associated with a particular form of histological cholangitis principally affecting the canals of Hering.[27] Affected ductules are dilated and filled with inspissated bile. Neutrophils accumulate around and

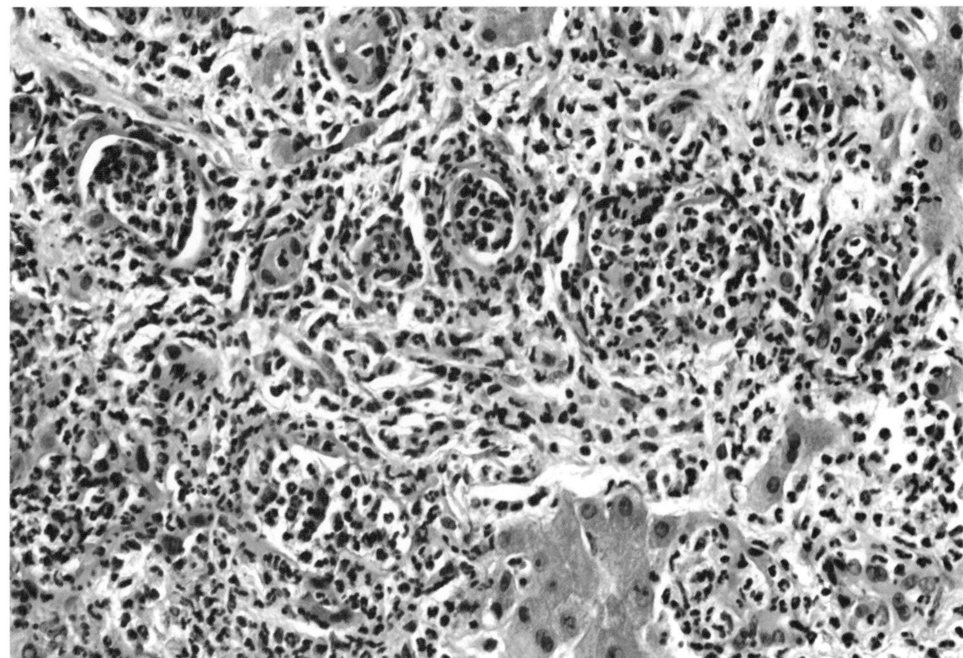

Figure 5.13 *Acute cholangitis.* Many neutrophil leucocytes are seen in the walls and dilated lumens of the bile ducts and in the surrounding connective tissue. (Wedge biopsy, H&E).

sometimes within them. Larger ducts may be affected, as may the periportal parenchyma in which bile is seen in dilated bile canaliculi. These changes are easily confused with those of large bile-duct obstruction, but in obstruction the inspissated bile in the canals of Hering is not a feature unless there is concomitant sepsis. Sepsis can also give rise to widespread canalicular cholestasis, with or without the ductular lesions. In the toxic shock syndrome the appearances of the small bile ducts can closely mimic ascending bacterial cholangitis.[28]

PRIMARY SCLEROSING CHOLANGITIS (PSC)

This condition is characterised by inflammation, strictures and saccular dilatations in the biliary tree. Typically found in adults with ulcerative colitis, it is also seen in neonates and children[29] and in the absence of inflammatory bowel disease. In a few cases, the latter is Crohn's disease, rather than ulcerative colitis.[30] Any part of the biliary tree may be affected and involvement of the gallbladder[31] and pancreas[32] has been reported. The gallbladder shows intramural lymphoplasmacytic infiltrates and lymphoid aggregates.[33] Patients do not necessarily have symptoms referable to the liver or abnormal liver function tests.[34] The disease may recur after liver transplantation.[35] Lesions similar to those of primary sclerosing cholangitis have been found in patients given arterial infusion of the anti-cancer drug fluorodeoxyuridine (FUDR) and other chemotherapeutic agents.[36,37] Obliteration or narrowing of hepatic arteries and portal vein branches suggests that in drug-related cases at least, the bile-duct damage may have an ischaemic origin.[38] Systemic

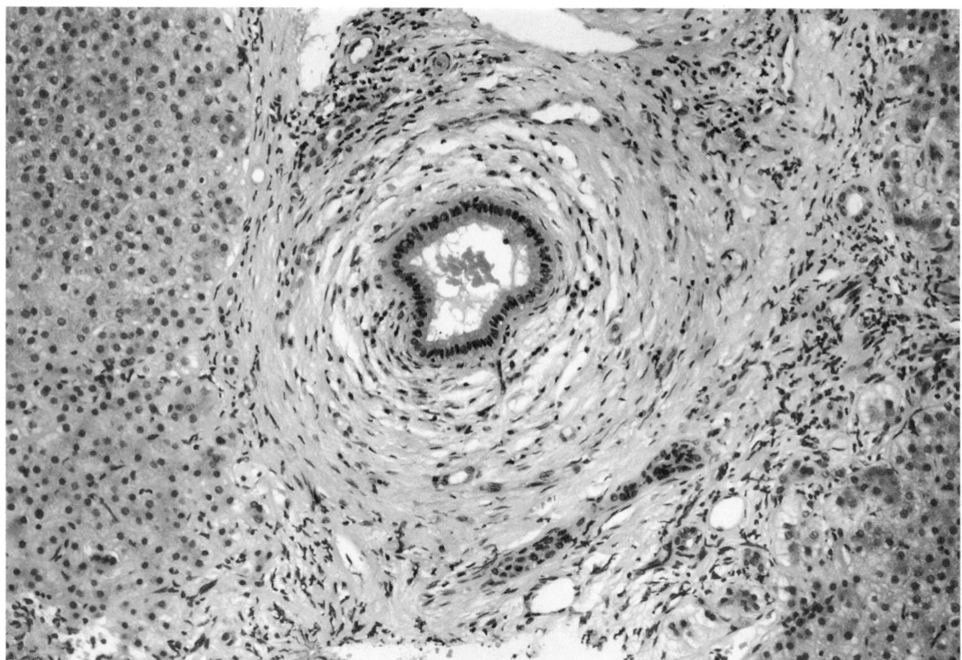

Figure 5.14 *Primary sclerosing cholangitis.* A bile duct is surrounded by a cuff of oedematous, inflamed fibrous tissue with an onion-skin appearance. (Needle biopsy, H&E).

vasculitis, liver transplantation-related hepatic artery thrombosis or chronic rejection vasculopathy and, rarely, septic shock[39] are other causes of ischaemic bile duct injury.[40]

Final diagnosis of primary sclerosing cholangitis normally rests on cholangiographic demonstration of the characteristic beading of bile ducts, but similar histological features, as described below, may be found in patients with normal cholangiograms. This can be explained on the basis of involvement of the smallest ducts, too small to be seen radiographically.[41] This **small-duct primary sclerosing cholangitis** corresponds approximately to the now obsolete label of 'pericholangitis', when applied to patients without cholangiographic abnormalities. Large- and small-duct forms of the disease frequently coexist.

The features seen on liver biopsy depend in part on the location of strictures in relation to the biopsy site. If the biopsy is taken from a part of the liver unaffected by the primary disease, but proximal to a stricture, then the changes, if any, will simply be those of bile-duct obstruction or cholangitis. If however, the biopsy site is affected by the primary disease, there may be one or more features suggesting the diagnosis. These include periduct oedema and concentric fibrosis (Fig. 5.14), ductular reaction, portal inflammation and atrophy or disappearance of the small ducts (Fig. 5.15). Loss of ducts is the commonest finding in the smallest portal tracts, while periduct fibrosis is typical of medium-sized tracts.[42] Major bile ducts, as seen for example in explanted livers at transplantation, may be inflamed, ulcerated or dilated. They may also rupture, producing a perihilar **xanthogranulomatous cholangitis.**[42a,42b]

Loss of interlobular bile ducts from the smallest portal tracts can be assessed only in biopsy samples of adequate size, that is to say containing several portal tracts. While interlobular ducts are not necessarily seen in all tracts because of the plane of section, arteries provide a useful guide; from 70–80%[43] to 92%[44] of arteries are normally accompanied by a duct lying near the centre of a portal tract. If there

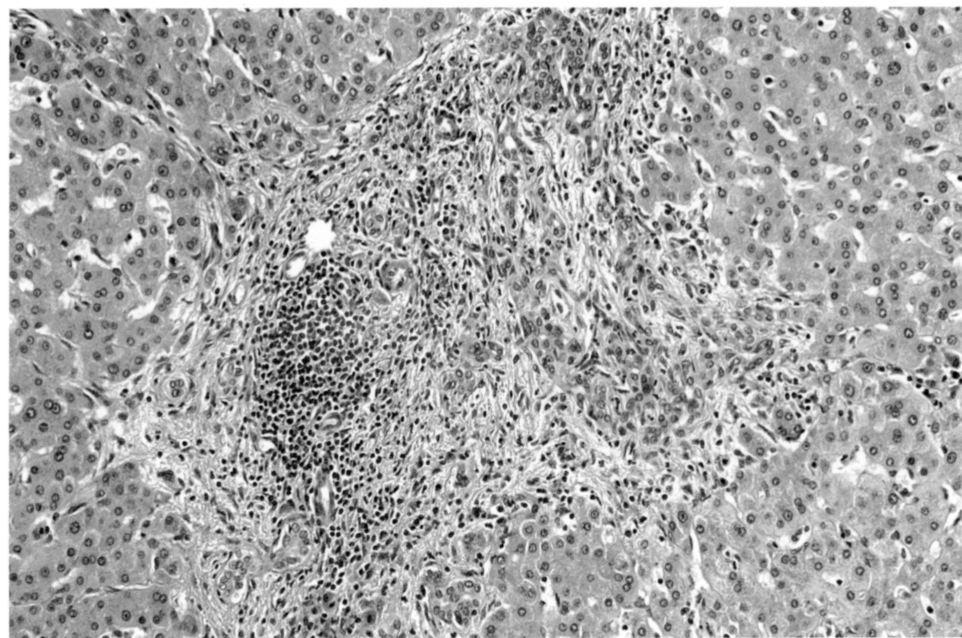

Figure 5.15 *Primary sclerosing cholangitis.* The inflamed portal tract lacks a bile duct. An aggregate of lymphocytes to the left of a small hepatic arteriole at the centre of the field is likely the former site of the duct. Inflammation extends into the adjacent parenchyma and there is interface hepatitis to the right of the portal tract. (Wedge biopsy, H&E).

is doubt, for instance because ducts are difficult to identify in an inflammatory infiltrate, immunostaining of duct-associated cytokeratins is helpful.[45] Suitable antibodies include AE-1 (Signet) and other antibodies against cytokeratins 7 and 19. In the presence of a ductular reaction, identification and counting of interlobular bile ducts is sometimes difficult.

The concentric fibrosis around medium-sized ducts is not entirely diagnostic, since it is occasionally found in other forms of biliary disease such as hepatolithiasis.[46] It is, however, a very helpful finding. The lamellar pattern of the fibrosis gives an 'onion-skin' appearance. The cuff of connective tissue around the duct may be oedematous and pale-staining or sclerotic, depending on the stage of the process. Inflammatory cells are seen in small numbers lying between the layers of collagen. The duct epithelium may show various degrees of atrophy and sometimes disappears entirely, leaving a characteristic rounded fibro-obliterative scar[47] (Fig. 5.16). Staining with diastase-PAS often reveals irregular or regular thickening of the basement membrane material around both scarred and unscarred ducts.[48] In long-standing or severe cases, portal fibrosis gradually increases, fibrous septa form and secondary biliary cirrhosis may develop. In some patients, on the other hand, the lesions remain mild and clinically insignificant for many years.[30,34] Portal tract fibrogenesis in sclerosing cholangitis and in primary biliary cirrhosis is in part attributed to an increased number of intrahepatic mast cells compared to other chronic liver diseases.[49] In fact, systemic mastocytosis has been associated with cholestasis[50] and a case of primary sclerosing cholangitis.[51]

Parenchymal changes in primary sclerosing cholangitis are usually less striking than the portal ones. Cholestasis may be seen as a result of large-duct obstruction or small-duct loss. In the later stages, the cholestasis is typically of the chronic type,

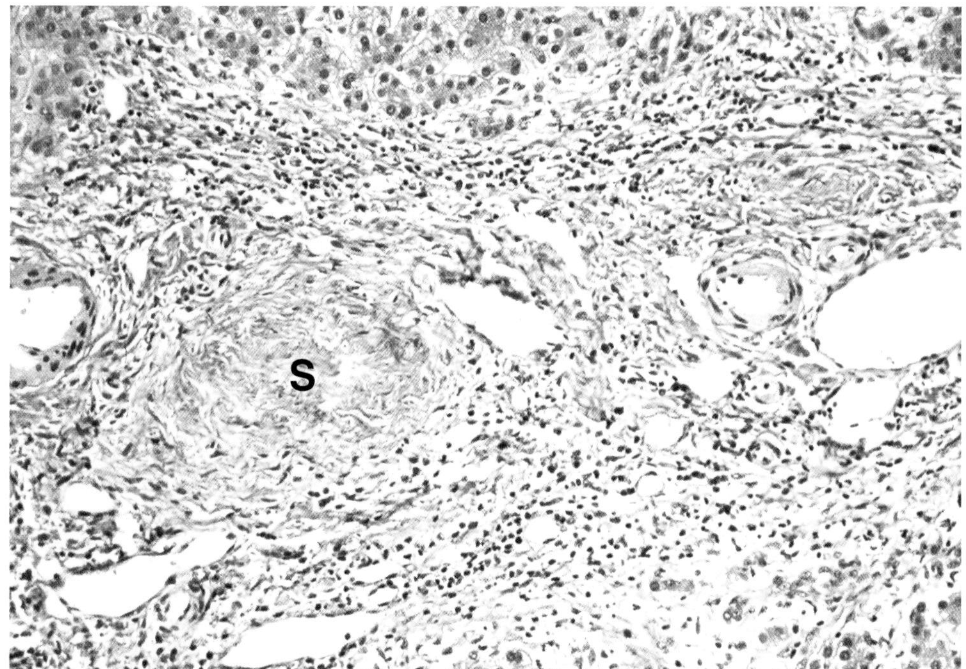

Figure 5.16 *Primary sclerosing cholangitis.* The bile duct in a large portal tract has been replaced by a fibrous scar (S). (Wedge biopsy, H&E).

with accumulation of copper and copper-associated protein. Extension of portal tract lymphoplasmacytic infiltrates into the periportal parenchyma (interface hepatitis) is common but not as a rule, severe (Fig. 5.15). However, more severe interface hepatitis may be seen in patients with an unfavourable clinical course[30] or in an overlap syndrome with autoimmune hepatitis. In children, the combination of autoimmune hepatitis and primary sclerosing cholangitis is well-recognised.[52] Liver cells may undergo hyperplasia, indicated by thickening of cell plates.

Histological assessment of liver biopsies in patients with an established diagnosis of primary sclerosing cholangitis is important for prognosis. Ludwig[41,53,54] has proposed a histological staging system based on essential and non-essential features. The stages correspond approximately to those of primary biliary cirrhosis: they are respectively designated portal, periportal, septal and cirrhotic.

There is an increased risk of carcinoma of the biliary tree in patients with sclerosing cholangitis[55] (Fig. 5.17) who may also have dysplasia of interlobular and septal bile ducts[56] (Fig. 5.18) and gallbladder,[57] including papillary bile duct dysplastic lesions.[58] The same risk of carcinoma does not appear to apply to the small duct form of PSC.[59]

The main **differential diagnosis** is from chronic hepatitis, primary biliary cirrhosis and other forms of chronic biliary tract disease. In **chronic hepatitis**, bile duct numbers are normal, periduct fibrosis is not seen and cholestasis is very uncommon. Stains for copper and copper-associated protein are negative or near-negative, unless cirrhosis has developed.[60] **Primary biliary cirrhosis** closely resembles primary sclerosing cholangitis in its later stages and firm diagnosis usually requires cholangiography and testing for antimitochondrial antibodies. However, the typical granulomatous cholangitis of primary biliary cirrhosis is not a feature of sclerosing cholangitis, although granulomas are very occasionally found in the liver. Substantial chronic

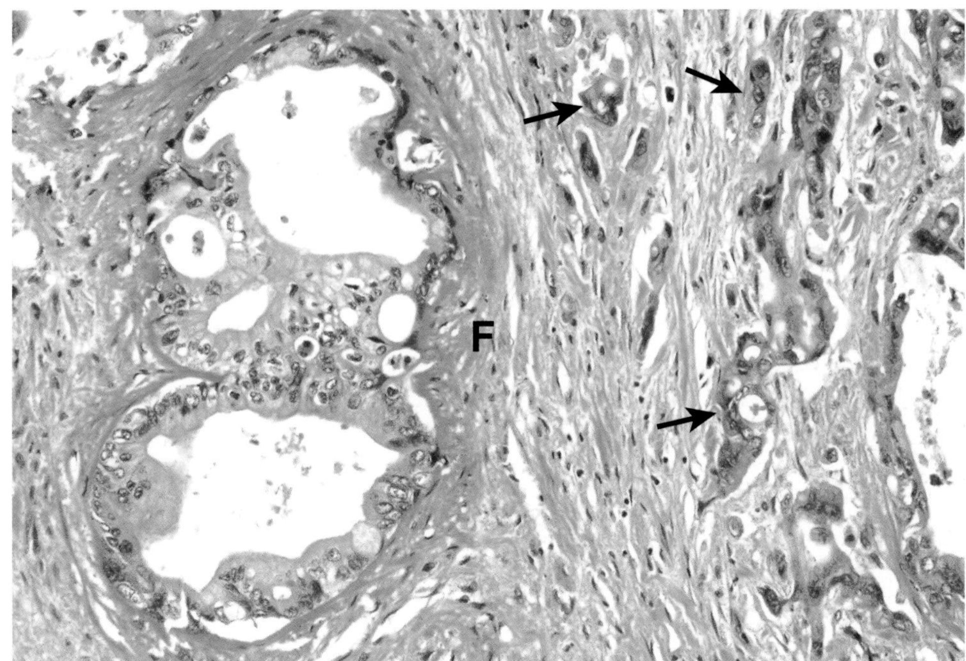

Figure 5.17 *Cholangiocarcinoma in primary sclerosing cholangitis.* Carcinoma has developed in the bile duct at left, still surrounded by periduct fibrosis (F). Invasive glands (arrows) are seen in the adjacent stroma. (Explanted liver, H&E).

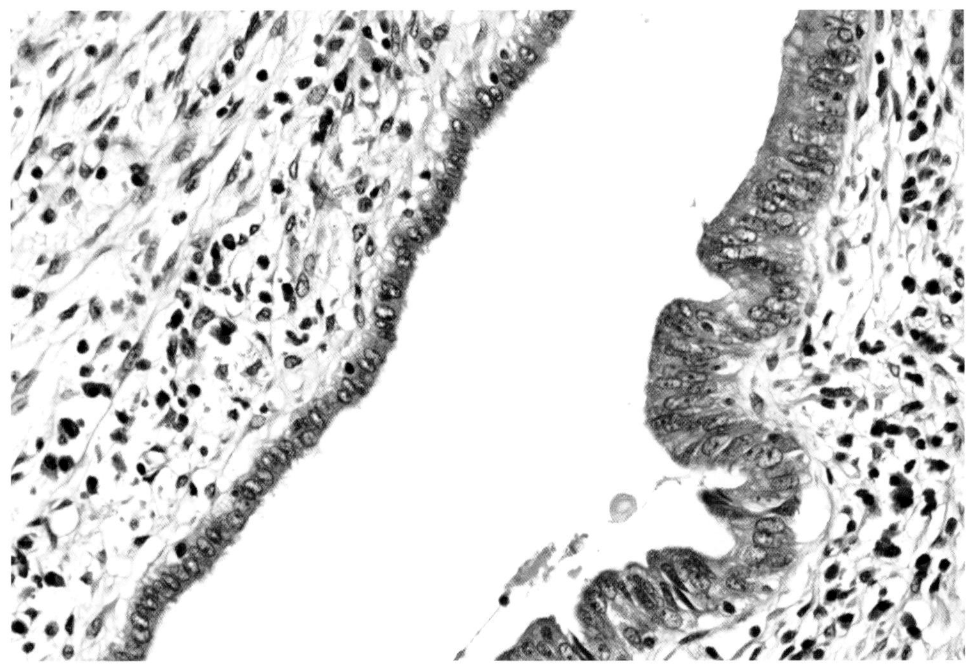

Figure 5.18 *Bile duct dysplasia in primary sclerosing cholangitis.* The epithelium of the right portion of the bile duct is crowded, adenomatous and shows nuclear atypia. (Operative specimen, H&E).

inflammation of portal tracts with or without lymphoid follicles favours primary biliary cirrhosis. Conversely, fibrous obliteration of ducts is much more characteristic of sclerosing cholangitis and there is often dense portal fibrosis with relatively little inflammation. The main difference from **other chronic biliary diseases** is the loss of ducts and interface hepatitis. There is occasionally confusion between the focal duct dilatations of **Caroli's disease** and the cholangiectases, which are typically seen in the large and medium-sized bile ducts in primary sclerosing cholangitis.[47,61]

PRIMARY BILIARY CIRRHOSIS

Primary biliary cirrhosis (PBC), generally regarded as an autoimmune disease, is characterised by a chronic non-suppurative destructive cholangitis, which can eventually lead to cirrhosis.[62] For much of its course, the term cirrhosis is not strictly applicable, but the name survives despite this inconsistency. However, some authors support the alternative term autoimmune cholangitis, as discussed on page 79. Primary biliary cirrhosis typically presents in middle life, but may also be found in the elderly, younger adults and uncommonly in adolescents.[63] Women are about ten times as commonly affected as men. In symptomatic patients, the onset is insidious, with itching as the commonest presenting symptom. Jaundice and histological cholestasis are usually absent in the early years of the disease. Characteristic findings on investigation of both symptomatic and asymptomatic patients include a raised serum alkaline phosphatase and the presence of antimitochondrial antibodies (AMA). The antibodies are specifically the M2 type, directed against inner mitochondrial membrane autoantigens which are members of the 2-oxo-acid dehydrogenase complex (2-OADC) of enzymes.[64,65] The most common of these antibodies reacts with the E2 subunit of the pyruvate dehydrogenase complex (PDC-E2). Antimitochondrial antibodies can be detected in more than 90% of patients. Current hypotheses suggest that expression of 2-OADC antigens on bile-duct epithelium together with appropriate class II histocompatibility antigens, production of antimitochondrial antibodies and T-lymphocyte response[66] mediate the bile duct damage in PBC.[65] Cross-reactivity of human antimitochondrial antibodies with bacterial antigens on *E. coli* and other organisms that may infect patients with PBC has been suggested in the 'molecular mimicry' hypothesis.[67]

Primary biliary cirrhosis is associated with a wide range of other conditions, many of them regarded as autoimmune in origin. The commonest association is with the sicca complex of dry eyes and mouth.[68] Others include scleroderma, thyroiditis, rheumatoid arthritis, membranous glomerulonephritis and coeliac disease.

Liver biopsy plays an important part in diagnosis throughout the often long course of the disease. Four histological stages have been described[53,62,69] (Table 5.2). These are not always easy to determine in needle biopsies, partly because the lesions of primary biliary cirrhosis are unevenly distributed within the liver and partly because the stages overlap. For example, Stage 1 bile duct lesions and granulomas are sometimes seen in an established cirrhosis. From a practical point of view, however, the pathologist is usually able to decide whether the disease appears to be still in Stage 1, with lesions more or less restricted to enlarged portal tracts, or whether it has extended to a significant degree into the adjacent parenchyma, with consequent alteration of lobular structure (the progressive lesion; Stages 2, 3 or 4). This is of some clinical importance, because Stage 1 often lasts for many years and

Table 5.2 Stages of primary biliary cirrhosis

1.	The florid duct lesion; portal hepatitis
2.	Ductular reaction and periportal hepatitis
3.	Scarring; bridging necrosis, septal fibrosis
4.	Cirrhosis

the prognosis is therefore relatively favourable, especially in patients without symptoms referable to the liver. Having established in other patients that the disease has progressed beyond Stage 1, the pathologist may also be able to determine with reasonable confidence that cirrhosis has developed. The patient is then at increased risk for hepatocellular carcinoma,[70,71] sometimes preceded by macroregenerative nodule formation.[72] However, other risk factors such as hepatitis C virus infection must be considered in patients with primary biliary cirrhosis who develop carcinoma.[73] Because different sets of differential diagnoses should be considered for the portal and the progressive lesion, these are considered separately in the following sections.

The portal lesion of primary biliary cirrhosis

The bile-duct damage characteristic of early primary biliary cirrhosis mainly affects the septal and larger interlobular ducts, while the smaller interlobular ducts remain intact until later. The epithelium of the affected ducts becomes irregular and is infiltrated with lymphocytes. The basement membrane becomes disrupted and the duct may rupture (Fig. 5.19). An inflammatory infiltrate is seen around or to one side of the duct. The denser parts of this infiltrate are mainly composed of lymphocytes, which may form aggregates or follicles with germinal centres (Fig. 5.20). Elsewhere, there is a mixture of plasma cells, often abundant, eosinophils and neutrophils. The eosinophils contribute to bile-duct damage, granuloma formation and other aspects of the inflammatory response by releasing mediators such as major basic protein and eosinophilic cationic protein, which are located within their granules.[74,75] The biochemical and/or histological improvement seen in certain patients treated with ursodeoxycholic acid appears to be attributable in part to inhibition of eosinophil degranulation.[74] Of the various histological features of the disease, interface hepatitis appears to be the most resistant to improvement with ursodeoxycholic acid.[76]

Granulomas are present in many patients, although they are not necessarily seen in small biopsies; their absence does not therefore exclude the diagnosis. They take a variety of forms,[77] ranging from well-defined granulomas like those of sarcoidosis or tuberculosis (Fig. 5.21), to small focal collections of histiocytoid cells. Alternatively there may be a substantial component of histiocytes or epithelioid cells within the inflammatory infiltrate, without formation of identifiable localised granulomas. A few lobular granulomas may also be present, but large numbers should suggest the diagnosis of other granulomatous diseases (see Ch. 15).

Not all liver biopsies from patients in this stage of the disease show the typical bile-duct lesions, so that a firm histological diagnosis cannot always be made. Small portal tracts may merely show 'non-specific' portal inflammation, in which case step sections may make the true diagnosis clear by revealing bile-duct lesions or

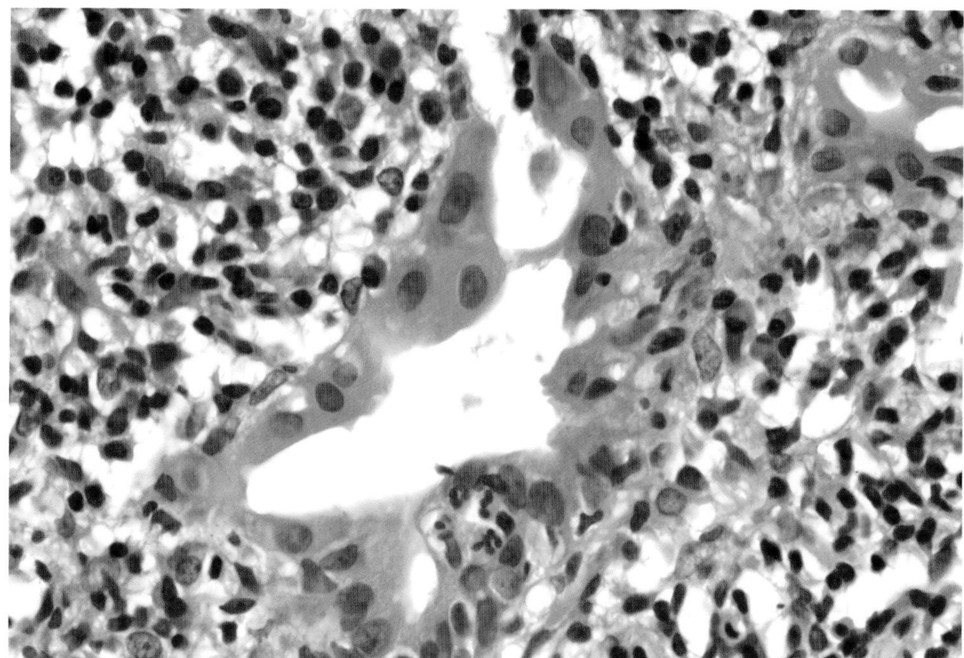

Figure 5.19 *Primary biliary cirrhosis*. A damaged large interlobular bile duct shows an irregular configuration, partly attenuated epithelium and intra-epithelial inflammatory cells. The surrounding infiltrate is rich in lymphocytes and plasma cells. (Wedge biopsy, H&E).

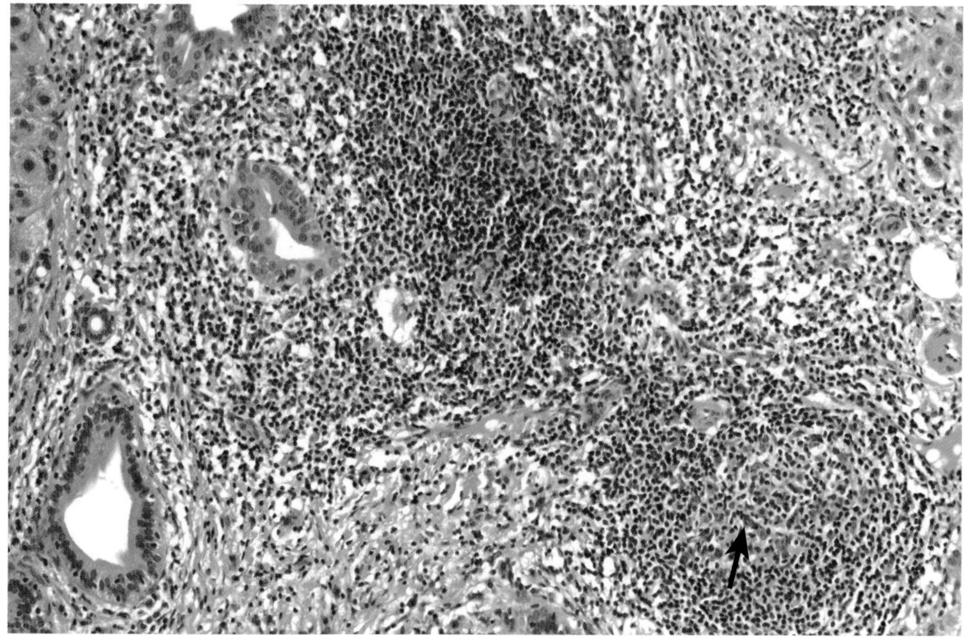

Figure 5.20 *Primary biliary cirrhosis*. A lymphoid aggregate and a follicle with a germinal centre (arrow), are seen near an inflamed duct with stratified epithelium. (Wedge biopsy, H&E).

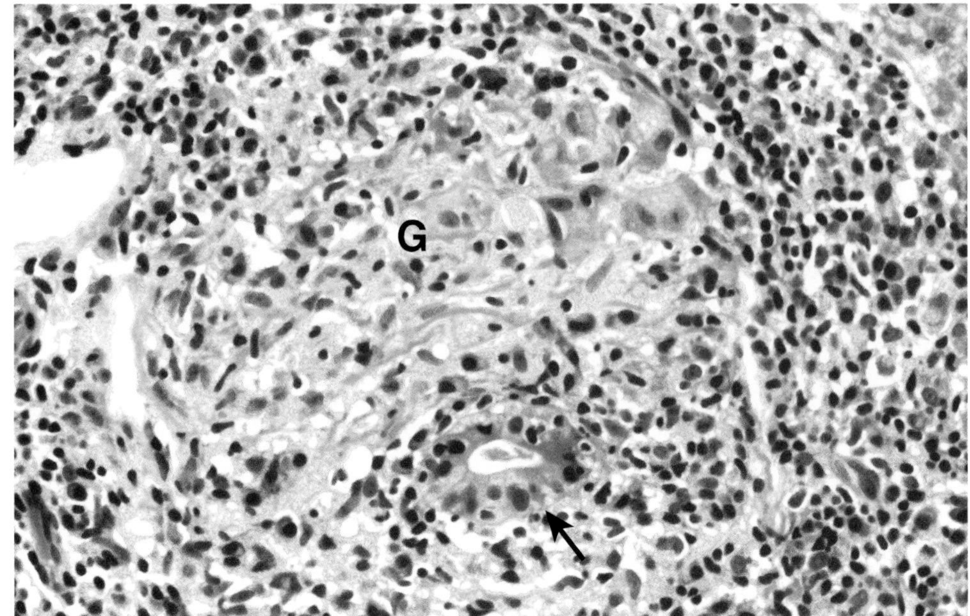

Figure 5.21 *Primary biliary cirrhosis.* A well-formed epithelioid-cell granuloma (G) has formed near a damaged bile duct (arrow). The background infiltrate contains many lymphocytes, plasma cells and scattered eosinophils. (Needle biopsy, H&E).

granulomas. In a small number of patients with the **premature ductopenic variant** of PBC,[78] widespread bile duct destruction and loss are accelerated at an early stage before the development of fibrosis or cirrhosis, with worse pruritus and clinical evidence of chronic cholestasis than would be anticipated.

Although in the first stage of primary biliary cirrhosis the lesions are by definition mainly portal, slight disruption of the limiting plate is common. Sinusoids may be infiltrated by lymphocytes, Kupffer cells are prominent and there may be focal necrosis[79] and thickening of liver-cell plates. Nodular regenerative hyperplasia, best recognised in reticulin preparations, is common even at this stage[80,81] and together with portal-vein narrowing[82] helps to explain the portal hypertension which frequently precedes the development of significant fibrosis or cirrhosis. Foci of small hepatocytes with basophilic cytoplasm and hyperchromatic nuclei (small-cell dysplasia) or hepatocytes with enlarged, pleomorphic nuclei (large-cell dysplasia) are occasionally found.[83]

Canalicular cholestasis is unusual in early primary biliary cirrhosis, unless there is a complicating factor such as steroid-induced jaundice. Cholestasis of the chronic type (cholate stasis) does not develop until later, although small amounts of copper-associated protein are occasionally seen in periportal hepatocytes.

The **differential diagnosis of early primary biliary cirrhosis** includes other causes of portal inflammation and of bile-duct damage. The differentiation from **primary sclerosing cholangitis** is discussed on page 67. In this disease duct atrophy and fibrosis predominate and granulomas are unusual. **Drug injury** occasionally leads to bile-duct damage, but the ducts affected are smaller than in early primary biliary cirrhosis, other parenchymal changes (fat, hepatocyte ballooning and apoptosis) are often present and the lesion is seen in the clinical context of an acutely jaundiced patient. Bile ducts are often abnormal in acute and chronic **viral hepatitis**, especially hepatitis C.[84] In hepatitis, the epithelium of the affected ducts may be abnormal in only part of its circumference (see Fig. 6.7) and is typically stratified and vacuolated.[85] The surrounding infiltrate is almost entirely composed of lymphocytes, with few plasma cells or segmented leucocytes and no granulomas. Large numbers of eosinophils, sometimes seen in primary biliary cirrhosis,[86] are rare. In doubtful cases the clinical context and laboratory investigations usually make the diagnosis clear. Because in viral hepatitis the duct damage is focal and does not lead to extensive duct loss, the clinical and biochemical picture is not necessarily cholestatic. Other causes of bile duct damage include **autoimmune hepatitis**,[87] **bile-duct obstruction with suppuration, graft-versus-host disease** and **rejection of a grafted liver**. The latter two situations are discussed in Chapter 16. Two rare causes of bile-duct damage associated with granulomas are **fascioliasis** and **sarcoidosis**, but in general this association strongly supports a diagnosis of primary biliary cirrhosis.

The progressive lesion of primary biliary cirrhosis

The disease now extends beyond the confines of the portal tracts and there is increasing fibrosis and alteration of lobular architecture. Bile-duct damage is less dramatic and granulomas are fewer, but there is a progressive fall in duct numbers. Duct numbers are best assessed in relation to arteries,[43] as already discussed in relation to primary sclerosing cholangitis. The sites of former ducts are marked by aggregates of lymphocytes (Fig. 5.22). These sometimes show compression artefact, with rupture of lymphocyte nuclei. The inflammatory reaction may also obliterate periductal capillaries.[88]

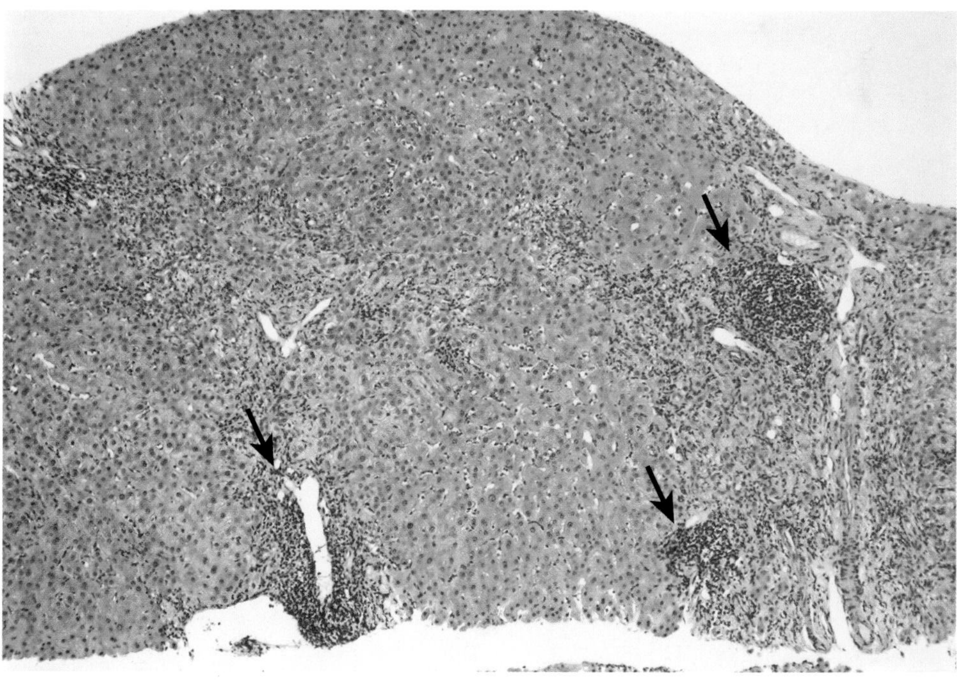

Figure 5.22 *Primary biliary cirrhosis.* Aggregates of lymphocytes (arrows) mark the former sites of bile ducts in this inflamed, fibrotic liver. The picture is very typical of the progressive phase of the disease. (Needle biopsy, H&E).

The portal tracts expand progressively as the inflammatory process begins to extend from them into the adjacent parenchyma. At this time two apparently separate processes affect the future course of the disease. The first comprises a combination of biliary and cholestatic features probably related to bile duct loss, while the second closely resembles the interface hepatitis of chronic hepatitis.[19,89] The earliest and often most obvious biliary feature is a ductular reaction (Fig. 5.23). For a time this allows bile to drain from the parenchyma into the main ducts in spite of destruction of the medium-sized ducts.[90] It is almost always associated with an infiltrate of neutrophils, so that it needs to be distinguished from the duct tortuosity and inflammation of mechanical bile-duct obstruction. The ductular reaction of primary biliary cirrhosis, and indeed of primary sclerosing cholangitis, is often focal, representing a system of bypass channels in relation to a local interruption of bile flow through the duct system. If the ductular structures are partly obscured by inflammation and fibrosis (Fig. 5.24), they can be highlighted by immunostaining for cytokeratin 7 or 19 (Fig. 5.25).

Loss of bile ducts also leads to the chronic form of cholestasis, marked by swelling of hepatocytes, bile staining, Mallory body formation and accumulation of copper (Fig. 5.26) and copper-associated protein (Fig. 5.27). Bile plugs are sometimes seen in canaliculi in the affected areas around portal tracts and septa, but more widespread canalicular cholestasis often reflects hepatocellular failure or associated sepsis. There may be many lipid-laden macrophages, forming diffuse or localised xanthomas.

In addition to the cholestatic features described above, interface hepatitis of the classical, lymphoplasmacytic type is common in the progressive stage of primary biliary cirrhosis.[19] The infiltrate is rich in activated T cells.[89,91,92] Because this hepatocellular component is a regular feature of PBC, the finding of interface

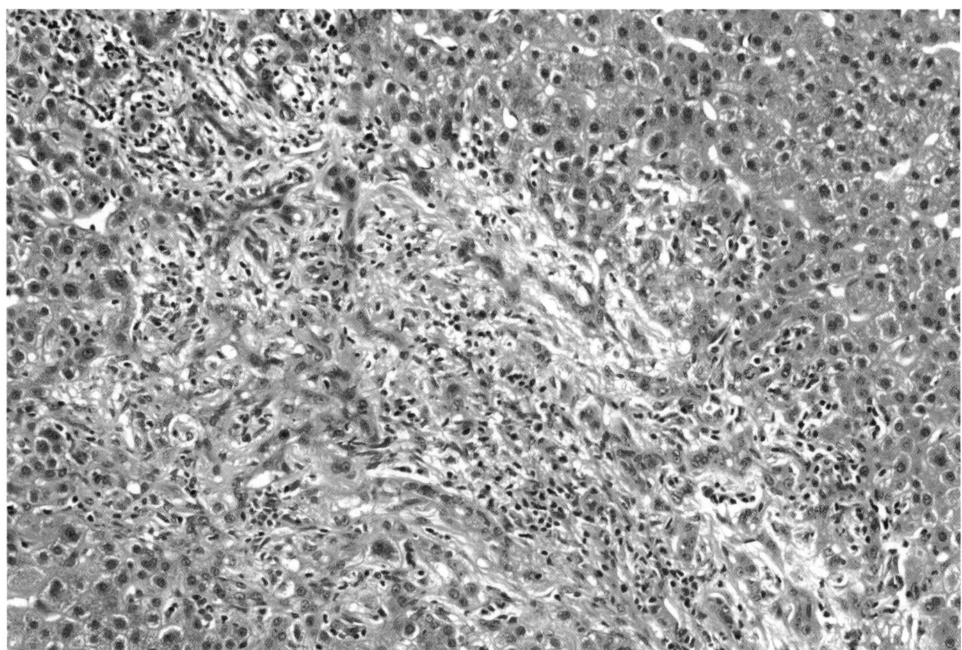

Figure 5.23 *Primary biliary cirrhosis.* A widened portal tract shows chronic inflammation and a ductular reaction, but no native bile duct. The margins of the tract are blurred by fibrosis and interface hepatitis. (Wedge biopsy, H&E).

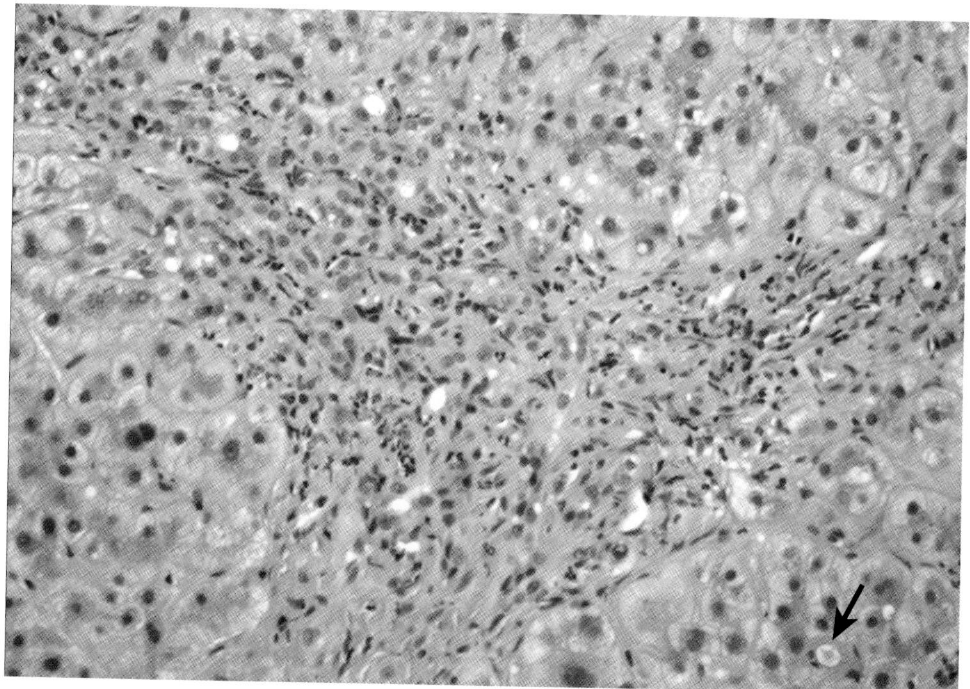

Figure 5.24 *Stage 3 primary biliary cirrhosis*. The portal tract is chronically inflamed and fibrotic, without a readily identified bile duct. A ductular reaction is present, but obscured by the inflammation and fibrosis. Cholestasis is present at the periphery of the lobule (arrow). (Needle biopsy, H&E).

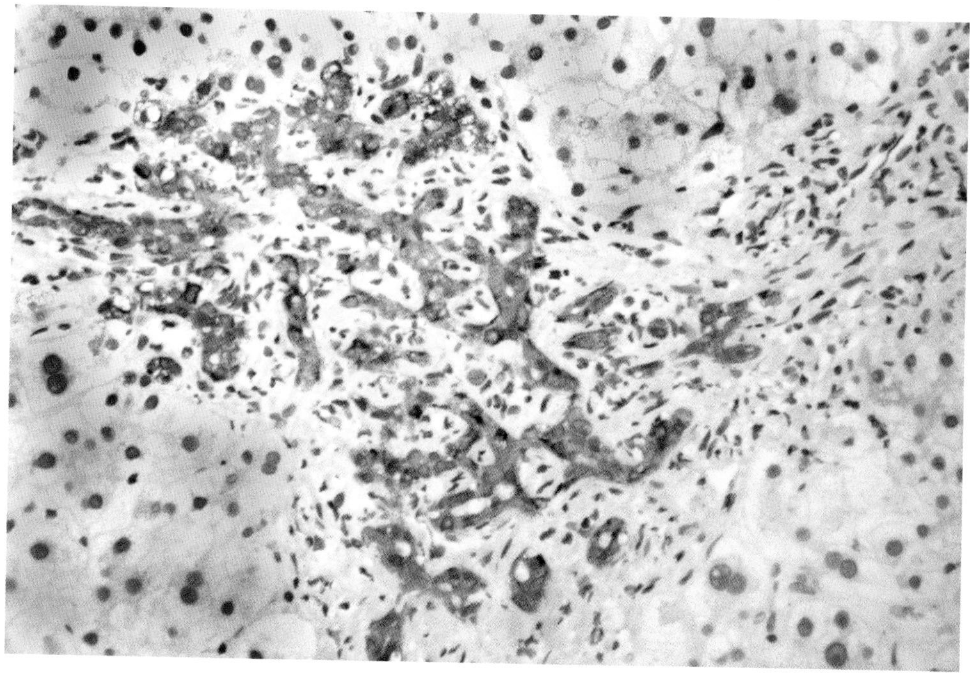

Figure 5.25 *Stage 3 primary biliary cirrhosis*. The ductular reaction is highlighted by cytokeratin 7 immunostaining of a serial section of the same biopsy shown in Figure 5.24. (Needle biopsy, specific immunoperoxidase).

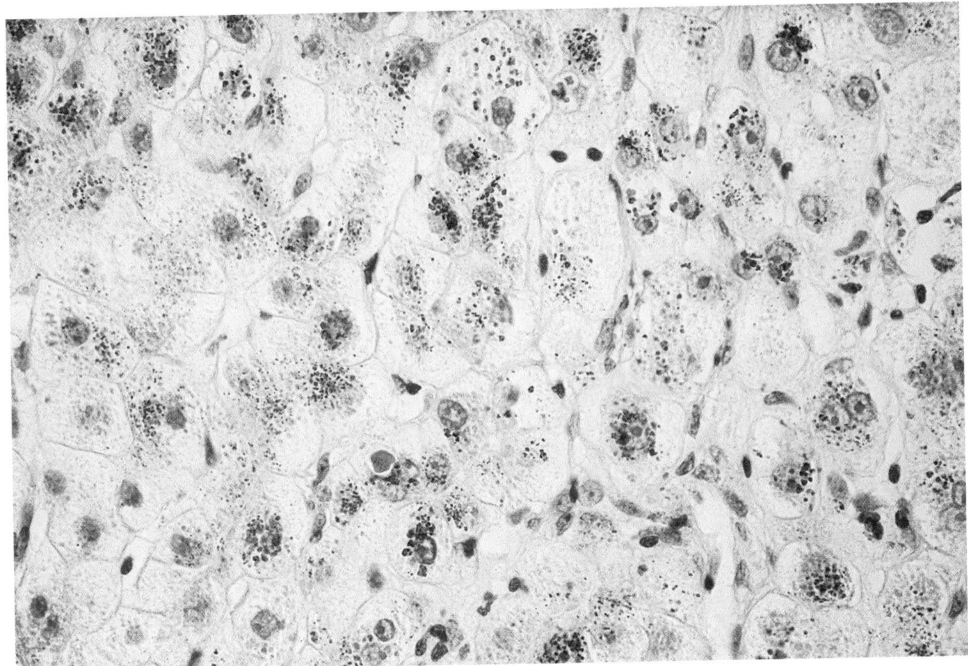

Figure 5.26 *Primary biliary cirrhosis.* Heavy accumulation of copper-rich granules is seen in hepatocytes. Note the different colour of the canalicular bile thrombus slightly below centre. (Needle biopsy, rhodanine).

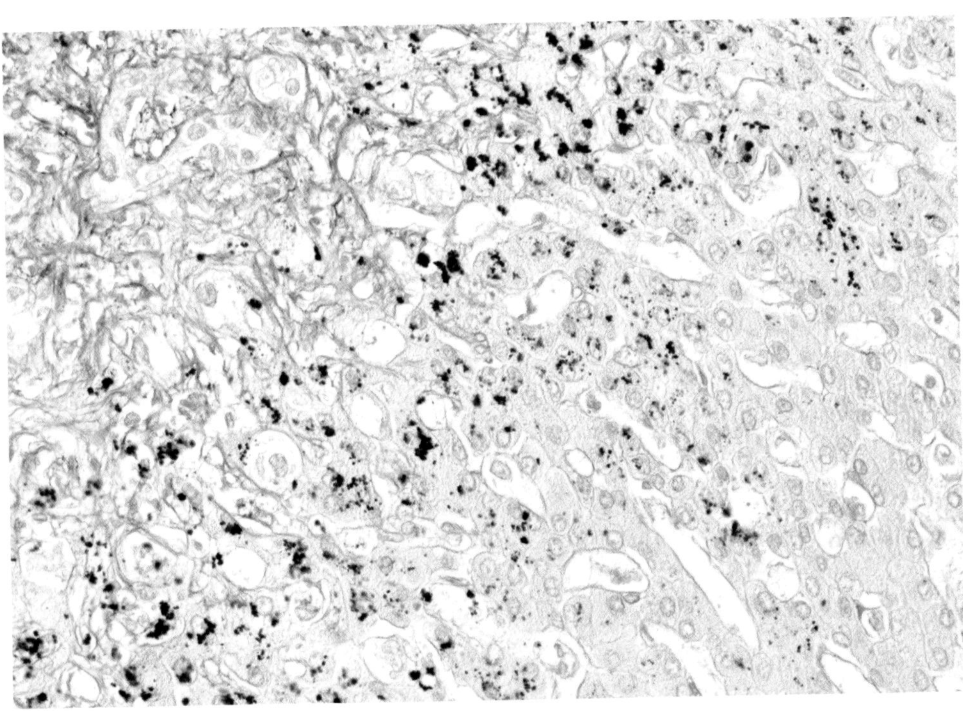

Figure 5.27 *Primary biliary cirrhosis.* Granular deposits of copper-associated protein have accumulated in hepatocytes near a fibrous septum (above left) at a late stage of the disease. (Needle biopsy, orcein).

hepatitis together with the biliary features of PBC should not by itself lead to the diagnosis of an overlap syndrome (see below). Lymphocytes also form bridge-like extensions into the lobules, and may be the forerunners of fibrous septa.[93] An increased number of intrahepatic mast cells is also present, which may contribute to portal tract fibrosis.[49] Necrosis of perivenular hepatocytes has been noted.[79] There is therefore a histological resemblance to hepatitis. Hepatocellular dysplasia of small- or large-cell type may be present.[83]

The combination of cholestatic and hepatitic processes leads to increasing fibrosis. Portal inflammation diminishes, but lymphoid aggregates continue to mark the former sites of bile ducts (Fig. 5.28). Septa extend from the portal tracts and eventually come to link portal tracts to each other and to terminal hepatic venules.[93] In patients in whom the biliary and cholestatic features predominate, the cirrhosis which ultimately develops is generally of the biliary type. When hepatitic features predominate, the cirrhosis tends to be of post-hepatitis type. All combinations of the two patterns may be seen.[94] Nodules often develop unevenly throughout the liver, so that nodular areas with the appearance of cirrhosis coexist with areas in which the lobular architecture remains preserved.

The **differential diagnosis of the progressive lesion** includes **primary sclerosing cholangitis** and **other forms of chronic biliary disease** on the one hand and **chronic hepatitis** on the other.[95] The differentiation from primary sclerosing cholangitis is discussed on page 67; in the later stages of the two diseases it is often impossible to make the distinction histologically. With respect to other forms of chronic biliary obstruction and chronic hepatitis, the most important observation is that bile duct numbers remain normal in both whereas they are characteristically reduced in primary biliary cirrhosis and in primary sclerosing cholangitis (Table 5.3).

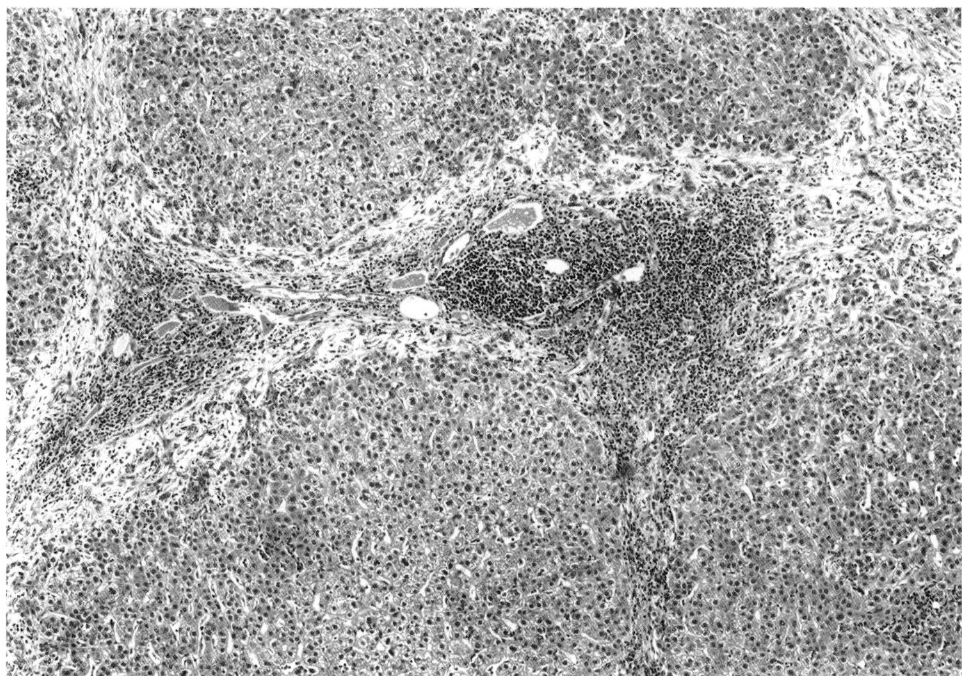

Figure 5.28 *Primary biliary cirrhosis*. There is extensive scarring without nodule formation. Aggregates of lymphocytes mark the former sites of bile ducts, as in Figure 5.23. (Post-mortem liver, H&E).

Table 5.3 Causes of bile-duct damage and loss

Loss of ducts	Little or no loss
Primary sclerosing cholangitis	Bile-duct obstruction
Primary biliary cirrhosis	Viral hepatitis
Idiopathic ductopenia	Drug jaundice
Graft-versus host disease	Parasitic duct disease
Chronic rejection of liver grafts	
Sarcoidosis	
Drug jaundice[a]	

[a]Note that while many drugs produce bile duct injury without loss, there are also well described cases where ductopenia and chronic cholestatic disease (sometimes requiring liver transplantation) are sequelae of drug hepatotoxicity.

Granulomas favour primary biliary cirrhosis over chronic hepatitis, as does chronic cholestasis particularly when it is seen in the absence of cirrhosis.[60] Difficulties remain even after these factors are taken into account, especially if the biopsy specimen is small or fragmented. They can usually be resolved by consideration of the clinical context and laboratory investigations; a middle-aged woman with itching, high serum alkaline phosphatase and antimitochondrial antibodies is unlikely to be suffering from chronic viral hepatitis. There are, however, unusual cases which present as overlap syndromes, discussed briefly below.

Overlap syndromes, transitional diseases and autoimmune cholangitis

Establishing a clearcut diagnosis of primary biliary cirrhosis or primary sclerosing cholangitis is occasionally problematic when an unusually severe degree of lymphoplasmacytic interface hepatitis is superimposed on otherwise typical histopathologic features of either disease (Fig. 5.29), raising the possibility of an **overlap syndrome**[96] with autoimmune hepatitis (AIH). Such patients may show a mix of serum autoantibodies (some of which may be merely non-specific markers of immune disease), further clouding the diagnosis. In some instances there appears to be a genetic predilection for the hepatitic component, as in certain cases of PBC where a specific histocompatibility profile is present.[97] Rendering a diagnosis of either PBC/AIH or PSC/AIH overlap syndrome therefore requires close consultation between pathologist and clinician, taking into account and appropriately weighting the biopsy features, serologic and biochemical data and cholangiographic findings.[52,96] Use of a clinicopathologic scoring system that was specifically developed for autoimmune hepatitis[98] may be helpful in some cases.[99]

The interrelatedness of PBC, PSC and AIH as disorders of cellular immunity[100] is further highlighted by descriptions of clinical **transition** from one form to another. Such examples include cases of autoimmune hepatitis which later progress to PSC,[101] paediatric PSC patients with autoimmune serologic and histopathologic features[102] and transplanted PBC patients who develop AIH in their allografts.[103]

A number of patients with typical biopsy features of primary biliary cirrhosis but no demonstrable serum antimitochondrial antibodies have been described as

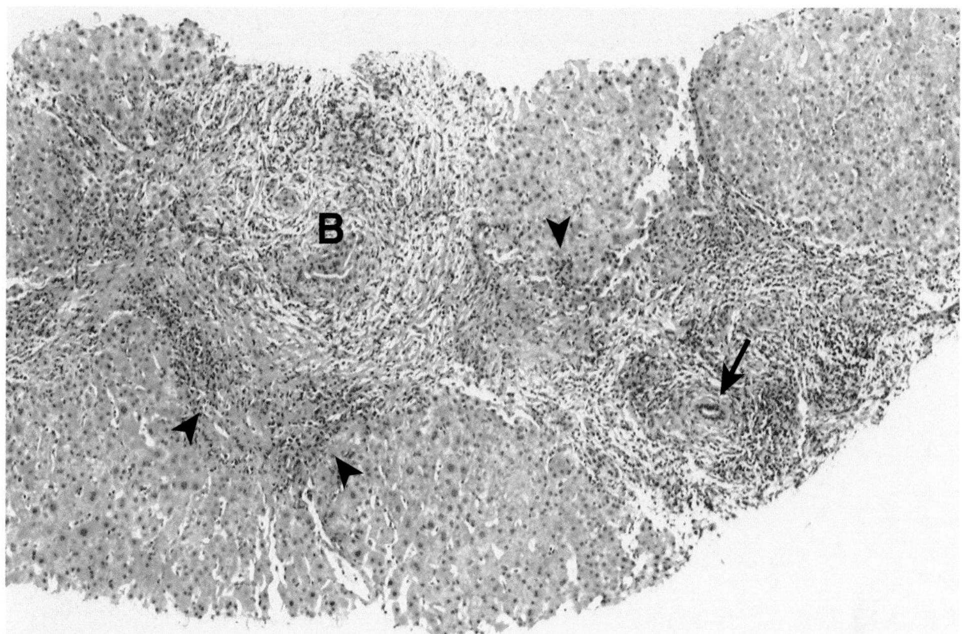

Figure 5.29 *Overlap syndrome.* Biopsy from a young patient with ulcerative colitis, but clinicopathological and serological features suggesting primary sclerosing cholangitis-autoimmune hepatitis overlap syndrome. The biopsy features of biliary disease include abnormal bile duct morphology (B), portal oedema and periduct fibrosis (arrow), while the extensive interface hepatitis (arrowheads) suggests an autoimmune component. (Needle biopsy, H&E).

cases of **autoimmune cholangitis** because of coexistent antinuclear or other autoantibodies, occasional corticosteroid responsiveness and other features that suggest an autoimmune clinical profile.[104] Such cases may reflect problems in the sensitivity of current mitochondrial antibody tests and are now usually considered to be examples of AMA-negative PBC.[96]

OTHER DISORDERS WITH INTRAHEPATIC BILE DUCT LOSS

As indicated earlier, the loss of significant numbers of intrahepatic bile ducts (ductopenia) can be seen not only in primary biliary cirrhosis and primary sclerosing cholangitis but also in several conditions listed in Table 5.3. In addition to these, there are patients in whom the pathogenesis of duct loss is poorly understood. Some of these may represent later stages of childhood **non-syndromatic paucity of intrahepatic bile ducts**.[105] In patients with **idiopathic adulthood ductopenia (IAD)**, predominantly males with cholestatic biochemical profiles, duct loss could also be the end result of small-duct primary sclerosing cholangitis or due to bile duct damage associated with chronic hepatitis C[106] or autoimmune cholangitis.[107] Rarely, IAD is familial.[108] Ductopenia due to the paraneoplastic effects of **Hodgkin's disease** was reported.[109] A group of asymptomatic patients with idiopathic ductopenia and elevated serum gamma glutamyl transferase activity has also been described.[110]

1 Jansen PLM, Sturm E. Genetic cholestasis, causes and consequences for hepatobiliary transport. *Liver Int* 2003; **23**: 315–322.
2 Vu TH, Tanji K, Holve SA, et al. Navajao neurohepatopathy: a mitochondrial DNA depletion syndrome? *Hepatology* 2001; **34**: 116–120.
3 Crawford JM, Boyer JL. Clinicopathology conferences: inflammation-induced cholestasis. *Hepatology* 1998; **28**: 253–260.
4 Turkish A, Levy J, Kato M, et al. Pancreatitis and probable paraneoplastic cholestasis as presenting manifestations of pancreatic lymphoma in a child. *J Pediatr Gastroenterol Nutrition* 2004: **39**: 552–556.
5 Christoffersen P, Poulsen H. Histological changes in human liver biopsies following extrahepatic biliary obstruction. *Acta Pathol Microbiol Scand* 1970; **212**: 150–157.
6 Roskams TA, Theise ND, Balabaud C, et al. Nomenclature of the finer branches of the biliary tree: canals, ductules, and ductular reactions in human livers. *Hepatology* 2004; **39**: 1739–1745.
7 LeSage G, Glaser S, Alpini G. Regulation of cholangiocyte proliferation. *Liver* 2001; **21**: 73–80.
8 Nijjar SS, Wallace L, Crosby HA, et al. Altered Notch ligand expression in human liver disease. Further evidence for a role of the Notch signaling pathway in hepatic neovascularization and biliary ductular defects. *Am J Pathol* 2002; **160**: 1695–1703.
9 Gaya DR, Thorburn KA, Oien KA, et al. Hepatic granulomas: a 10 year single centre experience. *J Clin Pathol* 2003; **56**: 850–853.
10 Sakamoto T, Ezure T, Yokomuro S, et al. Liver transplantation database (LTD) investigators. Interleukin-6, hepatocyte growth factor, and their receptors in biliary epithelial cells during a type I ductular reaction in mice: interactions between the periductal inflammatory and stromal cells and the biliary epithelium. *Hepatology* 1998; **28**: 1260–1268.
11 Gerber MA, Thung SN, Bodenheimer HC Jr., et al. Characteristic histologic triad in liver adjacent to metastatic neoplasm. *Liver* 1986; **6**: 85–88.
12 Wilson C, Auld CD, Schlinkert R, et al. Hepatobiliary complications in chronic pancreatitis. *Gut* 1989; **30**: 520–527.
13 Flinn WR, Olson DF, Oyasu R, et al. Biliary bacteria and hepatic histopathologic changes in gallstone disease. *Ann Surg* 1977; **185**: 593–597.
14 Sonzogni A, Colloredo G, Fabris L, et al. Isolated idiopathic bile ductular hyperplasia in patients with persistently abnormal liver function tests. *J Hepatol* 2004; **40**: 592–598.
15 Lewindon PJ, Pereira TN, Hoskins AC, et al. The role of hepatic stellate cells and transforming growth factor-beta-1 in cystic fibrosis liver disease. *Am J Pathol* 2002; **160**: 1705–1715.
16 Baumann U, Crosby HA, Ramani P, et al. Expression of the stem cell factor receptor c-kit in normal and diseased pediatric liver: identification of a human hepatic progenitor cell? *Hepatology* 1999; **30**: 112–117.
17 Harada K, Kono N, Tsuneyama K, et al. Cell-kinetic study of proliferating bile ductules in various hepatobiliary diseases. *Liver* 1998; **18**: 277–284.
18 Robrechts C, Vos R De, Heuvel M Van den, et al. Primary liver tumour of intermediate (hepatocyte-bile duct cell) phenotype: a progenitor cell tumour? *Liver* 1998; **18**: 288–293.
19 Portmann B, Popper H, Neuberger J, et al. Sequential and diagnostic features in primary biliary cirrhosis based on serial histologic study in 209 patients. *Gastroenterology* 1985; **88**: 1777–1790.
20 Weinbren K, Hadjis NS, Blumgart LH. Structural aspects of the liver in patients with biliary disease and portal hypertension. *J Clin Pathol* 1985; **38**: 1013–1020.
21 Hammel P, Couvelard A, O'Toole D, et al. Regression of liver fibrosis after biliary drainage in patients with chronic pancreatitis and stenosis of the common bile duct. *N Engl J Med* 2001; **344**: 418–423.
22 Carpenter HA. Bacterial and parasitic cholangitis. *Mayo Clin Proc* 1998; **73**: 473–478.
23 Shimada H, Nihmoto S, Matsuba A,

et al. Acute cholangitis: a histopathologic study. *J Clin Gastroenterol* 1988; **10**: 197–200.

24 Sasaki M, Nakanuma Y, Kim YS. Expression of apomucins in the intrahepatic biliary tree in hepatolithiasis differs from that in normal liver and extrahepatic biliary obstruction. *Hepatology* 1998; **27**: 46–53.

25 Bouche H, Housset C, Dumont J-L, et al. AIDS-related cholangitis: diagnostic features and course in 15 patients. *J Hepatol* 1993; **17**: 34–39.

26 Pol S, Romana CA, Richard S, et al. Microsporidia infection in patients with the human immunodeficiency virus and unexplained cholangitis. *N Engl J Med* 1993; **328**: 95–99.

27 Lefkowitch JH. Bile ductular cholestasis: an ominous histopathologic sign related to sepsis and 'cholangitis lenta'. *Hum Pathol* 1982; **13**: 19–24.

28 Ishak KG, Rogers WA. Cryptogenic acute cholangitis – association with toxic shock syndrome. *Am J Clin Pathol* 1981; **76**: 619–626.

29 Wilschanski M, Chait P, Wade JA, et al. Primary sclerosing cholangitis in 32 children: clinical, laboratory and radiographic features, with survival analysis. *Hepatology* 1995; **22**: 1415–1422.

30 Aadland E, Schrumpf E, Fausa O, et al. Primary sclerosing cholangitis: a long-term follow-up study. *Scand J Gastroenterol* 1987; **22**: 655–664.

31 Jeffrey GP, Reed DW, Carrello S, et al. Histological and immunohistochemical study of the gall bladder lesion in primary sclerosing cholangitis. *Gut* 1991; **32**: 424–429.

32 Kawaguchi K, Koike M, Tsuruta K, et al. Lymphoplasmacytic sclerosing pancreatitis with cholangitis: a variant of primary sclerosing cholangitis extensively involving pancreas. *Hum Pathol* 1991; **22**: 387–395.

33 Abraham SC, Cruz-Correa M, Argani P, et al. Lymphoplasmacytic chronic cholecystitis and biliary tract disease in patients with lymphoplasmacytic sclerosing pancreatitis. *Am J Surg Pathol* 2003; **27**: 441–451.

34 Broome U, Glaumann H, Hultcrantz R. Liver histology and follow up of 68 patients with ulcerative colitis and normal liver function tests. *Gut* 1990; **31**: 468–472.

35 Graziadei IW, Wiesner RH, Batts KP, et al. Recurrence of primary sclerosing cholangitis following liver transplantation. *Hepatology* 1999; **29**: 1050–1056.

36 Kemeny MM, Battifora H, Blayney DW, et al. Sclerosing cholangitis after continuous hepatic artery infusion of FUDR. *Ann Surg* 1985; **202**: 176–181.

37 Herrmann G, Lorenz M, Kirkowa-Reimann M, et al. Morphological changes after intra-arterial chemotherapy of the liver. *Hepatogastroenterology* 1987; **34**: 5–9.

38 Ludwig J, Kim CH, Wiesner RH, et al. Floxuridine-induced sclerosing cholangitis: an ischemic cholangiopathy? *Hepatology* 1989; **9**: 215–218.

39 Engler S, Elsing C, Flechtenmacher C, et al. Progressive sclerosing cholangitis after shock: a new variant of vanishing bile duct disorders. *Gut* 2003; **52**: 688–693.

40 Batts KP. Ischemic cholangitis. *Mayo Clin Proc* 1998; **73**: 380–385.

41 Ludwig J. Small-duct primary sclerosing cholangitis. *Semin Liver Dis* 1991; **11**: 11–17.

42 Harrison RF, Hubscher SG. The spectrum of bile duct lesions in end-stage primary sclerosing cholangitis. *Histopathology* 1991; **19**: 321–327.

42a Keaveny AP, Gordon FD, Goldar-Najafi A et al. Native liver xanthogranulomatous cholangiopathy in primary sclerosing cholangitis: impact on posttransplant outcome. *Liver Transplant* 2004; **10**: 115–122.

42b Khettry U, Keaveny A, Goldar-Najafi A et al. Liver transplantation for primary sclerong cholangitis: a long-term clinicopathologic study. *Hum Pathol* 2003; **34**: 1127–1136.

43 Nakanuma Y, Ohta G. Histometric and serial section observations of the intrahepatic bile ducts in primary biliary cirrhosis. *Gastroenterology* 1979; **76**: 1326–1332.

44 Crawford AR, Lin X-Z, Crawford JM. The normal adult human liver biopsy: a quantitative reference standard. *Hepatology* 1998; **28**: 323–331.

45 Eyken P Van, Sciot R, Desmet VJ. A cytokeratin immunohistochemical study of cholestatic liver disease: evidence that hepatocytes can express 'bile duct-type' cytokeratins. *Histopathology* 1989; **15**: 125–135.

46 Nakanuma Y, Yamaguchi K, Ohta G, et al. Pathological features of hepatolithiasis in Japan. *Hum Pathol* 1988; **19**: 1181–1186.
47 Ludwig J, MacCarty RL, LaRusso NF, et al. Intrahepatic cholangiectases and large-duct obliteration in primary sclerosing cholangitis. *Hepatology* 1986; **6**: 560–568.
48 Fleming KA. Interlobular bile duct basement membrane thickening – a specific marker for primary sclerosing cholangitis (PSC)? *J Pathol* 1993; **169 (Suppl)**: 199A–185A.
49 Farrell DJ, Hines JE, Walls AF, et al. Intrahepatic mast cells in chronic liver diseases. *Hepatology* 1995; **22**: 1175–1181.
50 Safyan EL, Veerabagu MP, Swerdlow SH, et al. Intrahepatic cholestasis due to systemic mastocytosis: a case report and review of literature. *Am J Gastroenterol* 1997; **92**: 1197–1200.
51 Baron TH, Koehler RE, Rodgers WH, et al. Mast cell cholangiopathy: another cause of sclerosing cholangitis. *Gastroenterology* 1995; **109**: 1677–1681.
52 Gregorio GV, Portmann B, Karani J, et al. Autoimmune hepatitis/sclerosing cholangitis overlap syndrome in childhood: a 16-year prospective study. *Hepatology* 2001; **33**: 544–553.
53 Ludwig J, Dickson ER, McDonald GS. Staging of chronic nonsuppurative destructive cholangitis (syndrome of primary biliary cirrhosis). *Virchows Arch Pathol Anat* 1978; **379**: 103–112.
54 Ludwig J, LaRusso NF, Wiesner RH. The syndrome of primary sclerosing cholangitis. In: Popper H, Shaffner F, ed. Progress in Liver Diseases, Vol. IX. Philadelphia PA: WB Saunders, 1990: 555.
55 Bergquist A, Ekbom A, Olsson R, et al. Hepatic and extrahepatic malignancies in primary sclerosing cholangitis. *J Hepatol* 2002; **36**: 321–327.
56 Fleming KA, Boberg KM, Glaumann H, et al. Biliary dysplasia as a marker of cholangiocarcinoma in primary sclerosing cholangitis. *J Hepatol* 2001; **34**: 360–365.
57 Haworth AC, Manley PN, Groll A, et al. Bile duct carcinoma and biliary tract dysplasia in chronic ulcerative colitis. *Arch Pathol Lab Med* 1989; **113**: 434–436.
58 Ludwig J, Wahlstrom HE, Batts KP, et al. Papillary bile duct dysplasia in primary sclerosing cholangitis. *Gastroenterology* 1992; **102**: 2134–2138.
59 Broomé U, Glaumann H, Lindstöm E, et al. Natural history and outcome in 32 Swedish patients with small duct primary sclerosing cholangitis (PSC). *J Hepatol* 2002; **36**: 586–589.
60 Guarascio P, Yentis F, Cevikbas U, et al. Value of copper-associated protein in diagnostic assessment of liver biopsy. *J Clin Pathol* 1983; **36**: 18–23.
61 Ludwig J. Surgical pathology of the syndrome of primary sclerosing cholangitis. *Am J Surg Pathol* 1989; **13 (Suppl 1)**: 43–49.
62 Rubin E, Schaffner F, Popper H. Primary biliary cirrhosis. Chronic non-suppurative destructive cholangitis. *Am J Pathol* 1965; **46**: 387–407.
63 Dahlan Y, Smith L, Simmonds D, et al. Pediatric-onset primary biliary cirrhosis. *Gastroenterology* 2003; **125**: 1476–1479.
64 Kaplan MM. Primary biliary cirrhosis. *N Engl J Med* 1996; **335**: 1570–1580.
65 Leung PSC, Coppel RL, Ansari A, et al. Antimitochondrial antibodies in primary biliary cirrhosis. *Semin Liver Dis* 1997; **17**: 61–69.
66 Jones DEJ. Pathogenesis of primary biliary cirrhosis. *J Hepatol* 2003; **39**: 639–648.
67 Neuberger J. Antibodies and primary biliary cirrhosis – piecing together the jigsaw. *J Hepatol* 2002; **36**: 126–129.
68 Culp KS, Fleming CR, Duffy J, et al. Autoimmune associations in primary biliary cirrhosis. *Mayo Clin Proc* 1982; **57**: 365–370.
69 Scheuer P. Primary biliary cirrhosis. *Proc R Soc Med* 1967; **60**: 1257–1260.
70 Nakanuma Y, Terada T, Doishita K, et al. Hepatocellular carcinoma in primary biliary cirrhosis: an autopsy study. *Hepatology* 1990; **11**: 1010–1016.
71 Jones DEJ, Metcalf JV, Collier JD, et al. Hepatocellular carcinoma in primary biliary cirrhosis and its impact on outcomes. *Hepatology* 1997; **26**: 1138–1142.
72 Terada T, Kurumaya H, Nakanuma Y, et al. Macroregenerative nodules of the liver in primary biliary cirrhosis: report of two autopsy cases. *Am J Gastroenterol* 1989; **84**: 418–421.
73 Floreani A, Baragiotta A, Baldo V, et al. Hepatic and extrahepatic malignancies in primary biliary cirrhosis. *Hepatology* 1999; **29**: 1425–1428.

74 Yamazaki K, Suzuki K, Nakamura A, et al. Ursodeoxycholic acid inhibits eosinophil degranulation in patients with primary biliary cirrhosis. *Hepatology* 1999; **30**: 71–78.
75 Neuberger J. Eosinophils and primary biliary cirrhosis – stoking the fire? *Hepatology* 1999; **30**: 335–337.
76 Degott C, Zafrani ES, Callard P, et al. Histopathological study of primary biliary cirrhosis and the effect of ursodeoxycholic acid treatment on histology progression. *Hepatology* 1999; **29**: 1007–1012.
77 Nakanuma Y, Ohta G. Quantitation of hepatic granulomas and epithelioid cells in primary biliary cirrhosis. *Hepatology* 1983; **3**: 423–427.
78 Vleggaar FP, Buuren HR van, Zondervan PE, et al. Jaundice in non-cirrhotic primary biliary cirrhosis: the premature ductopenic variant. *Gut* 2001; **49**: 276–281.
79 Nakanuma Y. Necroinflammatory changes in hepatic lobules in primary biliary cirrhosis with less well-defined cholestatic changes. *Hum Pathol* 1993; **24**: 378–383.
80 McMahon RF, Babbs C, Warnes TW. Nodular regenerative hyperplasia of the liver. CREST Syndr primary biliary cirrhosis: an overlap syndrome? *Gut* 1989; **30**: 1430–1433.
81 Colina F, Pinedo F, Solís A, et al. Nodular regenerative hyperplasia of the liver in early histological stages of primary biliary cirrhosis. *Gastroenterology* 1992; **102**: 1319–1324.
82 Nakanuma Y, Ohta G, Kobayashi K, et al. Histological and histometric examination of the intrahepatic portal vein branches in primary biliary cirrhosis without regenerative nodules. *Am J Gastroenterol* 1982; **77**: 405–413.
83 Nakanuma Y, Hirata K. Unusual hepatocellular lesions in primary biliary cirrhosis resembling but unrelated to hepatocellular neoplasms. *Virchows Arch (A)* 1993; **422**: 17–23.
84 Bach N, Thung SN, Schaffner F. The histological features of chronic hepatitis C and autoimmune chronic hepatitis: a comparative analysis. *Hepatology* 1992; **15**: 572–577.
85 Christoffersen P, Poulsen H, Scheuer PJ. Abnormal bile duct epithelium in chronic aggressive hepatitis and primary biliary cirrhosis. *Hum Pathol* 1972; **3**: 227–235.
86 Terasaki S, Nakanuma Y, Yamazaki M, et al. Eosinophilic infiltration of the liver in primary biliary cirrhosis: a morphological study. *Hepatology* 1993; **17**: 206–212.
87 Czaja AJ, Carpenter HA. Autoimmune hepatitis with incidental histologic features of bile duct injury. *Hepatology* 2001; **34**: 659–665.
88 Washington K, Clavien P-A, Killenberg P. Peribiliary vascular plexus in primary sclerosing cholangitis and primary biliary cirrhosis. *Hum Pathol* 1997; **28**: 791–795.
89 Nakanuma Y, Saito K, Unoura M. Semiquantitative assessment of cholestasis and lymphocytic piecemeal necrosis in primary biliary cirrhosis: a histologic and immunohistochemical study. *J Clin Gastroenterol* 1990; **12**: 357–362.
90 Yamada S, Howe S, Scheuer PJ. Three-dimensional reconstruction of biliary pathways in primary biliary cirrhosis: a computer-assisted study. *J Pathol* 1987; **152**: 317–323.
91 Leon MP, Bassendine MF, Gibbs P, et al. Immunogenicity of biliary epithelium: study of the adhesive interaction with lymphocytes. *Gastroenterology* 1997; **112**: 968–977.
92 Dienes HP, Lohse AW, Gerken G, et al. Bile duct epithelia as target cells in primary biliary cirrhosis and primary sclerosing cholangitis. *Virchows Arch* 1997; **431**: 119–124.
93 Nakanuma Y. Pathology of septum formation in primary biliary cirrhosis: a histological study in the non-cirrhotic stage. *Virchows Arch (A)* 1991; **419**: 381–387.
94 Scheuer PJ. Pathologic features and evolution of primary biliary cirrhosis and primary sclerosing cholangitis. *Mayo Clin Proc* 1998; **73**: 179–183.
95 Williamson JM, Chalmers DM, Clayden AD, et al. Primary biliary cirrhosis and chronic active hepatitis: an examination of clinical, biochemical, and histopathological features in differential diagnosis. *J Clin Pathol* 1985; **38**: 1007–1012.
96 Woodward J, Neuberger J. Autoimmune overlap syndromes. *Hepatology* 2001; **33**: 994–1002.

97 Lohse AW. Meyer zum Büschenfelde K-H, Franz B, et al. Characterization of the overlap syndrome of primary biliary cirrhosis (PBC) and autoimmune hepatitis: evidence for it being a hepatitic form of PBC in genetically susceptible individuals. *Hepatology* 1999; **29**: 1078–1084.
98 Alvarez F, Berg PA, Biandin FB, et al. International Autoimmune Hepatitis Group report: review of criteria for diagnosis of autoimmune hepatitis. *J Hepatol* 1999; **31**: 929–938.
99 Kaya M, Angulo P, Lindor KD. Overlap of autoimmune hepatitis and primary sclerosing cholangitis: an evaluation of a modified scoring system. *J Hepatol* 2000; **33**: 537–542.
100 Kita H, Mackay IR, Water J Van de, et al. The lymphoid liver: considerations on pathways to autoimmune injury. *Gastroenterology* 2001; **120**: 1485–1501.
101 Abdo AA, Bain VG, Kichian K, Lee SS. Evolution of autoimmune hepatitis to primary sclerosing cholangitis: a sequential syndrome. *Hepatology* 2002; **36**: 1393–1399.
102 Feldstein AE, Perrault J, El-Youssif M, et al. Primary sclerosing cholangitis in children: a long-term follow-up study. *Hepatology* 2003; **38**: 210–217.
103 Jones DE, James OF, Portmann B, et al. Development of autoimmune hepatitis following liver transplantation for primary biliary cirrhosis. *Hepatology* 1999; **30**: 53–57.
104 Brunner G, Klinge O. Ein der chronisch-destruierenden nicht-eitrigen Cholangitis ähnliches Krankheitsbild mit antinjukleären Antikörpern (Immuncholangitis). *Dtsch Med Wochenschr* 1987; **112**: 1454–1458.
105 Bruguera M, Llach J, Rodés J. Nonsyndromic paucity of intrahepatic bile ducts in infancy and idiopathic ductopenia in adulthood: the same syndrome? *Hepatology* 1992; **15**: 830–834.
106 Dural AT, Genta RM, Goodman ZD, et al. Idiopathic adulthood ductopenia associated with hepatitis C virus. *Dig Dis Sci* 2002; **47**: 1625–1626.
107 Ludwig J. Idiopathic adulthood ductopenia: an update. *Mayo Clin Proc* 1998; **73**: 285–291.
108 Burak KW, Pearson DC, Swain MG, et al. Familial idiopathic adulthood ductopenia: a report of five cases in three generations. *J Hepatol* 2000; **32**: 159–163.
109 Crosbie OM, Crown JP, Nolan NPM, et al. Resolution of paraneoplastic bile duct paucity following successful treatment of Hodgkin's disease. *Hepatology* 1997; **26**: 5–8.
110 Moreno A, Carreño CA, González C. Idiopathic biliary ductopenia in adults without symptoms of liver disease. *N Engl J Med* 1997; **336**: 835–838.

GENERAL READING

Portmann BC, Nakanuma Y. Diseases of the bile ducts. In: MacSween RNM, Anthony PP, Scheuer PJ, et al., eds. Pathology of the Liver, 4th edn. Edinburgh: Churchill Livingstone, 2002: 435–506.

Li MK, Crawford JM. The pathology of cholestasis. *Semin Liver Dis* 2004; **24**: 21–42.

Crawford JM. Development of the intrahepatic biliary tree. *Semin Liver Dis* 2002; **22**: 213–226.

Roskams T, Desmet VJ. Ductular reaction and its diagnostic significance. *Semin Diagn Pathol* 1998; **15**: 259–269.

Roskams TA, Theise ND, Balabaud C, et al. Nomenclature of the finer branches of the biliary tree: canals, ductules, and ductular reactions in human livers. *Hepatology* 2004; **39**: 1739–1745.

Roberts SK, Ludwig J, LaRusso NF. The pathobiology of biliary epithelia. *Gastroenterology* 1997; **112**: 269–279.

Neuberger J. Antibodies and primary biliary cirrhosis – piecing together the jigsaw. *J Hepatol* 2002; **36**: 126–129.

Woodward J, Neuberger J. Autoimmune overlap syndromes. *Hepatology* 2001; **33**: 994–1002.

Kim WR, Ludwig J, Lindor KD. Variant forms of cholestatic diseases involving small bile ducts in adults. *Am J Gastroenterol* 2000; **95**: 1130–1138.

Jansen PLM, Muller M, Sturm E. Genes and cholestasis. *Hepatology* 2001; **34**: 1067–1074.

ACUTE VIRAL HEPATITIS

INTRODUCTION

Acute hepatitis is not usually an indication for liver biopsy. There are, however, at least three reasons why pathologists sometimes receive liver biopsy samples from patients with acute hepatitis. First, there may be doubt about the clinical diagnosis, or even a mistaken working diagnosis. Second, a diagnosis of hepatitis may be well-established but the clinician needs information on the stage of the disease or its severity. Third, the patient may have received a liver transplant and the pathologist is being asked to help decide if symptoms or biochemical abnormalities are due to recurrent (or new) viral hepatitis or to some other cause such as rejection. For all these reasons, a knowledge of the pathology of acute hepatitis is essential. There is a further reason, no less important than the others: without a knowledge of acute hepatitis, the pathologist cannot hope to understand chronic hepatitis and cirrhosis, together the cause of most liver disease in the world. This chapter describes acute viral hepatitis and its immediate sequelae in the immunocompetent patient. The specific problems of diagnosing hepatitis in an immunosuppressed patient after transplantation are reviewed in Chapter 16.

The hepatitis viruses are listed in Table 6.1. While several other candidates have been extensively investigated in recent years, none has so far been established as a definite cause of viral hepatitis and most episodes of acute and chronic hepatitis can be attributed to one of the viruses listed, to autoimmune hepatitis (Ch. 9) or to a hepatotoxic agent (Ch. 8). An exception to this statement is fulminant hepatitis, the cause of which cannot currently be established in a substantial minority of patients.[1–3] Occasionally, a virus more often associated with infection of other organs,

Table 6.1 The hepatitis viruses

Virus	Type	Spread and disease
Hepatitis A (HAV)	RNA hepatovirus	Faecal–oral, acute
Hepatitis B (HBV)	DNA hepadnavirus	Parenteral, acute or chronic
Hepatitis C (HCV)	RNA hepacivirus	Parenteral or sporadic; acute, more often chronic
Hepatitis D (HDV)	RNA deltavirus, defective	Pathogenic when combined with HBV
Hepatitis E (HEV)	RNA virus	Faecal–oral, epidemic or sporadic acute disease

such as one of the herpes viruses[4–6] or an adenovirus[7,8], gives rise to a severe hepatitis. These agents are further discussed in Chapter 15. Mild acute hepatitis has been reported in patients infected with the SARS virus (severe acute respiratory syndrome-associated coronavirus).[9]

PATHOLOGICAL FEATURES

The essential components of the acute phase of hepatitis are inflammatory-cell infiltration and hepatocellular damage. Other features include cholestasis, Kupffer-cell activation, endotheliitis, bile duct damage, the ductular reaction and hepatocellular regeneration.

Hepatocellular damage

Changes seen under the light microscope range from minor degrees of cell swelling to cell death. They are accompanied by the inflammatory infiltration described below, reflecting the important role of cellular immunity in the pathogenesis of most forms of hepatitis. Both hepatocellular damage and inflammation are usually most severe in perivenular areas, giving rise to a characteristic histological pattern (Fig. 6.1). A periportal pattern of necrosis and inflammation, sometimes seen in hepatitis A, is less common.

The mildest and probably reversible change is cell swelling. The cytoplasm of affected cells is rarified, granular and sometimes finely vacuolated. The more severe degrees of cell swelling are called ballooning degeneration (Fig. 6.2). This differs from the feathery degeneration of cholestasis, in which the cytoplasm has a reticular pattern (see Fig. 5.3). Other hepatocytes undergo apoptosis, which is thought to be an important method of cell death in hepatitis.[10] Shrinkage and increased staining of the cytoplasm, sometimes called acidophilic change or degeneration, is probably a precursor of apoptosis, in which the hepatocytes shrink further, become very dense and undergo fragmentation. The apoptotic bodies seen lying free in the sinusoids represent the largest fragments or entire unfragmented apoptotic cells (Fig. 6.2). They are often called acidophil bodies or Councilman bodies, Councilman having first described them in yellow fever.[11] Apoptotic bodies sometimes contain pyknotic nuclear remnants and often appear to bulge beyond the plane of the section. Another form of hepatocellular damage in acute hepatitis is focal (spotty) necrosis, in which liver cell plates are disrupted or replaced by small groups of lymphocytes and macrophages. Whether these mark a site of necrosis or of apoptosis is not clear; the damage to hepatocytes is deduced from their absence rather than seen. Whatever its mechanism, loss of hepatocytes or liver-cell drop out, coupled with focal regeneration, leads to a characteristic irregularity of the liver-cell plates which usually allows acute hepatitis to be distinguished from hepatocellular damage secondary to cholestasis. The loss of hepatocytes also leads to condensation of the extracellular matrix, best seen in reticulin preparations (Fig. 6.3).

Hepatocyte nuclei show prominent nucleoli and increased variation in size and may be multiple. When syncytial giant hepatocytes are very prominent, the term

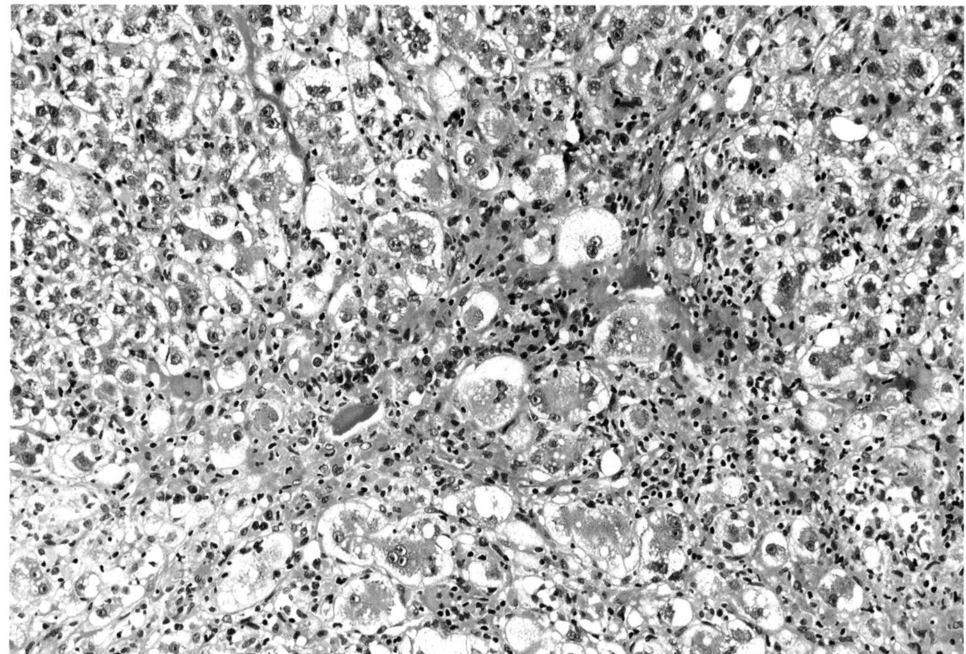

Figure 6.1 *Acute viral hepatitis*. Surviving hepatocytes in the perivenular area in the centre of the field are swollen and the area is infiltrated by inflammatory cells. (Needle biopsy, H&E).

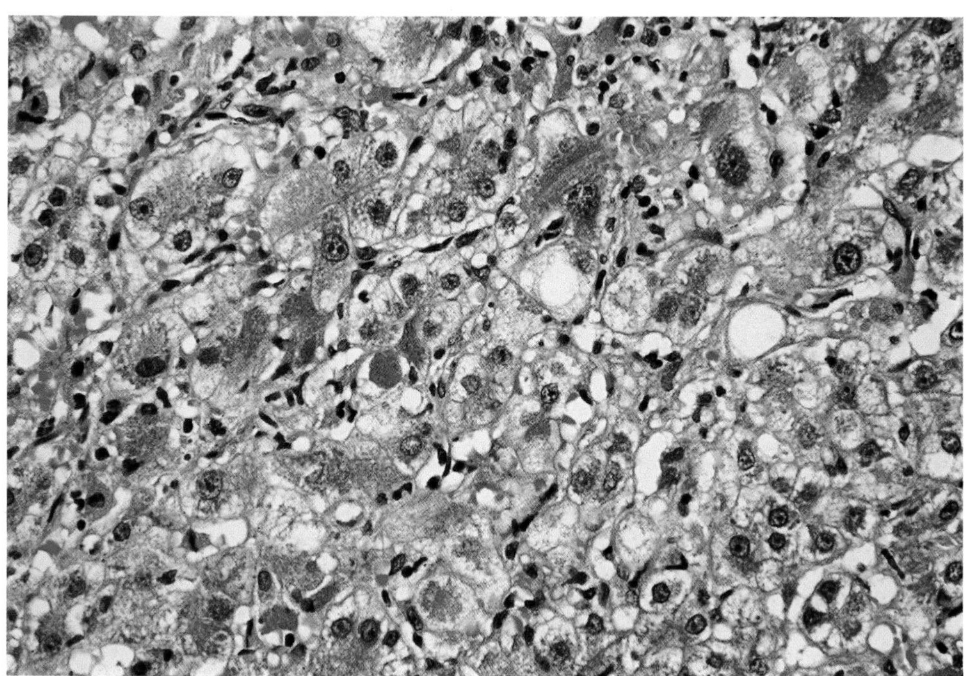

Figure 6.2 *Acute viral hepatitis*. Normal liver-cell plate structure is disrupted. Hepatocytes vary in size and some are ballooned and vacuolated. An apoptotic hepatocyte is seen left of centre. (Needle biopsy, H&E).

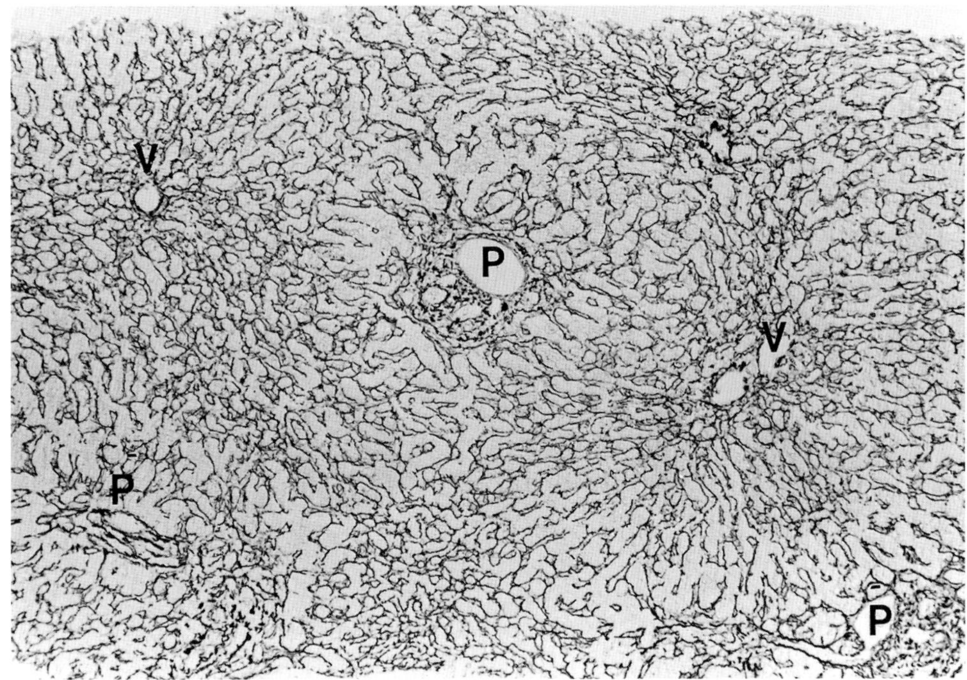

Figure 6.3 *Acute viral hepatitis.* The reticulin framework is condensed near the efferent venules (V), but not immediately around the portal tracts (P). (Needle biopsy, reticulin).

giant cell hepatitis is appropriate.[12,13] This is only rarely of proven viral origin and is also more characteristic of acute hepatitis in neonates. In adults, autoimmune hepatitis is an important association.[14–17]

Cholestasis in the form of bile thrombi in canaliculi is common in acute hepatitis but rare in chronic hepatitis, which is diagnostically helpful. It is a result of damage to the bile secretory apparatus of the hepatocytes, but may also result from interference with bile flow at the level of the portal tracts.[18] The term cholestatic hepatitis is best kept as a clinical description of patients with a prolonged cholestatic course. Mild hepatocellular siderosis or steatosis is occasionally seen.

The inflammatory infiltrate

Unlike classic acute inflammation, hepatitis is characterised by a mainly lymphocytic infiltrate within the parenchyma and portal tracts. In acute hepatitis, the most conspicuous inflammation is usually perivenular. The extent of portal inflammation is very variable and portal tracts may be either normal in size or expanded. The larger conducting tracts are often spared. The edges of small portal tracts may be well defined or blurred by outward extension of the infiltrate. This so-called spillover resembles the interface hepatitis of chronic hepatitis (Ch. 9) and may be difficult to distinguish from it. The parenchymal changes, clinical history and virological findings usually make the correct diagnosis clear.

While most of the infiltrating cells in acute hepatitis are small T lymphocytes,[19] plasma cells may also be prominent[20] and there are often a few neutrophils and eosinophils. The plasma cells do not necessarily indicate autoimmune hepatitis, nor do a few eosinophils prove a diagnosis of drug injury. Kupffer cells and other macrophages accumulate and enlarge, many of them forming discrete clumps together with lymphocytes. They may contain yellow-brown ceroid pigment, staining with PAS after diastase digestion (Fig. 6.4). They may also contain stainable iron (Fig. 6.5), but this is less common.

Sinusoidal and venular endothelial cells also take part in the hepatitic process. Sinusoidal endothelial cells become swollen and may contain dense iron-positive granules[21] (Fig. 6.5). Terminal hepatic venules may show disruption of the endothelium and lymphocytic infiltration.

Portal changes

In contrast to chronic hepatitis the parenchymal changes dominate the picture, but there is always some portal inflammation, affecting most or all small portal tracts (Fig. 6.6). The density of the infiltrate varies. Interlobular bile ducts may show abnormalities including irregularity, crowding and stratification of the epithelium, cytoplasmic vacuolation and infiltration by lymphocytes (Fig. 6.7). These changes, together with lymphoid follicle formation, are most often seen in hepatitis C. Bile duct loss (ductopenia) is very rare.

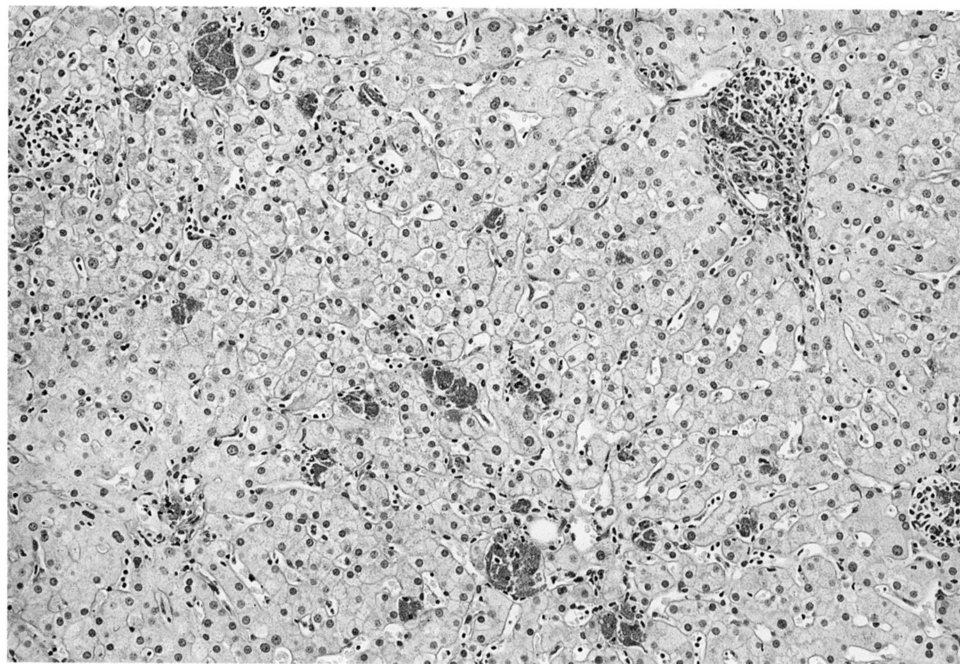

Figure 6.4 *Acute viral hepatitis*. Macrophages contain diastase PAS-positive material. (Needle biopsy, diastase-PAS).

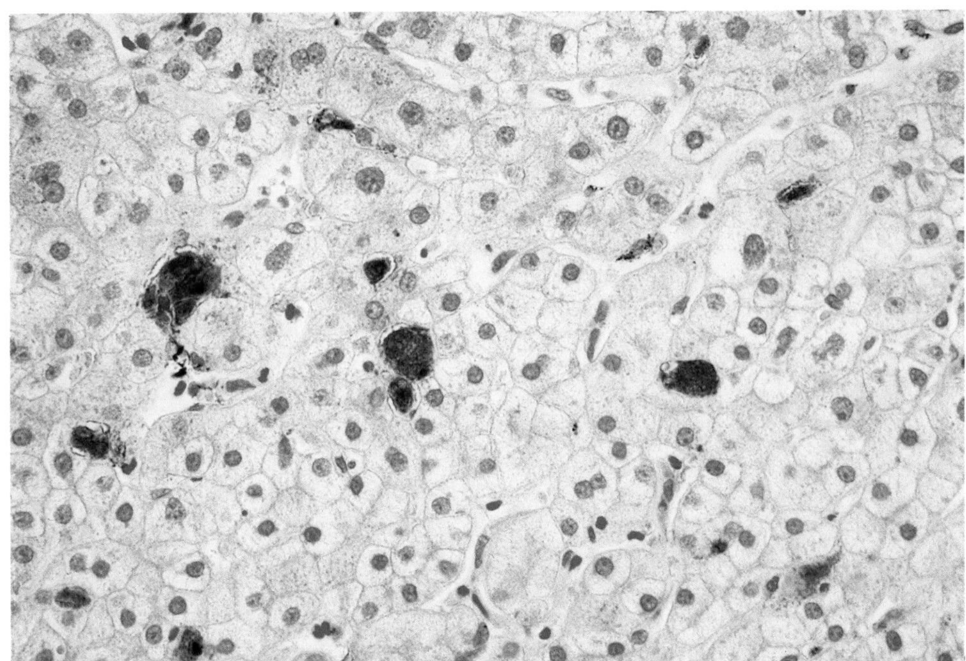

Figure 6.5 *Acute viral hepatitis*. Enlarged macrophages are strongly iron-positive. Some endothelial cells also contain dense Perls-positive granules. (Section kindly provided by Dr Susan Davies). (Needle biopsy, Perls' stain).

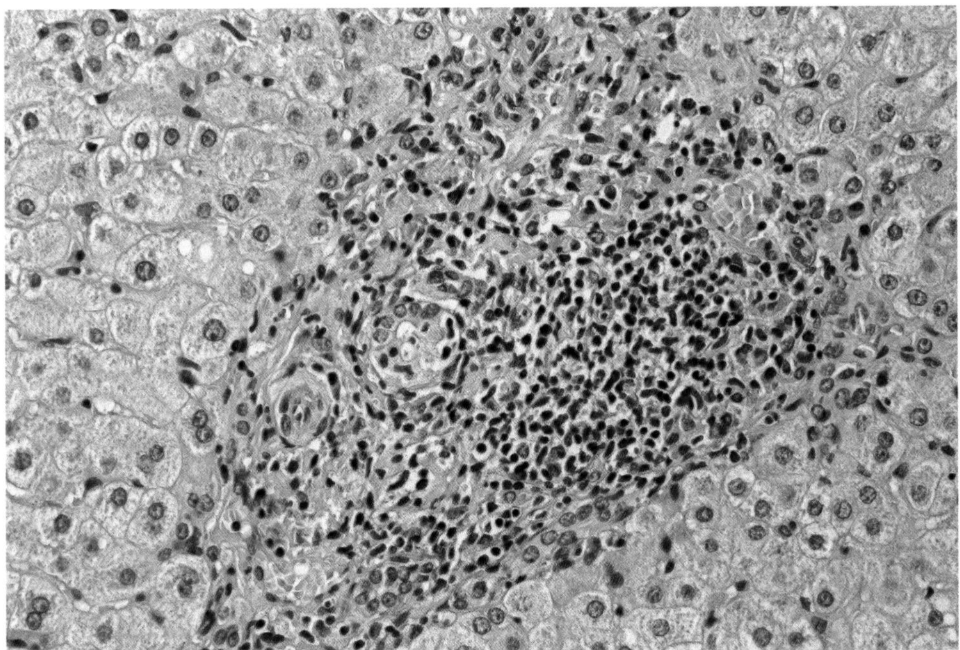

Figure 6.6 *Acute viral hepatitis*. A portal tract is infiltrated by inflammatory cells, mainly lymphocytes. In places the infiltrate extends a short way into the adjacent parenchyma. (Needle biopsy, H&E).

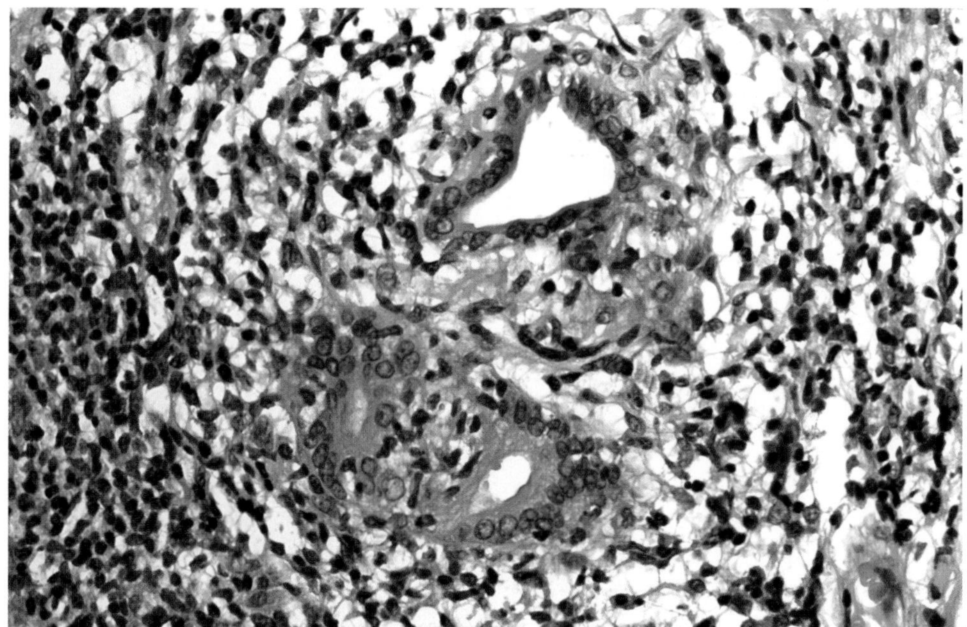

Figure 6.7 *Acute viral hepatitis*. Bile-duct epithelium is irregular and infiltrated by lymphocytes. The upper duct profile shows epithelial atrophy and dilatation. (Wedge biopsy, H&E).

Histological variants

The histological changes in acute hepatitis are infinitely variable, but a few patterns deserve special mention. These are confluent necrosis, bridging necrosis, necrosis of entire lobules and periportal necrosis.

Confluent necrosis signifies death of a substantial area of the parenchyma. Focal as opposed to zonal areas of confluent necrosis haphazardly distributed in relation to lobular zones are more likely to be due to causes other than acute viral hepatitis; possibilities to be considered include opportunistic infections with herpes simplex or zoster viruses and lymphoma. **Bridging necrosis** (Figs 6.8, 6.9 and Fig. 4.2) is the term given to confluent necrosis linking terminal venules to portal tracts. A possible explanation for this location is that it represents the entire zone 3 of an acinus, a view supported by the curved shape of many bridges. Bridging necrosis is a manifestation of severe acute hepatitis but its distribution even within a single biopsy may be irregular. Necrosis and inflammation linking adjacent portal tracts without involvement of terminal venules should not strictly be called bridging because it almost certainly has different pathogenetic significance; it results from widening of portal tracts, with or without periportal necrosis.

Bridges of confluent necrosis with subsequent collapse may be mistaken for the septa of chronic liver disease. In making the important distinction between them, the pathologist is often helped by stains for elastic tissue. Unlike stains for collagens, these normally give negative results in the parenchyma, but elastic tissue accumulates as septa age.[22] Recent collapse is therefore negative (Fig. 6.10), whereas old septa are positive. Substantial amounts of elastic tissue take months or years to accumulate, but small amounts can be detected by sensitive methods such as Victoria blue as early as 1 or 2 months after onset of hepatitis.[23]

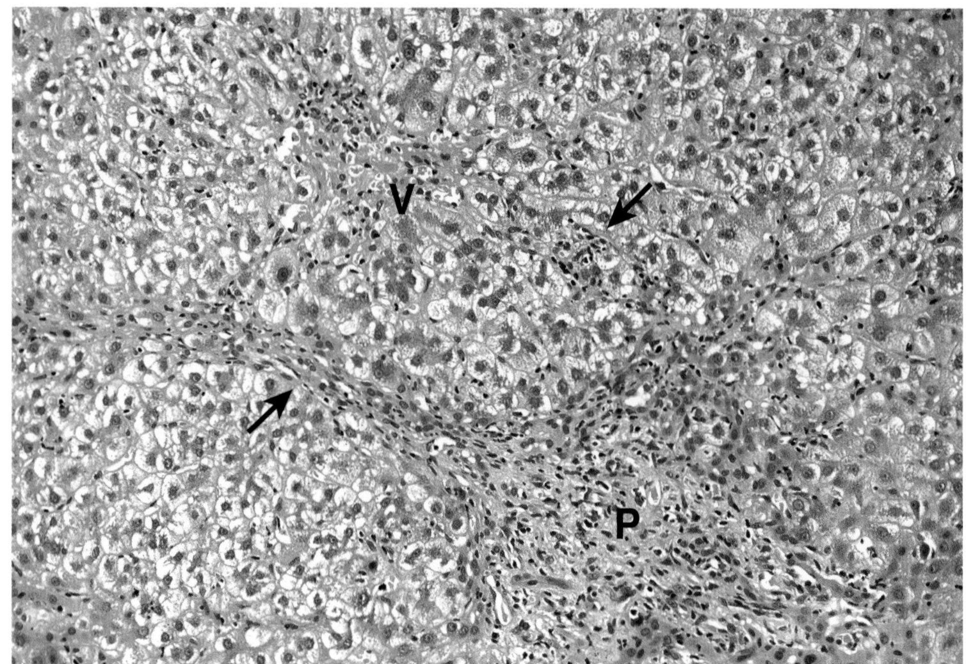

Figure 6.8 *Acute viral hepatitis: bridging necrosis*. Two curved lines of collapse (arrows) extend from a portal tract (P). An efferent venule (V) is seen top centre. (Needle biopsy, H&E).

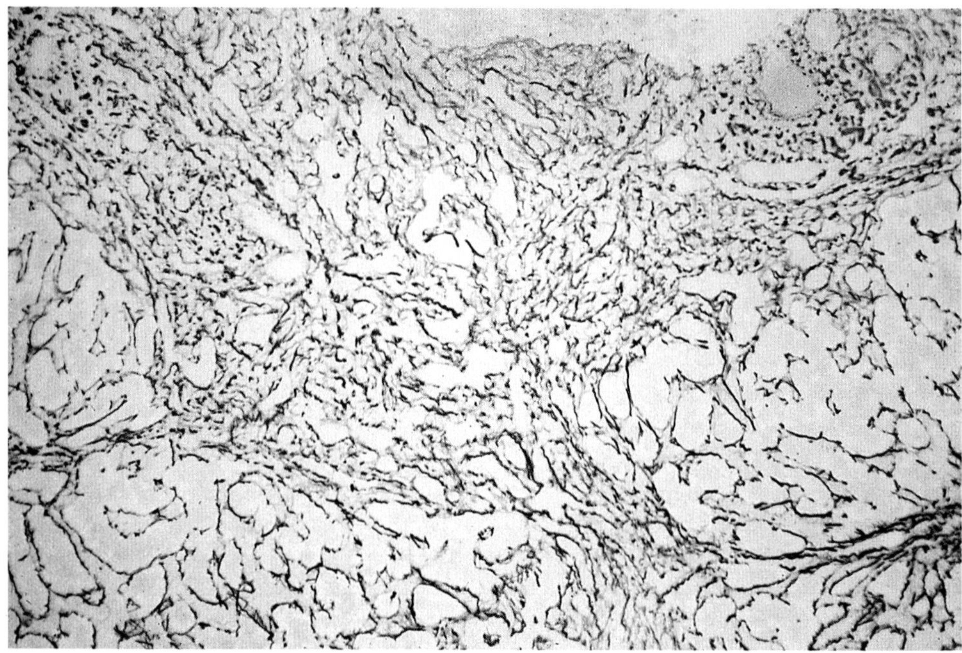

Figure 6.9 *Acute viral hepatitis: bridging necrosis*. Recent collapse following confluent necrosis is seen as condensation of reticulin, mimicking fibrosis. (Needle biopsy, reticulin).

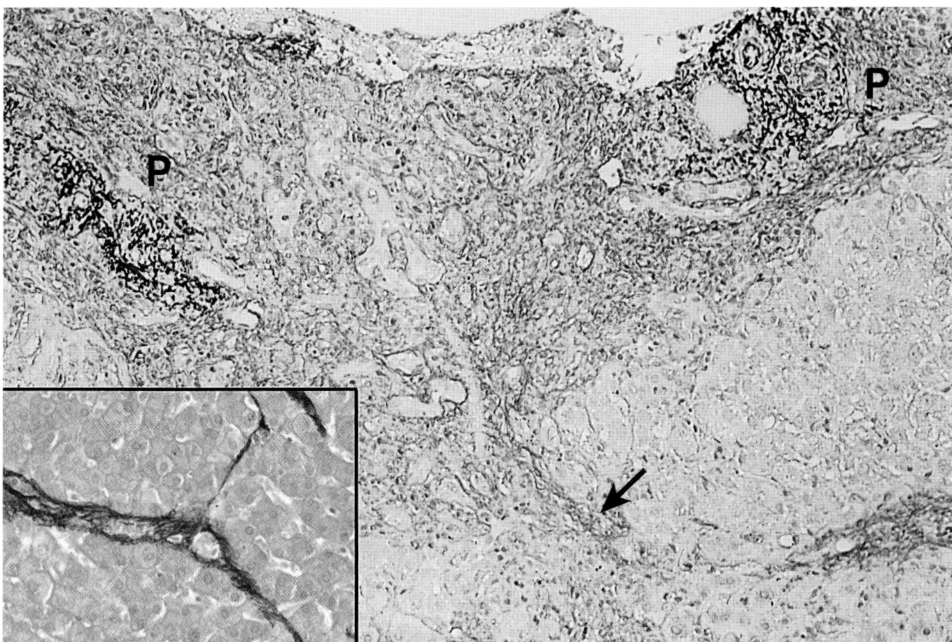

Figure 6.10 *Acute hepatitis: bridging necrosis*. The field is the same as that shown in Figure 6.9. A stain for elastic fibres is positive in two portal tracts (P) but not in the intervening area of collapse. A necrotic bridge (arrow) is also negative. *Inset*: This contrasts with an elastic fibre-rich septum in chronic liver disease. (Needle biopsy, orcein).

In a minority of patients with acute viral hepatitis confluent necrosis extends throughout entire lobules or acini (**panlobular or panacinar necrosis**) or several adjacent ones (**multilobular or multiacinar necrosis**). This is a common feature in patients with fulminant hepatitis. The term massive necrosis is also sometimes used, but can be misleading in so far as a needle biopsy specimen may not be representative of the liver as a whole and can lead to over- or under-estimation of the true extent of liver damage.[24] This throws doubt on the usefulness of liver biopsy as a means of assessing prognosis in severe acute hepatitis. Sometimes multilobular necrosis involves only the subcapsular zone and a small needle specimen may then give a falsely pessimistic picture (see Fig. 1.3). In multilobular necrosis the parenchyma is replaced by collapsed stroma, inflammatory cells and activated macrophages (Fig. 6.11). Around the surviving portal tracts, there are prominent duct-like structures, some of which probably represent proliferation of pluripotential progenitor cells[25,26] (see Fig. 4.6d). Late-onset hepatic failure is a term used for patients developing encephalopathy between 8 and 24 weeks after onset of symptoms.[27] Study of liver biopsies and explanted livers from these patients has shown a consistent pattern of map-like necrosis together with areas of nodular regeneration.

Periportal rather than the more usual perivenular necrosis is a feature in some patients with hepatitis A (below).

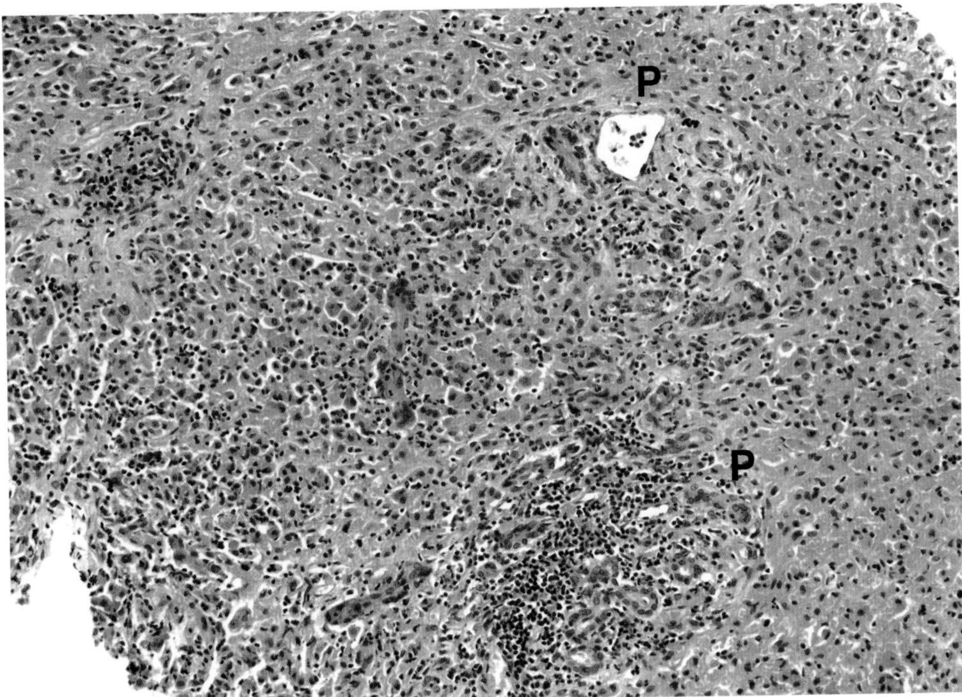

Figure 6.11 *Acute viral hepatitis: multilobular necrosis.* Portal tracts (P) can be identified but the parenchyma has been replaced by inflammatory cells, necrotic debris and duct-like structures. (Needle biopsy, H&E).

INDIVIDUAL CAUSES OF VIRAL HEPATITIS

There are more similarities than differences between hepatitis A, B, C, D and E, but certain patterns are more common in one type than another and are described here. They do not allow the pathologist to identify the cause of the hepatitis on histological appearances alone. The picture may be confused by the presence of more than one virus, or by additional damage resulting from alcohol abuse.

Hepatitis A

Two main patterns are described, occurring separately or together.[28–30] One is a histological picture of perivenular cholestasis with little liver-cell damage or inflammation, easily mistaken for other causes of cholestasis (Fig. 6.12). The second is a hepatitis with periportal necrosis and a dense portal infiltrate which includes abundant, often aggregated plasma cells (Fig. 6.13). These two patterns may be related, the cholestasis resulting from interruption of bile flow by the periportal necrosis.[18] Other patterns of hepatitis as described above are also found, but fulminant hepatitis with multilobular necrosis is rare. Extensive microvesicular change of hepatocytes, previously described in hepatitis D infection, has been seen also in severe acute hepatitis A (Fig. 6.14). Fibrin-ring granulomas have been reported.[31,32] A chronic course[33] is very rare.

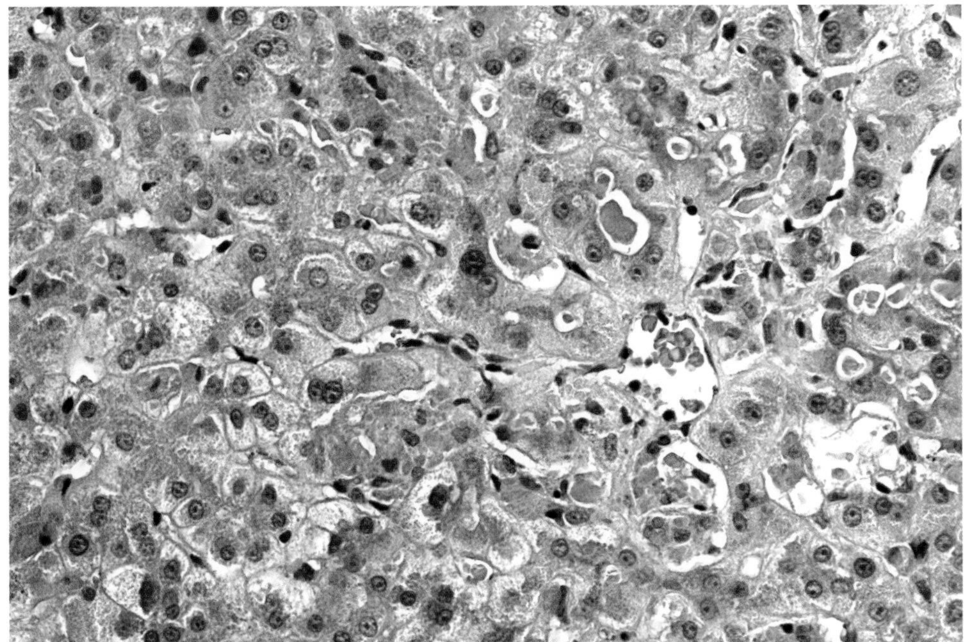

Figure 6.12 *Hepatitis A.* Perivenular area showing irregularity of liver-cell plates and cholestasis, but only mild inflammatory infiltration. (Needle biopsy, H&E).

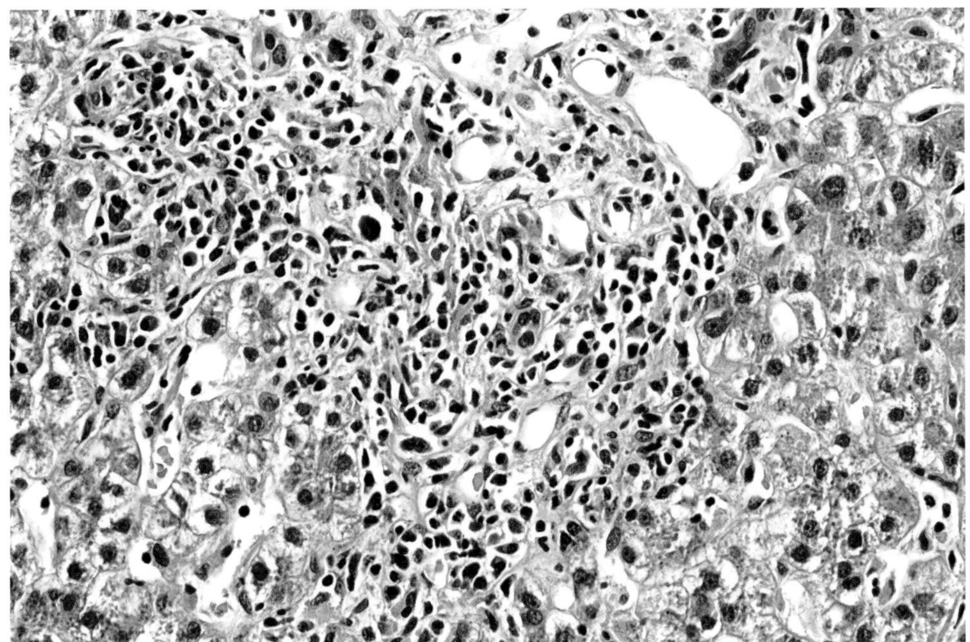

Figure 6.13 *Hepatitis A.* A portal area is heavily infiltrated by lymphocytes and plasma cells, some of which extend into the adjacent parenchyma. The limiting plate is irregular. The picture resembles that of chronic hepatitis with interface hepatitis. (Needle biopsy, H&E).

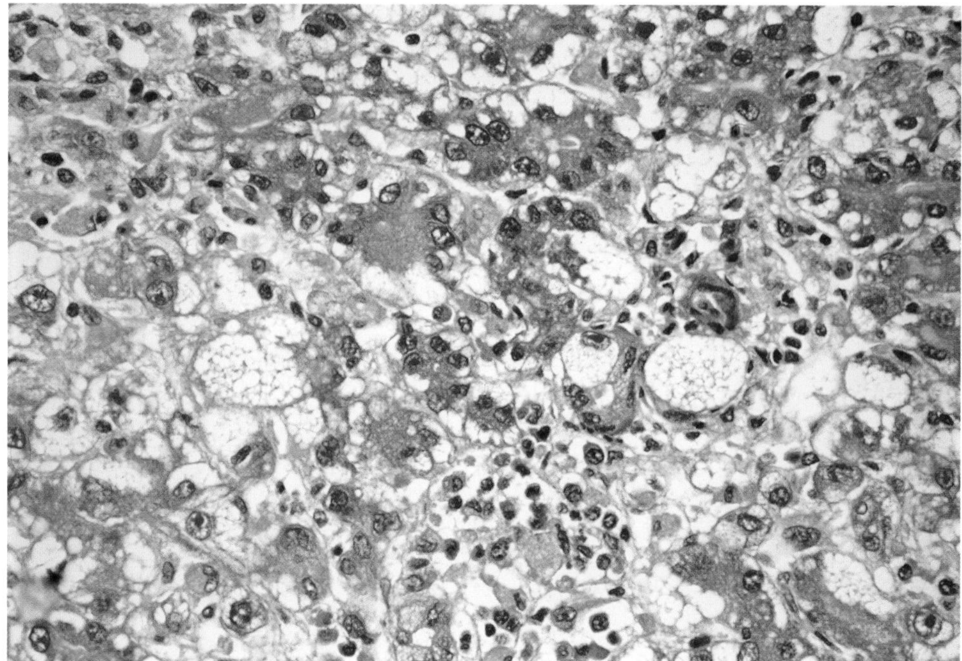

Figure 6.14 *Hepatitis A.* In this patient with a clinical picture of fulminant hepatitis, hepatocytes are swollen and microvesicular. There is cholestasis and a lymphocytic infiltrate. (Needle biopsy, H&E).

Hepatitis B

The histological appearances are broadly similar to those of other forms of viral hepatitis. Some of the differences reported in the literature may well reflect patient selection rather than features specific for HBV infection. However, lymphocytes and macrophages sometimes lie in close contact with hepatocytes (peripolesis) or even invaginate them deeply (emperipolesis), which probably reflects the immunological nature of the cell damage. In a comparative study, periportal inflammation tended to be more severe in acute hepatitis B than in hepatitis C.[34] Liver cells and their nuclei may show a moderate degree of pleomorphism. In most cases of acute hepatitis, the hepatitis B core and surface antigens (HBcAg and HBsAg) are either not demonstrable or very sparse, but in one study of livers infected with a hepatitis B virus mutant[35] HBsAg could be demonstrated by immunostaining in over half the patients and HBcAg in a minority. The presence of ground-glass hepatocytes (Ch. 9) or positive staining of surface material with Victoria blue or orcein indicates chronic disease. Recurrence of HBV infection after liver transplantation is an exception to this rule, both antigens being found in large amounts (see Ch. 16). In parenterally-transmitted hepatitis, including types B and C, birefringent spicules of talc may be found in portal tracts as a result of intravenous drug abuse.[36]

Following clinical recovery of acute hepatitis B, occult infection and mild histological abnormalities including portal inflammation, focal necrosis, apoptosis and fibrosis may persist for at least a decade.[37]

Hepatitis C

Usually the histological features are those of any acute hepatitis, but two distinguishing features have been noted in acute hepatitis C. First, there may be prominent infiltration of sinusoids by lymphocytes in the absence of severe liver-cell damage,[38] giving rise to a picture reminiscent of infectious mononucleosis (Fig. 6.15). Second, lymphoid follicles and bile-duct damage, features also associated with chronic hepatitis, may be seen within a few weeks or months of onset.[39] There may be cholestasis. The common finding of steatosis in hepatitis C is discussed in Chapter 9. Fulminant hepatitis C is very rare in the Western world[3] but may be commoner in parts of Asia.[40]

Hepatitis D (delta hepatitis)

Coinfection or superinfection with the hepatitis D virus (HDV) alters the course of type B hepatitis. It encourages chronicity and enhances severity,[41–43] except after liver transplantation. The antigen, HDAg, can easily be demonstrated immunohistochemically in paraffin sections and is mainly found in hepatocyte nuclei (Fig. 6.16). These may have finely granular eosinophilic centres (so-called 'sanded' nuclei[44]). Cytoplasmic and membrane-associated staining is also sometimes seen.

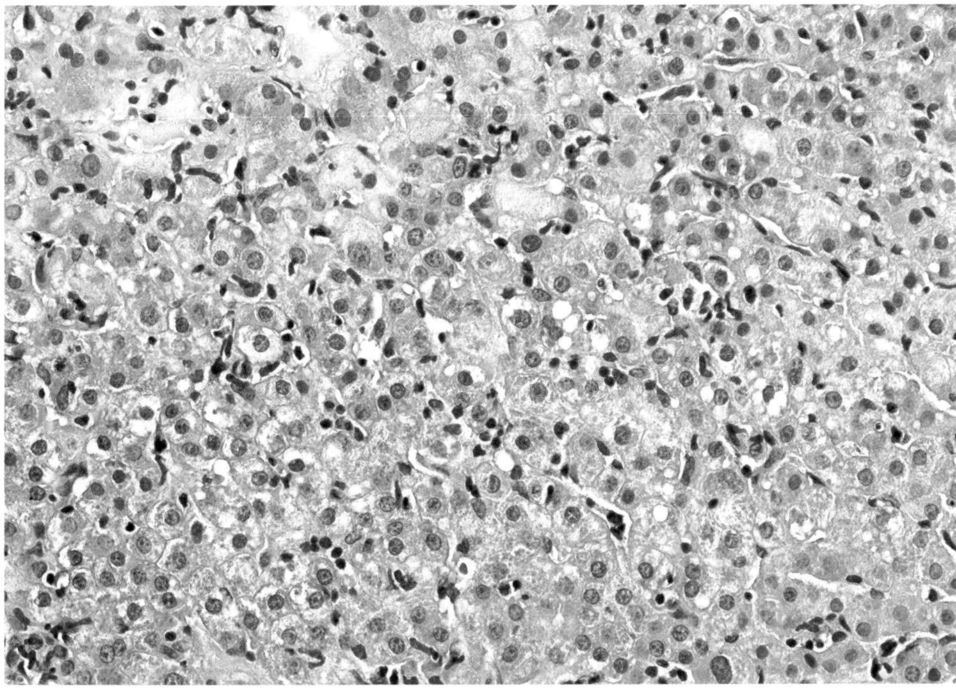

Figure 6.15 *Acute hepatitis C.* In this example the main abnormality is infiltration of sinusoids by lymphocytes. (Needle biopsy, H&E).

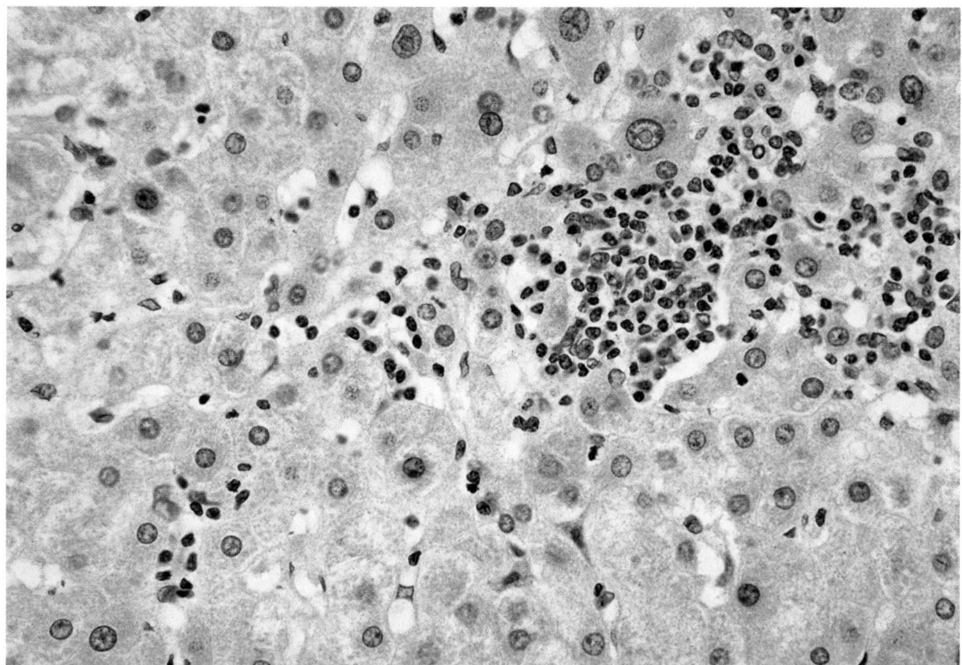

Figure 6.16 *Delta (HDV) hepatitis.* Some hepatocyte nuclei contain the delta antigen and are stained red. There is a substantial lymphocytic infiltrate. (Needle biopsy, specific immunostain, alkaline phosphatase method).

Severe acute hepatitis in a patient with markers of HBV infection may be due to superinfection by HDV of a chronic HBV carrier.[45] In an outbreak of HDV infection among Venezuelan Indians, notable features included early small-droplet fatty change, sparse lymphocytes and abundant macrophages in the parenchyma and substantial portal infiltration.[46] Later in the attack, there was extensive necrosis and collapse. Microvesicular fatty change and acidophilic necrosis of hepatocytes have been reported from Colombia[47] and North America.[48] In non-immunosuppressed patients with current HDV infection, liver biopsy is likely to show substantial necrosis and inflammation. Following liver transplantation, on the other hand, HDV without HBV is sometimes demonstrable in the absence of hepatitic changes, indicating that HDV can survive in the absence of HBV. It does not then appear, however, to be capable of causing liver damage.[49]

Hepatitis E

This is the result of infection by the enteric route with an RNA virus.[50] The disease causes epidemics in Asia and has also been found in Africa and North America. In the Western world, it is most often seen in travellers (Fig. 6.17). Infection does not appear to lead to chronic disease, but may cause severe decompensation of pre-existing chronic liver disease due to other causes.[51,52] There is little detailed information on the pathological changes of hepatitis E virus infection in man. In a small number of patients studied, the appearances were like those of hepatitis A, with prominent cholestasis and a predominantly portal and periportal inflammatory

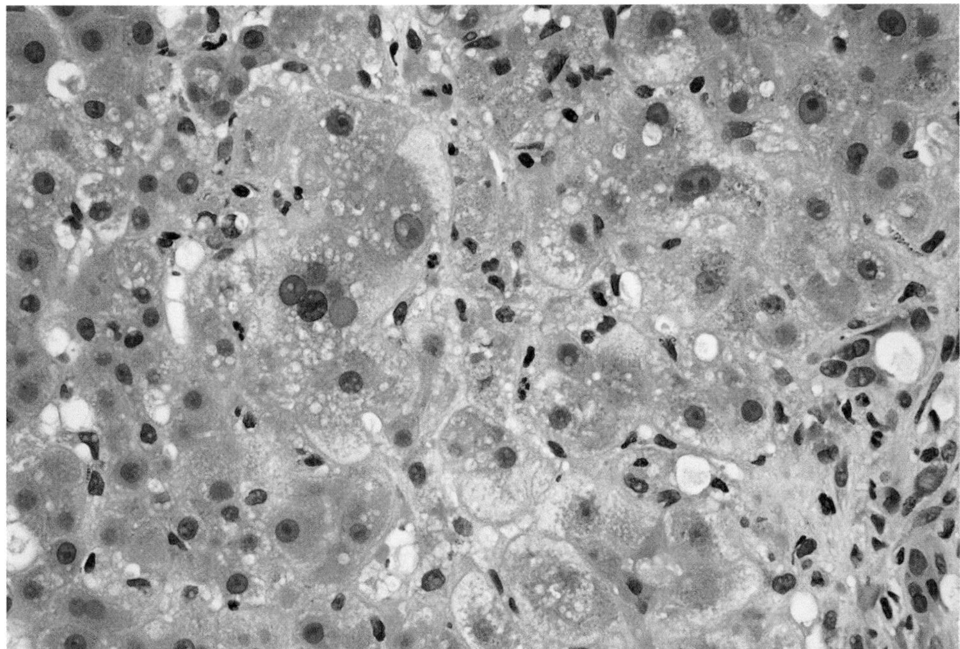

Figure 6.17 *Hepatitis E.* Hepatocytes are vacuolated and one to the left of centre is greatly enlarged and multinucleated. There is a mixed infiltrate and macrophages contain brown ceroid pigment. (Needle biopsy, H&E).

infiltrate.[53] Histological cholestasis has been described in an elderly patient with a prolonged cholestatic clinical course.[54] The liver of a pregnant woman with fatal hepatitis E showed little portal inflammation, much cholestasis and prominent phlebitis, and virus particles were seen in bile ductules by electron microscopy.[55]

DIFFERENTIAL DIAGNOSIS OF ACUTE VIRAL HEPATITIS

The distinction of acute hepatitis from **bile-duct obstruction** rests mainly on the finding of typical hepatitic changes in the parenchyma. **Drug-related hepatitis** may be indistinguishable from viral hepatitis and should always be suspected if the cause of the hepatitis is in doubt. Features more common in drug-induced than in viral hepatitis include sharply-defined perivenular necrosis, granulomas, abundant neutrophils or eosinophils and a poorly developed portal inflammatory reaction. Cholestasis may overshadow the hepatitic features. **Autoimmune hepatitis** may have a clinically acute onset, histologically indistinguishable from viral hepatitis or alternatively with histological features of chronic disease. This is discussed more fully in Chapter 9. In **steatohepatitis** there is usually conspicuous fatty change. Mallory bodies may be present in ballooned hepatocytes and the infiltrate typically includes neutrophils. The key to the diagnosis is the presence of pericellular fibrosis in affected areas. The differentiation of acute from **chronic hepatitis** is briefly discussed in the section on bridging necrosis above. While the parenchymal changes predominate in acute hepatitis, especially in perivenular areas, portal and periportal changes predominate in chronic disease. The distinction is sometimes difficult to make, especially when extensive lobular changes are found during an exacerbation of chronic hepatitis.

FATE AND MORPHOLOGICAL SEQUELAE OF ACUTE VIRAL HEPATITIS

Resolution

As far as can be deduced from the available evidence, most examples of hepatitis A, B and E are followed by complete or near-complete resolution and a return of the liver to normal. A chronic course is probably more common when hepatitis B is complicated by delta infection than otherwise, and in hepatitis C the risk of chronicity is high. Even in patients whose hepatitis resolves, some residual changes may persist for many months after clinical recovery (Figs 6.18, 6.19).

Scarring

Localised collapse, scarring and regeneration following severe hepatitis with bridging or panlobular necrosis sometimes produce a histological picture indistinguishable from cirrhosis.

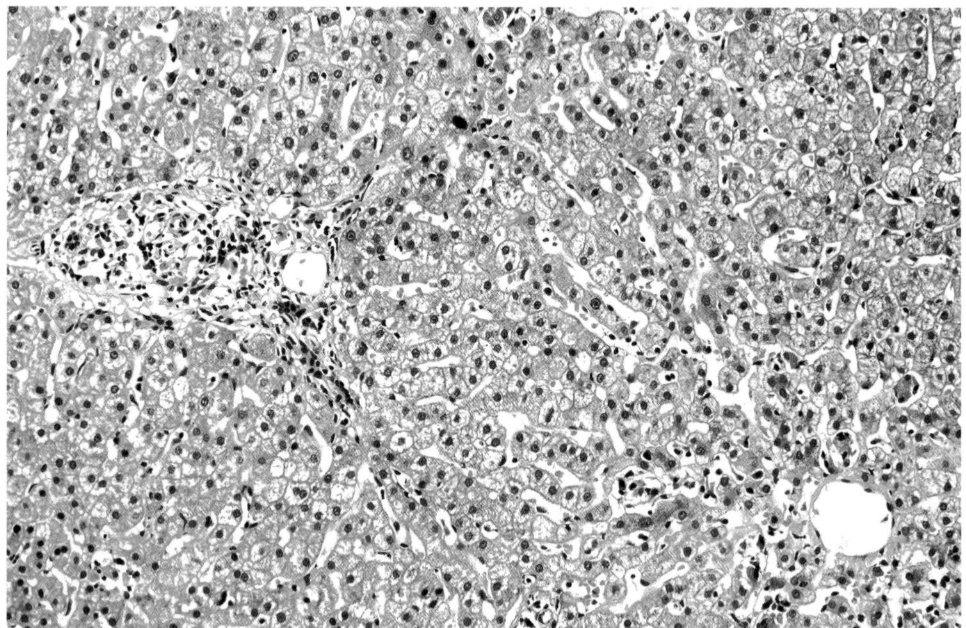

Figure 6.18 *Acute viral hepatitis: residual changes.* Short septa extend from the mildly inflamed portal tract to the left. Minimal inflammation and irregular liver-cell plates are seen around the efferent venule below right. (Needle biopsy, H&E).

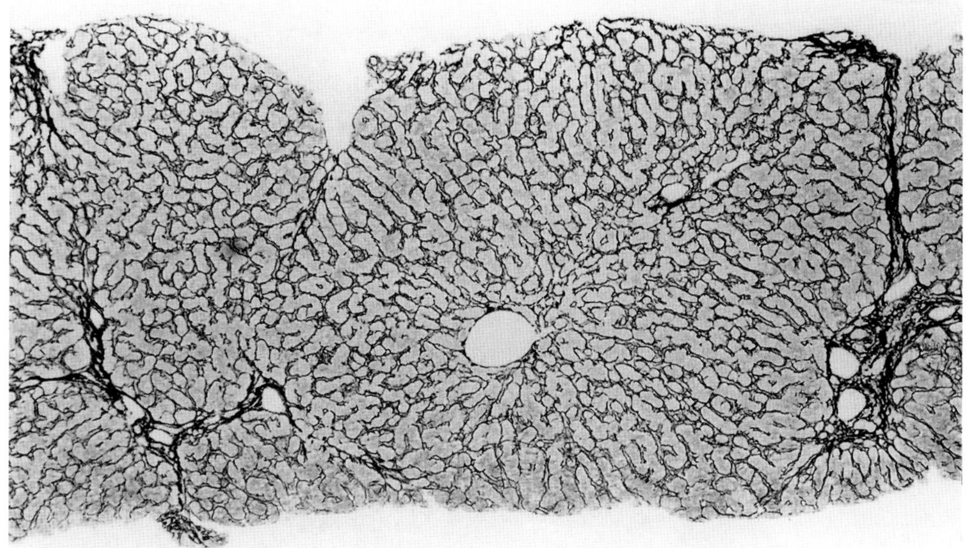

Figure 6.19 *Acute viral hepatitis: residual changes*. Slender septa link portal tracts (left and right), but the perivenular area (centre) is unaffected and architectural relationships are preserved. (Needle biopsy, reticulin).

Fatal outcome or need for liver transplantation

Necrosis is usually severe. Regenerative hyperplasia of surviving hepatocytes or progenitor cells may be seen.

Chronic hepatitis

Most individuals with hepatitis C virus infection develop chronic hepatitis. This has substantial impact on daily liver biopsy practice. Chronic hepatitis also develops in many patients with hepatitis B.

Cirrhosis

Cirrhosis resulting from infection with a hepatitis virus almost always follows a period of chronic hepatitis, with repeated or continuous hepatocellular necrosis and regeneration. Occasionally it may follow directly after a single episode of severe acute hepatitis.

Hepatocellular carcinoma

This may develop on the basis of cirrhosis in patients infected with HBV or HCV. Occasionally, however, hepatocellular carcinoma is found in the absence of cirrhosis. Usually after a prolonged period of chronic liver disease.[56]

REFERENCES

1 Ben Ari Z, Samuel D, Zemel R, et al. Fulminant non-A-G viral hepatitis leading to liver transplantation. *Arch Intern Med* 2000; **160**: 388–392.

2 Petrovic LM, Arkadopoulos N, Demetriou AA. Activation of hepatic stellate cells in liver tissue of patients with fulminant liver failure after treatment with bioartificial liver. *Hum Pathol* 2001; **32**: 1371–1375.

3 Schiødt FV, Davern TJ, Shakil AO, et al. Viral hepatitis-related acute liver failure. *Am J Gastroenterol* 2003; **98**: 448–453.

4 Peters DJ, Greene WH, Ruggiero F, et al. Herpes simplex-induced fulminant hepatitis in adults: a call for empiric therapy. *Dig Dis Sci* 2000; **45**: 2399–2404.

5 Pinna AD, Rakela J, Demetris AJ, et al. Five cases of fulminant hepatitis due to herpes simplex virus in adults. *Dig Dis Sci* 2002; **47**: 750–754.

6 Collin L, Moulin P, Jungers M, et al. Epstein-Barr virus (EBV)-induced liver failure in the absence of extensive liver-cell necrosis: a case for cytokine-induced liver dysfunction? *J Hepatol* 2004; **41**: 174–175.

7 Wang WH, Wang HL. Fulminant adenovirus hepatitis following bone marrow transplantation. A case report and brief review of the literature. *Arch Pathol Lab Med* 2003; **127**: e246–e248.

8 Longerich T, Haferkamp K, Tox U, et al. Acute liver failure in a renal transplant patient caused by adenoviral hepatitis superimposed on a fibrosing cholestatic hepatitis B. *Hum Pathol* 2004; **35**: 894–897.

9 Chau TN, Lee KC, Yao H, et al. SARS-associated viral hepatitis caused by a novel coronavirus: Report of three cases. *Hepatology* 2004; **39**: 302–310.

10 Lau JYN, Xie X, Lai MMC, et al. Apoptosis and viral hepatitis. *Semin Liver Dis* 1998; **18**: 169–176.

11 Klotz O, Belt TH. The pathology of the liver in yellow fever. *Am J Pathol* 1930; **6**: 663–689.

12 Phillips MJ, Blendis LM, Poucell S, et al. Syncytial giant-cell hepatitis. Sporadic hepatitis with distinctive pathological features, a severe clinical course and paramyxoviral features. *N Engl J Med* 1991; **324**: 455–460.

13 Fimmel CJ, Guo L, Compans RW, et al. A case of syncytial giant cell hepatitis with features of a paramyxoviral infection. *Am J Gastroenterol* 1998; **93**: 1931–1937.

14 Devaney K, Goodman ZD, Ishak KG. Postinfantile giant-cell transformation in hepatitis. *Hepatology* 1992; **16**: 327–333.

15 Lau JYN, Koukoulis G, Mieli-Vergani G, et al. Syncytial giant-cell hepatitis – a specific disease entity? *J Hepatol* 1992; **15**: 216–219.

16 Protzer U, Dienes HP, Bianchi L, et al. Post-infantile giant cell hepatitis in patients with primary sclerosing cholangitis and autoimmune hepatitis. *Liver* 1996; **16**: 274–282.

17 Ben Ari Z, Broida E, Monselise Y, et al. Syncytial giant-cell hepatitis due to autoimmune hepatitis type II (LKM1+) presenting as subfulminant hepatitis. *Am J Gastroenterol* 2000; **95**: 799–801.

18 Sciot R, Van Damme B , Desmet VJ. Cholestatic features in hepatitis A. *J Hepatol* 1986; **3**: 172–181.

19 Volpes R, van den Oord JJ, Desmet VJ. Memory T cells represent the predominant lymphocyte subset in acute and chronic liver inflammation. *Hepatology* 1991; **13**: 826–829.

20 Mietkiewski JM, Scheuer PJ. Immunoglobulin-containing plasma cells in acute hepatitis. *Liver* 1985; **5**: 84–88.

21 Bardadin KA, Scheuer PJ. Endothelial cell changes in acute hepatitis. A light and electron microscopic study. *J Pathol* 1984; **144**: 213–220.

22 Scheuer PJ, Maggi G. Hepatic fibrosis and collapse: histological distinction by orcein staining. *Histopathology* 1980; **4**: 487–490.

23 Thung SN, Gerber MA. The formation of elastic fibers in livers with massive hepatic necrosis. *Arch Pathol Lab Med* 1982; **106**: 468–469.

24 Hanau C, Munoz SJ, Rubin R. Histopathological heterogeneity in fulminant hepatic failure. *Hepatology* 1995; **21**: 345–351.

25 Demetris AJ, Seaberg EC, Wennerberg A, et al. Ductular reaction after submassive necrosis in humans. Special emphasis on analysis of ductular hepatocytes. *Am J Pathol* 1996; **149**: 439–448.

26 Roskams T, De Vos R, van Eyken P, et al. Hepatic OV-6 expression in human liver disease and rat experiments: evidence for hepatic progenitor cells in man. *J Hepatol* 1998; **29**: 455–463.

27 Ellis AJ, Saleh M, Smith H, et al. Late-onset hepatic failure: clinical features, serology and outcome following transplantation. *J Hepatol* 1995; **23**: 363–372.

28 Teixeira MR Jr., Weller IVD, Murray AM, et al. The pathology of hepatitis A in man. *Liver* 1982; **2**: 53–60.

29 Abe H, Beninger PR, Ikejiri N, et al. Light microscopic findings of liver biopsy specimens from patients with hepatitis type A and comparison with type B. *Gastroenterology* 1982; **82**: 938–947.

30 Okuno T, Sano A, Deguchi T, et al. Pathology of acute hepatitis A in humans. Comparison with acute hepatitis B. *Am J Clin Pathol* 1984; **81**: 162–169.

31 Ponz E, Garcia-Pagan JC, Bruguera M, et al. Hepatic fibrin-ring granulomas in a patient with hepatitis A. *Gastroenterology* 1991; **100**: 268–270.

32 Ruel M, Sevestre H, Henry-Biabaud E, et al. Fibrin ring granulomas in hepatitis A. *Dig Dis Sci* 1992; **37**: 1915–1917.

33 Inoue K, Yoshiba M, Yotsuyanagi H, et al. Chronic hepatitis A with persistent viral replication. *J Med Virol* 1996; **50**: 322–324.

34 Chu CW, Hwang SJ, Luo JC, et al. Comparison of clinical, virologic and pathologic features in patients with acute hepatitis B and C. *J Gastroenterol Hepatol* 2001; **16**: 209–214.

35 Uchida T, Shimojima S, Gotoh K, et al. Pathology of livers infected with 'silent' hepatitis B virus mutant. *Liver* 1994; **14**: 251–256.

36 Molos MA, Litton N, Schubert TT. Talc liver. *J Clin Gastroenterol* 1987; **9**: 198–203.

37 Yuki N, Nagaoka T, Yamashiro M, et al. Long-term histologic and virologic outcomes of acute self-limited hepatitis B. *Hepatology* 2003; **37**: 1172–1179.

38 Bamber M, Murray A, Arborgh BA, et al. Short incubation non-A, non-B hepatitis transmitted by factor VIII concentrates in patients with congenital coagulation disorders. *Gut* 1981; **22**: 854–859.

39 Kobayashi K, Hashimoto E, Ludwig J, et al. Liver biopsy features of acute hepatitis C compared with hepatitis A, B and non-A, non-B, non-C. *Liver* 1993; **13**: 69–73.

40 Chu CM, Sheen IS, Liaw YF. The role of hepatitis C virus in fulminant viral hepatitis in an area with endemic hepatitis A and B. *Gastroenterology* 1994; **107**: 189–195.

41 Govindarajan S, De-Cock KM, Redeker AG. Natural course of delta superinfection in chronic hepatitis B virus-infected patients: histopathologic study with multiple liver biopsies. *Hepatology* 1986; **6**: 640–644.

42 Verme G, Amoroso P, Lettieri G, et al. A histological study of hepatitis delta virus liver disease. *Hepatology* 1986; **6**: 1303–1307.

43 Lin H-H, Liaw Y-F, Chen T-J, et al. Natural course of patients with chronic type B hepatitis following acute hepatitis delta virus superinfection. *Liver* 1989; **9**: 129–134.

44 Moreno A. Ramón y Cahal S, Marazuela M et al. Sanded nuclei in delta patients. *Liver* 1989; **9**: 367–371.

45 Smedile A, Farci P, Verme G, et al. Influence of delta infection on severity of hepatitis B. *Lancet* 1982; **ii**: 945–947.

46 Popper H, Thung SN, Gerber MA, et al. Histologic studies of severe delta agent infection in Venezuelan Indians. *Hepatology* 1983; **3**: 906–912.

47 Buitrago B, Popper H, Hadler SC, et al. Specific histologic features of Santa Marta hepatitis: a severe form of hepatitis delta-virus infection in northern South America. *Hepatology* 1986; **6**: 1285–1291.

48 Lefkowitch JH, Goldstein H, Yatto R, et al. Cytopathic liver injury in acute delta virus hepatitis. *Gastroenterology* 1987; **92**: 1262–1266.

49 Davies SE, Lau JYN, O'Grady JG, et al. Evidence that hepatitis D virus needs hepatitis B virus to cause hepatocellular damage. *Am J Clin Pathol* 1992; **98**: 554–558.

50 Aggarwal R, Krawczynski K, Hepatitis E. An overview and recent advances in clinical and laboratory research. *J Gastroenterol Hepatol* 2000; **15**: 9–20.

51 Hamid SS, Atiq M, Shehzad F, et al. Hepatitis E virus superinfection in patients with chronic liver disease. *Hepatology* 2002; **36**: 474–478.

52 Ramachandran J, Eapen CE, Kang G, et al. Hepatitis E superinfection produces severe decompensation in patients with chronic liver disease. *J Gastroenterol Hepatol* 2004; **19**: 134–138.
53 Dienes HP, Hütteroth T, Bianchi L, et al. Hepatitis A-like non-A, non-B hepatitis: light and electron microscopic observations of three cases. *Virchows Arch [A]* 1986; **409**: 657–667.
54 Mechnik L, Bergman N, Attali M, et al. Acute hepatitis E virus infection presenting as a prolonged cholestatic jaundice. *J Clin Gastroenterol* 2001; **33**: 421–422.
55 Asher LVS, Innis BL, Shrestha MP, et al. Virus-like particles in the liver of a patient with fulminant hepatitis and antibody to hepatitis E virus. *J Med Virol* 1990; **31**: 229–233.
56 Grando-Lemaire V, Guettier C, Chevret S, Beaugrand M, Trinchet JC. Hepatocellular carcinoma without cirrhosis in the West: epidemiological factors and histopathology of the non-tumorous liver. Groupe d'Etude et de Traitement du Carcinome Hepatocellulaire. *J Hepatol* 1999; **31**:508-513.

GENERAL READING

Aggarwal R, Krawczynski K, Hepatitis E. An overview and recent advances in clinical and laboratory research. *J Gastroenterol Hepatol* 2000; **15**: 9–20.
Jaeschke H, Gujral J, Bajt M. Apoptosis and necrosis in liver disease. *Liver Int* 2004; **24**: 85–89.
Lavanchy D. Hepatitis B virus epidemiology, disease burden, treatment and current and emerging prevention and control measures. *J Viral Hepat* 2004; **11**: 97–107.
Penin F, Dubuisson J, Rey FA, et al. Structural biology of hepatitis C virus. *Hepatology* 2004; **39**: 5–19.
Schmid R. History of viral hepatitis: a tale of dogmas and misinterpretations. *J Gastroenterol Hepatol* 2001; **16**: 718–722.

CHAPTER 7

STEATOSIS AND STEATOHEPATITIS

STEATOSIS

Steatosis (fatty change, fatty liver) is the accumulation of abnormal amounts of lipid in hepatocytes. Most steatosis is of the macrovesicular type, in which a single large fat vacuole or several smaller ones occupy the greater part of the cell, pushing the nucleus to the periphery (Fig. 7.1). The less common and often more serious type is microvesicular steatosis (Fig. 7.2). The fat in this type is finely divided and the nucleus remains central. The two types of steatosis are sometimes found together.

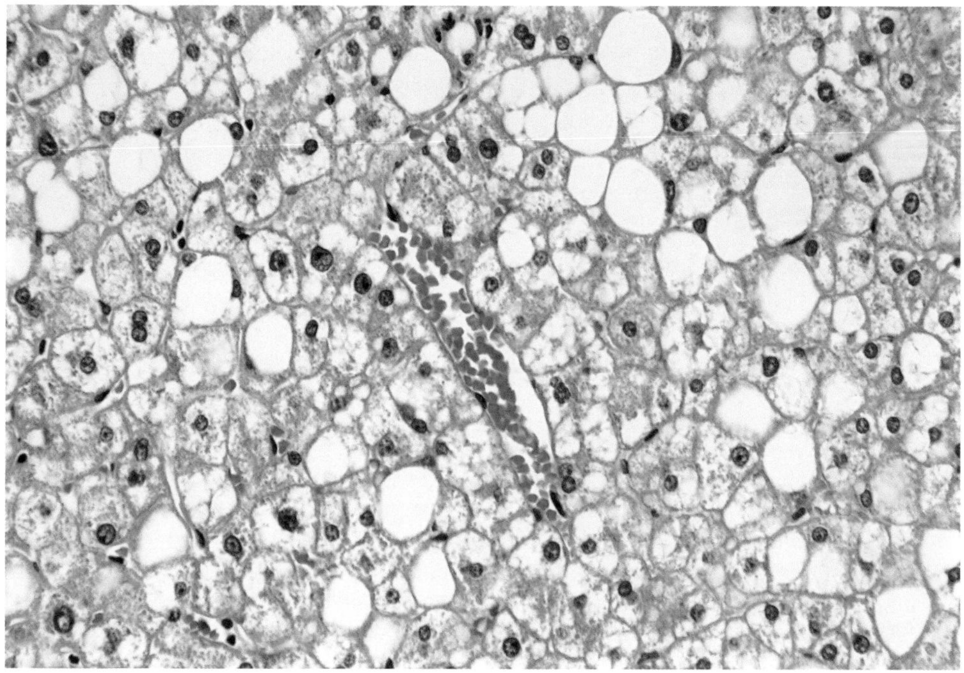

Figure 7.1 *Macrovesicular steatosis*. There are large fat vacuoles in perivenular hepatocytes, displacing the nuclei to the edges of the cells. (Needle biopsy, H&E).

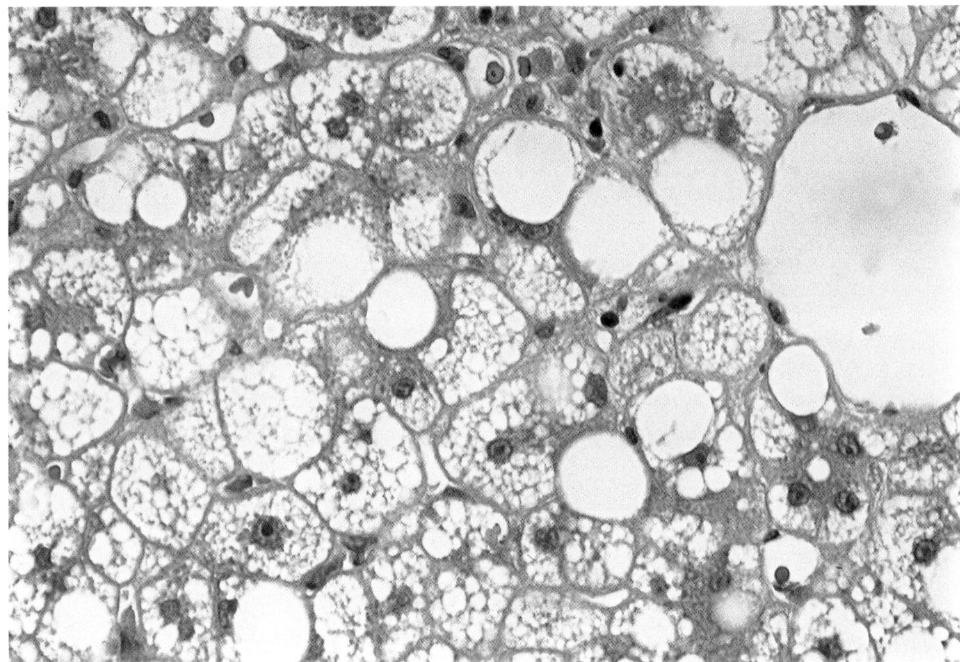

Figure 7.2 *Microvesicular steatosis.* Swollen hepatocytes near an efferent venule (right) contain numerous small vacuoles. The nuclei have maintained their central position. Some large fat vacuoles are also present. (Needle biopsy, H&E).

Table 7.1 Common causes of macrovesicular steatosis

Obesity and diabetes mellitus
Protein-calorie malnutrition
Total parenteral nutrition
Drugs and toxins (e.g. alcohol)
Metabolic disorders (e.g. Wilson's disease)
Infections (e.g. hepatitis C)

Macrovesicular steatosis

Macrovesicular steatosis is common. It is frequently apparent by non-invasive imaging and may be accompanied by moderate abnormalities of serum aminotransferases, alkaline phosphatase and gamma glutamyl transpeptidase. There are many causes, of which the most common are listed in Table 7.1. It is usually not possible to determine the cause of uncomplicated macrovesicular steatosis from histological examination alone. However, the location of the fat may give a clue; most steatosis is perivenular but periportal steatosis is sometimes seen in AIDS (Fig. 7.3), in patients on parenteral nutrition and in kwashiorkor. In patients with diabetes mellitus, glycogen vacuolation of hepatocyte nuclei is common[1] (Fig. 7.4). Hepatomegaly in diabetics is not always attributable to steatosis; rarely, diabetics who are poorly controlled may develop **Mauriac syndrome**, in which massive accumulation of glycogen in hepatocytes gives rise to a picture closely resembling inherited glycogen storage disease.[2]

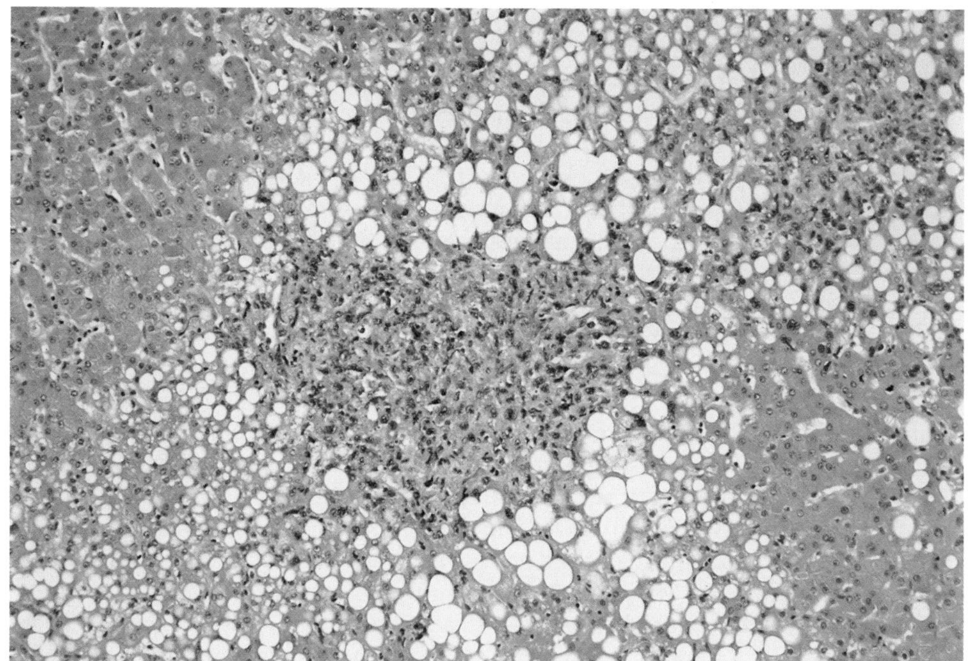

Figure 7.3 *Periportal steatosis.* Liver biopsy from a patient with AIDS and portal tract infiltration by large-cell lymphoma. Periportal hepatocytes contain large fat vacuoles. (Needle biopsy, H&E).

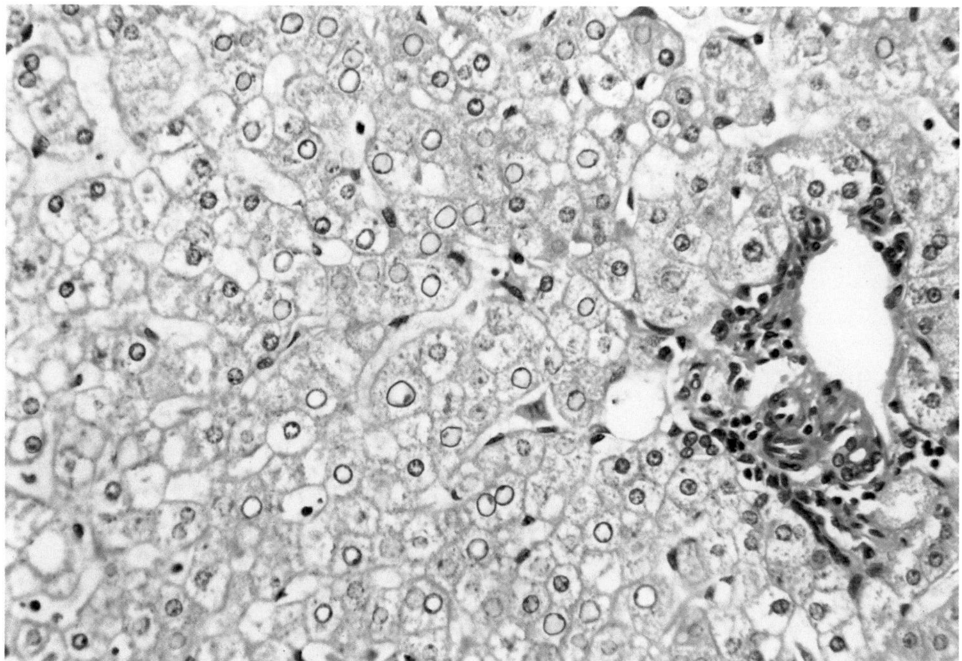

Figure 7.4 *Diabetes mellitus.* Glycogen vacuolation is seen in the nuclei of most periportal hepatocytes. (Needle biopsy, H&E).

In **focal fatty change**[3] more or less rounded foci of steatosis are seen in an otherwise normal liver and may be mistaken for neoplasms on imaging.

The lipid in macrovesicular steatosis accumulates in hepatocytes because of increased triglyceride synthesis or decreased excretion.[4] Increased synthesis results from availability of excess free fatty acids and fatty acid precursors and from reduced fatty acid oxidation. Reduced excretion is a result of diminished apoprotein production, seen for example in protein malnutrition and alcohol abuse.

Occasionally lipid-laden hepatocytes rupture and the fat is then taken up by macrophages. The resulting lesion is a **lipogranuloma** (Fig. 7.5). Lipogranulomas are situated within the lobules, often near terminal venules. Serial sectioning may be needed to identify the fat in the centre of the lesion. Lipogranulomas may undergo fibrosis, but this does not appear to contribute to progressive liver disease and must be distinguished from the more important pericellular fibrosis characteristic of steatohepatitis (see below). Globules within portal tracts are usually the result of uptake of ingested or injected mineral oils by macrophages, rather than uptake of lipids[5] (Fig. 7.6). Lipopeliosis, the formation of large fat cysts following release of lipid from hepatocytes after transplantation, is described in Chapter 16.

The differential diagnosis of macrovesicular steatosis includes microvesicular steatosis. The presence of several fat vacuoles in one hepatocyte has to be distinguished from true microvesicular steatosis (below) in which vacuoles are generally less than 1 μm in diameter and may even be invisible in paraffin sections by light microscopy. The distinction is clinically important. The location of the nucleus helps to differentiate the two conditions. A second differential diagnosis is from stellate cell hyperplasia (Fig. 7.7) in which the vacuoles are not in hepatocytes but in parasinusoidally-located stellate cells.[6] Their nuclei are compressed into a crescentic shape by the vitamin A-rich globules. Stellate cell hyperplasia may be

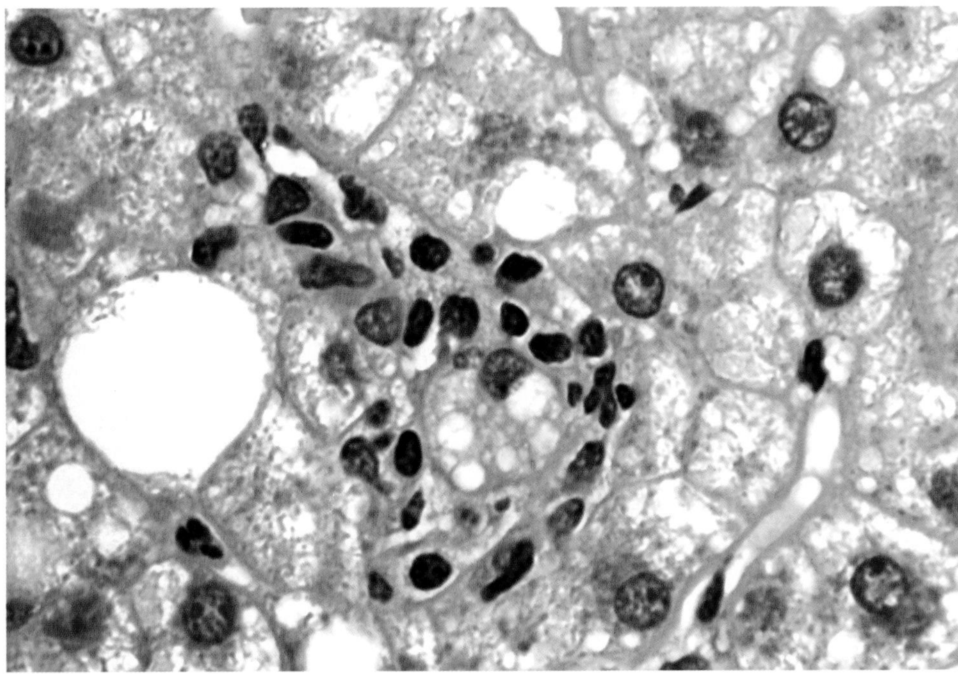

Figure 7.5 *Lipogranuloma.* A group of inflammatory cells surrounds a cluster of small fat vacuoles. (Needle biopsy, H&E).

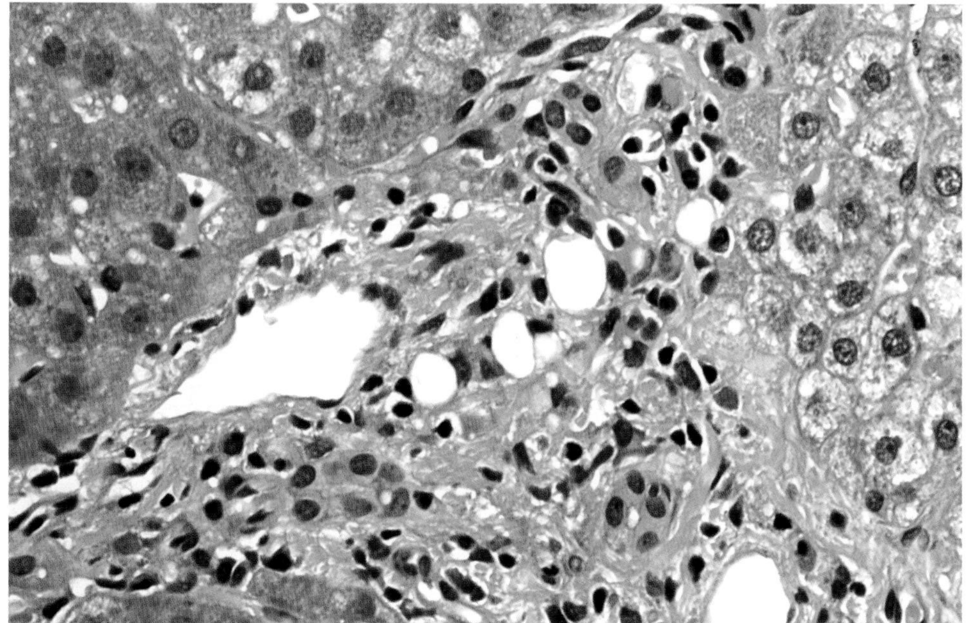

Figure 7.6 *Mineral oil globules*. A row of vacuoles within macrophages is seen to the right of a portal venule. (Needle biopsy, H&E).

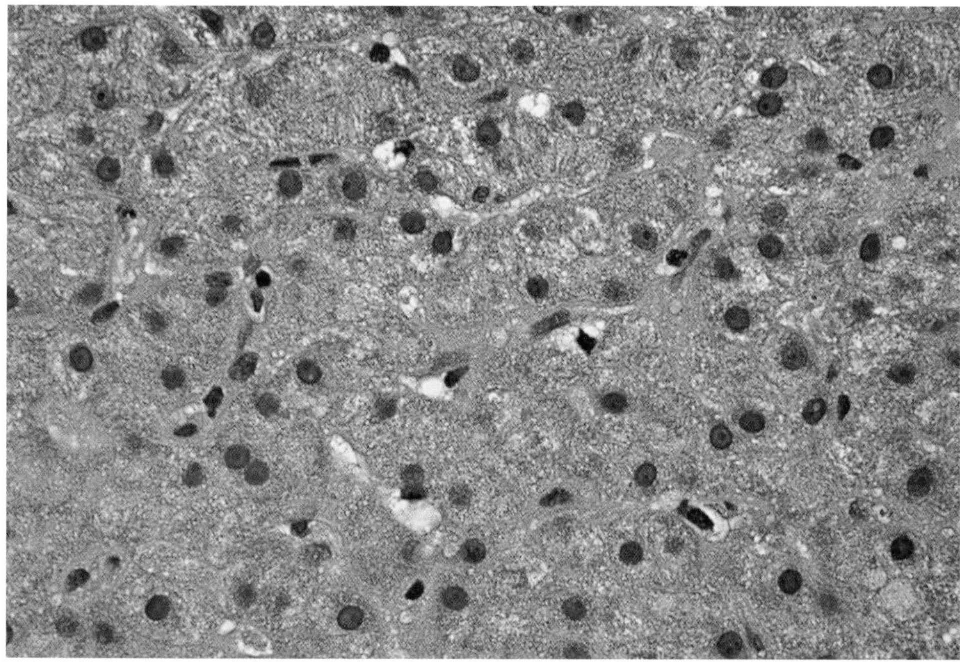

Figure 7.7 *Stellate cell hyperplasia*. Stellate cells with single or multiple lipid vacuoles lie in the space of Disse between hepatocytes. Stellate-cell nuclei are small, intensely basophilic and indented by the cytoplasmic vacuoles. Hepatocyte nuclei are larger, less dense and rounded. (Needle biopsy, H&E).

unexplained, but should lead to investigation of possible abuse of vitamin A or other retinoids.

While macrovesicular steatosis is not in itself a clinically serious lesion, it provides the background on which the important lesions of alcoholic and non-alcoholic steatohepatitis develop.[7] However, in a recent study of over 200 patients with simple steatosis without hepatitis, progression to cirrhosis, common in alcoholics, was very rare in obese non-drinkers.[8]

Microvesicular steatosis

In this serious and sometimes fatal condition, finely-divided fat accumulates in hepatocyte cytoplasm as a result of mitochondrial damage leading to impaired β-oxidation. Causes include acute fatty liver of pregnancy (Ch. 15), hepatotoxic drugs such as valproate and nucleoside analogues (Ch. 8), foamy degeneration in the alcoholic (see below) and total parenteral nutrition (Table 7.2). Another cause, Reye's syndrome, has declined sharply in incidence in recent years. Viral infections occasionally give rise to similar changes.[9]

Histologically, the cytoplasmic lipid is seen to be very finely divided and is not always obvious in paraffin sections. It can be stained with oil red O in frozen sections. The affected hepatocytes are often swollen. Their nuclei remain central (Fig. 7.2).

The differential diagnosis is from macrovesicular steatosis (above) and from conditions in which hepatocytes are swollen for other reasons, such as hepatitis. As discussed in Chapter 13, phospholipids and sphingolipids accumulate in various metabolic disorders. Cholesterol esters accumulate in hepatocytes in Wolman's disease and cholesterol ester storage disease, and glycogen accumulates in glycogen storage disease.

STEATOHEPATITIS, ALCOHOLIC (ASH) AND NON-ALCOHOLIC (NASH)

In some patients with steatosis an inflammatory and fibrosing lesion, steatohepatitis, develops. This may then lead to cirrhosis. Most patients with steatohepatitis are alcohol abusers, overweight or diabetic, or have a combination of these attributes.

Table 7.2 Main causes of microvesicular steatosis

Acute fatty liver of pregnancy
Alcoholic foamy degeneration
Drugs (e.g. nucleoside analogues, valproate)
Toxins (e.g. in Jamaican vomiting disease)
Total parenteral nutrition
Inborn errors of metabolism (e.g. urea cycle disorders)
Reye's syndrome
Infections

The terms **alcoholic steatohepatitis (ASH)** and **non-alcoholic steatohepatitis (NASH)** are used accordingly. In a minority of patients NASH is associated with other factors, listed later in this chapter. The terms **alcoholic fatty liver disease (AFLD)** and **non-alcoholic fatty liver disease (NAFLD)** are used to describe the complete range of changes from uncomplicated steatosis to steatohepatitis and cirrhosis.

Pathological features of steatohepatitis

The changes in ASH and NASH are very similar, and the two conditions cannot usually be distinguished on histological grounds alone.[10] The main pathological features comprise hepatocellular damage, inflammation and fibrosis (Table 7.3). The following description is of the fully developed lesion.

Hepatocellular damage is generally most severe in or even restricted to perivenular areas (Fig. 7.8). It takes the form of cell swelling and clearing of the cytoplasm, together with the appearance of Mallory bodies (Mallory's hyalin). The affected cells often do not contain obvious fat vacuoles, but these are visible in other parts of the parenchyma. The Mallory bodies consist of clumps and skeins of dense eosinophilic material, which sometimes forms a ring around the nucleus. When they are difficult to identify, positive immunostaining for p62 or ubiquitin is helpful (Fig. 7.9).[11,12] Hepatocytes may also contain megamitochondria, rounded or elongated eosinophilic bodies from 2 μm to 10 μm across (Fig. 7.10). These can be distinguished from Mallory bodies by their more definite outline and by red staining with Chromotrope aniline blue; Mallory bodies usually stain blue with the latter. Megamitochondria can be found in both ASH and NASH as well as in the livers of alcohol abusers in the absence of steatohepatitis.[13–15] Apoptotic hepatocytes are usually not a prominent feature in routine sections, but specific methods for apoptosis have shown it to be important in both ASH[16,17] and NASH.[18]

The inflammatory infiltrate is characteristically rich in neutrophils but lymphocytes are also present. These are mainly T cells of CD4 and CD8 phenotype, and are found both in areas of steatohepatitis and in portal tracts.[19] Neutrophils surround or even infiltrate ballooned, Mallory body-containing hepatocytes (Fig. 7.11). Macrophages and other sinusoidal cells take part in the process. Kupffer cells may contain fat vacuoles.[19] Both macrophages and sinusoidal endothelial cells

Table 7.3 Main pathological features of steatohepatitis

Main pathological features of steatohepatitis
Steatosis
Hepatocyte ballooning
Hepatocyte apoptosis
Mallory body formation
Inflammatory infiltration
Neutrophils
Lymphocytes
Sinusoidal cells
Fibrosis
Pericellular
Other

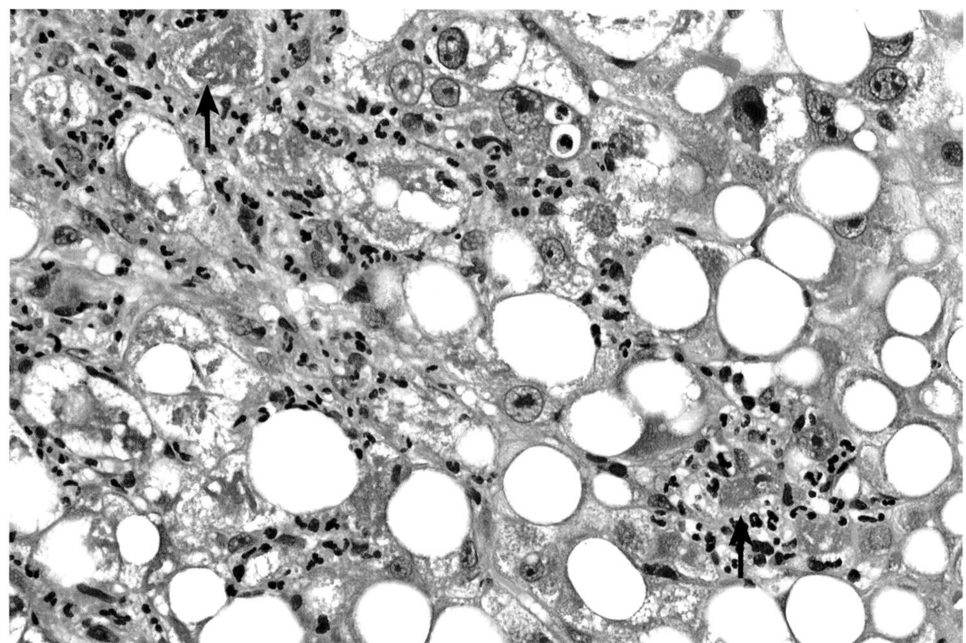

Figure 7.8 *Alcoholic steatohepatitis*. Inflammatory cells, mainly neutrophils, are clustered around and within hepatocytes, some of which contain densely-stained Mallory bodies (arrows). Many hepatocytes contain large fat vacuoles. (Needle biopsy, H&E).

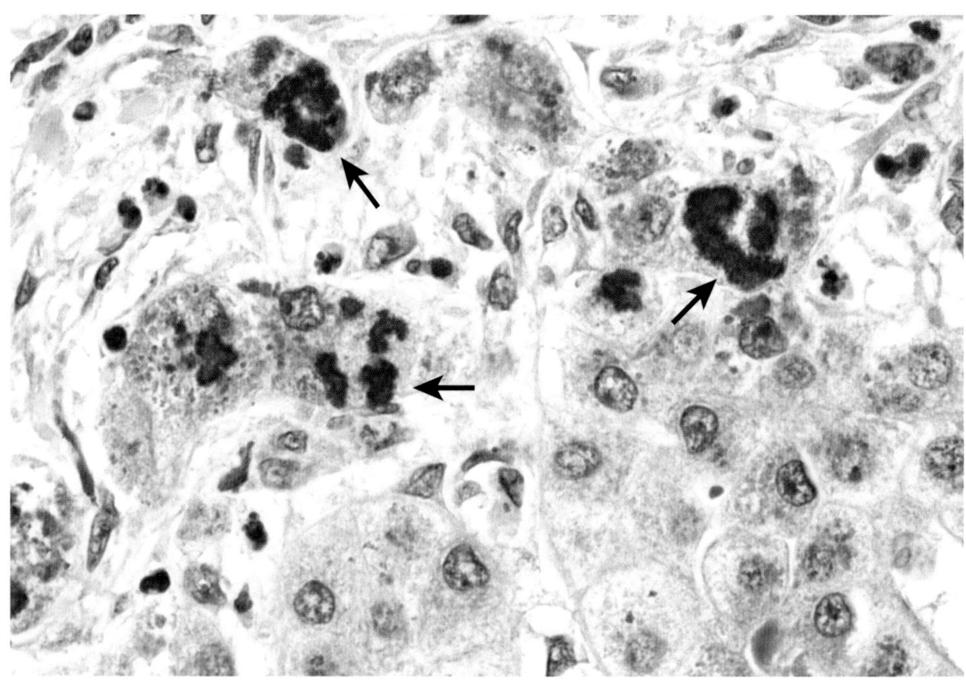

Figure 7.9 *Mallory bodies*. The Mallory bodies in this example of steatohepatitis stain strongly for ubiquitin (arrows). (Needle biopsy, specific immunostain for ubiquitin).

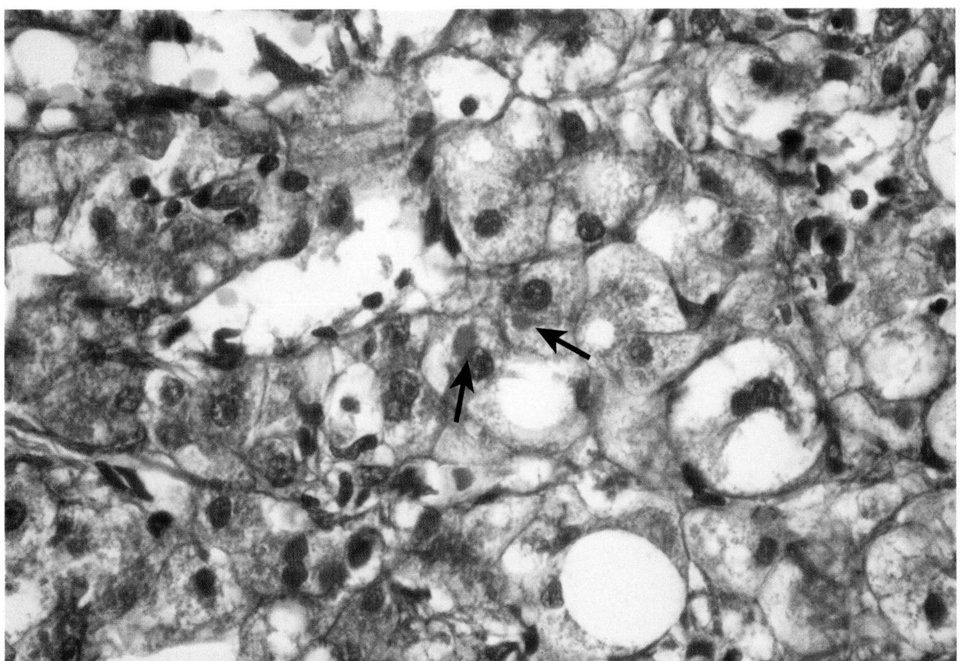

Figure 7.10 *Alcoholic steatohepatitis*. Two bright red giant mitochondria are marked with arrows. Collagen fibres, stained blue, are seen around ballooned hepatocytes. (Needle biopsy, CAB).

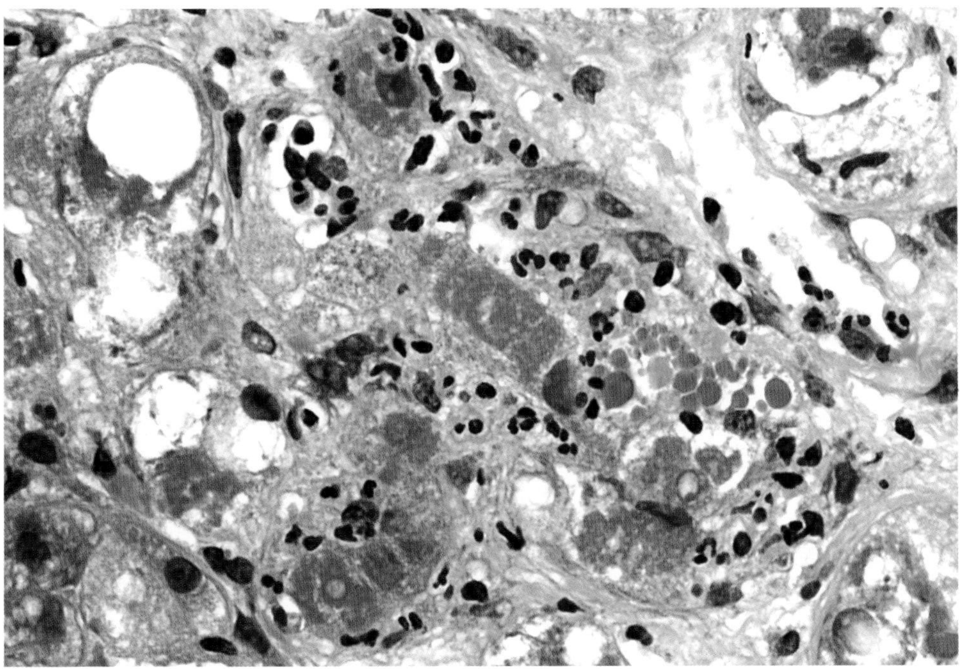

Figure 7.11 *Alcoholic steatohepatitis*. Hepatocytes contain abundant Mallory bodies and neutrophils. (Needle biopsy, H&E).

may contain stainable iron.[20] Large amounts of iron in hepatocytes are an indication for further investigation to exclude coexisting hereditary haemochromatosis.

Fibrosis is an integral part of the lesion of steatohepatitis. The most characteristic form of fibrosis is pericellular ('chicken-wire' fibrosis). Delicate or thicker strands of collagen surround ballooned hepatocytes to form a network well seen with trichrome stains (Fig. 7.12) and less easy to detect in reticulin preparations. The location corresponds to that of the cell damage and inflammation. In severe steatohepatitis, the fibrosis extends to the portal tracts as well as between perivenular areas, forming fibrous bridges (Fig. 7.13). Portal fibrosis is sometimes seen in the absence of the pericellular component.

These are the histological features of a classic, fully-developed steatohepatitis. Like all pathological processes, however, steatohepatitis is an evolving lesion, which also varies in severity. For these reasons liver biopsy may show less obvious changes, not readily recognised as part of the spectrum. Mallory bodies may be absent or not demonstrable in the biopsy sample. The inflammatory infiltrate may be predominantly lymphocytic, and pericellular fibrosis may be slight or undetectable. In a small minority of patients the only indication of a probable steatohepatitis is a finding of a few swollen, Mallory body-containing hepatocytes without associated inflammation. This should always be reported and regarded as a sign that the patient may be at risk of progressive disease, which is more important from the point of view of patient management than the definition of minimal diagnostic criteria. Another feature of probable significance is the finding of pericellular fibrosis without any of the other changes of steatohepatitis, possibly the result of past steatohepatitis. However, Latry and colleagues[21] reported an increase in stellate cells, collagen and basement membrane material in the space of Disse in diabetics, suggesting the possibility of fibrosis as a primary event.

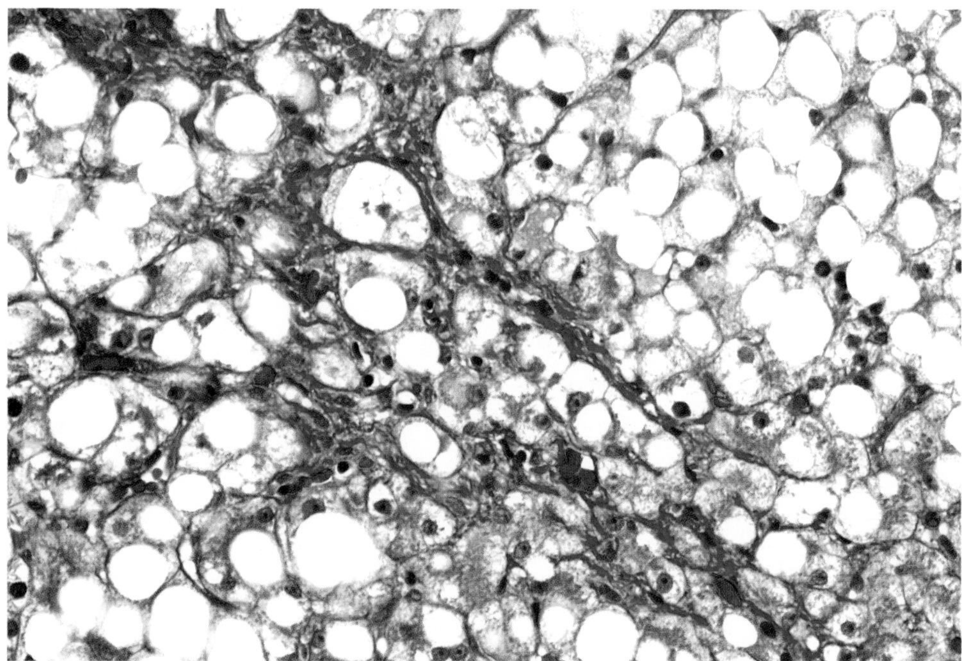

Figure 7.12 *Pericellular fibrosis.* Collagen fibres, stained blue, form a meshwork in this example of steatohepatitis. (Needle biopsy, CAB).

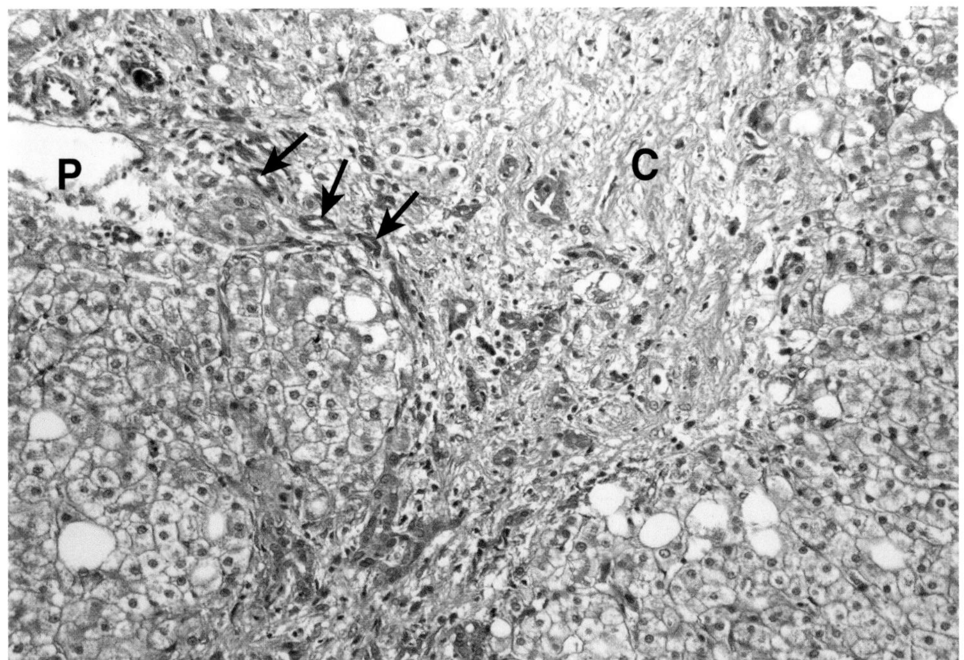

Figure 7.13 *Fibrosis in alcoholic steatohepatitis.* Abundant collagen (C) has been laid down in a perivenular area, linked to a portal tract (P) by a fibrous bridge with ductular reaction (arrows). (Needle biopsy, Martius scarlet blue).

Histological differential diagnosis

The histological differential diagnosis of steatohepatitis includes other forms of hepatitis. In viral and autoimmune hepatitis the infiltrating cells are lymphocytes and plasma cells rather than neutrophils. In acute viral hepatitis there is collapse of the reticulin framework but the 'chicken-wire' pattern of pericellular fibrosis is not seen. There may be steatosis in patients with chronic hepatitis C (Ch. 9), but the other features of steatohepatitis are absent. The fibrosis of venous outflow obstruction is usually linear and parasinusoidal rather than pericellular, but sometimes the hepatic fibrosis of long-standing cardiac disease can resemble that of steatohepatitis. The presence of congestion and absence of other features of steatohepatitis should make the diagnosis clear.

In chronic cholestasis with or without cirrhosis, hepatocytes near fibrous septa are typically ballooned and may contain Mallory bodies as well as bilirubin. Neutrophils are also seen. The correct diagnosis is made by attention to the location of the lesion and to clinical circumstances. Ballooning and Mallory bodies are also features of Wilson's disease; again, confusion with steatohepatitis is unlikely.

Because steatohepatitis is common in some populations, it is quite often found together with the changes of another liver disease in the same biopsy. Documented diseases coexisting with steatohepatitis include chronic hepatitis, primary biliary cirrhosis, iron storage disorders, drug-induced liver injury and metabolic disorders.[22] The pathologist should therefore consider whether all the changes seen in a biopsy can be explained by steatohepatitis alone.

OTHER ALCOHOL-RELATED LIVER LESIONS

The pathological features of **alcoholic steatohepatitis (ASH)** have been described above. A wide variety of other changes may be found in liver biopsies from drinkers (Table 7.4). In some alcohol abusers the liver is histologically **normal** or shows only mild macrovesicular steatosis. Portal tracts may contain lymphocytic infiltrates in the absence of other features of hepatitis.[23]

Steatosis

Steatosis in drinkers is usually most severe in perivenular areas. Foci of microvesicular steatosis may be present in addition. The cause of simple macrovesicular steatosis cannot be determined histologically and it is important that all causes of steatosis should be considered by pathologist and clinician.

Alcoholic foamy degeneration

Alcoholic foamy degeneration[24] is a relatively rare, potentially life-threatening condition characterised by extensive microvesicular steatosis in perivenular areas. Macrovesicular fat may be seen elsewhere. There may be cholestasis, fine fibrosis and scanty Mallory bodies, but inflammation is minimal or absent and the condition is thus distinct from ASH. Biochemical and histological features of cholestasis have been described.[25]

Table 7.4 Liver lesions in the alcoholic

- Steatosis
  - Macrovesicular
  - Microvesicular (foamy degeneration)
- Steatohepatitis
- Megamitochondria
- Siderosis
- Fibrosis
  - Pericellular
  - Perivenular
  - Portal
- Cirrhosis
- Hepatocellular carcinoma
- Effects of non-hepatic alcohol-related diseases

Fibrosis

Fibrosis is occasionally seen in drinkers in the absence of severe steatosis or steatohepatitis. When the fibrosis is **portal** (Fig. 7.14), the possibility of associated biliary disease, alcoholic pancreatitis or coexisting viral hepatitis should be considered. **Perivenular** fibrosis (Fig. 7.15) may be found with or without steatosis or steatohepatitis. The collagenous wall of one or more hepatic venules appears thickened, but this is difficult to interpret because of normal variation in the width of the wall. **Pericellular** fibrosis is an important component of steatohepatitis as already noted, and should always be looked for with the help of a collagen stain. When it is found in the absence of the other features of steatohepatitis it may represent the remnant of a previous episode of this lesion. As such, it is a warning that the patient may be at risk of progressive disease if the cause is not removed.

Siderosis

Siderosis is quite common in the livers of drinkers, but is usually mild and involves Kupffer cells as well as hepatocytes. Substantial amounts of iron in hepatocytes should always lead to investigation of possible hereditary haemochromatosis.

Fetal alcohol syndrome

In the fetal alcohol syndrome, children of mothers abusing alcohol during pregnancy have fatty livers together with perisinusoidal and portal fibrosis.[26]

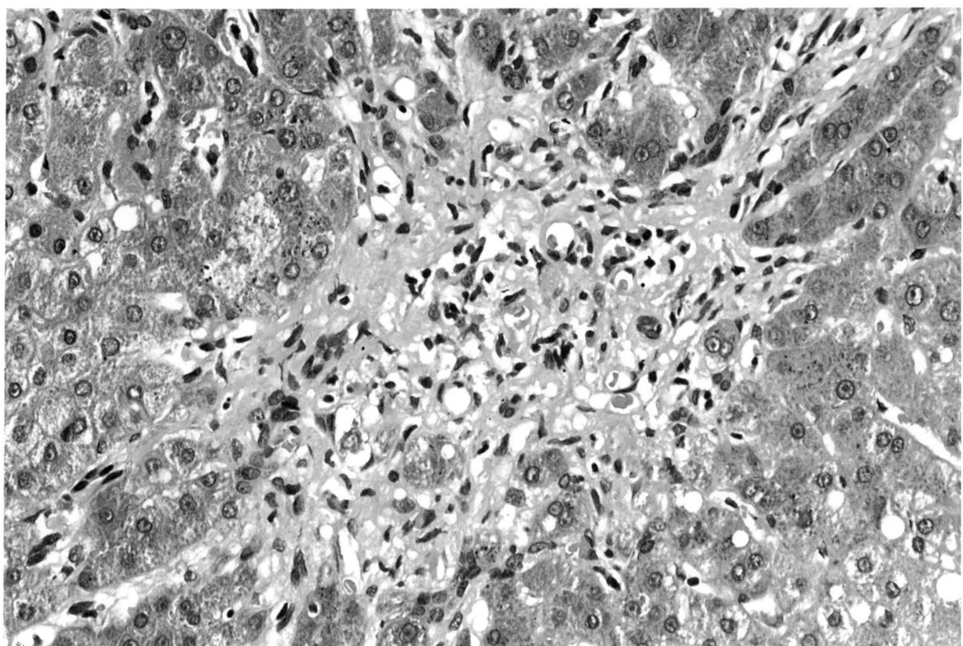

Figure 7.14 *Portal fibrosis in an alcoholic.* A small portal tract has undergone fibrosis to produce a stellate outline. (Needle biopsy, H&E).

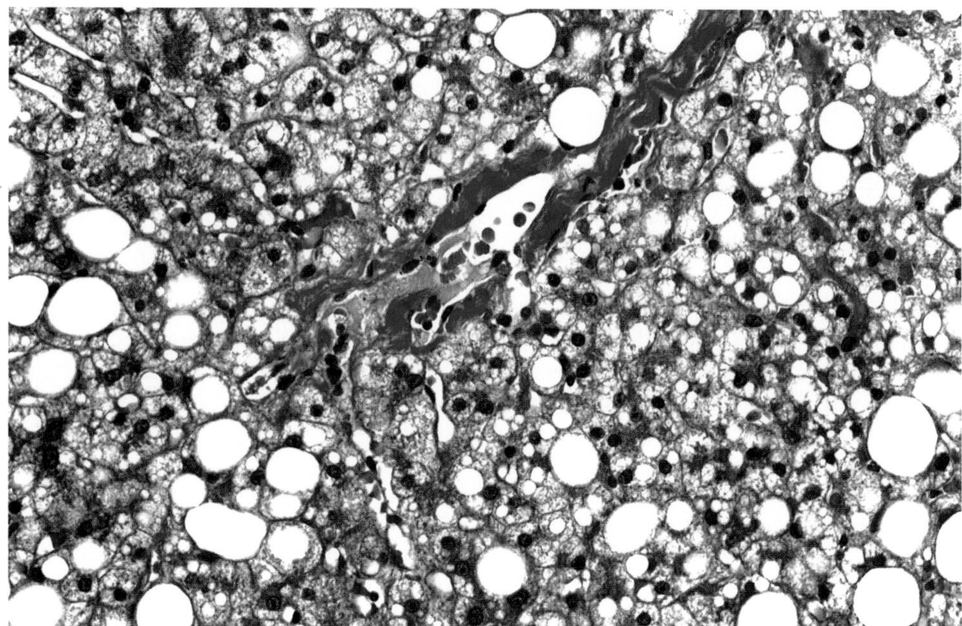

Figure 7.15 *Perivenular fibrosis in an alcoholic.* In this steatotic liver the wall of an efferent venule is irregularly thickened by collagen. Pericellular fibrosis is not evident. (Needle biopsy, CAB).

Cirrhosis

Cirrhosis in the alcoholic develops as a result of increasing fibrosis in steatohepatitis, together with nodular regeneration of the surviving parenchyma. There may also be other routes to cirrhosis, not involving steatohepatitis, but these are difficult to prove. Because steatohepatitis tends to involve all lobules, the cirrhosis is usually micronodular at first (see Figs 10.12, 10.13). As the regeneration nodules enlarge, the cirrhosis remodels to a macronodular pattern and the original cause of the cirrhosis becomes more difficult or even impossible to establish on histological grounds. Venous occlusion is common,[27,28] and may be missed unless stains for collagen or elastic tissue are examined. **Hepatocellular carcinoma** may develop within the cirrhotic liver.

Other Lesions

Alcohol-related lesions affecting organs other than the liver may cause liver changes. Chronic alcoholic pancreatitis has already been cited as a cause of portal fibrosis.[29] In patients with alcoholic cardiomyopathy the changes of right-sided heart failure may be found.

Finally, alcohol-related liver disease may coexist with other, non alcohol-related liver diseases. Alcohol consumption appears to accelerate the progression of fibrosis in hepatitis C.[30]

Non-alcoholic steatohepatitis (NASH) has assumed increasing importance in recent years, both because of the increased prevalence of obesity in Western populations and as a result of greater awareness of the condition. The diagnosis is now a major clinical consideration when liver function tests are abnormal but viral markers are negative. The main clinical associations are listed in Table 7.5. It is important to note that while obesity, diabetes and the metabolic syndrome are common associations with NASH, patients are not all obese,[32] and hyperlipidaemia and other disorders of lipid metabolism may need to be investigated. NASH can affect men, women and also children.[33] In the latter, a histological picture of steatosis, portal fibrosis with or without fibrous septa and a mainly lymphocytic infiltrate is sometimes found.

There is an extensive literature on the pathogenesis of NASH, some of it cited under 'General Reading' at the end of this chapter. The exact mechanisms have not been fully elucidated, but many of the important factors involved have been defined. These include insulin resistance,[34,35] excess of free fatty acids in hepatocytes, lipid peroxidation[36] and oxidative stress.[37] Venous obstruction may be important in the progression to cirrhosis.[38] An element of genetic predisposition is likely[39,40] and NASH has been reported in kindreds.[41] Some of the above factors, such as excess of free fatty acids and oxidative stress, are common to NASH and ASH and help to explain their similarity.

The histological lesion of NASH (Fig. 7.16) is as described above under steatohepatitis, but it is rarely very severe compared with ASH. The presence of abundant neutrophils and Mallory bodies should therefore lead to a suspicion of alcohol abuse. Glycogen vacuolation of nuclei is common in NASH.[10] Occasionally the lobular changes appear to be periportal rather than perivenular[42] but this may reflect the difficulty of accurate localisation in two-dimensional sections. The pericellular fibrosis of NASH is very like that of ASH and is illustrated in Figure 8.8. It is associated with hepatocellular injury, as shown by ballooning degeneration and Mallory body formation.[43] In some patients fibrosis is confined to the portal areas.[44] A bile ductular reaction may be present.

Progression of the lesion to cirrhosis is variable but often slow.[45] Like other forms of cirrhosis it carries the risk of liver failure and hepatocellular carcinoma.[46,47] Clinical features associated with NASH are also common in patients with cryptogenic cirrhosis, suggesting that the latter is frequently the end result of NASH.[48–51]

A scoring system for NASH has been devised, allowing semi-quantitative assessment and reporting of liver biopsy changes.[52,53] Separate scores are allotted for the severity of the hepatocyte damage and inflammation on the one hand, and for

Table 7.5 Main causes and associations of NASH

Obesity
Diabetes mellitus
Metabolic syndrome
Hyperlipidaemia
Gastrointestinal surgery for obesity
Drugs and chemicals (e.g. amiodarone, tamoxifen, petrochemicals[31])

fibrosis and cirrhosis on the other (Table 7.6). The system has recently been further refined as a research tool.[54] As in the case of scoring in chronic viral hepatitis (Ch. 9), the resulting numbers must be regarded as categories rather than measurements.

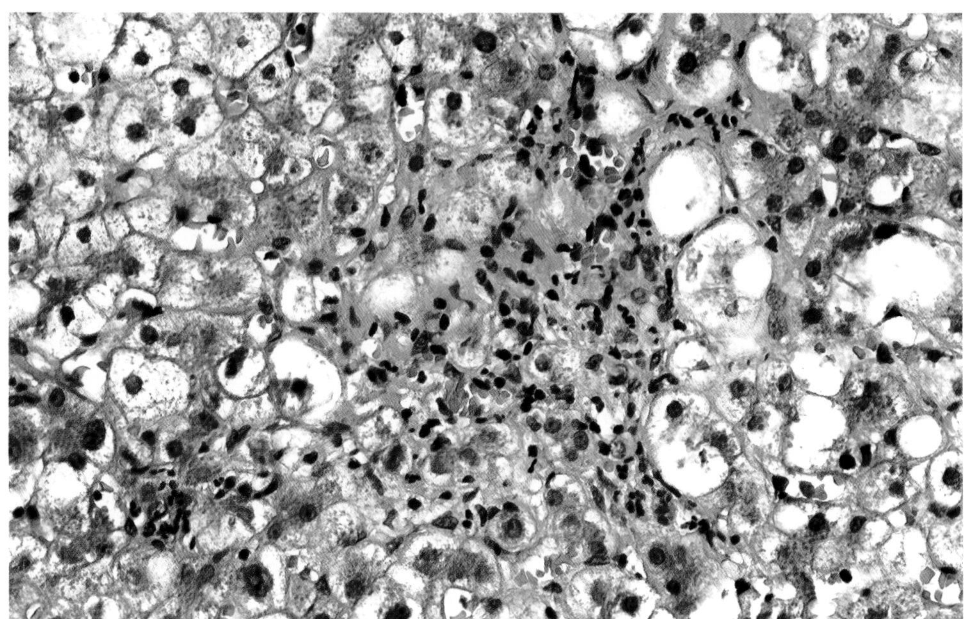

Figure 7.16 *Non-alcoholic steatohepatitis.* There is steatosis, hepatocellular ballooning and infiltration by neutrophils, as in the alcoholic counterpart. (Needle biopsy, H&E).

Table 7.6 A scoring system for steatohepatitis

Necroinflammatory grading	
Grade 1 (mild)	Steatosis (mainly macrovesicular) involving up to 66% of lobules; occasional ballooned perivenular hepatocytes; scattered neutrophils with or without lymphocytes; no or mild chronic portal inflammation
Grade 2 (moderate)	Steatosis of any degree; obvious ballooning (mainly perivenular); intralobular neutrophils, may be associated with perivenular pericellular fibrosis if evident; mild to moderate portal and intralobular chronic inflammation
Grade 3 (severe)	Panlobular steatosis; obvious perivenular ballooning and disarray; marked lobular inflammation; neutrophils may be concentrated in perivenular areas of ballooning and in areas of pericellular fibrosis if evident. Portal inflammation mild or moderate
Fibrosis staging	
Stage 1	Pericellular fibrosis in perivenular areas, focal or extensive
Stage 2	As above, plus focal or extensive periportal fibrosis
Stage 3	Bridging fibrosis, focal or extensive
Stage 4	Cirrhosis

Adapted from Brunt[52,53] with permission from Blackwell Publishing and Elsevier Ltd.

REFERENCES

1 Abraham S, Furth EE. Receiver operating characteristic analysis of glycogenated nuclei in liver biopsy specimens: quantitative evaluation of their relationship with diabetes and obesity. *Hum Pathol* 1994; **25**: 1063–1068.
2 Chatila R, West AB. Hepatomegaly and abnormal liver tests due to glycogenosis in adults with diabetes. *Medicine (Baltimore)* 1996; **75**: 327–333.
3 Wanless IR. Benign liver tumors. *Clin Liver Dis* 2002; **6**: 513–526.
4 Burt AD, Mutton A, Day CP. Diagnosis and interpretation of steatosis and steatohepatitis. *Sem Diagn Pathol* 1998; **15**: 246–258.
5 Wanless IR, Geddie WR. Mineral oil lipogranulomata in liver and spleen. A study of 465 autopsies. *Arch Pathol Lab Med* 1985; **109**: 283–286.
6 Levine PH, Delgado Y, Theise ND, et al. Stellate-cell lipidosis in liver biopsy specimens. Recognition and significance. *Am J Clin Pathol* 2003; **119**: 254–258.
7 Day CP, James OFW. Steatohepatitis: a tale of two 'hits'? *Gastroenterology* 1998; **114**: 842–845.
8 Dam-Larsen S, Franzmann M, Andersen IB, et al. Long term prognosis of fatty liver: risk of chronic liver disease and death. *Gut* 2004; **53**: 750–755.
9 Aita K, Jin Y, Irie H, et al. Are there histopathologic characteristics particular to fulminant hepatic failure caused by human herpesvirus-6 infection? A case report and discussion. *Hum Pathol* 2001; **32**: 887–889.
10 Itoh S, Yougel T, Kawagoe K. Comparison between nonalcoholic steatohepatitis and alcoholic hepatitis. *Am J Gastroenterol* 1987; **82**: 650–654.
11 Banner BF, Savas L, Zivny J, et al. Ubiquitin as a marker of cell injury in nonalcoholic steatohepatitis. *Am J Clin Pathol* 2000; **114**: 860–866.
12 Denk H, Stumptner C, Zatloukal K. Mallory bodies revisited. *J Hepatol* 2000; **32**: 689–702.
13 Caldwell SH, Swerdlow RH, Khan EM, et al. Mitochondrial abnormalities in non-alcoholic steatohepatitis. *J Hepatol* 1999; **31**: 430–434.
14 Sanyal AJ, Campbell-Sargent C, Mirshahi F, et al. Nonalcoholic steatohepatitis: association of insulin resistance and mitochondrial abnormalities. *Gastroenterology* 2001; **120**: 1183–1192.
15 Le TH, Caldwell SH, Redick JA, et al. The zonal distribution of megamitochondria with crystalline inclusions in nonalcoholic steatohepatitis. *Hepatology* 2004; **39**: 1423–1429.
16 Natori S, Rust C, Stadheim LM, et al. Hepatocyte apoptosis is a pathologic feature of human alcoholic hepatitis. *J Hepatol* 2001; **34**: 248–253.
17 Ziol M, Tepper M, Lohez M, et al. Clinical and biological relevance of hepatocyte apoptosis in alcoholic hepatitis. *J Hepatol* 2001; **34**: 254–260.
18 Feldstein AE, Canbay A, Angulo P, et al. Hepatocyte apoptosis and fas expression are prominent features of human nonalcoholic steatohepatitis. *Gastroenterology* 2003; **125**: 437–443.
19 Lefkowitch JH, Haythe JH, Regent N. Kupffer cell aggregation and perivenular distribution in steatohepatitis. *Mod Pathol* 2002; **15**: 699–704.
20 Turlin B, Mendler MH, Moirand R, et al. Histologic features of the liver in insulin resistance-associated iron overload. A study of 139 patients. *Am J Clin Pathol* 2001; **116**: 263–270.
21 Latry P, Bioulac-Sage P, Echinard E, et al. Perisinusoidal fibrosis and basement membrane-like material in the livers of diabetic patients. *Hum Pathol* 1987; **18**: 775–780.
22 Brunt EM, Ramrakhiani S, Cordes BG, et al. Concurrence of histologic features of steatohepatitis with other forms of chronic liver disease. *Mod Pathol* 2003; **16**: 49–56.
23 Colombat M, Charlotte F, Ratziu V, et al. Portal lymphocytic infiltrate in alcoholic liver disease. *Hum Pathol* 2002; **33**: 1170–1174.
24 Uchida T, Kao H, Quispe-Sjogren M, et al. Alcoholic foamy degeneration – a pattern of acute alcoholic injury of the liver. *Gastroenterology* 1983; **84**: 683–692.
25 Suri S, Mitros FA, Ahluwalia JP. Alcoholic foamy degeneration and a markedly elevated GGT: a case report and literature review. *Dig Dis Sci* 2003; **48**: 1142–1146.

26 Lefkowitch JH, Rushton AR, Feng-Chen KC. Hepatic fibrosis in fetal alcohol syndrome. Pathologic similarities to adult alcoholic liver disease. *Gastroenterology* 1983; **85**: 951–957.
27 Goodman ZD, Ishak KG. Occlusive venous lesions in alcoholic liver disease. A study of 200 cases. *Gastroenterology* 1982; **83**: 786–796.
28 Burt AD, MacSween RN. Hepatic vein lesions in alcoholic liver disease: retrospective biopsy and necropsy study. *J Clin Pathol* 1986; **39**: 63–67.
29 Morgan MY, Sherlock S, Scheuer PJ. Portal fibrosis in the livers of alcoholic patients. *Gut* 1978; **19**: 1015–1021.
30 Poynard T, Ratziu V, Benhamou Y, et al. Natural history of HCV infection. *Best Pr Res Clin Gastroenterol* 2000; **14**: 211–228.
31 Cotrim HP, De Freitas LAR, Freitas C, et al. Clinical and histopathological features of NASH in workers exposed to chemicals with or without associated metabolic conditions. *Liver Int* 2004; **24**: 131–135.
32 Bacon BR, Farahvash MJ, Janney CG, et al. Nonalcoholic steatohepatitis: an expanded clinical entity. *Gastroenterology* 1994; **107**: 1103–1109.
33 Rashid M, Roberts EA. Nonalcoholic steatohepatitis in children. *J Pediatr Gastroenterol Nutr* 2000; **30**: 48–53.
34 Dixon JB, Bhathal PS, O'Brien PE. Nonalcoholic fatty liver disease: predictors of nonalcoholic steatohepatitis and liver fibrosis in the severely obese. *Gastroenterology* 2001; **121**: 91–100.
35 Day CP. Pathogenesis of steatohepatitis. *Best Pr Res Clin Gastroenterol* 2002; **16**: 663–678.
36 Macdonald GA, Bridle KR, Ward PJ, et al. Lipid peroxidation in hepatic steatosis in humans is associated with hepatic fibrosis and occurs predominately in acinar zone 3. *J Gastroenterol Hepatol* 2001; **16**: 599–606.
37 Seki S, Kitada T, Yamada T, et al. In situ detection of lipid peroxidation and oxidative DNA damage in non-alcoholic fatty liver diseases. *J Hepatol* 2002; **37**: 56–62.
38 Wanless IR, Shiota K. The pathogenesis of nonalcoholic steatohepatitis and other fatty liver diseases: a four-step model including the role of lipid release and hepatic venular obstruction in the progression to cirrhosis. *Semin Liver Dis* 2004; **24**: 99–106.
39 Valenti L, Fracanzani AL, Dongiovanni P, et al. Tumor necrosis factor alpha promoter polymorphisms and insulin resistance in nonalcoholic fatty liver disease. *Gastroenterology* 2002; **122**: 274–280.
40 Namikawa C, Shu-Ping Z, Vyselaar JR, et al. Polymorphisms of microsomal triglyceride transfer protein gene and manganese superoxide dismutase gene in non-alcoholic steatohepatitis. *J Hepatol* 2004; **40**: 781–786.
41 Struben VM, Hespenheide EE, Caldwell SH. Nonalcoholic steatohepatitis and cryptogenic cirrhosis within kindreds. *Am J Med* 2000; **108**: 9–13.
42 Nagore N, Scheuer PJ. The pathology of diabetic hepatitis. *J Pathol* 1988; **156**: 155–160.
43 Gramlich T, Kleiner DE, McCullough AJ, et al. Pathologic features associated with fibrosis in nonalcoholic fatty liver disease. *Hum Pathol* 2004; **35**: 196–199.
44 Abrams GA, Kunde SS, Lazenby AJ, et al. Portal fibrosis and hepatic steatosis in morbidly obese subjects: A spectrum of nonalcoholic fatty liver disease. *Hepatology* 2004; **40**: 475–483.
45 Fassio E, Álvarez E, Dominguez N, Landeira G, Longo C. Natural history of nonalcoholic steatohepatitis: a longitudinal study of repeat liver biopsies. *Hepatology* 2004; **40**: 820–826.
46 Shimada M, Hashimoto E, Taniai M, et al. Hepatocellular carcinoma in patients with non-alcoholic steatohepatitis. *J Hepatol* 2002; **37**: 154–160.
47 Hui JM, Kench JG, Chitturi S, et al. Long-term outcomes of cirrhosis in nonalcoholic steatohepatitis compared with hepatitis C. *Hepatology* 2003; **38**: 420–427.
48 Caldwell SH, Oelsner DH, Iezzoni JC, et al. Cryptogenic cirrhosis: clinical characterization and risk factors for underlying disease. *Hepatology* 1999; **29**: 664–669.
49 Poonawala A, Nair SP, Thuluvath PJ. Prevalence of obesity and diabetes in patients with cryptogenic cirrhosis: a case–control study. *Hepatology* 2000; **32**: 689–692.
50 Bugianesi E, Leone N, Vanni E, et al. Expanding the natural history of

nonalcoholic steatohepatitis: from cryptogenic cirrhosis to hepatocellular carcinoma. *Gastroenterology* 2002; **123**: 134–140.

51 Clark JM, Diehl AM. Nonalcoholic fatty liver disease: an underrecognized cause of cryptogenic cirrhosis. *JAMA* 2003; **289**: 3000–3004.

52 Brunt EM, Janney CG, Di Bisceglie AM, et al. Nonalcoholic steatohepatitis: a proposal for grading and staging the histological lesions. *Am J Gastroenterol* 1999; **94**: 2467–2474.

53 Brunt EM, Tiniakos DG. Pathology of steatohepatitis. *Best Pr Res Clin Gastroenterol* 2002; **16**: 691–707.

54 Brunt EM, Neuschwander-Tetri BA, Oliver D, et al. Nonalcoholic steatohepatitis: Histologic features and clinical correlations with 30 blinded biopsy specimens. *Hum Pathol* 2004; **35**: 1070–1082.

GENERAL READING

Adams LA, Sanderson S, Lind KD, Angulo P. The histological course of nonalcoholic fatty liver disease: a longitudinal study of 103 patients with sequential liver biopsies. *J Hepatol* 2005; 42:132–138.

Arteel G, Marsano L, Mendez C, et al. Advances in alcoholic liver disease. *Best Pr Res Clin Gastroenterol* 2003; **17**: 625–647.

Browning JD, Horton JD. Molecular mediators of hepatic steatosis and liver injury. *J Clin Invest* 2004; **114**: 147–152.

Brunt EM. Nonalcoholic steatohepatitis. *Semin Liver Dis* 2004; **24**: 3–20.

Denk H, Stumptner C, Zatloukal K. Mallory bodies revisited. *J Hepatol* 2000; **32**: 689–702.

Farrell GC, George J, Hall P de la M, McCullough AJ, eds. Fatty Liver Disease: NASH and Related Disorders. Oxford: Blackwell Publishing, 2005.

Mofrad P, Contos MJ, Haque M, et al. Clinical and histologic spectrum of nonalcoholic fatty liver disease associated with normal ALT values. *Hepatology* 2003; **37**: 1286–1292.

Reuben A. Pearls of pathology. *Hepatology* 2003; **37**: 715–718.

Zafrani ES. Non-alcoholic fatty liver disease: an emerging pathological spectrum. *Virchows Arch* 2004; **444**: 3–12.

CHAPTER

8 DRUGS AND TOXINS

INTRODUCTION

This chapter deals with the pathology of the important liver lesions attributed to drugs and toxins, with their recognition and with their differential diagnosis. There are many hundreds of hepatotoxic drugs and other chemicals and new reports of adverse drug reactions appear regularly in the literature. Details of the lesions attributed to each of the many individual drugs are not considered appropriate for a bench book of this kind. If required, the information can be found in one of several comprehensive reviews.[1–4] There is also a regularly updated bibliography in the French literature.[5] The pathologist reporting a liver biopsy should, however, bear in mind that a drug cannot be exonerated simply because an adverse reaction has not been reported; there is always a first time.

Chemical injury is not confined to drugs listed in pharmacopoeias. Herbal medicines,[6] illicit drugs,[7–15] criminally administered poisons,[16] industrial chemicals,[17–20] vitamins[21,22] and foods[23,24] have all been held responsible for liver disease. Drugs used for the treatment of liver disease have themselves been suspected of causing liver damage.[25]

In his foreword to the second edition of Stricker's Drug-induced Hepatic Injury,[1] Zimmerman writes: '... virtually all known acute and chronic hepatic lesions can result from drug injury'. This important observation implies that drugs should be considered as a possible cause of any liver lesion found on biopsy, but some lesions are more often produced by drugs than others. Hepatocellular necrosis, hepatitis and cholestasis in particular should arouse a greater degree of suspicion, especially if no other cause has been found. Also, some groups of drugs are associated with particular kinds of injury; non-steroidal anti-inflammatory drugs (NSAIDs), for example, are often associated with hepatocellular injury, while neuroleptic drugs mostly cause cholestasis. However, these are generalisations and a drug which causes a dose-related hepatocellular necrosis in one patient may cause non-dose related hepatitis, cholestasis or granulomas in another.[26,27]

The diagnostic pathologist should be aware of the potential of drugs and other substances to cause this wide variety of acute and chronic liver lesions and to know which lesions are most likely to be drug-induced. He or she should be familiar with their likely course and outcome and the main points of similarity and difference from other, non drug-related liver diseases. Finally, the pathologist should know where to look up the effects of individual drugs.

CLASSIFICATION AND MECHANISMS

Drugs may be regarded as producing liver injury in two main ways (Table 8.1). **Intrinsic (predictable) hepatotoxins** are those which predictably produce liver damage when taken in sufficient quantities. The type of damage is often characteristic of a particular drug; for example, the typical result of paracetamol (acetaminophen) overdose is hepatocellular necrosis and steatosis. Intrinsic hepatotoxicity can often be studied in laboratory animals. This type of hepatotoxicity is also frequently **zonal** in distribution; examples of this are the perivenular lesions of paracetamol and carbon tetrachloride and the periportal necrosis seen in phosphorus toxicity. The mechanism of intrinsic hepatotoxicity can be **direct** or **indirect**; in the former, the chemical or its metabolites causes structural damage to cells and organelles, while in indirect intrinsic hepatotoxicity the chemical interferes with a specific metabolic pathway or cell component.

The commoner kind of drug-related liver damage is **idiosyncratic (unpredictable)**. Only a small proportion of patients on a particular drug is affected, so that the adverse reaction is not detected in initial human trials. Many different mechanisms for idiosyncratic hepatotoxicity have now been elucidated. They include individual genetic variation in the metabolism of drugs and the development of immune reactions to a drug or its metabolites.[28] The immune reactions may be directed to neoantigens produced by the binding of reactive metabolites to hepatic drug metabolising enzymes of the P450 system.[29,30] In some instances, the distinction between an idiosyncratic and intrinsic drug reaction is difficult to make. Typical idiosyncratic damage may follow a small dose of the offending drug and cannot easily be studied in the laboratory. With the exception of a few drugs shown to cause liver damage in patients using a particular metabolic pathway, idiosyncratic drug injury is unpredictable in the sense that the susceptibility of individual patients cannot be tested before the drug is given.

Most intrinsic hepatotoxins produce liver damage within a few hours or days, whereas in the idiosyncratic type of injury, there is often a latent period of many days, weeks or months[31] before liver disease becomes apparent. The latent period tends to shorten with repeated administration of the drug. Because of the latent period and the tendency for idiosyncratic injury to mimic non-drug-related liver

Table 8.1 Examples of liver lesions due to drugs and toxins

Lesion	Example of substance
Intrinsic hepatotoxicity	
Microvesicular steatosis	Valproate
Phospholipidosis	Amiodarone
Hepatocellular necrosis	Paracetamol (acetaminophen)
Fibrosis	Vitamin A
Cholestasis	Contraceptive steroids
Venous occlusion	Pyrrolizidine alkaloids
Angiosarcoma	Vinyl chloride
Idiosyncratic hepatotoxicity	
Hepatitis	Isoniazid
Cholestasis	Amoxicillin-clavulanic acid
Granuloma formation	Allopurinol

diseases, clinician and pathologist need to be alert to the possibility of idiosyncratic drug injury if diagnostic errors are to be avoided. The clinician may be helped by a clinical scale or scoring system,[32] and the pathologist by a suspicious or characteristic pattern of injury. Conclusive proof that a particular drug or combination of drugs is responsible is often impossible to obtain, although re-challenge (usually inadvertent) can provide strong circumstantial evidence. Liver injury may follow inadvertent re-challenge many years after a first episode.[33] Biochemical evidence of improvement after drug withdrawal is occasionally supported by a return to normal histology.[31]

MORPHOLOGICAL CATEGORIES

The categories described below represent the main changes attributed to drugs and toxins, apart from alcohol-related liver damage (Ch. 7), neoplasms (Ch. 11) and vascular lesions (Ch. 12). A mixture of lesions may be found in the same liver; amiodarone, for example, produces both phospholipidosis and steatohepatitis, but by different mechanisms.[34] As already indicated, a single drug may give rise to different forms of hepatotoxicity in different patients. Phenylbutazone, for example, can cause necrosis, cholestasis, granuloma formation or combinations of these[35] while the non-steroidal anti-inflammatory drugs nimesulfide and diclofenac can cause either severe hepatitis or cholestasis.[36,37]

Adaptation

Not all changes seen under the microscope necessarily represent liver damage. The increase in endoplasmic reticulum produced by long-term treatment with anti-convulsant drugs is commonly regarded as an adaptive phenomenon.[38,39] By light microscopy, this increase is seen as an abundance of pale-staining cytoplasm in hepatocytes (Fig. 8.1), difficult to distinguish from simple abundance of glycogen on an H&E stained section.

Non-hepatitic liver-cell damage

One of the most common manifestations of intrinsic hepatotoxicity is **steatosis**. As discussed in Chapter 7, this may be macrovesicular or microvesicular. Macrovesicular steatosis, in which the nucleus of the hepatocyte is displaced by one or more fat vacuoles easily visible by light microscopy, is produced for example by chlorinated hydrocarbons and methotrexate. It is common in patients on total parenteral nutrition,[40,41] although underlying disease may also contribute to the liver changes.[42] In patients treated with gold compounds for rheumatoid arthritis, intralobular lipogranulomas, focal accumulations of lipid-containing macrophages, have been found to contain gold pigment in the form of fine black or brown granules. These were also seen within portal lipid droplets.[43]

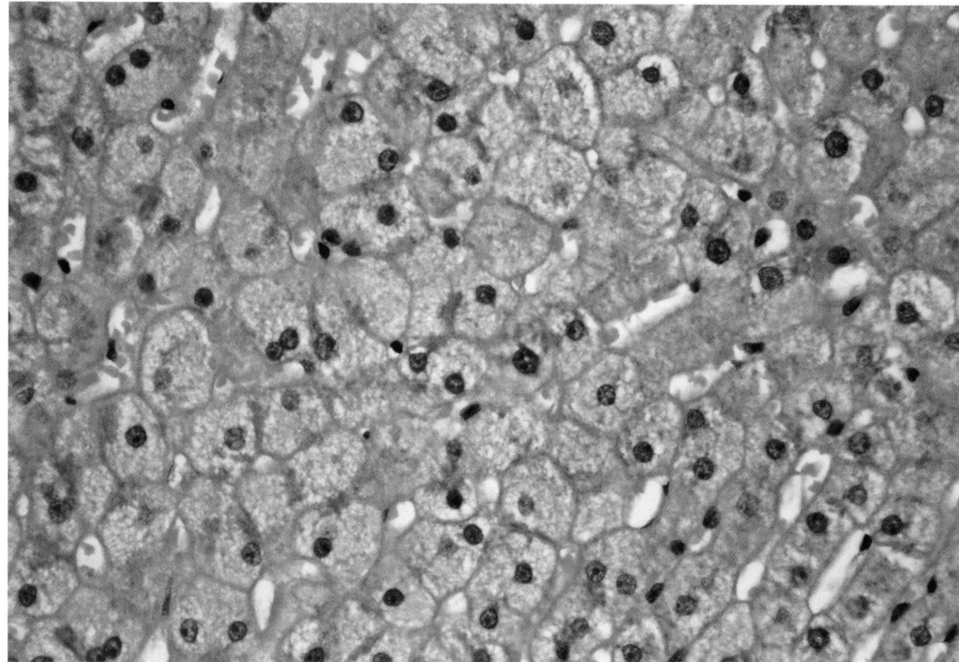

Figure 8.1 *Adaptation.* Hepatocytes in this biopsy from a patient on anti-epileptic drugs are enlarged and have abundant pale-staining cytoplasm. (Needle biopsy, H&E).

Causes of the more serious microvesicular steatosis[44] (Fig. 8.2) include treatment with the anticonvulsant drug valproate[45] and with the nucleoside analogue fialuridine.[46] This leads to the combination of microvesicular steatosis with mitochondrial abnormalities found also in Reye's syndrome (see Ch. 13). Similar changes are reported after zidovudine,[47] didanosine (Fig. 8.3) and other nucleoside reverse transcriptase inhibitors in highly active anti-retroviral therapy (HAART) for AIDS.[48,49] In the microvesicular form of steatosis, the fat within the hepatocytes is finely divided and is not always obvious with conventional stains. The hepatocyte nuclei remain in their normal central location, in contrast to macrovesicular steatosis. There is a variable degree of associated hepatocellular necrosis.

Several drugs, among them amiodarone[34] and trimethoprim-sulfamethoxazole (co-trimoxazole),[50] are causes of acquired **phospholipidosis**. Similar changes have been reported in patients receiving total parenteral nutrition.[51] Lamellar inclusions are seen within hepatocytes and other cells by electron microscopy (see Fig. 17.3). Light microscopy of conventionally-stained sections is not diagnostic.

In acute arsenic intoxication, a striking increase in hepatocyte mitoses has been reported, accompanied by ballooning, cholestasis and mild inflammation.[16] Markers of cell proliferation were also markedly increased.

An unusual form of cell injury is produced by cyanamide, used in alcohol aversion therapy.[52–54] Periportal hepatocytes contain large, pale-staining **cytoplasmic inclusion bodies**, giving the cells a superficial resemblance to the ground-glass cells of chronic type B hepatitis (see Fig. 9.10). The inclusions are, however, orcein-negative and diastase-PAS-positive.

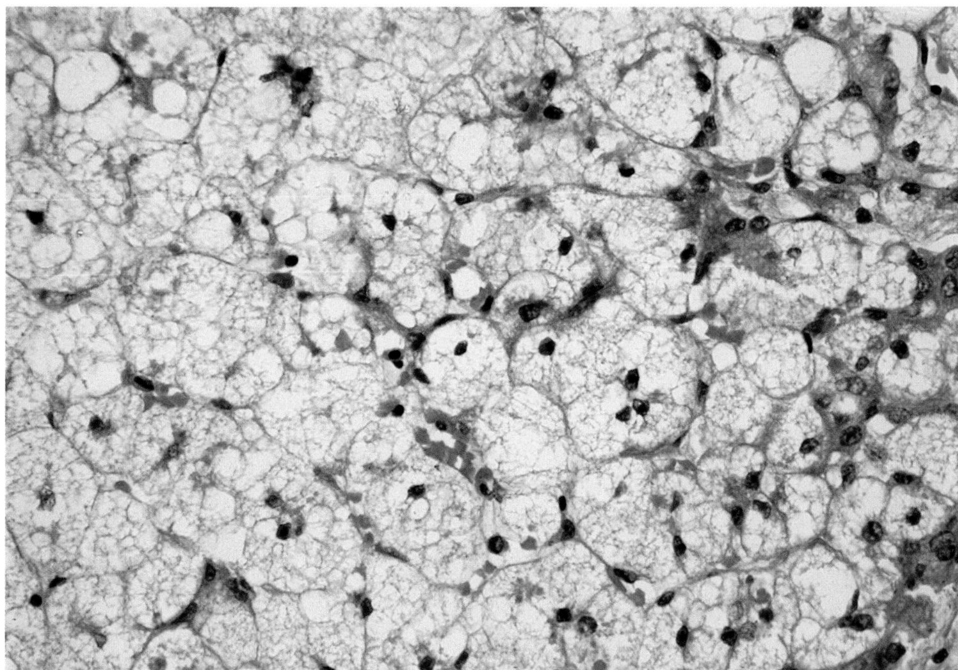

Figure 8.2 *Microvesicular steatosis.* In this example of valproate toxicity the hepatocytes are swollen and finely vacuolated. The section was kindly provided by Professor BC Portmann. (Recipient liver at transplantation, H&E).

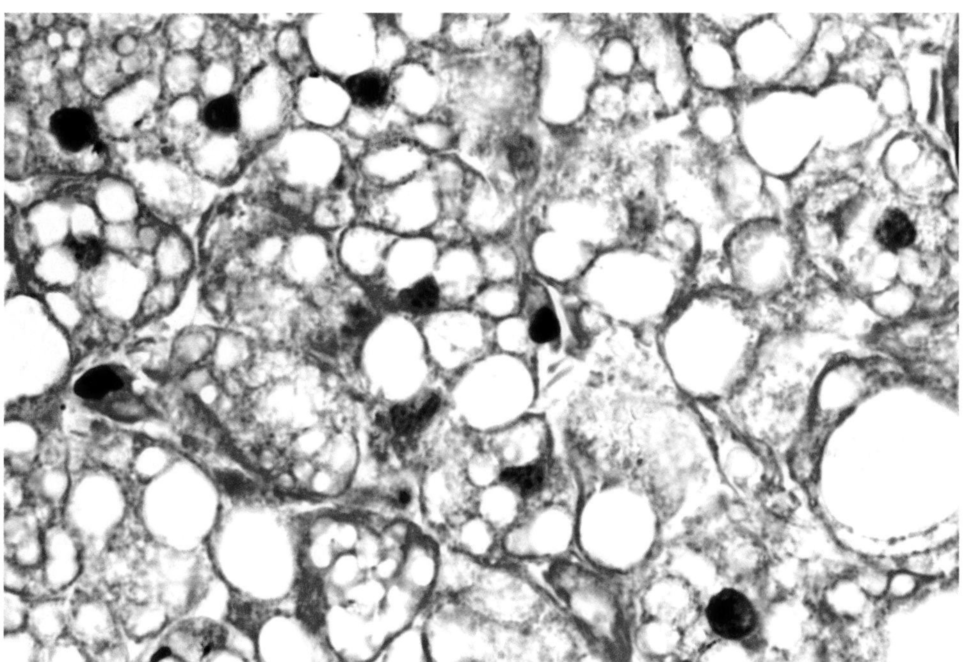

Figure 8.3 *Didanosine-induced microvesicular steatosis.* Small droplet fat vacuoles are prominent in hepatocytes, most of which show nuclei maintained in a central position. (Needle biopsy, H&E).

Hepatocellular necrosis

Hepatocellular necrosis without the diffuse inflammatory lesion of hepatitis is usually a consequence of the intrinsic type of hepatotoxicity. A common example is suicidal or accidental overdose with the analgesic paracetamol (acetaminophen).[55] Jaundice develops after an interval of days, during which available glutathione, which reacts with a toxic metabolite, is used up. The necrosis, like that of shock or heat-stroke (see Fig. 12.2), is most severe in perivenular regions (acinar zone 3) and is accompanied by little or no inflammation (Fig. 8.4). Kupffer cells contain brown ceroid pigment. Portal tracts usually remain normal. Complete recovery is possible. While most paracetamol-induced necrosis follows suicidal overdose, it is occasionally found in habitual drinkers taking large doses in the high therapeutic range.[56]

Hepatocellular necrosis, sometimes accompanied by steatosis, is also a feature of cocaine intoxication,[7,9,11] of glue sniffing and of solvent abuse.[12,57] In most instances the necrosis is perivenular and mid-zonal (in acinar zones 3 and 2), but periportal (zone 1) necrosis has been reported in a cocaine user.[58] 'Ecstasy' (3,4 methylenedioxy-methamphetamine, MDMA) can cause a hepatitic lesion of the kind described in the next section,[13,14,59] but there may also be confluent hepatocellular necrosis as a result of concurrent hyperthermia.[15] Other agents capable of causing confluent necrosis include industrial hydrochlorofluorocarbons.[17]

Acute drug-induced hepatitis

A large number of drugs of different chemical structure and with widely differing pharmacological actions occasionally give rise to acute hepatitis, and any drug

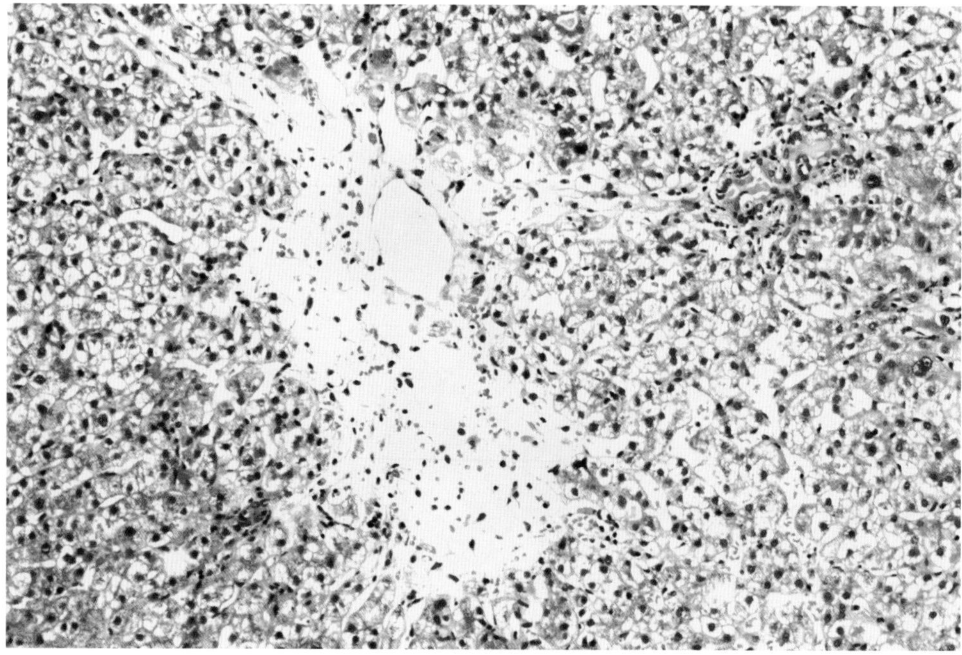

Figure 8.4 *Hepatocellular necrosis due to paracetamol (acetaminophen).* Confluent necrosis with little inflammation is seen in a perivenular area. (Needle biopsy, H&E).

should be regarded as a potential offender. Acute drug-induced hepatotoxicity is of the idiosyncratic type. The histological lesion is very like that of acute viral hepatitis, and often indistinguishable from it (Figs 8.5, 8.6). Incriminated substances include antituberculous drugs,[60] non-steroidal anti-inflammatory drugs, anaesthetics,[61,62] herbal remedies[6] and many others.

In the idiosyncratic injury of hepatitic type the latent period between exposure to the drug and clinically-evident liver disease ranges from a few days to several months, a long latent period sometimes making diagnosis difficult. However, correct diagnosis of idiosyncratic drug-induced hepatitis is most important, because inadvertent re-challenge may have serious consequences.

The hepatitis ranges in severity from a mild inflammatory lesion, sometimes combined with a cholestatic reaction (see under Cholestasis, below), to severe and even fatal disease.[63] In milder cases, removal of the drug usually leads to rapid improvement.

Differential diagnosis

The possibility of drug idiosyncrasy should be considered in all patients with acute hepatitis, because in many cases the histological appearances are identical to those of viral hepatitis. A higher than usual degree of suspicion should be aroused when the hepatitis is histologically unusual (Table 8.2). Well-demarcated centrilobular confluent necrosis (Fig. 8.5) is common. There may be a very mild lobular hepatitis together with canalicular cholestasis. The portal inflammatory reaction may be poorly developed or even absent. Conversely, the portal infiltrate may be unusually rich in neutrophils or eosinophils, although the latter are neither proof of drug

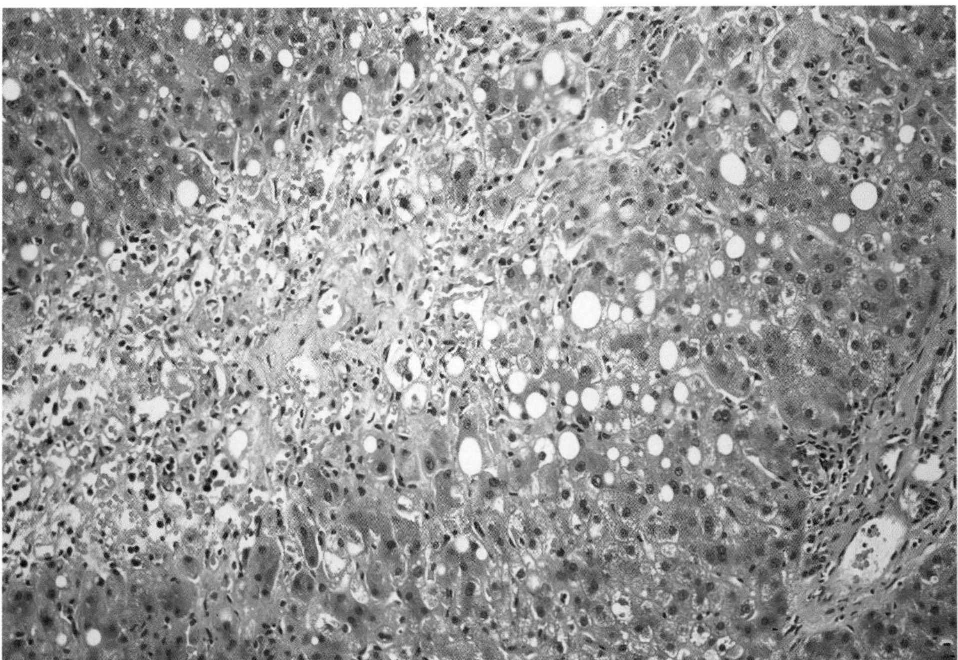

Figure 8.5 *Drug jaundice: hepatitic type.* In this acute hepatitis attributed to indomethacin, necrosis in acinar zone 3 is well-demarcated from the remaining parenchyma. The latter shows steatosis. Note the very mild portal inflammation (below right). (Needle biopsy, H&E).

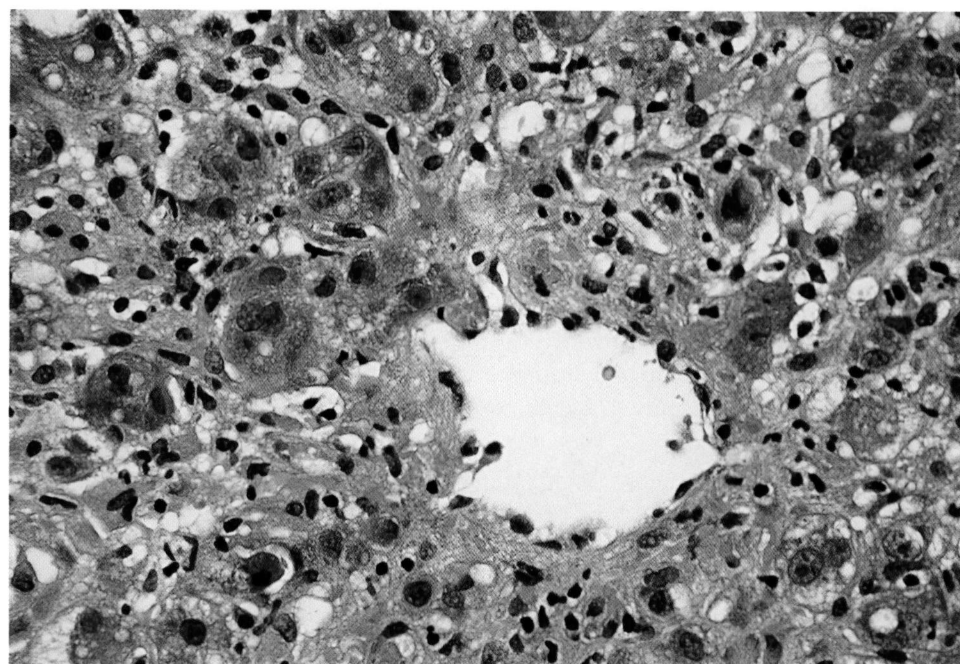

Figure 8.6 *Drug jaundice: hepatitic type.* There is a severe lobular hepatitis with disruption of liver-cell plates and apoptosis, attributed to ecstasy (3,4-methylenedioxymetamphetamine). The patient is the second of the two reported by Fidler and colleagues.[20] (Needle biopsy, H&E).

Table 8.2 Features sometimes associated with drug-induced hepatitis

Demarcated perivenular (acinar zone 3) necrosis
Minimal hepatitis with canalicular cholestasis
Poorly-developed portal inflammatory reaction
Abundant neutrophils
Abundant eosinophils
Epithelioid-cell granulomas

aetiology nor necessary for its diagnosis. The presence of epithelioid-cell granulomas increases the likelihood that drug idiosyncrasy is the correct diagnosis.

Chronic drug-induced hepatitis

In some patients, drug-induced hepatitis becomes chronic after prolonged or repeated exposure. A chronic course proved to be unexpectedly common in a recent follow-up study.[64] A high degree of suspicion of possible drug aetiology is particularly important because of the possibility of improvement after withdrawal of the drug. The histological pattern is that of chronic hepatitis with or without cirrhosis (Fig. 8.7). In patients still taking the offending drug there is usually substantial

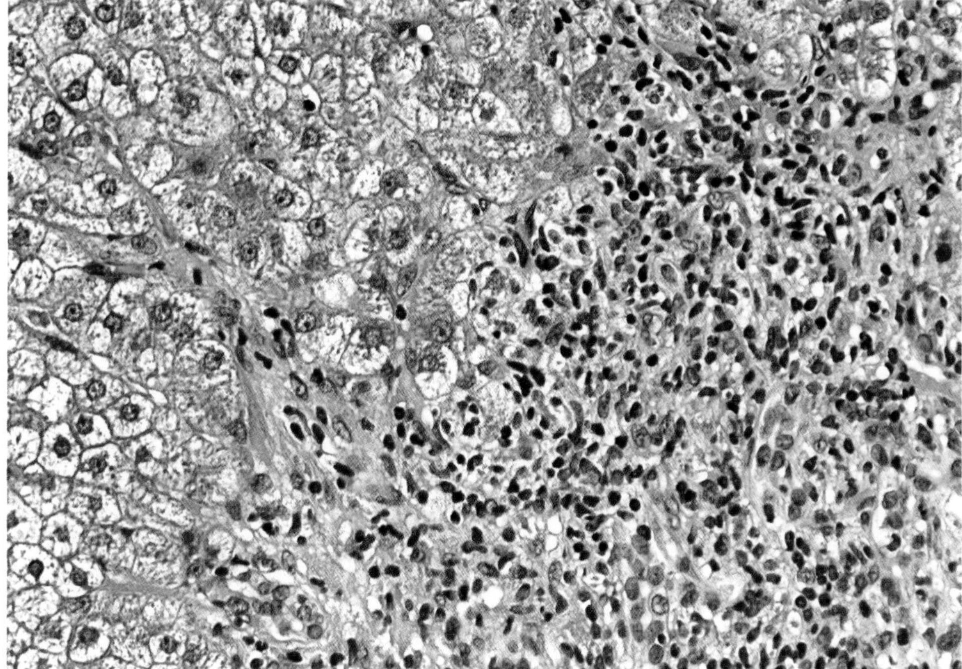

Figure 8.7 *Drug-induced chronic hepatitis.* Liver damage, here attributed to methyldopa, has taken the form of extensive interface hepatitis. There is a heavy lymphoplasmacytic infiltrate. (Needle biopsy, H&E).

necrosis and inflammation; inflammation confined to portal tracts is not a common pattern of drug injury. Drugs considered to be responsible for chronic hepatitis include such widely used agents as nitrofurantoin[65,66] and phenytoin.[67] Among other incriminated substances is the Chinese herbal product Jin Bu Huan.[68] Autoantibodies may be present in the serum of patients with drug-induced chronic hepatitis, leading to potential confusion with non-drug-related autoimmune hepatitis.[69] Drugs have indeed been cited as a possible trigger of autoimmune hepatitis.[70,71] The tetracycline derivative minocycline can itself give rise to a chronic hepatitis closely resembling autoimmune hepatitis clinically, immunologically and histologically.[72,73]

Differential diagnosis

The appearances of drug-induced chronic hepatitis are indistinguishable from those of chronic hepatitis of viral or autoimmune aetiology.

Steatohepatitis

Steatohepatitis refers to a specific form of hepatic injury characterised by steatosis, hepatocellular ballooning, Mallory body formation, inflammation and pericellular fibrosis, sometimes progressing to cirrhosis. The commonest cause is alcohol abuse. Drugs are among the causes of non-alcoholic steatohepatitis (NASH). Incriminated agents include synthetic oestrogens,[74] amiodarone[34,75] and tamoxifen[76–78] (Fig. 8.8).

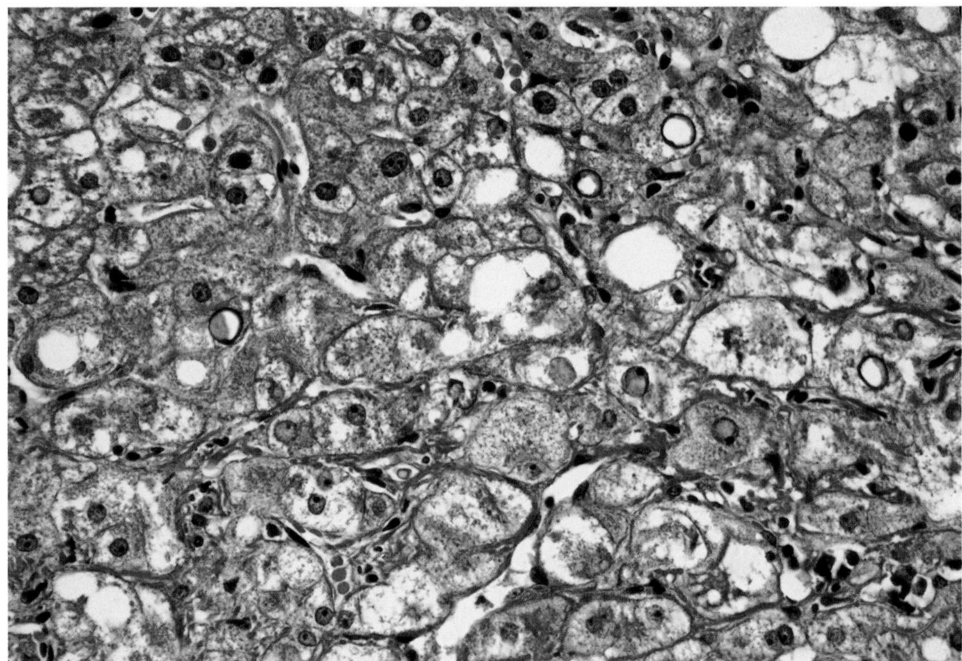

Figure 8.8 *Steatohepatitis attributed to tamoxifen toxicity.* Hepatocytes in the lower part of the field are swollen and surrounded by collagen, stained blue. There is also steatosis and nuclear vacuolation. The patient is the third of the three reported by Pinto and colleagues.[78] (The biopsy was kindly provided by Professor Amelia Baptista).

Similar changes are sometimes seen in patients on parenteral nutrition[40] and in industrial workers exposed to volatile petrochemical products.[18] In the case of amiodarone steatosis itself may be mild or absent,[79] but otherwise there is a close resemblance to other forms of NASH and to alcoholic steatohepatitis, including the potential for cirrhosis. However, amiodarone-related steatohepatitis has a periportal predilection in contrast to the perivenular distribution seen with other causes of steatohepatitis. It is interesting to note that some patients with reported drug-related steatohepatitis were also obese,[78] which raises the possibility of an interaction between drug and other factors.

Fibrosis and cirrhosis

As already stated, cirrhosis may result from chronic drug-induced hepatitis. Progressive fibrosis and portal hypertension in a non-hepatitic setting are known complications of long-term exposure to arsenic or vinyl chloride. Excess intake of vitamin A (hypervitaminosis A) affects hepatic stellate cells, which may appear unusually prominent (Fig. 8.9). Perisinusoidal fibrosis, veno-occlusive disease and cirrhosis[22] are other consequences.

Pathologists are sometimes asked to report on liver biopsies from patients given or about to receive long-term methotrexate for psoriasis or rheumatoid arthritis. Although methotrexate was initially considered to be a potent hepatotoxin, doubt has more recently been thrown on its potential to cause serious liver disease in the

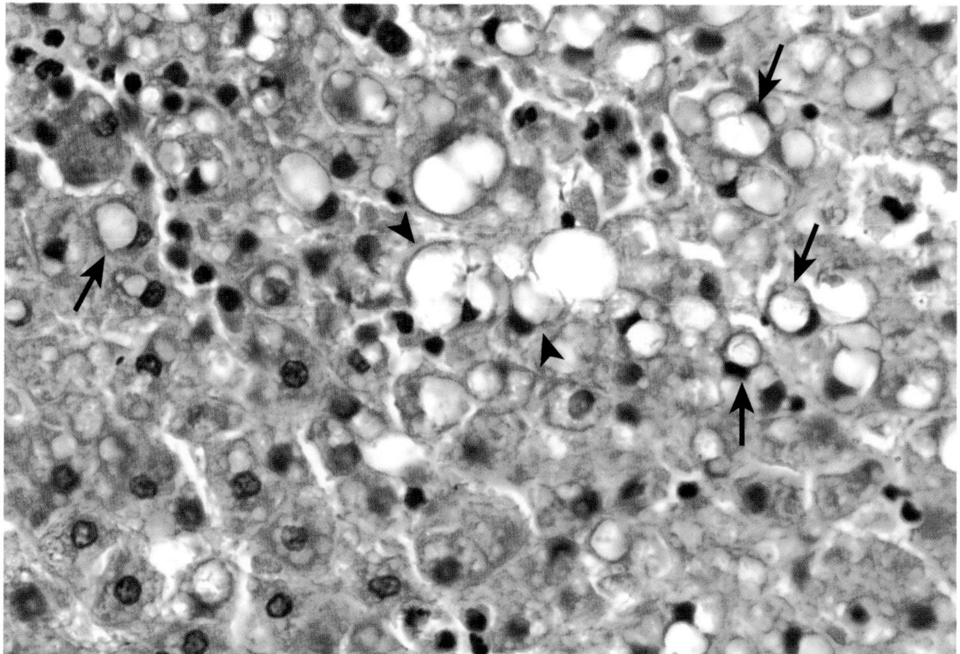

Figure 8.9 *Hypervitaminosis A.* Prominent, hypertrophied stellate cells with lipid vacuoles and peripheral dark, compressed nuclei are seen between hepatocytes, in perisinusoidal spaces (arrows). Some of the stellate cells are multivesicular (arrowheads). (Needle biopsy, H&E).

absence of additional risk factors.[80] These include regular or heavy alcohol intake[81] and obesity.[82] Significant liver injury is reputedly less common in patients with rheumatoid arthritis than in those with psoriasis. Histological abnormalities attributed to methotrexate include steatosis, hepatocyte pleomorphism, portal fibrosis and inflammation, formation of fibrous septa extending from the portal tracts (Fig. 8.10) and cirrhosis. A grading system for methotrexate liver injury was developed by Roenigk and colleagues, which scores the degree of fat, inflammation and fibrosis.[83] Minor changes such as focal necrosis and steatosis are common in baseline pre-treatment biopsies, and are presumably related to the underlying disease (e.g. psoriasis) or to additional risk factors. Periportal septum formation is more likely to be due to methotrexate, whereas fibrosis mainly in perivenular regions should lead to suspicion of alcohol abuse or non-alcoholic steatohepatitis.

Cholestasis

Steroid-induced cholestasis

Steroid-induced cholestasis[84] lies on the borderline between intrinsic and idiosyncratic hepatotoxicity. On the one hand, it is reproducible in laboratory animals and some steroids cause biochemical abnormalities in man in a predictable and dose-dependent manner. On the other hand, clinical liver disease cannot be predicted in the individual patient and is seen in only a small proportion of patients

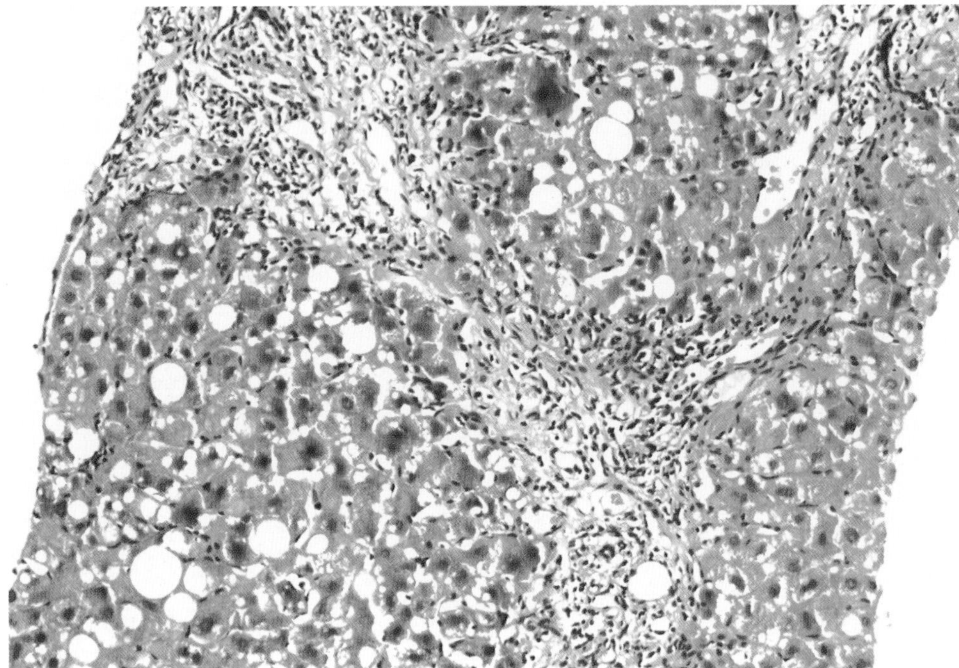

Figure 8.10 *Liver damage attributed to methotrexate.* Two portal tracts in this field show chronic inflammation and fibrosis extending outwards. The parenchyma shows steatosis. (Needle biopsy, H&E).

receiving anabolic or contraceptive steroids. Patients susceptible to contraceptive steroid-induced jaundice are also prone to develop cholestasis in late pregnancy.

The histological picture is one of canalicular cholestasis in perivenular areas, with little or no necrosis or inflammation beyond that attributable to the cholestasis itself. Isolated hepatocytes may undergo feathery degeneration and in prolonged cholestasis, liver-cell rosettes are a common finding (as seen in Fig. 4.4). Portal tracts usually remain normal but may be minimally inflamed. Because of the lack of necrosis and inflammation, this type of lesion is sometimes known as pure or bland cholestasis.

Differential diagnosis

The differential diagnosis is from other causes of bland cholestasis such as benign recurrent intrahepatic cholestasis (BRIC) and is discussed in detail in Chapter 5.

Idiosyncratic drug-induced cholestasis

Idiosyncratic drug-induced cholestasis, typified by chlorpromazine jaundice[85] but also caused by many other drugs, differs from bland cholestasis in that some degree of portal inflammation is usually present (Fig. 8.11). There is sometimes inflammatory infiltration of the lobules and evidence of hepatocellular damage. Zimmerman and Ishak[4] therefore refer to this type of lesion as hepatocanalicular. The portal infiltrate often includes eosinophils and these are occasionally abundant, but their absence does not exclude a diagnosis of drug-induced hepatocanalicular cholestasis. Small interlobular ducts often show abnormalities such as irregular distribution of epithelial cell nuclei, cytoplasmic vacuolation, variation in nuclear

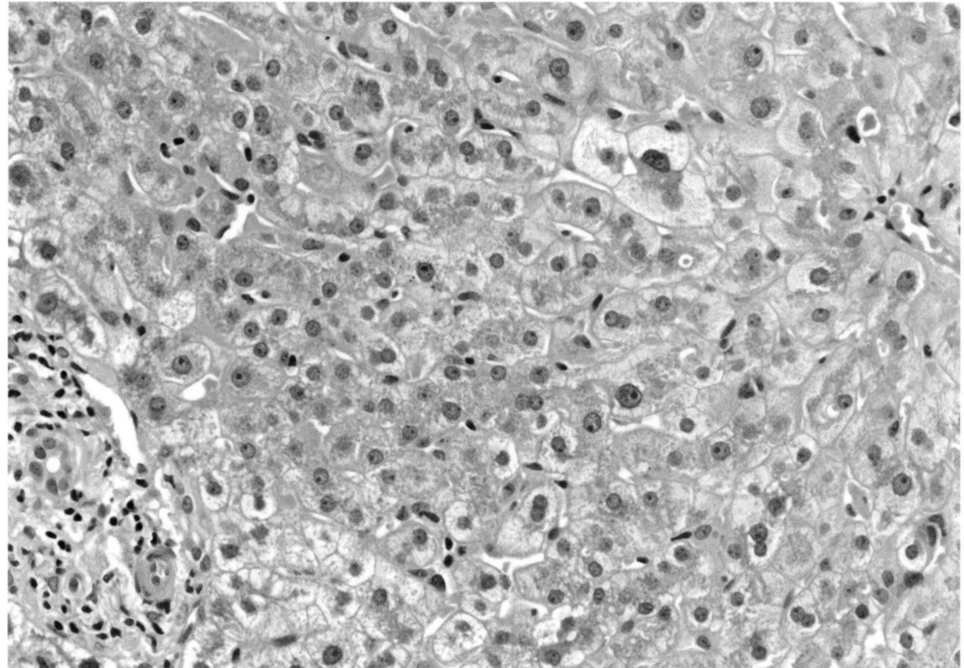

Figure 8.11 *Drug jaundice: cholestatic type.* In this patient with jaundice following chlorpromazine therapy there is mild inflammation of the portal tract (lower left) and swelling of hepatocytes, especially in the perivenular area (above, centre and right). (Needle biopsy, H&E).

size and infiltration by lymphocytes. These changes are usually mild, but occasionally more severe (Fig. 8.12), even leading to ductopenia (see **vanishing bile duct syndrome**, below). The lobular changes (Fig. 8.11) are as in bland cholestasis, except for the additional element of inflammation and necrosis which is sometimes found, as mentioned above. There is therefore a spectrum of appearances in this type of cholestasis, from an almost bland cholestatic lesion to one resembling mild acute viral hepatitis. Even in the absence of necrosis and inflammation, hepatocellular changes are seen which possibly result from prolonged cholestasis itself but which may also include an element of adaptive proliferation of the smooth endoplasmic reticulum. These changes include prominent hepatocellular swelling, abundant pale-staining cytoplasm and, commonly, multinucleation. Mitotic figures may be evident.[85]

Differential diagnosis

The differential diagnosis of idiosyncratic drug-induced cholestasis is from bile-duct obstruction, acute viral or drug-induced hepatitis and cholestasis of the bland type. Portal oedema, prominent neutrophils, marked ductular reaction and absence of lobular inflammation favour the first. In the absence of substantial portal inflammation, the distinction between idiosyncratic drug jaundice and bland steroid-induced cholestasis becomes difficult to make and requires clinical information. In such circumstances, bile-duct obstruction cannot be completely ruled out. The differential diagnosis also includes other causes of bland cholestasis, such as benign recurrent cholestasis. Severe liver-cell damage and inflammation favour viral hepatitis or the drug injury of hepatitic type already discussed.

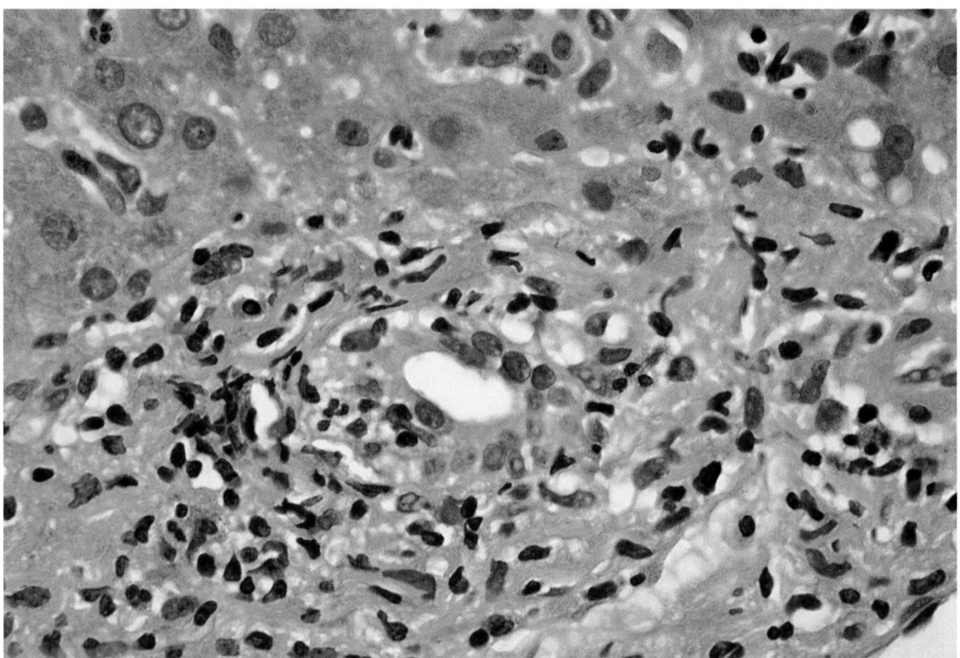

Figure 8.12 *Drug jaundice: cholestatic type.* An inflamed portal tract from a patient with jaundice attributed to Augmentin (amoxicillin and clavulanic acid). The epithelium of an interlobular bile-duct is irregular, vacuolated and infiltrated by lymphocytes. Biopsy kindly provided by Dr Karin Oien. (Needle biopsy, H&E).

The clinical course of idiosyncratic drug jaundice varies. In most patients, removal of the offending drug leads to rapid improvement. Occasionally the cholestasis is slow to improve but liver biopsy shows cholestasis only, with no fibrosis or other evidence of progressive disease. In rare instances, true chronic disease develops on the basis of severe bile-duct damage and duct loss, with consequent fibrosis and other features of chronic biliary disease. The clinical picture resembles primary biliary cirrhosis. This **vanishing bile duct syndrome** has been reported after a number of drugs[86,87] including chlorpromazine,[85] a combination of chlorpropamide with erythromycin ethylsuccinate,[88] prochlorperazine,[89] gold salts,[90] ciprofloxacin,[91] haloperidol,[92] ajmaline[93] glycyrrhizin[94] and amoxicillin and flucloxacillin[95] among others. Augmentin (amoxicillin and clavulanic acid) (see Fig. 8.12) is a well-documented cause of cholestasis, with striking focal destruction of bile ducts in some biopsies.[96–99] This is occasionally associated with granuloma formation. Prolonged cholestasis may be the result of the duct damage and, in some patients, of duct loss.

More acute bile duct injury is seen in poisoning with the herbicide paraquat.[100] Zimmerman and Ishak[4] designate this type of injury as ductal or cholangio-destructive, in contrast to canalicular and hepatocanalicular cholestasis.

Long-term parenteral nutrition, already noted in relation to steatosis and steatohepatitis in adults, may in infants and children be associated with a progressive form of liver injury, typified by cholestasis, hepatocellular damage, ductular reaction, fibrosis and even cirrhosis.[40,41,101] Whether the parenteral nutrition itself is responsible for all these changes is not proven.[41,42] The lesion may mimic bile-duct obstruction[102] (see Fig. 13.18).

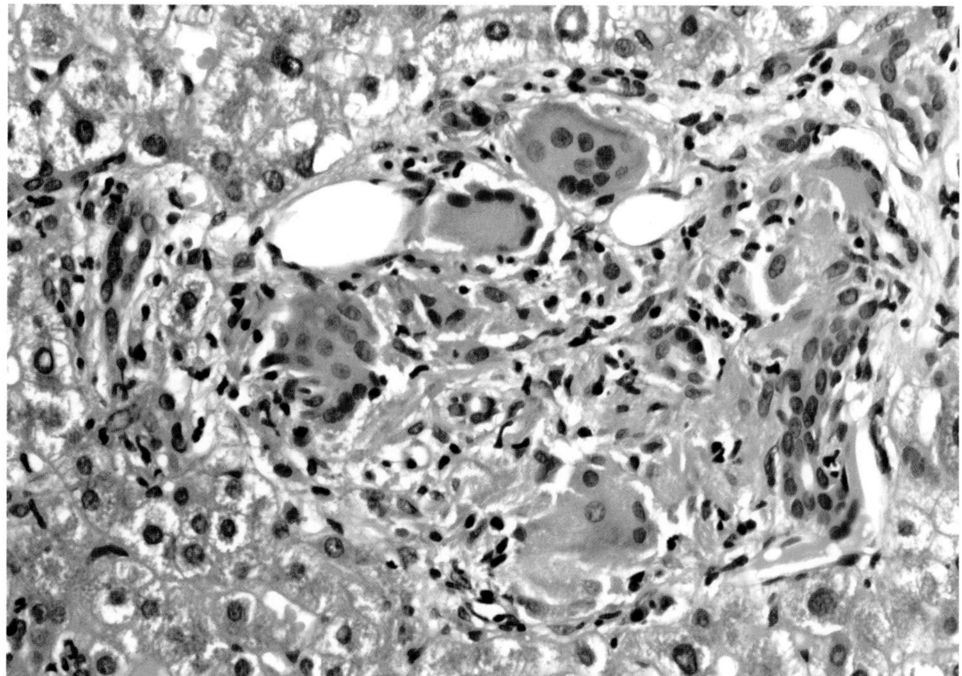

Figure 8.13 *Drug-induced granuloma formation.* A portal tract contains a granuloma with many multinucleated giant cells. The patient became jaundiced after taking phenylbutazone. (Needle biopsy, H&E).

Granulomas

Drugs are an important cause of otherwise unexplained granulomas. They are sometimes the only or main manifestation of a drug reaction, but can also form part of a cholestatic or hepatitis picture.[75] The granulomas may be portal (Fig. 8.13), parenchymal, or both. They usually show little or no necrosis and are infiltrated by a variety of inflammatory cells including plasma cells and eosinophils. Allopurinol has been reported to cause granulomas of the fibrin-ring type.[103] The list of drugs associated with hepatic granulomas is small compared with the list of those causing hepatitis or cholestasis, but it is nevertheless substantial.[4,104,105]

REFERENCES

1 Stricker BHC. Drug-induced Hepatic Injury. Amsterdam: Elsevier Science; 1992:

2 Farrell GC. Drug-induced Liver Disease. Edinburgh: Churchill Livingstone, 1994.

3 Pessayre D, Larrey D, Biour M. Drug-induced liver injury. In: Bircher J, Benhamou J-P, McIntyre N, et al., eds. Oxford Textbook of Clinical Hepatology, 2nd edn. Oxford: Oxford University Press, 1999: 1261.

4 Zimmerman HJ, Ishak KG. Hepatic injury due to drugs and toxins. In: MacSween RNM, Burt AD, Portmann BC, et al., eds. Pathology of the Liver, 4th edn. Edinburgh: Churchill Livingstone, 2002: 621.

5 Biour M, Poupon R, Grange JD, et al. Drug-induced hepatotoxicity. The 13th updated edition of the bibliographic database of drug-related liver injuries and responsible drugs. *Gastroenterol Clin Biol* 2000; **24**: 1052–1091.

6 Fogden E, Neuberger J. Alternative medicines and the liver. *Liver Int* 2003; **23**: 213–220.

7 Kanel GC, Cassidy W, Shuster L, et al. Cocaine-induced liver cell injury: comparison of morphological features in man and in experimental models. *Hepatology* 1990; **11**: 646–651.

8 Trigueiro de Araújo MS, Gerard F, Chossegros P et al. Vascular hepatotoxicity related to heroin addiction. *Virchows Arch (A)* 1990; **417**: 497–503.

9 Wanless IR, Dore S, Gopinath N, et al. Histopathology of cocaine hepatotoxicity. Report of four patients. *Gastroenterology* 1990; **98**: 497–501.

10 Mallat A, Dhumeaux D. Cocaine and the liver. *J Hepatol* 1991; **12**: 275–278.

11 Silva MO, Roth D, Reddy KR, et al. Hepatic dysfunction accompanying acute cocaine intoxication. *J Hepatol* 1991; **12**: 312–315.

12 McIntyre AS, Long RG. Fatal fulminant hepatic failure in a 'solvent abuser'. *Postgrad Med J* 1992; **68**: 29–30.

13 Ellis AJ, Wendon JA, Portmann B, et al. Acute liver damage and ecstasy ingestion. *Gut* 1996; **38**: 454–458.

14 Fidler H, Dhillon A, Gertner D, et al. Chronic ecstasy (3,4-methylenedioxy-metamphetamine) abuse: a recurrent and unpredictable cause of severe acute hepatitis. *J Hepatol* 1996; **25**: 563–566.

15 Milroy CM, Clark JC, Forrest ARW. Pathology of deaths associated with 'ecstasy' and 'eve' misuse. *J Clin Pathol* 1996; **49**: 149–153.

16 Brenard R, Laterre P-F, Reynaert M, et al. Increased hepatocyte mitotic activity as a diagnostic marker of acute arsenic intoxication. A report of two cases. *J Hepatol* 1996; **25**: 218–220.

17 Hoet P, Graf MLM, Bourdi M, et al. Epidemic of liver disease caused by hydrochlorofluorocarbons used as ozone-sparing substitutes of chlorofluorocarbons. *Lancet* 1997; **350**: 556–559.

18 Cotrim HP, Andrade ZA, Parana R, et al. Nonalcoholic steatohepatitis: a toxic liver disease in industrial workers. *Liver* 1999; **19**: 299–304.

19 Kahl R. Toxic liver injury. In: Bircher J, Benhamou J-P, McIntyre N, et al., eds. Oxford Textbook of Clinical Hepatology, 2nd edn. Oxford: Oxford University Press, 1999: 1319.

20 Kahl R. Liver injury in man ascribed to non-drug chemicals and natural toxins. In: Bircher J, Benhamou J-P, McIntyre N, et al., eds. Oxford Textbook of Clinical Hepatology, 2nd edn. Oxford: Oxford University Press, 1999: 2083.

21 Bioulac-Sage P, Quinton A, Saric J, et al. Chance discovery of hepatic fibrosis in patient with asymptomatic hypervitaminosis A. *Arch Pathol Lab Med* 1988; **112**: 505–509.

22 Jorens PG, Michielsen PP, Pelckmans PA, et al. Vitamin A abuse: development of cirrhosis despite cessation of vitamin A. A six-year clinical and histopathologic follow-up. *Liver* 1992; **12**: 381–386.

23 Galler GW, Weisenberg E, Brasitus TA. Mushroom poisoning: the role of orthotopic liver transplantation. *J Clin Gastroenterol* 1992; **15**: 229–232.

24 Nagai K, Hosaka H, Kubo S, et al. Vitamin A toxicity secondary to excessive intake of yellow-green vegetables, liver and laver. *J Hepatol* 1999; **31**: 142–148.

25 Silva MO, Reddy KR, Jeffers LJ, et al. Interferon-induced chronic active hepatitis? *Gastroenterology* 1991; **101**: 840–842.

26 Lindgren A, Aldenborg F, Norkrans G, et al. Paracetamol-induced cholestatic and granulomatous liver injuries. *J Int Med* 1997; **241**: 435–439.

27 Andrade RJ, Lucena MI, Garcia-Escaño MD, et al. Sever idiosyncratic acute hepatic injury caused by paracetamol. *J Hepatol* 1998; **28**: 1078–.

28 Kenna JG. Immunoallergic drug-induced hepatitis: lessons from halothane. *J Hepatol* 1997; **26 (Suppl 1)**: 5–12.

29 Robin M-A, Le Roy M, Descatoire V, et al. Plasma membrane cytochromes P450 as neoantigens and autoimmune targets in drug-induced hepatitis. *J Hepatol* 1997; **26(Suppl 1)**: 23–30.

30 Eliasson E. Stãl POA, Lytton S. Expression of autoantibodies to specific cytochromes P450 in a case of

disulfiram hepatitis. *J Hepatol* 1998; **29**: 819–825.
31 Grieco A, Vecchio FM, Greco AV, et al. Cholestatic hepatitis due to ticlopidine: clinical and histological recovery after drug withdrawal. Case report and review of the literature. *J Hepatol* 1998; **10**: 713–715.
32 Aithal GP, Rawlins MD, Day CP. Clinical diagnostic scale: a useful tool in the evaluation of suspected hepatotoxic adverse drug reactions. *J Hepatol* 2000; **33**: 949–952.
33 Paiva LA, Wright PJ, Koff RS. Long-term hepatic memory for hypersensitivity to nitrofurantoin. *Am J Gastroenterol* 1992; **87**: 891–893.
34 Lewis JH, Mullick F, Ishak KG, et al. Histopathologic analysis of suspected amiodarone hepatotoxicity. *Hum Pathol* 1990; **21**: 59–67.
35 Benjamin SB, Ishak KG, Zimmerman HJ, et al. Phenylbutazone liver injury: a clinical-pathologic survey of 23 cases and review of the literature. *Hepatology* 1981; **1**: 255–263.
36 Banks AT, Zimmerman HJ, Ishak KG, et al. Diclofenac-associated hepatotoxicity: analysis of 180 cases reported to the Food and Drug Administration as adverse reactions. *Hepatology* 1995; **22**: 820–827.
37 Steenbergen W Van, Peeters P, Bondt J De, et al. Nimesulfide-induced acute hepatitis: evidence from six cases. *J Hepatol* 1998; **29**: 135–141.
38 Jezequel AM, Librari ML, Mosca P, et al. Changes induced in human liver by long-term anticonvulsant therapy. Functional and ultrastructural data. *Liver* 1984; **4**: 307–317.
39 Pamperl H, Gradner W, Fridrich L, et al. Influence of long-term anticonvulsant treatment on liver ultrastructure in man. *Liver* 1984; **4**: 294–300.
40 Klein S, Nealon WH. Hepatobiliary abnormalities associated with total parenteral nutrition. *Semin Liver Dis* 1988; **8**: 237–246.
41 Quigley EM, Marsh MN, Shaffer JL, et al. Hepatobiliary complications of total parenteral nutrition. *Gastroenterology* 1993; **104**: 286–301.
42 Wolfe BM, Walker BK, Shaul DB, et al. Effect of total parenteral nutrition on hepatic histology. *Arch Surg* 1988; **123**: 1084–1090.
43 Landas SK, Mitros FA, Furst DE, et al. Lipogranulomas and gold in the liver in rheumatoid arthritis. *Am J Surg Pathol* 1992; **16**: 171–174.
44 Fromenty B, Berson A, Pessayre D. Microvesicular steatosis and steatohepatitis: role of mitochondrial dysfunction and lipid peroxidation. *J Hepatol* 1997; **26 (Suppl 1)**: 13–22.
45 Zimmerman HJ, Ishak KG. Valproate-induced hepatic injury: analyses of 23 fatal cases. *Hepatology* 1982; **2**: 591–597.
46 Kleiner DE, Gaffey MJ, Sallie R, et al. Histopathologic changes associated with fialuridine hepatotoxicity. *Mod Pathol* 1997; **10**: 192–199.
47 Chariot P, Drogou I, Lacroix-Szmania I de, et al. Zidovudine-induced mitochondrial disorder with massive liver steatosis, myopathy, lactic acidosis, and mitochondrial DNA depletion. *J Hepatol* 1999; **30**: 156–160.
48 Spengler U, Lichterfeld M, Rockstroh JK. Antiretroviral drug toxicity – a challenge for the hepatologist? *J Hepatol* 2002; **36**: 283–294.
49 Clark SJ, Creighton S, Portmann B, et al. Acute liver failure associated with antiretroviral treatment for HIV: a report of six cases. *J Hepatol* 2002; **36**: 295–301.
50 Muñoz SJ, Martinez-Hernandez A, Maddrey WC. Intrahepatic cholestasis and phospholipidosis associated with the use of trimethoprim-sulfamethoxazole. *Hepatology* 1990; **12**: 342–347.
51 Degott C, Messing B, Moreau D, et al. Liver phospholipidosis induced by parenteral nutrition: histologic, biochemical, and ultrastructural investigations. *Gastroenterology* 1988; **95**: 183–191.
52 Vazquez JJ, Guillen FJ, Zozaya J, et al. Cyanamide-induced liver injury. A predictable lesion. *Liver* 1983; **3**: 225–230.
53 Bruguera M, Lamar C, Bernet M, et al. Hepatic disease associated with ground-glass inclusions in hepatocytes after cyanamide therapy. *Arch Pathol Lab Med* 1986; **110**: 906–910.
54 Yokoyama A, Sato S, Maruyama K, et al. Cyanamide-associated alcoholic liver disease: a sequential histological evaluation. *Alcohol Clin Exp Res* 1995; **19**: 1307–1311.

55 Portmann B, Talbot IC, Day DW, et al. Histopathological changes in the liver following a paracetamol overdose: correlation with clinical and biochemical parameters. *J Pathol* 1975; **117**: 169–181.
56 Maddrey WC. Hepatic effects of acetaminophen. Enhanced toxicity in alcoholics. *J Clin Gastroenterol* 1987; **9**: 180–185.
57 Baerg RD, Kimberg DV. Centrilobular hepatic necrosis and acute renal failure in 'solvent sniffers'. *Ann Intern Med* 1970; **73**: 713–720.
58 Perino LE, Warren GH, Levine JS. Cocaine-induced hepatotoxicity in humans. *Gastroenterology* 1987; **93**: 176–180.
59 Andreu V, Mas A, Bruguera M, et al. Ecstasy: a common cause of severe acute hepatotoxicity. *J Hepatol* 1998; **29**: 394–397.
60 Mitchell I, Wendon J, Fitt S, et al. Antituberculous therapy and acute liver failure. *Lancet* 1995; **345**: 555–556.
61 Neuberger J. Halothane hepatitis. *Eur J Gastro Hepatol* 1998; **10**: 631–633.
62 Lo SK, Wendon J, Mieli-Vergani G, et al. Halothane-induced acute liver failure: continuing occurrence and use of liver transplantation. *Eur J Gastro Hepatol* 1998; **10**: 635–639.
63 Paterson D, Kerlin P, Walker N, et al. Piroxicam induced submassive necrosis of the liver. *Gut* 1992; **33**: 1436–1438.
64 Aithal PG, Day CP. The natural history of histologically proved drug induced liver disease. *Gut* 1999; **44**: 731–735.
65 Sharp JR, Ishak KG, Zimmerman HJ. Chronic active hepatitis and severe hepatic necrosis associated with nitrofurantoin. *Ann Intern Med* 1980; **92**: 14–19.
66 Stricker BH, Blok AP, Claas FH, et al. Hepatic injury associated with the use of nitrofurans: a clinicopathological study of 52 reported cases. *Hepatology* 1988; **8**: 599–606.
67 Roy AK, Mahoney HC, Levine RA. Phenytoin-induced chronic hepatitis. *Dig Dis Sci* 1993; **38**: 740–743.
68 Picciotto A, Campo N, Brizzolara R, et al. Chronic hepatitis induced by Jin Bu Huan. *J Hepatol* 1998; **28**: 165–167.
69 Scully LJ, Clarke D, Barr RJ. Diclofenac induced hepatitis. Three cases with features of autoimmune chronic active hepatitis. *Dig Dis Sci* 1993; **38**: 744–751.
70 Kamiyama T, Nouchi T, Kojima S, et al. Autoimmune hepatitis triggered by administration of an herbal medicine. *Am J Gastroenterol* 1997; **92**: 703–704.
71 Sterling MJ, Kane M, Grace ND. Pemoline-induced autoimmune hepatitis. *Am J Gastroenterol* 1996; **91**: 2233–2234.
72 Gough A, Chapman S, Wagstaff K, et al. Minocycline induced autoimmune hepatitis and systemic lupus erythematosus-like syndrome. *Br Med J* 1996; **312**: 169–172.
73 Malcolm A, Heap TR, Eckstein RP, et al. Minocycline-induced liver injury. *Am J Gastroenterol* 1996; **91**: 1641–1643.
74 Seki K, Minami Y, Nishikawa M, et al. 'Nonalcoholic steatohepatitis' induced by massive doses of synthetic estrogen. *Gastroenterol Jap* 1983; **18**: 197–203.
75 Harrison RF, Elias E. Amiodarone-associated cirrhosis with hepatic and lymph node granulomas. *Histopathology* 1993; **22**: 80–82.
76 Hoof M Van, Rahier J, Horsmans Y. Tamoxifen-induced steatohepatitis [letter]. *Ann Intern Med* 1996; **124**: 855–856.
77 Cai Q, Bensen M, Greene R, et al. Tamoxifen-induced transient multifocal hepatic fatty infiltration. *Am J Gastroenterol* 2000; **95**: 277–279.
78 Pinto HC, Baptista A, Camilo ME, et al. Tamoxifen-associated steatohepatitis – report of three cases. *J Hepatol* 1995; **23**: 95–97.
79 Chang C-C, Petrelli M, Tomashefski JFJ, et al. Severe intrahepatic cholestasis caused by amiodarone toxicity after withdrawal of the drug. A case report and review of the literature. *Arch Pathol Lab Med* 1999; **123**: 251–256.
80 Tang H, Neuberger J. Review article: methotrexate in gastroenterology – dangerous villain or simply misunderstood? *Aliment Pharmacol Ther* 1996; **10**: 851–858.
81 Whiting OK, Fye KH, Sack KD. Methotrexate and histologic hepatic abnormalities: a meta-analysis. *Am J Med* 1991; **90**: 711–716.
82 Newman M, Auerbach R, Feiner H, et al. The role of liver biopsies in psoriatic patients receiving long-term

methotrexate treatment. Improvement in liver abnormalities after cessation of treatment. *Arch Dermatol* 1989; **125**: 1218–1224.

83 Roenigk HH Jr, Auerbach R, Maibach HI et al. Methotrexate guidelines – revised. *J Am Acad Derm* 1982; **6**: 145–155.

84 Ishak KG. Hepatic lesions caused by anabolic and contraceptive steroids. *Semin Liver Dis* 1981; **1**: 116–128.

85 Ishak KG, Irey NS. Hepatic injury associated with the phenothiazines. Clinicopathologic and follow-up study of 36 patients. *Arch Pathol* 1972; **93**: 283–304.

86 Degott C, Feldmann G, Larrey D, et al. Drug-induced prolonged cholestasis in adults: a histological semi-quantitative study demonstrating progressive ductopenia. *Hepatology* 1992; **15**: 244–251.

87 Desmet VJ. Vanishing bile duct syndrome in drug-induced liver disease. *J Hepatol* 1997; **26 (Suppl 1)**: 31–35.

88 Geubel AP, Nakad A, Rahier J, et al. Prolonged cholestasis and disappearance of interlobular bile ducts following chlorpropamide and erythromycin ethylsuccinate. Case drug interaction? *Liver* 1988; **8**: 350–353.

89 Lok ASF, Ng IOL. Prochlorperazine-induced chronic cholestasis. *J Hepatol* 1988; **6**: 369–373.

90 Basset C, Vadrot J, Denis J, et al. Prolonged cholestasis and ductopenia following gold salt therapy. *Liver Int* 2003; **23**: 89–93.

91 Bataille L, Rahier J, Geubel A. Delayed and prolonged cholestatic hepatitis with ductopenia after long-term ciprofloxacin therapy for Crohn's disease. *J Hepatol* 2002; **37**: 696–699.

92 Dincsoy HP, Saelinger DA. Haloperidol-induced chronic cholestatic liver disease. *Gastroenterology* 1982; **83**: 694–700.

93 Larrey D, Pessayre D, Duhamel G, et al. Prolonged cholestasis after ajmaline-induced acute hepatitis. *J Hepatol* 1986; **2**: 81–87.

94 Ishii M, Miyazaki M, Yamamoto T, et al. A case of drug-induced ductopenia resulting in fatal biliary cirrhosis. *Liver* 1993; **13**: 227–231.

95 Davies MH, Harrison RF, Elias E, et al. Antibiotic-associated acute vanishing bile duct syndrome: a pattern associated with severe, prolonged, intrahepatic cholestasis. *J Hepatol* 1994; **20**: 112–116.

96 Richardet J-P, Mallat A, Zafrani ES, et al. Prolonged cholestasis with ductopenia after administration of amoxicillin/clavulanic acid. *Dig Dis Sci* 1999; **44**: 1997–2000.

97 O'Donohue J, Oien KA, Donaldson P, et al. Co-amoxiclav jaundice: clinical and histological features and HLA class II association. *Gut* 2000; **47**: 717–720.

98 Hautekeete ML, Horsmans Y, Waeyenberge C Van, et al. HLA association of amoxicillin-clavulanate-induced hepatitis. *Gastroenterology* 1999; **117**: 1181–1186.

99 Ryley NG, Fleming KA, Chapman RWG. Focal destructive cholangiopathy associated with amoxycillin/clavulinic acid (Augmentin). *J Hepatol* 1995; **23**: 278–282.

100 Mullick FG, Ishak KG, Mahabir R, et al. Hepatic injury associated with paraquat toxicity in humans. *Liver* 1981; **1**: 209–221.

101 Baker AL, Rosenberg IH. Hepatic complications of total parenteral nutrition. *Am J Med* 1987; **82**: 489–497.

102 Body JJ, Bleiberg H, Bron D, et al. Total parenteral nutrition-induced cholestasis mimicking large bile duct obstruction. *Histopathology* 1982; **6**: 787–792.

103 Vanderstigel M, Zafrani ES, Lejonc JL, et al. Allopurinol hypersensitivity syndrome as a cause of hepatic fibrin-ring granulomas. *Gastroenterology* 1986; **90**: 188–190.

104 Ishak KG, Zimmerman HJ. Drug-induced and toxic granulomatous hepatitis. *Baillières Clin Gastroenterol* 1988; **2**: 463–480.

105 James DG, Scheuer PJ. Hepatic granulomas. In: Bircher J, Benhamou J-P, McIntyre N, et al., eds. Oxford Textbook of Clinical Hepatology, 2nd edn. Oxford: Oxford University Press, 1999: 1099.

GENERAL READING

Aithal PG, Day CP. The natural history of histologically proved drug induced liver disease. *Gut* 1999; **44**: 731–735.

Goodman ZD. Drug hepatotoxicity. *Clin Liver Dis* 2002; **6**: 381–398.

Larrey D. Drug-induced liver diseases. *J Hepatol* 2000; **32 (Suppl 1)**: 77–88.

Pirmohamed M, Breckenridge AM, Kitteringham NR, Park BK. Adverse drug reactions. *BMJ* 1998; **316**: 1295–1298.

Vial T, Biour M, Descotes J, Trepo C. Antibiotic-associated hepatitis: update from 1990. *Ann Pharmacother* 1997; **31**: 204–220.

Biour M, Poupon R, Grange JD, Chazouilleres O. Drug-induced hepatotoxicity. The 13(th) updated edition of the bibliographic database of drug-related liver injuries and responsible drugs. *Gastroenterol Clin Biol* 2000; **24**: 1052–1091.

Zimmerman HJ, Ishak KG. Hepatic injury due to drugs and toxins. In: MacSween RNM, Burt AD, Portmann BC, Ishak KG, Scheuer PJ, Anthony PP, eds. Pathology of the Liver, 4th edn. Edinburgh, UK: Churchill Livingstone, 2002: 621–709.

Lee WM. Drug-induced hepatotoxicity. *N Engl J Med* 2003; **349**: 474–485.

CHAPTER 9

CHRONIC HEPATITIS

DEFINITION AND CAUSES

Chronic hepatitis is a common reason for persistently abnormal liver function tests[1] and forms the background for the development of much cirrhosis[2] and hepatocellular carcinoma. It is defined as persistence of liver injury with raised aminotransferase levels or viral markers for more than 6 months.[3] This definition, though artificial, helps to establish a borderline in studies of acute and chronic hepatitis. In practice, however, this borderline is not always easy to draw, because acute self-limiting hepatitis is sometimes prolonged beyond 6 months and because chronic hepatitis may have an acute or indefinable onset.

Many chronic liver diseases have an inflammatory component, but the term chronic hepatitis is often restricted to a limited number of causes (Table 9.1). Some of the histological features of this group, such as interface hepatitis and lymphocytic infiltration, are also found in other conditions (Table 9.2) not included in this chapter. For the sake of clarity, a diagnosis of chronic hepatitis should therefore include the probable cause whenever possible.

Table 9.1 Classic causes of chronic hepatitis

Hepatitis B, with or without HDV infection
Hepatitis C
Autoimmune hepatitis
Drug-induced hepatitis
Chronic hepatitis of unknown cause

Table 9.2 Conditions sharing pathological features with classic forms of chronic hepatitis

Wilson's disease
α_1-Antitrypsin deficiency
Primary biliary cirrhosis
Primary sclerosing cholangitis

CLASSIFICATION AND NOMENCLATURE

In 1994, two international working parties recommended the replacement of the old histological classification into chronic active, chronic persistent and chronic lobular hepatitis by a predominantly aetiological classification supplemented by semi-quantitative scoring.[4,5] This reflected the fact that the cause of a chronic hepatitis could, by 1994, be determined in most patients and appropriate treatment given. Also, it had become apparent that the future course of a chronic hepatitis could not after all be accurately predicted from the histological appearances.

Because of the growing importance of the semi-quantitative scoring, particularly in clinical trials of new therapies, this aspect of chronic hepatitis is discussed in detail at the end of the chapter.

USE OF LIVER BIOPSY IN CHRONIC HEPATITIS

Opinion is divided on the need for biopsy in the diagnosis and management of patients with chronic hepatitis.[6,7] Histology continues to play a central role in the assessment of new treatment regimes, however, and is used by many physicians to establish a diagnosis and to guide management.[8,9] Criteria used by physicians for the latter include the severity of the hepatitis (grading), the extent of progression towards cirrhosis (staging) and individual features such as steatosis and iron deposition. In the case of autoimmune hepatitis, liver biopsy plays an important part in the decision to stop treatment.[10] In patients with multiple aetiological agents, biopsy may help to establish their relative importance; an example of this is the patient with thalassaemia and viral hepatitis. Large-cell and small-cell change (dysplasia), possible predictors of hepatocellular carcinoma, are sometimes found before cirrhosis develops but will be discussed with the latter, in Chapter 10. Table 9.3 lists the possible reasons for liver biopsy in chronic hepatitis.

Table 9.3 Uses of liver biopsy in chronic hepatitis

Establishment of the diagnosis
Diagnosis of incidental lesions
Assessment of histological activity (grading)
Evaluation of types of necrosis
Evaluation of structural changes (staging)
Clues to aetiology and possible superinfection
Immunohistochemical assessment of viral antigens
Monitoring of therapy

Portal changes

Most small portal tracts are infiltrated to a variable extent by lymphocytes together with smaller numbers of plasma cells and occasional segmented leucocytes. Lymphoid aggregates and lymphoid follicles with germinal centres are common in, but not exclusive to, hepatitis C. Larger conducting tracts are less affected than small terminal tracts and this has to be taken into account in assessing the severity of a hepatitis.

In the mildest forms of chronic hepatitis, the infiltrate is confined to portal tracts (Fig. 9.1) and the margins of the tracts remain regular. In the more severe forms, infiltration extends into the adjacent parenchyma, as described below. In mild chronic hepatitis, the tracts are often enlarged and short fibrous spurs may be seen extending from them (Fig. 9.2). These and other structural changes are most easily evaluated in reticulin or collagen stains.

Interlobular bile ducts may be damaged, as shown by irregularity of the epithelial wall, vacuolation and infiltration by lymphocytes. Increased ductular profiles are sometimes seen, probably reflecting progenitor-cell activity (see Chapter 4).

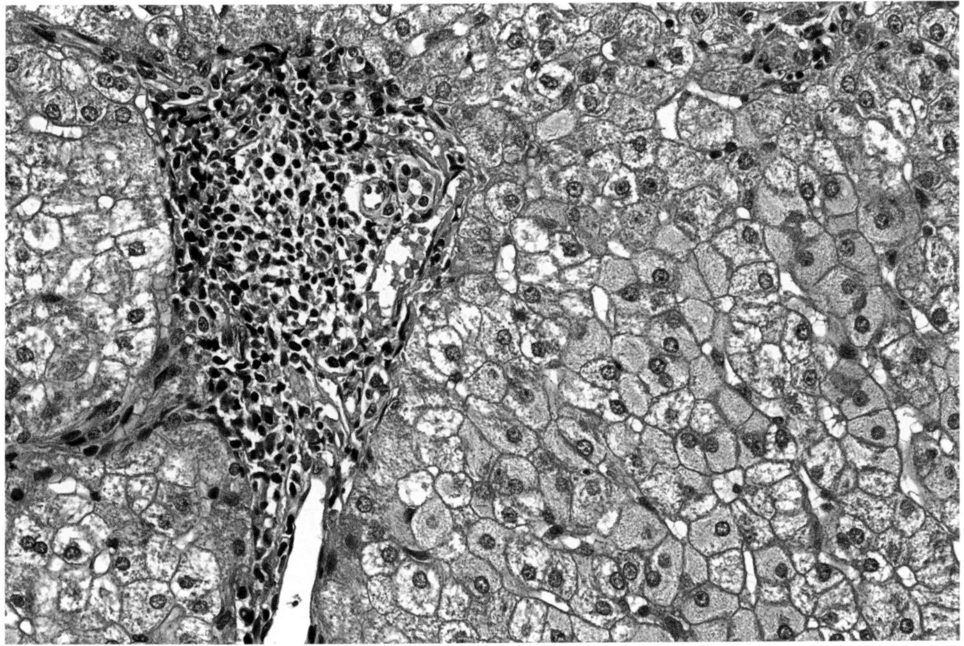

Figure 9.1 *Chronic hepatitis B, mild.* The portal tract is heavily infiltrated with lymphocytes. These do not extend beyond the margins of the tract, the limiting plate of hepatocytes is intact and interface hepatitis is absent. Some hepatocytes have a ground-glass appearance. (Needle biopsy, H&E).

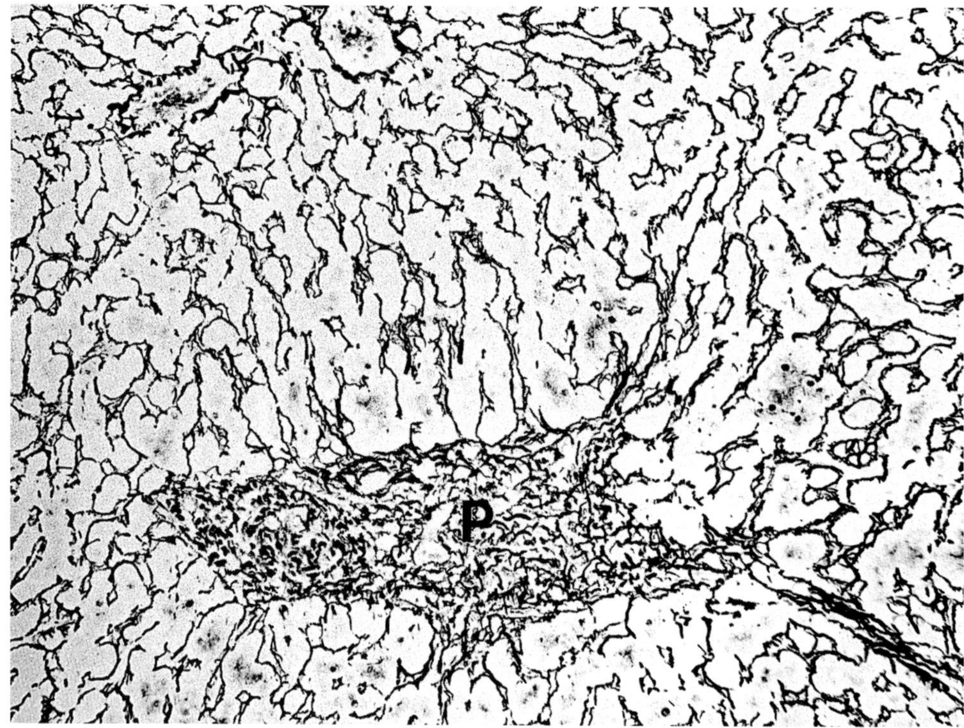

Figure 9.2 *Chronic hepatitis*. Short septa extend from the slightly enlarged portal tract (P) but normal architectural relationships are preserved. (Needle biopsy, reticulin).

Parenchymal changes

The periportal lesion: interface hepatitis

In all but the mildest forms of chronic hepatitis, the inflammatory infiltrate extends from the portal tracts into the adjacent parenchyma and there is destruction of hepatocytes (Figs 9.3, 9.4). This process of interface hepatitis or piecemeal necrosis is most easily identified by the irregularity of the limiting plates of hepatocytes around the portal tracts. The term interface hepatitis is now often preferred to the older term piecemeal necrosis because there is evidence to suggest that apoptosis rather than necrosis may be involved.[11,12] However, the relative roles played by apoptosis and necrosis in viral hepatitis are not yet entirely clear, because the two processes share several characteristics.[13]

Interface hepatitis at its mildest is recognised by lymphocytes in the periportal parenchyma, in association with hepatocellular damage. In more severe examples trapped surviving hepatocytes may be seen within the inflammatory infiltrate (Fig. 9.5) and fibrous septa extend from the portal tract (Fig. 9.6). In cirrhotic livers the process is seen at the edges of nodules and septa rather than immediately around portal tracts (see Fig. 10.19); in either case, however, the hepatitic process involves the interface between connective tissue and parenchyma. Interface hepatitis varies not only in severity but also in the extent of involvement of the interface, whatever its exact location. This is taken into consideration in some grading systems.

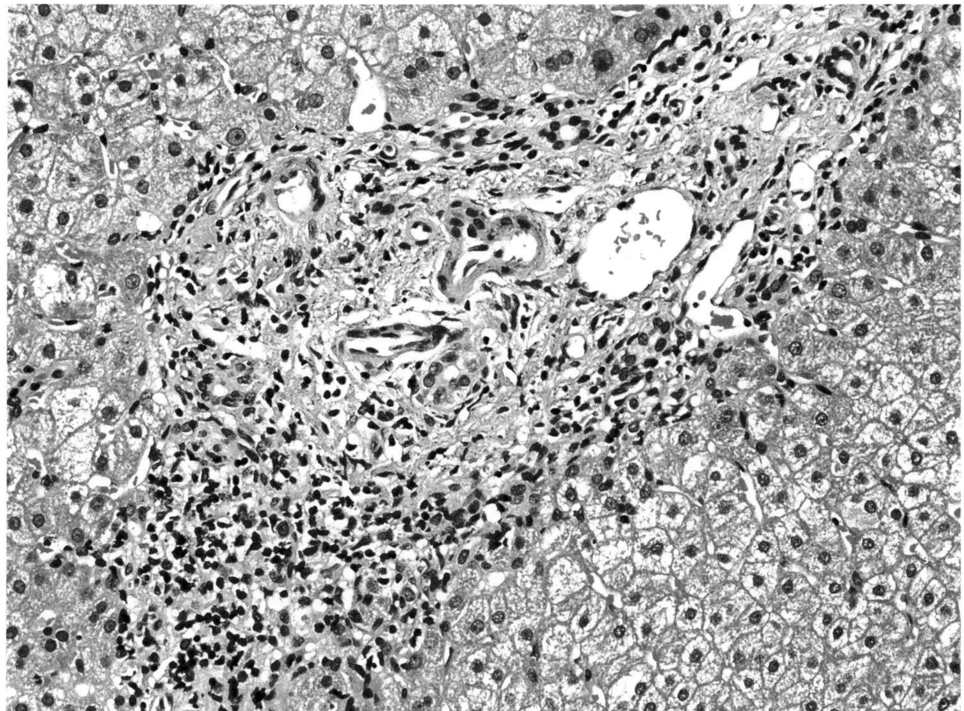

Figure 9.3 *Interface hepatitis.* In contrast to the upper margin of this portal tract, the edges of the lower margin are blurred by inflammatory infiltration and hepatocyte loss. (Needle biopsy, H&E).

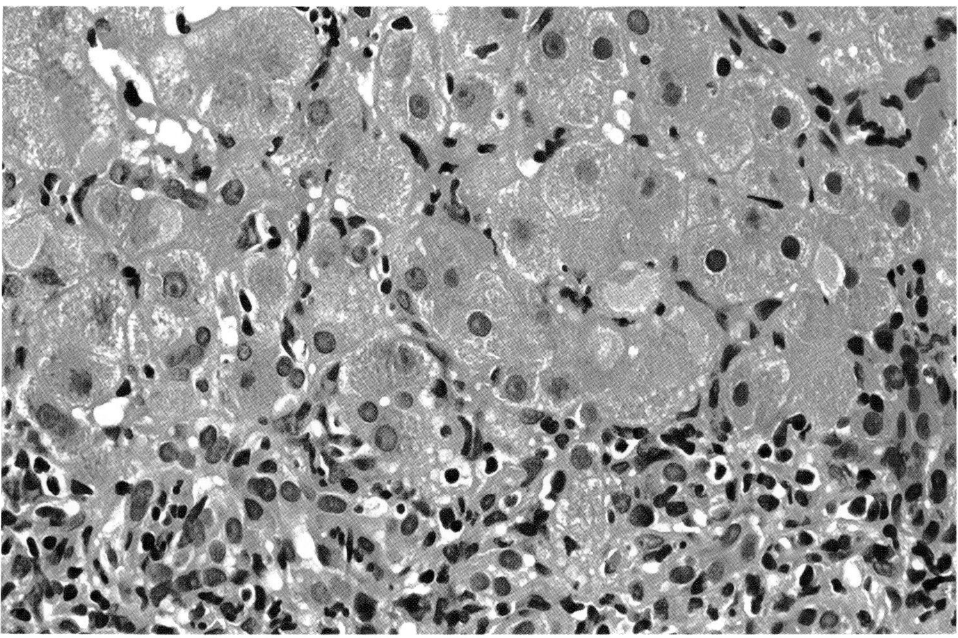

Figure 9.4 *Interface hepatitis.* At a higher magnification than Figure 9.3, lymphocytes are seen infiltrating between surviving hepatocytes. The interface between inflamed portal tract and parenchyma is irregular. (Needle biopsy, H&E).

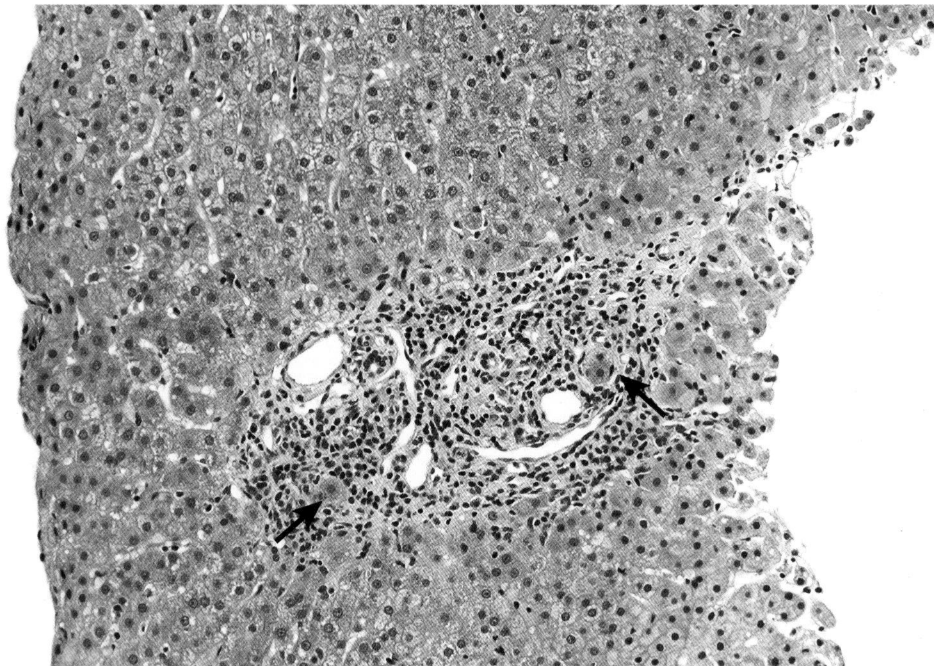

Figure 9.5 *Chronic hepatitis, mild to moderate*. The lower edge of the portal tract shows interface hepatitis, with trapping of hepatocytes in the infiltrate (arrows). (Needle biopsy, H&E).

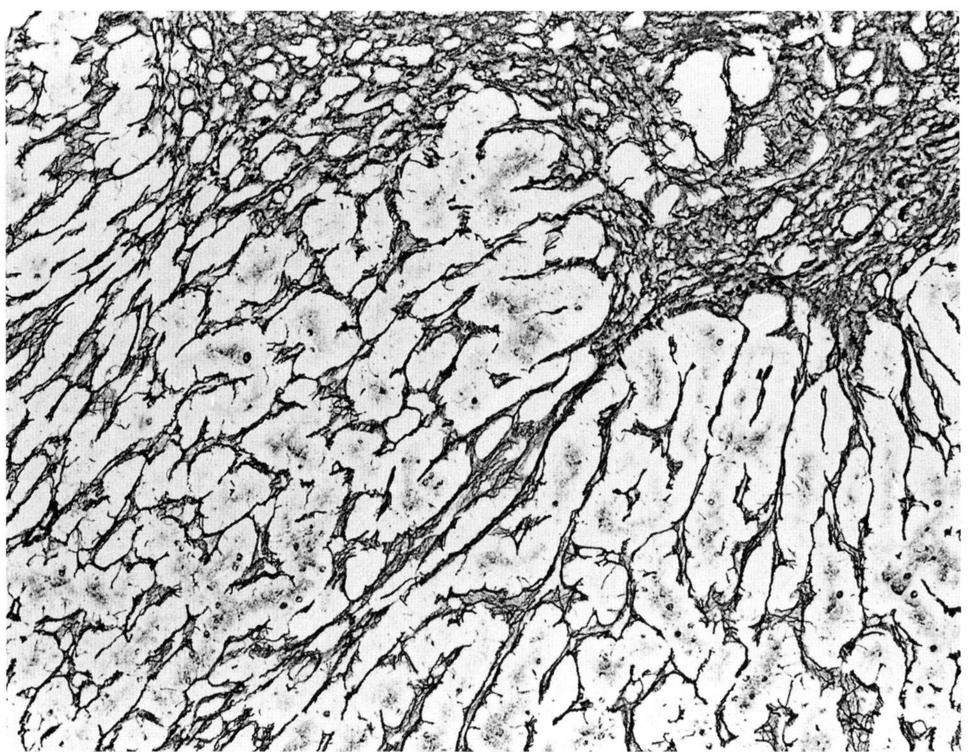

Figure 9.6 *Chronic hepatitis with fibrosis*. Fibrosis extends from the portal tract above into the parenchyma. (Needle biopsy, reticulin).

The lobular lesion

Deeper within the parenchyma there are varying degrees of hepatocellular damage and inflammation, sometimes called the lobular component or lobular hepatitis. Most commonly, this takes the form of focal necrosis, but confluent and bridging necrosis may also be seen. Panlobular necrosis is rare in chronic hepatitis. Also uncommon is the finding of severe lobular hepatitis in the absence of substantial portal and periportal inflammation.[14] The severity of lobular hepatitis correlates with the accumulation of progenitor cells.[15]

Focal (spotty) necrosis is seen as areas of hepatocyte loss with infiltration by lymphocytes, macrophages and other cells. Each area covers the space normally occupied by up to about four or five hepatocytes (Fig. 9.7). Larger areas of hepatocyte loss are referred to as confluent necrosis. However, the borderline between focal and confluent necrosis has not to our knowledge been accurately defined in the literature and the above distinction represents the personal view of the authors. As in acute hepatitis, bridging necrosis refers to confluent necrosis and collapse linking vascular structures and is usually restricted to bridges linking portal tracts to terminal hepatic venules.

Severe lobular hepatitis is often accompanied by the formation of small rounded or ovoid gland-like clusters of surviving hepatocytes, so-called hepatitic rosettes (Fig. 9.8). Unlike cholestatic rosettes (Ch. 4), these are embedded in connective tissue and probably form as a result of hyperplasia of hepatocytes trapped in a collapsed and inflamed area of parenchyma.

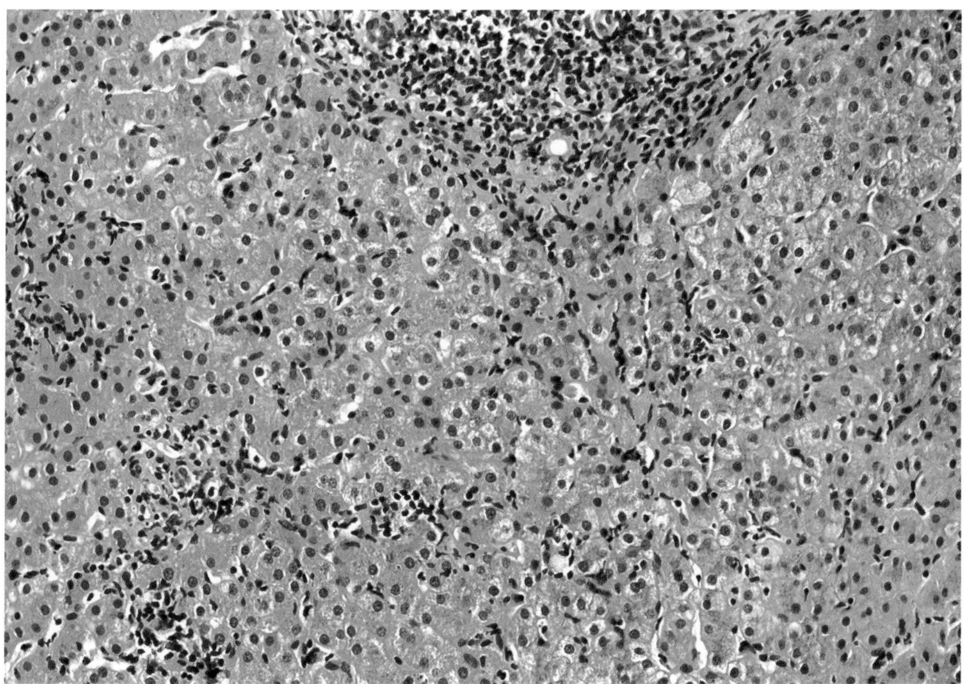

Figure 9.7 *Chronic hepatitis with lobular activity.* Clumps of inflammatory cells, some of them associated with hepatocyte loss, extend through the parenchyma. The portal tract above is inflamed. (Needle biopsy, H&E).

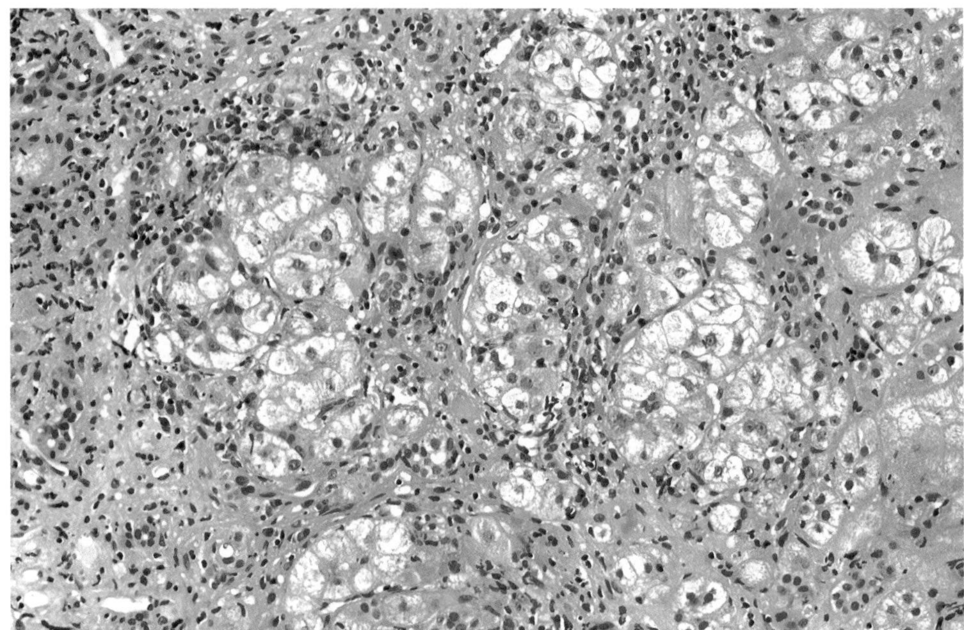

Figure 9.8 *Chronic hepatitis, severe, with rosette formation*. Parenchymal architecture has been completely disrupted. Surviving hepatocytes have formed gland-like rosettes, which are separated by bridges of collapse and inflammation. (Needle biopsy, H&E).

In a minority of patients with chronic hepatitis some of the hepatocytes fuse to form multinucleated giant cells like those of neonatal hepatitis (Fig. 9.9). Suggested trigger mechanisms include cholestasis and autoimmune hepatitis,[16] but giant cell formation is occasionally seen in hepatitis of virtually any cause.

Other hepatocyte changes seen in chronic hepatitis include steatosis, iron deposition and oncocytic change. Steatosis is commonest in chronic hepatitis C and is further discussed under that heading below, as is siderosis. Iron deposits are sometimes focal.[17] Substantial hepatocellular siderosis should always lead to consideration of possible hereditary haemochromatosis, but siderosis is not necessarily related to an HFE gene mutation.[18] Oncocytic change results from the accumulation of large numbers of closely-packed mitochondria in hepatocytes, giving them a granular, densely eosinophilic appearance[19,20] (Fig. 9.9). These cells are most common within hepatitic rosettes. Their significance is uncertain. Finally, the appearance of bile thrombi in dilated canaliculi is most unusual in chronic hepatitis. While this type of cholestasis could result from an acute exacerbation of chronic disease, alternative explanations such as drug hepatotoxicity should be considered.

In some patients with chronic viral or autoimmune hepatitis, distinctive eosinophilic and diastase PAS-positive inclusions are seen in sinusoidal endothelial cells[21] (Fig. 9.10). The inclusions have been shown to contain immunoglobulins.[22]

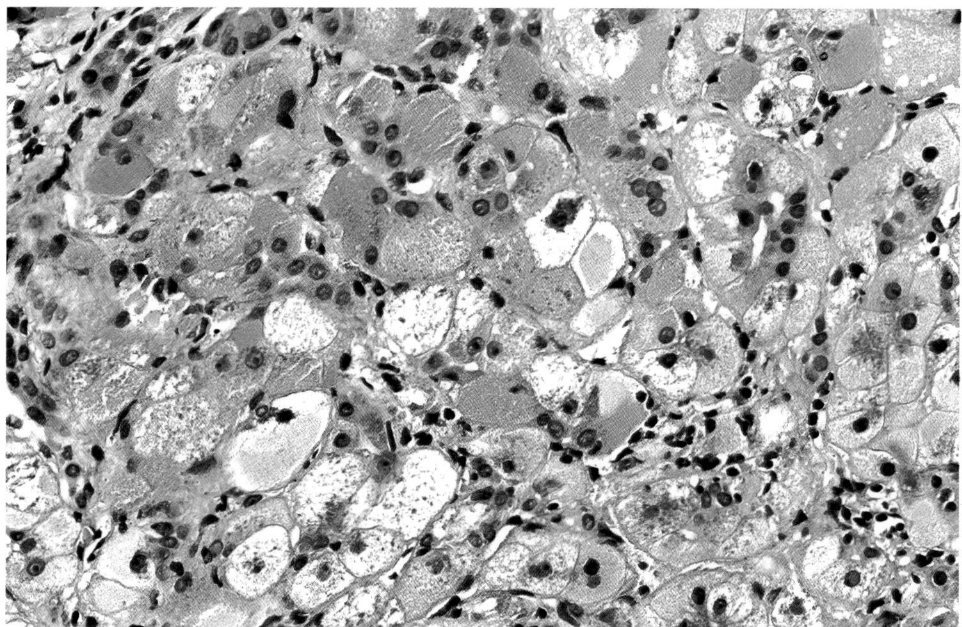

Figure 9.9 *Oncocyte formation in chronic hepatitis*. Some of the hepatocytes in this severe chronic hepatitis have intensely eosinophilic granular cytoplasm. Others have a ground-glass appearance. Many of the hepatocytes are multinucleated. (Needle biopsy, H&E).

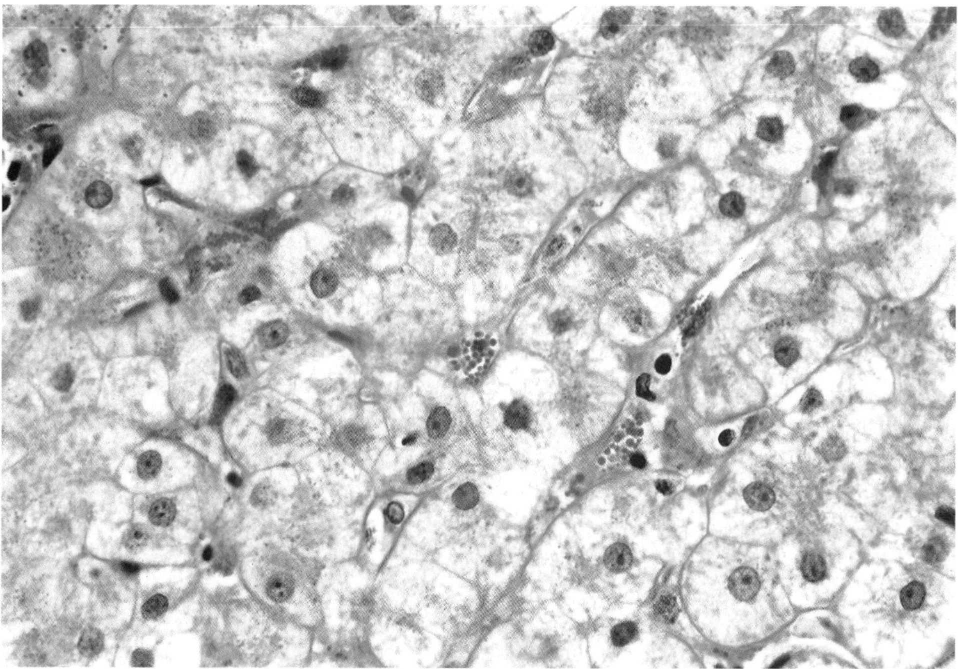

Figure 9.10 *Sinusoidal inclusion-containing endothelial cells*. In this example of chronic hepatitis C, multiple small granular inclusions are seen in the endothelium. (Needle biopsy, diastase-PAS).

Chronic hepatitis B and D

Chronic hepatitis B infection in both adults and children[23,24] goes through a series of phases marked by different serological, histological and immunocytochemical findings.[25] It begins with a period of immune tolerance, in which there are high levels of HBV-DNA in serum. HBeAg is positive and anti-HBe negative. Histological activity varies, and both interface hepatitis and lobular hepatitis may be seen on liver biopsy. However, low levels of activity are more common. The surface antigen, HBsAg, can be demonstrated immunohistochemically. It is most abundant in the characteristic **ground-glass hepatocytes** (Fig. 9.11), but can also be seen in a membranous or submembranous location in hepatocytes without a ground-glass pattern. The ground-glass cells are typically scattered singly throughout the parenchyma at this stage of infection. Their name derives from the finely granular appearance of the central part of the cytoplasm, which is rich in endoplasmic reticulum and hepatitis B surface material. Other organelles are located at the cell periphery and often appear to be separated from the ground-glass area by a pale halo. The differential diagnosis of ground-glass hepatocytes is from the oncocytic cells described in the previous section, from drug-induced hypertrophy of the endoplasmic reticulum (Fig. 8.1) and from inclusion-containing hepatocytes in cyanamide toxicity (Ch. 8), Lafora's disease and fibrinogen storage disease.[26] Clinical circumstances together with immunostaining for HBsAg make confusion unlikely.

The core antigen, HBcAg, is also demonstrable by immunostaining. It is mainly located in hepatocyte nuclei, but also, when necro-inflammatory activity is high, in cytoplasm (Fig. 1.9). Positive nuclear staining correlates with viral load.[27] Nuclei

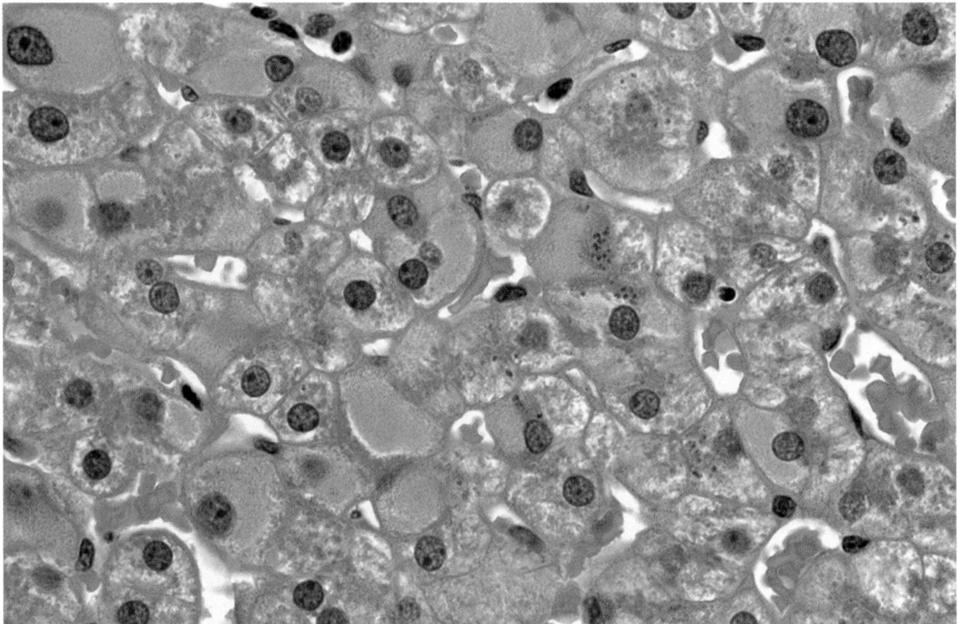

Figure 9.11 *Chronic hepatitis B with ground-glass hepatocytes.* In many hepatocytes the central part of the cytoplasm has a homogeneous ground-glass appearance. A paler-staining halo is seen around the ground-glass areas in some cells. (Needle biopsy, H&E).

which contain large amounts of core protein sometimes have a pale, homogeneous appearance on H&E-stained section and have been described as 'sanded'.[28]

The immunotolerant phase of chronic HBV infection is followed by immune clearance and seroconversion to a non-replicative phase in which HBeAg disappears from serum to be replaced by anti-HBe. During the phase of immune clearance, of very variable length, histological activity is typically high.

In the third, non-replicative phase, histological activity is usually considered to be low, as are markers of viral replication. However, in a large study of liver biopsies from patients in this phase, about one third showed varying degrees of interface hepatitis, sometimes in the presence of normal aminotransferase levels.[29] Lobular activity was not necessarily accompanied by portal and periportal inflammation. Ground-glass hepatocytes may be aggregated in focal accumulations in the non-replicative phase.

Reactivation of virus replication and histological activity are common and are sometimes associated with the emergence of viral mutants. In some of these mutants, expression of HBeAg is defective and histological activity is unexpectedly high, in spite of the negative HBeAg and presence of anti-HBe.

Finally, in a minority of patients with chronic HBV infection, HBsAg becomes negative and anti-HBs appears in the serum. HBV-DNA may still be detectable in small amounts in serum and liver.

This complex evolution, not always as orderly as the above simplified description might suggest, is marked by a very variable degree of fibrosis, depending on the severity and timing of the hepatitic process. Cirrhosis may develop at any stage, especially in patients whose HBV infection is complicated by infection with other viruses such as HCV and HDV.[30]

Apart from the presence of ground-glass hepatocytes and HBV antigens, there are other features which characterise chronic hepatitis B. Marked variation in the size and appearance of hepatocyte nuclei has been described,[31] as has close contact between hepatocytes and lymphocytes,[32] in keeping with the immunological nature of the hepatitis. The lymphocytes are usually of CD8+ type, in contrast to the portal infiltrate which is rich in CD4+ lymphocytes, B lymphocytes and dendritic cells.[33] Lymphoid follicles are occasionally found in portal tracts but are less common and less prominent than in hepatitis C.[34]

Infection with the delta virus (HDV) modifies infection with the hepatitis B virus, as already noted in Chapter 6. Its presence is associated with relatively high histological activity except after liver transplantation. Inflammation is rarely restricted to portal tracts, and there is likely to be substantial inflammation in periportal areas as well as deeper within the lobules. Positive immunostaining for HDV (see Fig. 6.16) denotes active infection. A 'sanded' appearance similar to that produced by hepatitis core protein may be seen when there is abundant HDV in hepatocyte nuclei.[35] In the presence of HDV infection there is a greater risk of chronicity than with HBV alone, and liver-associated mortality is increased.[36] Once cirrhosis has developed in patients with hepatitis B, HDV infection confers a greater risk of developing hepatocellular carcinoma and a higher mortality.[37]

Chronic hepatitis C

Chronic hepatitis C affects more than 170 million persons worldwide.[38] It is not usually life-threatening until cirrhosis develops, typically several decades after onset of the hepatitis. Factors associated with faster progression to cirrhosis include older age,[39] male sex, fibrosis on initial biopsy,[40] high necro-inflammatory activity on initial biopsy,[41] iron deposition (see Pathological features, below), alcohol consumption, previous HBV infection[42] and HIV infection.[43] There are six different genotypes of the virus,[44] affecting disease severity and response to specific treatment,[45] patients with genotypes 2 and 3 responding best to specific therapy.

The use of liver biopsy in the management of patients with HCV infection has been the subject of extensive discussion. There are serious efforts to replace biopsy to some extent with formulae based on biochemical findings,[46,47] but these fail to predict histological findings accurately.[8,9] Repeatedly normal or near-normal serum aminotransferases suggest mild histological changes,[48] yet a substantial proportion of such patients has been found to have serious liver damage and even cirrhosis.[49,50] The consensus view appears to be that liver biopsy currently continues to provide useful information not obtainable in other ways.[7,51,52]

Pathological features

The histological features of chronic hepatitis C, although not completely diagnostic in themselves, are very characteristic[34,53] (Table 9.4). The portal infiltrate is rich in lymphocytes which often form aggregates or follicles, some of them with prominent germinal centres (Fig. 9.12). These follicles are easily identified in reticulin preparations (Fig. 9.13). Follicles are not restricted to hepatitis C and can also be found in hepatitis B, autoimmune hepatitis and primary biliary cirrhosis, but in hepatitis C they are particularly common and prominent. Within, or to one side of the lymphoid infiltrates, damaged interlobular bile ducts may be seen, as in acute hepatitis. The damage takes the form of vacuolation, stratification and crowding of epithelial cells, and infiltration by lymphocytes.[54] The virus has been demonstrated in bile-duct epithelium and in bile.[55] Bile-duct damage is occasionally but by no means always associated with a clinically cholestatic course, and rare ductopenia has been reported.[56,57]

The intralobular changes typically include acidophilic degeneration of hepatocytes and formation of acidophil bodies, already described in Chapter 6. Confluent necrosis is uncommon. Sinusoids are focally or diffusely infiltrated by lymphocytes, giving rise in some biopsies to a striking beaded appearance reminiscent of infectious mononucleosis. Epithelioid-cell granulomas are occasionally found in lobules or portal tracts[58,59] and clumped material somewhat

Table 9.4 Histological features of chronic type C hepatitis

Histological features
Difficult to distinguish from acute hepatitis C
Often mild, but cirrhosis commonly develops
Lymphoid follicles in portal tracts
Damaged interlobular bile ducts
Lobular activity including acidophil bodies
Large-droplet steatosis
Lymphocytes in sinusoids
Granulomas

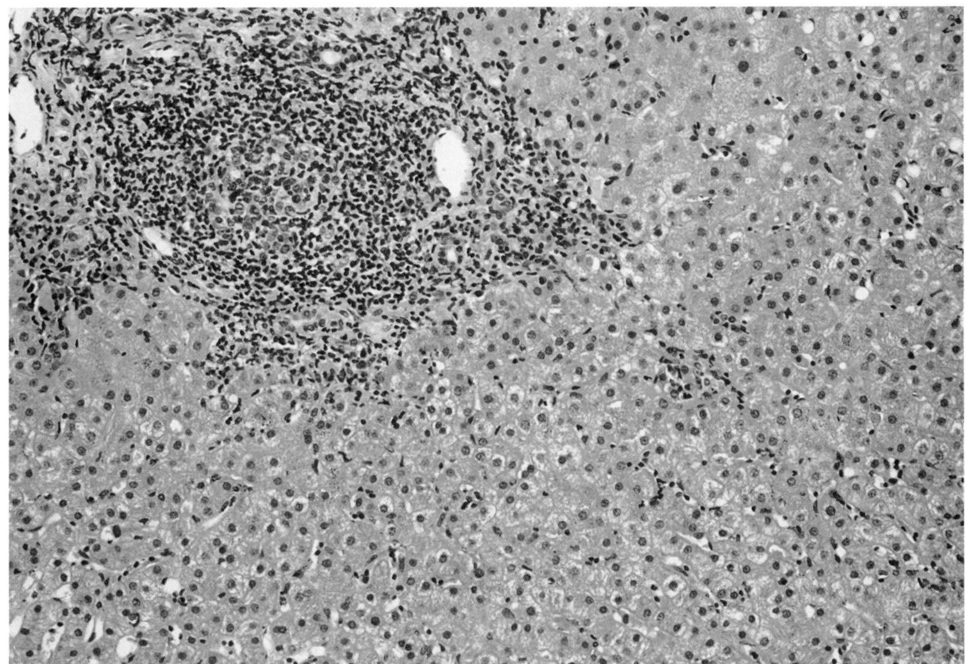

Figure 9.12 *Chronic hepatitis C.* The portal tract top left is heavily infiltrated by lymphocytes, which extend irregularly into the adjacent tissue. A lymphoid follicle with germinal centre has formed. (Needle biopsy, H&E). (Colour version of a half-tone figure in Scheuer PJ, Ashrafzadeh P, Sherlock S, et al.[34] with permission from the publishers).

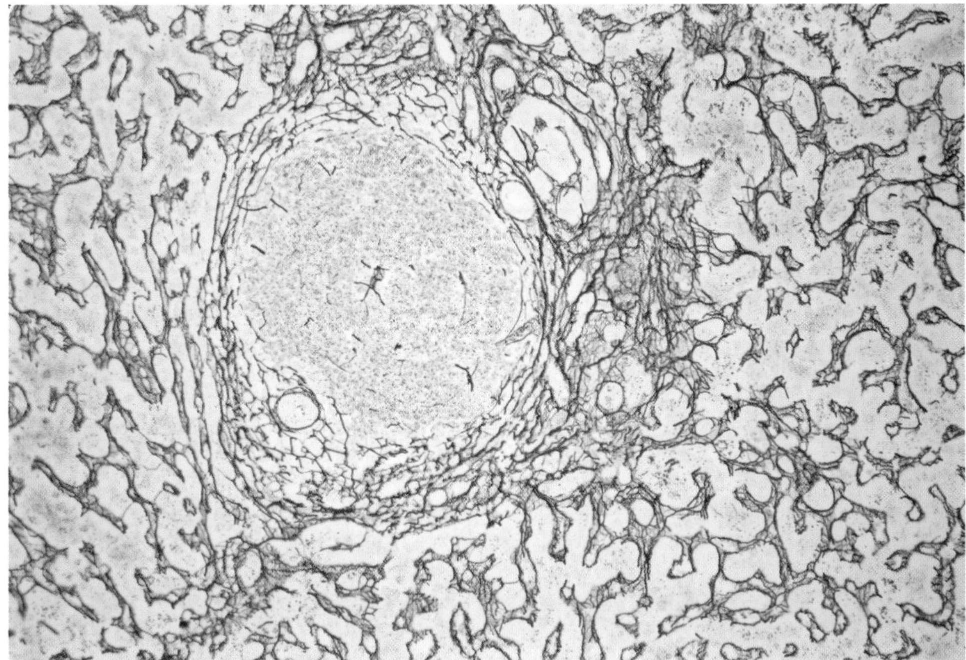

Figure 9.13 *Chronic hepatitis C.* The prominent pale area in the portal tract is the site of a lymphoid follicle. (Needle biopsy, reticulin).

like Mallory bodies has been reported in periportal hepatocytes.[60] The presence of talc crystals in liver tissue, seen by polarised light microscopy, is a specific, but insensitive marker of intravenous drug abuse.[61]

Iron deposition is common even in the absence of the frequently found HFE mutations of hereditary haemochromatosis and may influence progression of the disease.[62,63] Iron is seen not only in hepatocytes, but also in macrophages, endothelial cells and portal tracts.[64,65]

There is an extensive recent literature on the significance of steatosis in chronic hepatitis C. As already noted, steatosis is more common in hepatitis C than in other forms of chronic hepatitis and may be quite severe. It is a risk factor for progression,[66,67] and can interfere with therapy. The steatosis is often associated with obesity, diabetes or alcohol consumption.[68–71] However, in infection with HCV genotype 3[72,73] and very occasionally other genotypes,[74] the virus appears to have a direct effect and the steatosis improves after successful treatment.[75,76] The mechanism for the steatosis may be interference by the viral core protein with lipoprotein assembly and secretion.[77] In addition to steatosis, features of steatohepatitis such as pericellular fibrosis have been reported.[78]

The development of reliable and clinically useful methods for detecting viral proteins by immunohistochemistry has been hampered by the small amounts of virus present in each cell, at least in immunocompetent patients. Immunohistochemical staining with a monoclonal antibody against an envelope protein of the virus (HCV-E2) has recently proved successful in both frozen and paraffin-embedded material.[79] Finely granular positivity in the cytoplasm of hepatocytes was obtained with a sensitivity of 96% and specificity of 91%. The technique may have practical application in evaluating early graft infection after liver transplantation and in evaluating the effects of therapy.

In biopsies taken early in the course of the disease, the hepatitis is often mild, with little interface hepatitis or fibrosis. With time, fibrous septa extend from expanded portal tracts and link vascular structures. Fibrosis linking portal tracts has the appearance of web-like membranes on three-dimensional reconstruction.[80] A pericellular pattern of fibrosis in perivenular areas has been reported in children.[81] Spontaneous clearance of virus[82] or specific treatment of the infection[83] may bring about dramatic improvement of the fibrosis and structural changes.

Autoimmune hepatitis

Autoimmune hepatitis (AIH) is diagnosed mainly on the basis of serum autoantibodies and absence of evidence for other causes of chronic hepatitis. The autoantibody profile is the basis for subclassification into different types.[84] Histological evidence is important not only for confirming the diagnosis, but also as a means of detecting other conditions with which AIH may be confused. Histology is therefore one component of a scoring system, originally designed as a research tool but also now used in clinical practice.[85]

While there are no pathognomonic histological features of AIH, there is a characteristic picture in many patients before treatment. Biopsy shows active disease, with much hepatocellular damage and a heavy infiltrate of lymphocytes and plasma cells in portal tracts, at the interface and deep within the parenchyma (Figs 9.14, 9.15). Eosinophils may also be present.[86] Lymphoid follicles are less prominent than in hepatitis C. Bridging necrosis is common and surviving hepatocytes often form

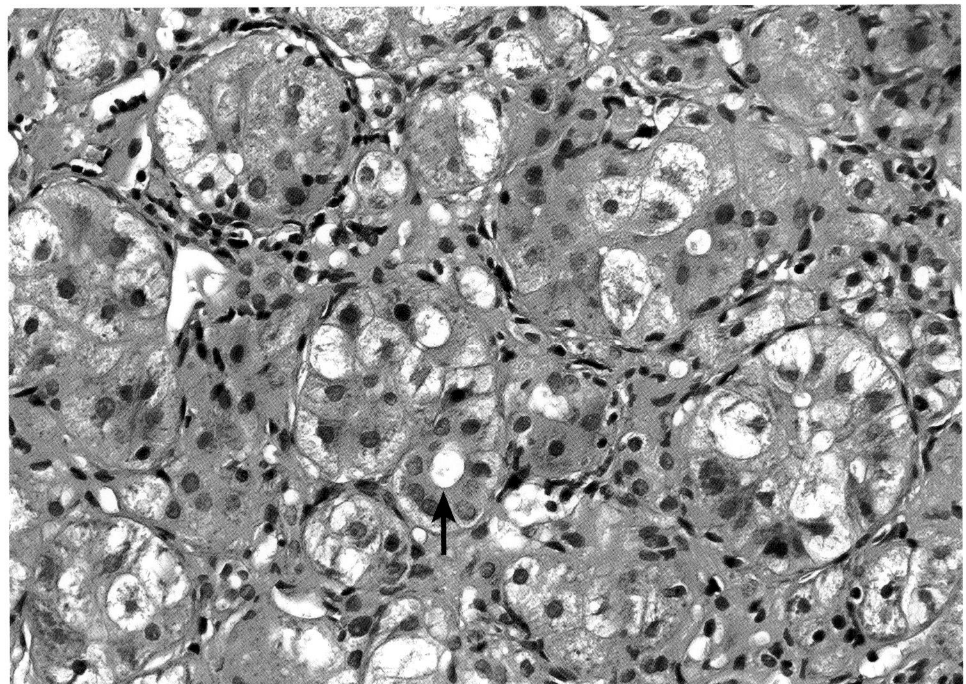

Figure 9.14 *Autoimmune hepatitis with rosette formation.* Rounded hepatitic rosettes, some with visible lumen (arrow), are surrounded by compressed sinusoids, fibrous tissue and inflammatory cells. (Needle biopsy, H&E).

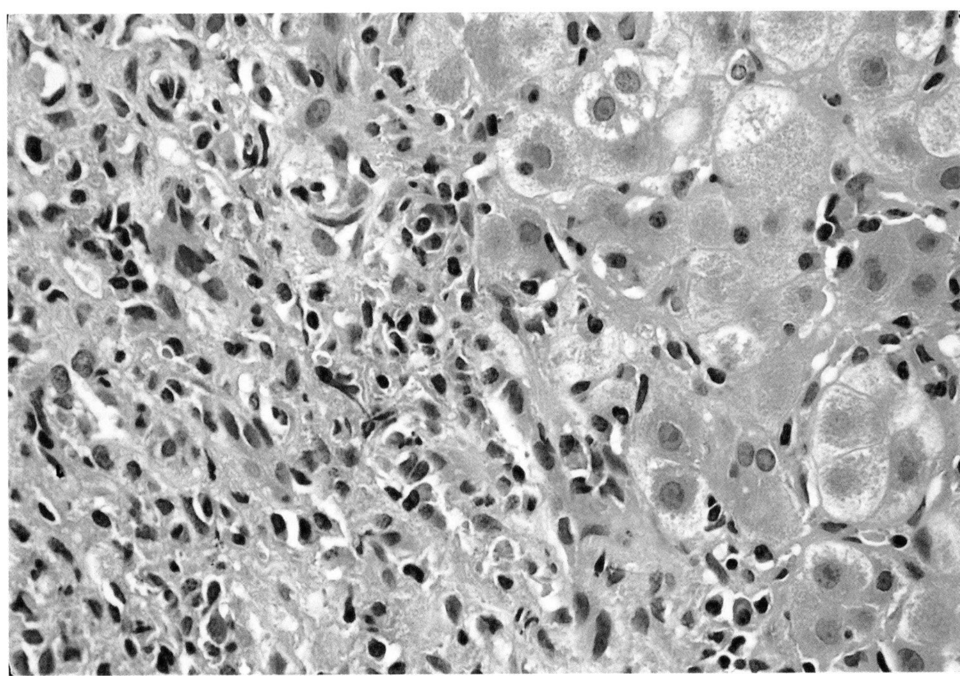

Figure 9.15 *Autoimmune hepatitis.* Inflammatory cells including plasma cells extend from the portal tract (left) into the parenchyma as part of the process of interface hepatitis. (Needle biopsy, H&E).

hepatitic rosettes (Fig. 9.14). Prominent syncytial giant hepatocytes in an adult hepatitis, while not diagnostic, should always raise the possibility of AIH.[87,88]

This classic histological picture is not, however, the only one seen in AIH and communication between pathologist and clinician is important to ensure a correct diagnosis.[89] Plasma cells are not always present in large numbers. In some patients the hepatitis is much milder, and in some there may be cholestasis, bile-duct damage or even ductopenia.[90,91] In adults, this has to be distinguished from the bile-duct lesions of primary biliary cirrhosis and the relatively uncommon overlap syndromes (Ch. 5). In children, AIH is often associated with an autoimmune form of sclerosing cholangitis.[92,93]

Autoimmune hepatitis is regarded as a chronic disease in all patients, but the clinical onset is sometimes acute. In a study of 26 patients biopsied within 6 months of onset,[94] most showed evidence of chronicity and a few had cirrhosis. However, careful analysis of connective tissue septa with the help of several connective tissue stains (Ch. 6) sometimes suggests recent onset with rapid development of nodules. Furthermore there are a few patients with AIH in whom the principal features on presentation are confluent necrosis and inflammation in perivenular areas, as in an acute hepatitis[95–98] (Fig. 9.16).

Patients with AIH usually respond rapidly to corticosteroid therapy. Biopsy following treatment shows varying degrees of resolution of the necro-inflammatory process and sometimes dramatic improvement in fibrosis and structural changes.[99,100] Liver biopsy helps to determine when corticosteroid treatment can safely be withdrawn.[10] The degree of plasma cell infiltration is a predictor of relapse,[101] and worsening histological activity appears to correlate with progression of fibrosis.[102] Biopsy therefore continues to play an important role in patient management.

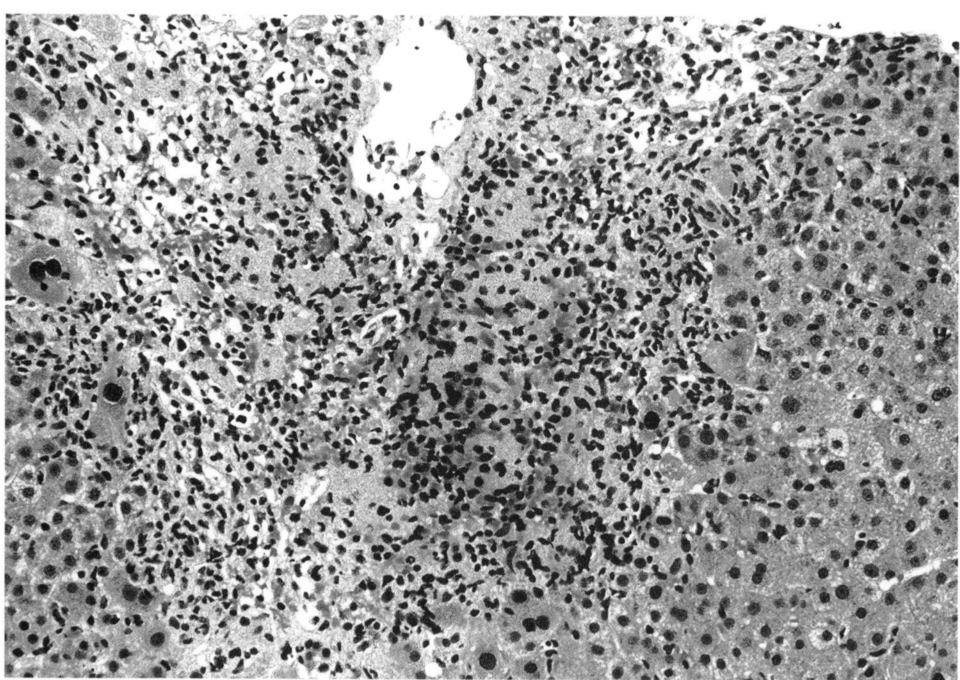

Figure 9.16 *Autoimmune hepatitis with confluent perivenular necrosis.* The parenchyma around an efferent venule (top centre) has been almost completely replaced by necrotic debris and inflammatory cells. (Needle biopsy, H&E).

DIFFERENTIAL DIAGNOSIS OF CHRONIC HEPATITIS

In biopsies with inflammation confined to portal tracts, other possibilities to be considered include **resolving acute hepatitis, non-specific inflammation near a focal lesion, primary biliary cirrhosis** and **lymphoma**. The nature of the infiltrate and involvement of most or all portal tracts in chronic hepatitis should resolve the issue in most cases, but clinical information is also needed.

More severe chronic hepatitis needs to be distinguished from **acute hepatitis**, which is sometimes difficult. As discussed in Chapter 6, staining for elastic fibres may enable recently-formed bridges to be distinguished from old fibrous septa. Canalicular cholestasis, common in acute hepatitis, is not often found in chronic hepatitis. In HBV infection in an immunocompetent patient the presence of HBsAg-containing ground-glass hepatocytes indicates chronic disease.

Other diseases to be considered in the more severe forms include **chronic biliary diseases**, especially primary biliary cirrhosis and primary sclerosing cholangitis, **α_1-antitrypsin deficiency, Wilson's disease, lymphoma** and **drug injury**. Loss of bile ducts and periportal accumulation of copper-associated protein suggest biliary disease rather than chronic hepatitis. α_1-Antitrypsin deficiency can be diagnosed by appropriate staining (Ch. 13), while Wilson's disease (Ch. 14) should be established principally by clinical features and biochemical findings. The infiltrates of various lymphomas are usually extensive and irregular and may undergo necrosis. Drugs sometimes cause a liver disease closely resembling AIH, or may act as a trigger, unmasking latent autoimmunity.[103] As in all liver diseases, correlation of clinical and histological findings reduces the risk of diagnostic error.

SEMI-QUANTITATIVE SCORING: GRADING AND STAGING

Scoring is now widely used to evaluate liver biopsies before treatment, to monitor the effects of treatment and to assess the effects of new therapies in clinical trials. It consists of two components, their names borrowed from oncology: **grading** and **staging**. Grading refers to the scoring of the necro-inflammatory lesion of a hepatitis, including the various types and degrees of hepatocellular damage and the location and extent of the inflammatory process. Staging records the extent of fibrosis and of changes in structure, including the development of cirrhosis. In many scoring systems, grading is subdivided into categories such as portal inflammation, interface hepatitis and lobular hepatitis, while staging is expressed as a single scale.

Assessment of fibrosis can also be carried out using morphometric measurement of collagen.[104,105] This gives an accurate measurement of the amount of fibrous tissue per unit area, but does not take structural changes such as nodule formation into account. Staging and morphometry should therefore be viewed as complementary to each other and not as alternatives.

Scoring is semi-quantitative rather than quantitative in the sense that, while scores are usually expressed as numbers, they do not represent measurements. Scoring involves subjective assessment of the various relevant histological features in a biopsy, and the scores allotted will inevitably vary somewhat from observer to observer depending on experience and personal bias. For this reason, comparison of scores allotted at different times or by different observers cannot be directly compared. This limits the usefulness of scoring as a routine reporting procedure.

Before embarking on scoring, the pathologist should consider carefully why the scores are required. This will help to determine the most suitable system for the particular purpose or project. For example, if what is needed is a decision as to whether the chronic hepatitis in a particular patient is mild, moderate or severe, a simple system will suffice, and will usually have the advantage over more complex systems in so far as the latter tend to be associated with greater intra- and inter-observer variation and are also more time-consuming. If, on the other hand, the purpose is to evaluate a group of biopsies in a clinical trial of a new treatment regime, then a complex system is more appropriate. A complex system would allow analysis not only of the overall severity of the changes, but also of individual features such as interface hepatitis and lobular activity. Examples of two simple systems are given in Table 9.5[106] and Table 9.6.[107] The simple staging system proposed by the METAVIR group[108] is given in Table 9.7, and the more complex and widely used Ishak system,[109] derived from the earlier Knodell Histology Activity Index,[110] in Table 9.8.

The results of a particular study can be compared in a general way with those of another, but because of the subjective nature of scoring, the numbers themselves cannot be directly compared or combined. Each study therefore stands on its own to some extent and the observers are free to modify a published scoring system to suit a particular purpose. For instance, a scoring range for steatosis, siderosis or bile-duct damage could be devised and added if required.

Reproducibility of scoring is improved when it is performed by more than one observer.[108] There should then be an initial discussion using a multi-headed microscope in order to ensure that all observers agree on the criteria used to score each feature. At the end of a study, discrepancies between observers can be resolved by joint discussion at the microscope. In a clinical trial, it may be helpful to re-assess

Table 9.5 A simple scoring system for chronic hepatitis

1. Grade
   - A. Portal inflammation and interface hepatitis
     - 0 Absent or minimal
     - 1 Portal inflammation only
     - 2 Mild or localised interface hepatitis
     - 3 Moderate or more extensive interface hepatitis
     - 4 Severe and widespread interface hepatitis
   - B. Lobular activity
     - 0 None
     - 1 Inflammatory cells but no hepatocellular damage
     - 2 Focal necrosis or apoptosis
     - 3 Severe hepatocellular damage
     - 4 Damage includes bridging confluent necrosis
2. Stage
   - 0 No fibrosis
   - 1 Fibrosis confined to portal tracts
   - 2 Periportal or portal–portal septa but intact vascular relationships
   - 3 Fibrosis with distorted structure but no obvious cirrhosis
   - 4 Probable or definite cirrhosis

Modified by permission from Elsevier from Scheuer.[106]

Table 9.6 The METAVIR algorithm

Interface hepatitis[a] (Piecemeal necrosis)		Lobular necrosis[b]		Overall histological activity[c]
0	+	0	=	0
0	+	1	=	1
0	+	2	=	2
1	+	0	=	1
1	+	1	=	1
1	+	2	=	2
2	+	0	=	2
2	+	1	=	2
2	+	2	=	3
3	+	0	=	3
3	+	1	=	3
3	+	2	=	3

[a]Interface hepatitis scored 0 (none), 1 (mild), 2 (moderate), 3 (severe).
[b]Lobular necrosis scored 0 (none or mild), 1 (moderate), 2 (severe).
[c]Histological activity scored 0 (none), 1 (mild), 2 (moderate), 3 (severe).
Modified by permission of Wiley-Liss, Inc., from Bedossa et al.[107]

Table 9.7 The METAVIR staging system

F0	No fibrosis
F1	Stellate enlargement of portal tracts but without septum formation
F2	Enlargement of portal tracts with rare septum formation
F3	Numerous septa without cirrhosis
F4	Cirrhosis

Modified by permission of Wiley-Liss, Inc., from Bedossa, et al.[108]

a proportion of biopsies in order to test intra-observer variation. The scoring should be performed by the same observer or observers throughout, and is usually done without knowledge of clinical data.

Interpretation of the results of scoring

When the scores from a group of biopsies are assessed, the statistical methods used to evaluate the results must be appropriate for categorical data. An example of a suitable method is that used by Lagging et al.[111] Some grading systems are divided into several categories. In the case of the Ishak score, these are interface hepatitis, confluent necrosis, lobular activity and portal inflammation. For each of these four categories the scale from 0 to 4 or 0 to 6 is not exactly linear and it is therefore not acceptable to add the four scores together and then to manipulate the result as if it were a true mathematical sum. To put the matter another way, a score of 2 for any particular feature does not denote exactly twice 1 or precisely half of 4, but simply a

Table 9.8 The Ishak scoring system

Category	Score
Grading	
A. Periportal or periseptal interface hepatitis	
Absent	0
Mild (focal, few portal areas)	1
Mild/moderate (focal, most portal areas)	2
Moderate (continuous around <50% of tracts or septa)	3
Severe (continuous around >50% of tracts or septa)	4
B. Confluent necrosis	
Absent	0
Focal	1
Zone 3 necrosis in some areas	2
Zone 3 necrosis in most areas	3
Zone 3 necrosis + occasional portal–central bridging	4
Zone 3 necrosis + multiple portal–central bridging	5
Panacinar or multiacinar necrosis	6
C. Focal (spotty) lytic necrosis, apoptosis and focal inflammation[a]	
Absent	0
<2 foci per 10 × objective	1
2–4 foci per 10 × objective	2
5–10 foci per 10 × objective	3
>10 foci per 10 × objective	4
D. Portal inflammation	
None	0
Mild, some or all portal areas	1
Moderate, some or all portal areas	2
Moderate/marked, all portal areas	3
Marked, all portal areas	4
Staging	
No fibrosis	0
Fibrous expansion of some portal areas, with or without short fibrous septa	1
Fibrous expansion of most portal areas, with or without short fibrous septa	2
Fibrous expansion of most portal areas with occasional portal–portal bridging	3
Fibrous expansion of portal areas with marked bridging (portal–portal and portal–central)	4
Marked bridging (portal–portal and/or portal–central) with occasional nodules (incomplete cirrhosis)	5
Cirrhosis, probable or definite	6

[a]Does not include diffuse sinusoidal infiltration by inflammatory cells.
Adapted by permission from Elsevier from Ishak K, et al.[109]

score somewhere between 1 and 3. Nevertheless, total grading scores are often used and published. In routine practice a total grading score gives an approximate indication of the severity of a patient's hepatitis, but no information on the relative contribution of each category. In clinical trials of new therapies, total grading scores are potentially misleading and the effect of the therapy on each individual grading category should be examined.

The possibility or indeed likelihood of sampling variation must also be kept in mind.[112] In chronic hepatitis C, there are differences between the findings in the left and the right lobe of the liver.[113] More important, small needle biopsy samples may be misleading. Recent studies have thrown light on this particular issue. In one study using image analysis to assess fibrosis, the ability of the image analysis to predict a METAVIR fibrosis score diminished progressively in specimens less than 25 mm long[104]. In another study, reducing the sample size optically led to underestimation of disease severity in samples less than 20 mm long and 1.4 mm wide.[114] According to this study, samples obtained with fine needles were considered unsatisfactory for scoring. Another group recommended that the use of fine needles in diffuse HCV-related liver disease should be restricted to early non-fibrotic lesions.[115] While not all investigators agree that fine-needle specimens are inadequate for grading and staging,[116] specimen size is clearly a critical issue.

In conclusion, many factors limit the accuracy of semi-quantitative scoring in chronic hepatitis.[117] Awareness of these factors, careful attempts to minimise observer variation and appropriate interpretation of the results should ensure the continued usefulness of grading and staging in clinical practice and research.

REFERENCES

1 Berasain C, Betes M, Panizo A, et al. Pathological and virological findings in patients with persistent hypertransaminasaemia of unknown aetiology. *Gut* 2000; **47**: 429–435.

2 Hano H, Takasaki S. Three-dimensional observations on the alterations of lobular architecture in chronic hepatitis with special reference to its angioarchitecture for a better understanding of the formal pathogenesis of liver cirrhosis. *Virchows Arch* 2003; **443**: 655–663.

3 Diseases of the Liver and Biliary Tract. Standardization of Nomenclature, Diagnostic Criteria, and Prognosis. New York: Raven Press, 1994.

4 Desmet VJ, Gerber M, Hoofnagle JH, et al. Classification of chronic hepatitis: diagnosis, grading and staging. *Hepatology* 1994; **19**: 1513–1520.

5 International Working Party. Terminology of chronic hepatitis, hepatic allograft rejection, and nodular lesions of the liver: summary of recommendations developed by an international working party, supported by the World Congresses of Gastroenterology, Los Angeles 1994. *Am J Gastroenterol* 1994; **89**: S177–S181.

6 Andriulli A, Festa V, Leandro G, et al. Usefulness of a liver biopsy in the evaluation of patients with elevated ALT values and serological markers of hepatitis viral infection: an AIGO study. *Dig Dis Sci* 2001; **46**: 1409–1415.

7 Saadeh S, Cammell G, Carey WD, et al. The role of liver biopsy in chronic hepatitis C. *Hepatology* 2001; **33**: 196–200.

8 Gebo KA, Herlong HF, Torbenson MS, et al. Role of liver biopsy in management of chronic hepatitis C: a systematic review. *Hepatology* 2002; **36**: S161–S172.

9 Bain VG, Bonacini M, Govindarajan S, et al. A multicentre study of the usefulness of liver biopsy in hepatitis C. *J Viral Hepat* 2004; **11**: 375–382.

10 Czaja AJ, Carpenter HA. Histological features associated with relapse after corticosteroid withdrawal in type 1 autoimmune hepatitis. *Liver Int* 2003; **23**: 116–123.

11 Lau JYN, Xie X, Lai MMC, et al. Apoptosis and viral hepatitis. *Semin Liver Dis* 1998; **18**: 169–176.

12 Oksuz M, Akkiz H, Isiksal F, et al. Expression of Fas antigen in liver tissue of patients with chronic hepatitis B and C. *Eur J Gastroenterol Hepatol* 2004; **16**: 341–345.

13 Jaeschke H, Gujral J, Bajt M. Apoptosis and necrosis in liver disease. *Liver Int* 2004; **24**: 85–89.
14 Liaw YF, Chu CM, Chen TJ, et al. Chronic lobular hepatitis: a clinicopathological and prognostic study. *Hepatology* 1982; **2**: 258–262.
15 Libbrecht L, Desmet V, Van Damme B, et al. Deep intralobular extension of human hepatic 'progenitor cells' correlates with parenchymal inflammation in chronic viral hepatitis: can 'progenitor cells' migrate? *J Pathol* 2000; **192**: 373–378.
16 Protzer U, Dienes HP, Bianchi L, et al. Post-infantile giant cell hepatitis in patients with primary sclerosing cholangitis and autoimmune hepatitis. *Liver* 1996; **16**: 274–282.
17 Lefkowitch JH, Yee HT, Sweeting J, et al. Iron-rich foci in chronic viral hepatitis. *Hum Pathol* 1998; **29**: 116–118.
18 Martinelli AL, Filho AB, Franco RF, et al. Liver iron deposits in hepatitis B patients: Association with severity of liver disease but not with hemochromatosis gene mutations. *J Gastroenterol Hepatol* 2004; **19**: 1036–1041.
19 Lefkowitch JH, Arborgh BA, Scheuer PJ. Oxyphilic granular hepatocytes. Mitochondrion-rich liver cells in hepatic disease. *Am J Clin Pathol* 1980; **74**: 432–441.
20 Gerber MA, Thung SN. Hepatic oncocytes. Incidence, staining characteristics, and ultrastructural features. *Am J Clin Pathol* 1981; **75**: 498–503.
21 Iwamura S, Enzan H, Saibara T, et al. Appearance of sinusoidal inclusion-containing endothelial cells in liver disease. *Hepatology* 1994; **20**: 604–610.
22 Iwamura S, Enzan H, Saibara T, et al. Hepatic sinusoidal endothelial cells can store and metabolize serum immunoglobulin. *Hepatology* 1995; **22**: 1456–1461.
23 Broderick AL, Jonas MM. Hepatitis B in children. *Semin Liver Dis* 2003; **23**: 59–68.
24 Boxall E, Sira J, Standish RA, et al. The natural history of hepatitis B in perinatally infected carriers. *Arch Dis Child Fetal Neonatal Ed* 2004; **89**: F456–F460.
25 Fattovich G. Natural history and prognosis of hepatitis B. *Semin Liver Dis* 2003; **23**: 47–58.
26 Callea F, De Vos R, Togni R, et al. Fibrinogen inclusions in liver cells: a new type of ground-glass hepatocyte. Immune light and electron microscopic characterization. *Histopathology* 1986; **10**: 65–73.
27 Serinoz E, Varli M, Erden E, et al. Nuclear localization of hepatitis B core antigen and its relations to liver injury, hepatocyte proliferation, and viral load. *J Clin Gastroenterol* 2003; **36**: 269–272.
28 Bianchi L, Gudat F. Sanded nuclei in hepatitis B: eosinophilic inclusions in liver cell nuclei due to excess in hepatitis B core antigen formation. *Lab Invest* 1976; **35**: 1–5.
29 Ter Borg F, ten Kate FJ, Cuypers HT, et al. A survey of liver pathology in needle biopsies from HBsAg and anti-HBe positive individuals. *J Clin Pathol* 2000; **53**: 541–548.
30 Mathurin P, Thibault V, Kadidja K, et al. Replication status and histological features of patients with triple (B, C, D) and dual (B, C) hepatic infections. *J Viral Hepat* 2000; **7**: 15–22.
31 Bianchi L, Gudat F. Chronic hepatitis. In: MacSween RNM, Anthony PP, Scheuer PJ, et al., eds. Pathology of the Liver, 3rd edn. Edinburgh: Churchill Livingstone, 1994: 349.
32 Dienes HP, Popper H, Arnold W, et al. Histologic observations in human hepatitis non-A, non-B. *Hepatology* 1982; **2**: 562–571.
33 van den Oord JJ , De Vos R, Facchetti F, et al. Distribution of non-lymphoid, inflammatory cells in chronic HBV infection. *J Pathol* 1990; **160**: 223–230.
34 Scheuer PJ, Ashrafzadeh P, Sherlock S, et al. The pathology of hepatitis C. *Hepatology* 1992; **15**: 567–571.
35 Moreno A, Ramón y Cahal S, Marazuela M, et al. Sanded nuclei in delta patients. *Liver* 1989; **9**: 367–371.
36 Abiad H, Ramani R, Currie JB, et al. The natural history of hepatitis D virus infection in Illinois state facilities for the developmentally disabled. *Am J Gastroenterol* 2001; **96**: 534–540.
37 Fattovich G, Giustina G, Christensen E, et al. Influence of hepatitis delta virus infection on morbidity and mortality in compensated cirrhosis type B. The

European Concerted Action on Viral Hepatitis (Eurohep). *Gut* 2000; **46**: 420–426.
38 Poynard T, Ratziu V, Benhamou Y, et al. Natural history of HCV infection. *Best Pr Res Clin Gastroenterol* 2000; **14**: 211–228.
39 Ghany MG, Kleiner DE, Alter H, et al. Progression of fibrosis in chronic hepatitis C. *Gastroenterology* 2003; **124**: 97–104.
40 Ryder SD. Progression of hepatic fibrosis in patients with hepatitis C: a prospective repeat liver biopsy study. *Gut* 2004; **53**: 451–455.
41 Fontaine H, Nalpas B, Poulet B, et al. Hepatitis activity index is a key factor in determining the natural history of chronic hepatitis C. *Hum Pathol* 2001; **32**: 904–909.
42 Giannini E, Ceppa P, Botta F, et al. Previous hepatitis B virus infection is associated with worse disease stage and occult hepatitis B virus infection has low prevalence and pathogenicity in hepatitis C virus-positive patients. *Liver Int* 2003; **23**: 12–18.
43 Poynard T, Mathurin P, Lai CL, et al. A comparison of fibrosis progression in chronic liver diseases. *J Hepatol* 2003; **38**: 257–265.
44 Webster G, Barnes E, Brown D, et al. HCV genotypes – role in pathogenesis of disease and response to therapy. *Best Pr Res Clin Gastroenterol* 2000; **14**: 229–240.
45 Roffi L, Redaelli A, Colloredo G, et al. Outcome of liver disease in a large cohort of histologically proven chronic hepatitis C: influence of HCV genotype. *Eur J Gastroenterol Hepatol* 2001; **13**: 501–506.
46 Imbert-Bismut F, Ratziu V, Pieroni L, et al. Biochemical markers of liver fibrosis in patients with hepatitis C virus infection: a prospective study. *Lancet* 2001; **357**: 1069–1075.
47 Afdhal NH. Diagnosing fibrosis in hepatitis C: is the pendulum swinging from biopsy to blood tests? *Hepatology* 2003; **37**: 972–974.
48 Persico M, Persico E, Suozzo R, et al. Natural history of hepatitis C virus carriers with persistently normal aminotransferase levels. *Gastroenterology* 2000; **118**: 760–764.
49 Nutt AK, Hassan HA, Lindsey J, et al. Liver biopsy in the evaluation of patients with chronic hepatitis C who have repeatedly normal or near-normal serum alanine aminotransferase levels. *Am J Med* 2000; **109**: 62–64.
50 Kyrlagkitsis I, Portmann B, Smith H, et al. Liver histology and progression of fibrosis in individuals with chronic hepatitis C and persistently normal ALT. *Am J Gastroenterol* 2003; **98**: 1588–1593.
51 Dienstag JL. The role of liver biopsy in chronic hepatitis C. *Hepatology* 2002; **36**: S152–S160.
52 Quereda C, Moreno S, Moreno L, et al. The role of liver biopsy in the management of chronic hepatitis C in patients infected with the human immunodeficiency virus. *Hum Pathol* 2004; **35**: 1083–1087.
53 Bach N, Thung SN, Schaffner F. The histological features of chronic hepatitis C and autoimmune chronic hepatitis: a comparative analysis. *Hepatology* 1992; **15**: 572–577.
54 Kaji K, Nakanuma Y, Sasaki M, et al. Hepatitic bile duct injuries in chronic hepatitis C: histopathologic and immunohistochemical studies. *Mod Pathol* 1994; **7**: 937–945.
55 Haruna Y, Kanda T, Honda M, et al. Detection of hepatitis C virus in the bile and bile duct epithelial cells of hepatitis C virus-infected patients. *Hepatology* 2001; **33**: 977–980.
56 Delladetsima JK, Makris F, Psichogiou M, et al. Cholestatic syndrome with bile duct damage and loss in renal transplant recipients with HCV infection. *Liver* 2001; **21**: 81–88.
57 Kumar KS, Saboorian MH, Lee WM. Cholestatic presentation of chronic hepatitis C: a clinical and histological study with a review of the literature. *Dig Dis Sci* 2001; **46**: 2066–2073.
58 Gaya DR, Thorburn D, Oien KA, et al. Hepatic granulomas: a 10 year single centre experience. *J Clin Pathol* 2003; **56**: 850–853.
59 Ozaras R, Tahan V, Mert A, et al. The prevalence of hepatic granulomas in chronic hepatitis C. *J Clin Gastroenterol* 2004; **38**: 449–452.
60 Lefkowitch JH, Schiff ER, Davis GL, et al. Pathological diagnosis of chronic

hepatitis C: a multicenter comparative study with chronic hepatitis B. *Gastroenterology* 1993; **104**: 595–603.
61 Sherman KE, Lewey SM, Goodman ZD. Talc in the liver of patients with chronic hepatitis C infection. *Am J Gastroenterol* 1995; **90**: 2164–2166.
62 Bonkovsky HL, Troy N, McNeal K, et al. Iron and HFE or TfR1 mutations as comorbid factors for development and progression of chronic hepatitis C. *J Hepatol* 2002; **37**: 848–854.
63 Martinelli AL, Ramalho LN, Zucoloto S. Hepatic stellate cells in hepatitis C patients: relationship with liver iron deposits and severity of liver disease. *J Gastroenterol Hepatol* 2004; **19**: 91–98.
64 Pirisi M, Scott CA, Avellini C, et al. Iron deposition and progression of disease in chronic hepatitis C. Role of interface hepatitis, portal inflammation, and HFE missense mutations. *Am J Clin Pathol* 2000; **113**: 546–554.
65 Metwally MA, Zein CO, Zein NN. Clinical significance of hepatic iron deposition and serum iron values in patients with chronic hepatitis C infection. *Am J Gastroenterol* 2004; **99**: 286–291.
66 Wyatt J, Baker H, Prasad P, et al. Steatosis and fibrosis in patients with chronic hepatitis C. *J Clin Pathol* 2004; **57**: 402–406.
67 Fartoux L, Chazoullières O, Wendum D, Poupon R, Serfaty L. Impact of steatosis on progression of fibrosis in patients with mild hepatitis C. *Hepatology* 2005; **41**: 82–87.
68 Adinolfi LE, Gambardella M, Andreana A, et al. Steatosis accelerates the progression of liver damage of chronic hepatitis C patients and correlates with specific HCV genotype and visceral obesity. *Hepatology* 2001; **33**: 1358–1364.
69 Monto A, Alonzo J, Watson JJ, et al. Steatosis in chronic hepatitis C: relative contributions of obesity, diabetes mellitus, and alcohol. *Hepatology* 2002; **36**: 729–736.
70 Sanyal AJ, Contos MJ, Sterling RK, et al. Nonalcoholic fatty liver disease in patients with hepatitis C is associated with features of the metabolic syndrome. *Am J Gastroenterol* 2003; **98**: 2064–2071.
71 Hu KQ, Kyulo NL, Esrailian E, et al. Overweight and obesity, hepatic steatosis, and progression of chronic hepatitis C: a retrospective study on a large cohort of patients in the United States. *J Hepatol* 2004; **40**: 147–154.
72 Rubbia-Brandt L, Quadri R, Abid K, et al. Hepatocyte steatosis is a cytopathic effect of hepatitis C virus genotype 3. *J Hepatol* 2000; **33**: 106–115.
73 Serfaty L, Andreani T, Giral P, et al. Hepatitis C virus induced hypobetalipoproteinemia: a possible mechanism for steatosis in chronic hepatitis C. *J Hepatol* 2001; **34**: 428–434.
74 Colloredo G, Sonzogni A, Rubbia-Brandt L, et al. Hepatitis C virus genotype 1 associated with massive steatosis of the liver and hypo-β-lipoproteinemia. *J Hepatol* 2004; **40**: 562–563.
75 Hofer H, Bankl HC, Wrba F, et al. Hepatocellular fat accumulation and low serum cholesterol in patients infected with HCV-3a. *Am J Gastroenterol* 2002; **97**: 2880–2885.
76 Kumar D, Farrell GC, Fung C, et al. Hepatitis C virus genotype 3 is cytopathic to hepatocytes: Reversal of hepatic steatosis after sustained therapeutic response. *Hepatology* 2002; **36**: 1266–1272.
77 Lonardo A, Adinolfi LE, Loria P, et al. Steatosis and hepatitis C virus: mechanisms and significance for hepatic and extrahepatic disease. *Gastroenterology* 2004; **126**: 586–597.
78 Clouston AD, Jonsson JR, Purdie DM, et al. Steatosis and chronic hepatitis C: analysis of fibrosis and stellate cell activation. *J Hepatol* 2001; **34**: 314–320.
79 Verslype C, Nevens F, Sinelli N, et al. Hepatic immunohistochemical staining with a monoclonal antibody against HCV-E2 to evaluate antiviral therapy and reinfection of liver grafts in hepatitis C viral infection. *J Hepatol* 2003; **38**: 208–214.
80 Hoofring A, Boitnott J, Torbenson M. Three-dimensional reconstruction of hepatic bridging fibrosis in chronic hepatitis C viral infection. *J Hepatol* 2003; **39**: 738–741.
81 Badizadegan K, Jonas MM, Ott MJ, et al. Histopathology of the liver in children with chronic hepatitis C infection. *Hepatology* 1998; **28**: 1416–1423.
82 Sugiyasu Y, Yuki N, Nagaoka T, et al. Histological improvement of chronic

liver disease after spontaneous serum hepatitis C virus clearance. *J Med Virol* 2003; **69**: 41–49.

83 Pol S, Carnot F, Nalpas B, et al. Reversibility of hepatitis C virus-related cirrhosis. *Hum Pathol* 2004; **35**: 107–112.

84 Al Khalidi JA, Czaja AJ. Current concepts in the diagnosis, pathogenesis, and treatment of autoimmune hepatitis. *Mayo Clin Proc* 2001; **76**: 1237–1252.

85 International Autoimmune Hepatitis Group. Review of criteria for diagnosis of autoimmune hepatitis. *J Hepatol* 1999; **31**: 929–938.

86 Goldstein NS, Soman A, Gordon SC. Portal tract eosinophils and hepatocyte cytokeratin 7 immunoreactivity helps distinguish early-stage, mildly active primary biliary cirrhosis and autoimmune hepatitis. *Am J Clin Pathol* 2001; **116**: 846–853.

87 Devaney K, Goodman ZD, Ishak KG. Postinfantile giant-cell transformation in hepatitis. *Hepatology* 1992; **16**: 327–333.

88 Lau JYN, Koukoulis G, Mieli-Vergani G, et al. Syncytial giant-cell hepatitis – a specific disease entity? *J Hepatol* 1992; **15**: 216–219.

89 Carpenter HA, Czaja AJ. The role of histologic evaluation in the diagnosis and management of autoimmune hepatitis and its variants. *Clin Liver Dis* 2002; **6**: 397–417.

90 Czaja AJ, Carpenter HA. Autoimmune hepatitis with incidental histologic features of bile duct injury. *Hepatology* 2001; **34**: 659–665.

91 Zolfino T, Heneghan MA, Norris S, et al. Characteristics of autoimmune hepatitis in patients who are not of European Caucasoid ethnic origin. *Gut* 2002; **50**: 713–717.

92 Gregorio GV, Portmann B, Karani J, et al. Autoimmune hepatitis/sclerosing cholangitis overlap syndrome in childhood: a 16-year prospective study. *Hepatology* 2001; **33**: 544–553.

93 Mieli-Vergani G, Vergani D. Autoimmune hepatitis in children. *Clin Liver Dis* 2002; **6**: 335–346.

94 Burgart LJ, Batts KP, Ludwig J, et al. Recent-onset autoimmune hepatitis. Biopsy findings and clinical correlations. *Am J Surg Pathol* 1995; **19**: 699–708.

95 Pratt DS, Fawaz KA, Rabson A, et al. A novel histological lesion in glucocorticoid-responsive chronic hepatitis. *Gastroenterology* 1997; **113**: 664–668.

96 Te HS, Koukoulis G, Ganger DR. Autoimmune hepatitis: a histological variant associated with prominent centrilobular necrosis. *Gut* 1997; **41**: 269–271.

97 Singh R, Nair S, Farr G, et al. Acute autoimmune hepatitis presenting with centrizonal liver disease: case report and review of the literature. *Am J Gastroenterol* 2002; **97**: 2670–2673.

98 Misdraji J, Thiim M, Graeme-Cook FM. Autoimmune hepatitis with centrilobular necrosis. *Am J Surg Pathol* 2004; **28**: 471–478.

99 Cotler SJ, Jakate S, Jensen DM. Resolution of cirrhosis in autoimmune hepatitis with corticosteroid therapy. *J Clin Gastroenterol* 2001; **32**: 428–430.

100 Czaja AJ, Carpenter HA. Decreased fibrosis during corticosteroid therapy of autoimmune hepatitis. *J Hepatol* 2004; **40**: 646–652.

101 Verma S, Gunuwan B, Mendler M, et al. Factors predicting relapse and poor outcome in type I autoimmune hepatitis: role of cirrhosis development, patterns of transaminases during remission and plasma cell activity in the liver biopsy. *Am J Gastroenterol* 2004; **99**: 1510–1516.

102 Czaja AJ, Carpenter HA. Progressive fibrosis during corticosteroid therapy of autoimmune hepatitis. *Hepatology* 2004; **39**: 1631–1638.

103 Goldstein NS, Bayati N, Silverman AL, et al. Minocycline as a cause of drug-induced autoimmune hepatitis. Report of four cases and comparison with autoimmune hepatitis. *Am J Clin Pathol* 2000; **114**: 591–598.

104 Bedossa P, Dargere D, Paradis V. Sampling variability of liver fibrosis in chronic hepatitis C. *Hepatology* 2003; **38**: 1449–1457.

105 Wright M, Thursz M, Pullen R, et al. Quantitative versus morphological assessment of liver fibrosis: semi-quantitative scores are more robust than digital image fibrosis area estimation. *Liver Int* 2003; **23**: 28–34.

106 Scheuer PJ. Classification of chronic viral hepatitis: a need for reassessment. *J Hepatol* 1991; **13**: 372–374.

107 Bedossa P, Poynard T and the METAVIR cooperative study group. An algorithm

for the grading of activity in chronic hepatitis C. *Hepatology* 1996; **24**: 289–293.

108 Bedossa P, Bioulac-Sage P, Callard P, et al. Intraobserver and interobserver variations in liver biopsy interpretation in patients with chronic hepatitis C. *Hepatology* 1994; **20**: 15–20.

109 Ishak K, Baptista A, Bianchi L, et al. Histological grading and staging of chronic hepatitis. *J Hepatol* 1995; **22**: 696–699.

110 Knodell RG, Ishak KG, Black WC, et al. Formulation and application of a numerical scoring system for assessing histological activity in asymptomatic chronic active hepatitis. *Hepatology* 1981; **1**: 431–435.

111 Lagging LM, Westin J, Svensson E, et al. Progression of fibrosis in untreated patients with hepatitis C virus infection. *Liver* 2002; **22**: 136–144.

112 Guido M, Rugge M. Liver biopsy sampling in chronic viral hepatitis. *Semin Liver Dis* 2004; **24**: 89–97.

113 Regev A, Berho M, Jeffers LJ, et al. Sampling error and intraobserver variation in liver biopsy in patients with chronic HCV infection. *Am J Gastroenterol* 2002; **97**: 2614–2618.

114 Colloredo G, Guido M, Sonzogni A, et al. Impact of liver biopsy size on histological evaluation of chronic viral hepatitis: the smaller the sample, the milder the disease. *J Hepatol* 2003; **39**: 239–244.

115 Brunetti F, Silini E, Pistorio A, et al. Coarse vs. fine needle aspiration biopsy for the assessment of diffuse liver disease from hepatitis C virus-related chronic hepatitis. *J Hepatol* 2004; **40**: 501–506.

116 Petz D, Klauck S, Rohl FW, et al. Feasibility of histological grading and staging of chronic viral hepatitis using specimens obtained by thin-needle biopsy. *Virchows Arch* 2003; **442**: 238–244.

117 Rousselet M-C, Michalak S, Dupré F, et al. Sources of variability in histological scoring of chronic hepatitis. *Hepatology* 2005; **41**: 257–264.

GENERAL READING

Carpenter HA, Czaja AJ. The role of histologic evaluation in the diagnosis and management of autoimmune hepatitis and its variants. *Clin Liver Dis* 2002; **6**: 397–417.

Czaja AJ. Autoimmune liver disease. *Curr Opin Gastroenterol* 2003; **19**: 232–242.

De Vos R, Verslype C, Depla E, et al. Ultrastructural visualization of hepatitis C virus components in human and primate liver biopsies. *J Hepatol* 2002; **37**: 370–379.

Fattovich G. Natural history and prognosis of hepatitis B. *Semin Liver Dis* 2003; **23**: 47–58.

Ganem D, Prince AM. Hepatitis B virus infection – natural history and clinical consequences. *N Engl J Med* 2004; **350**: 1118–1129.

Ishak KG. Pathologic features of chronic hepatitis. A review and update. *Am J Clin Pathol* 2000; **113**: 40–55.

Lai CL, Ratziu V, Yuen MF, et al. Viral hepatitis B. *Lancet* 2003; **362**: 2089–2094.

Lavanchy D. Hepatitis B virus epidemiology, disease burden, treatment, and current and emerging prevention and control measures. *J Viral Hepat* 2004; **11**: 97–107.

Marcellin P, Boyer N. Transition of care between paediatric and adult gastroenterology. Chronic viral hepatitis. *Best Pr Res Clin Gastroenterol* 2003; **17**: 259–275.

McFarlane IG. Definition and classification of autoimmune hepatitis. *Semin Liver Dis* 2002; **22**: 317–324.

Penin F, Dubuisson J, Rey FA, et al. Structural biology of hepatitis C virus. *Hepatology* 2004; **39**: 5–19.

Ramadori G, Saile B. Portal tract fibrogenesis in the liver. *Lab Invest* 2004; **84**: 153–159.

Scheuer PJ, Standish RA, Dhillon AP. Scoring of chronic hepatitis. *Clin Liver Dis* 2002; **6**: 335–347.

Seeff LB. Natural history of chronic hepatitis C. *Hepatology* 2004; **36**: S35–S46.

CHAPTER 10

CIRRHOSIS

INTRODUCTION

Cirrhosis is a diffuse process in which the normal lobules are replaced by architecturally abnormal nodules separated by fibrous tissue.[1,2] The nodules, which are most commonly the result of regenerative hyperplasia following hepatocellular injury, are functionally less efficient than normal hepatic parenchyma and there is a profound disturbance of vascular relationships.

Several different kinds of information can be obtained about the cirrhotic liver by means of liver biopsy (Table 10.1). The most important functions of biopsy are to establish a diagnosis, to assess the cause of the cirrhosis as far as possible and to detect hepatocellular carcinoma.

THE DIAGNOSIS OF CIRRHOSIS BY LIVER BIOPSY

The ease with which the pathologist can diagnose cirrhosis from a biopsy specimen depends on the sample as well as on the criteria used. The sample may be sufficiently big, and the nodules sufficiently small, to make the diagnosis obvious. However, a slender core from within a large cirrhotic nodule can be difficult to identify as such (see Fig. 1.4). There are occasions when the pathologist can do no more than hint at the possible diagnosis.

The type of biopsy needle used also influences the ease of diagnosis. Very narrow needles may be adequate to obtain tumour samples, but may be inadequate for the accurate diagnosis of medical conditions. For example, in staging chronic hepatitis, thin-needle biopsies obtained under computed tomographic guidance may

Table 10.1 Main information from liver biopsy in cirrhosis

Main information
Diagnosis of cirrhosis
Assessment of cause
Stage of development
Histological activity
Detection of hepatocellular carcinoma

under-diagnose cirrhosis for advanced bridging fibrosis.[3] Some clinicians prefer to use the Trucut type of needle when cirrhosis is suspected in order to lessen the risk of fragmentation,[4] but suitable samples can usually be obtained with needles of the aspiration type.[5,6] Transjugular biopsy is used when there is a risk of haemorrhage by other routes and provides samples which, though often small, are usually adequate for the diagnosis of cirrhosis.[7] The combination of biopsy with laparoscopy has been advocated.[8,9] Operative wedge biopsies of cirrhotic liver give an accurate idea of the relative proportions of parenchyma and stroma in the liver as a whole.[10]

The histological criteria for a diagnosis of cirrhosis are outlined in Table 10.2. The two fundamental criteria, nodularity and fibrosis, reflect the definition of cirrhosis. When there are well-defined rounded nodules surrounded by fibrous septa the diagnosis is easily established. The only likely confusion is with recent bridging necrosis, a problem which can be resolved by examination of stains for elastic fibres and by attention to clinical data. Occasionally, a nodular appearance just deep to the liver capsule is not representative of the whole liver but has resulted from transection of a tongue or peninsula extending from the main bulk of the parenchyma.

In many patients, the relative criteria listed in Table 10.2 are equally important. They allow a tentative diagnosis of cirrhosis to be reached, readily converted to a firm diagnosis when correlated with other data. A diagnosis of cirrhosis therefore requires communication between pathologist and clinician and cannot be exactly equated with a histological stage.[11]

Fragmentation

Fragmentation of the specimen, either at the time of biopsy or during processing in the laboratory, should itself suggest the possibility of cirrhosis (Fig. 10.1). The specimen is more likely to break into fragments when needles of the aspiration type (e.g. Menghini) are used. Other biopsy specimens that are likely to fragment are metastatic tumours surrounded by reactive fibrous tissue and hepatocellular carcinoma.

Table 10.2 Cirrhosis: diagnostic criteria

A. Fundamental
- Nodularity
- Fibrosis

B. Relative
- Fragmentation
- Abnormal structure
- Hepatocellular changes
  - Regenerative hyperplasia
  - Pleomorphism
  - Large-cell dysplasia (large-cell change)
  - Small-cell dysplasia (small-cell change)
  - Excess copper-associated protein

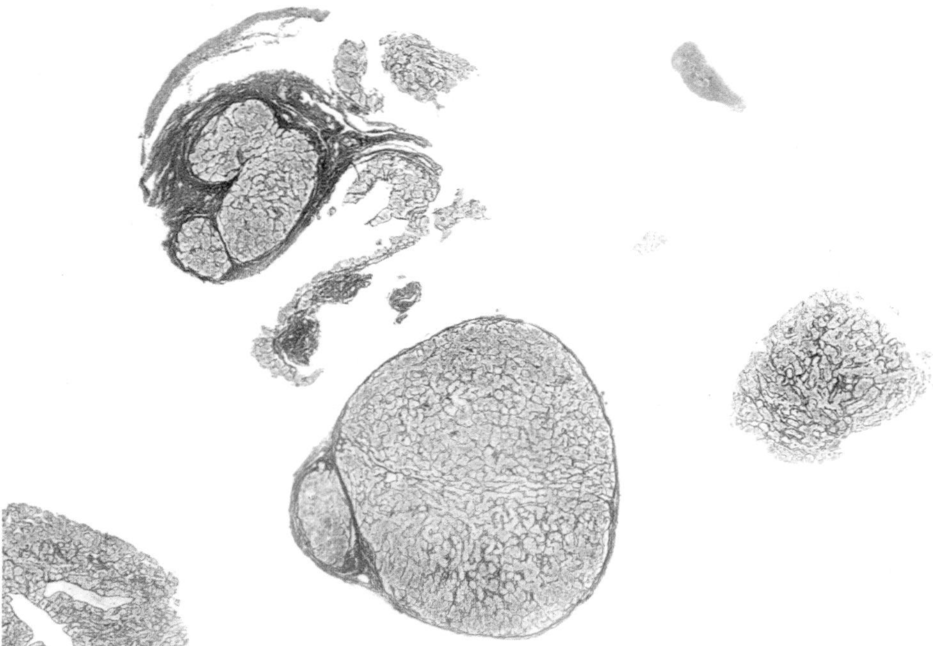

Figure 10.1 *Cirrhosis: fragmented sample.* A specimen obtained by the aspiration biopsy method has broken into rounded fragments peripherally circumscribed by fibrosis. (Needle biopsy, reticulin).

Abnormal structure

Structural changes should be assessed by means of a reticulin preparation, preferably not counterstained. This may show two features not readily seen with other stains. First, although nodules are readily cored out of the dense fibrous stroma of a cirrhotic liver during aspiration biopsy, a thin layer of connective tissue tends to adhere to the nodules over much of their surface (Fig. 10.2). This layer may be difficult to see even with the help of collagen stains and is easily missed in haematoxylin and eosin-stained sections (Fig. 10.3). Second, minor alterations of structure become apparent even in those nodules which closely mimic normal liver. Such alterations include abnormal orientation of reticulin fibres resulting from different patterns and rates of growth in different areas (Fig. 10.4) and approximation of portal tracts and terminal venules. The number of venules may be abnormally large in relation to the number of portal tracts (Fig. 10.5) and the latter are sometimes abnormally small and poorly formed (Fig. 1.4). A more obvious structural abnormality in cirrhosis is the presence of septa, linking central veins (terminal hepatic venules) to portal tracts. These septa must be distinguished from recently formed necrotic bridges.

In wedge biopsies, excess fibrous tissue in and near the capsule and crowding of vessels must be distinguished from the changes of cirrhosis. The latter extend through the specimen whereas the former are confined to the capsular and immediately subcapsular area.[7] Very occasionally a wedge biopsy of part of a large well-differentiated regeneration nodule fails to show the histological features of cirrhosis.

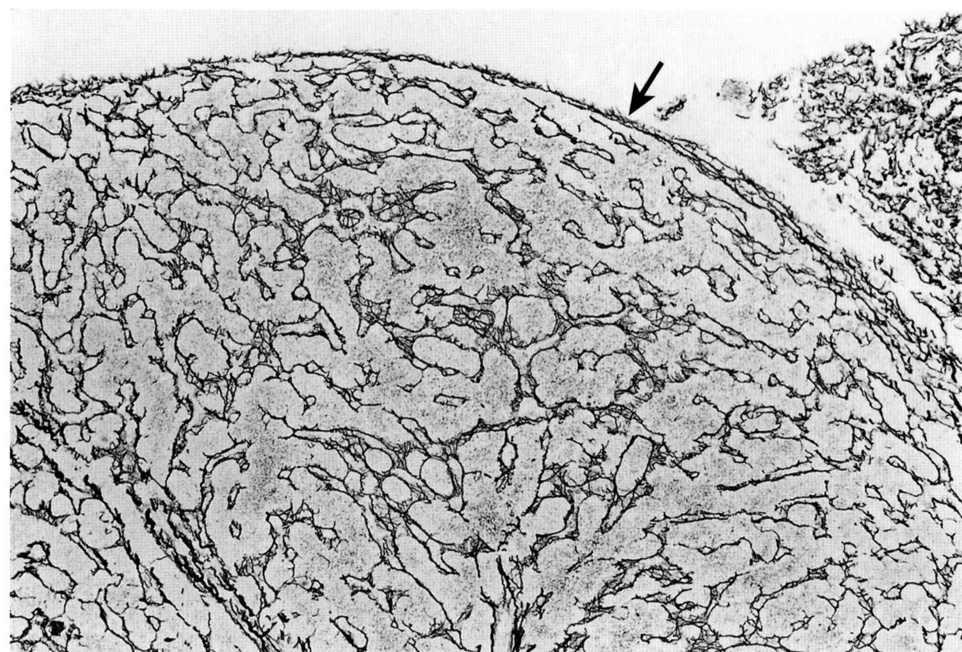

Figure 10.2 *Cirrhosis: selective sampling*. A nodule has been cored out of the connective tissue by the biopsy procedure, but a thin layer of connective tissue (arrow) has adhered to the nodule margin. (Needle biopsy, reticulin).

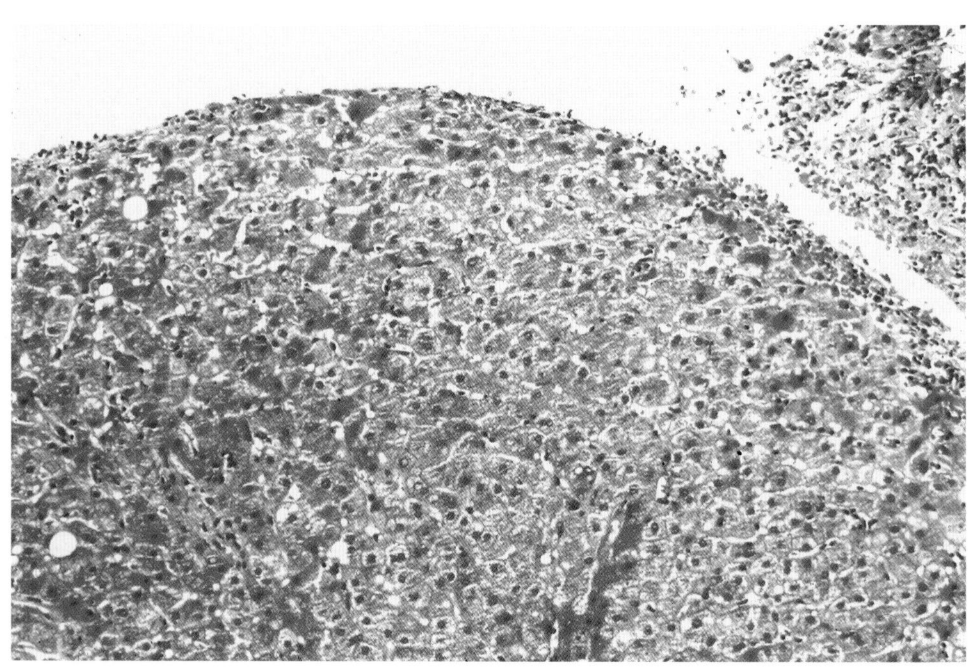

Figure 10.3 *Cirrhosis: selective sampling*. Same field as in Figure 10.2. In a haematoxylin and eosin preparation the thin layer of connective tissue is not easily seen. (Needle biopsy, H&E).

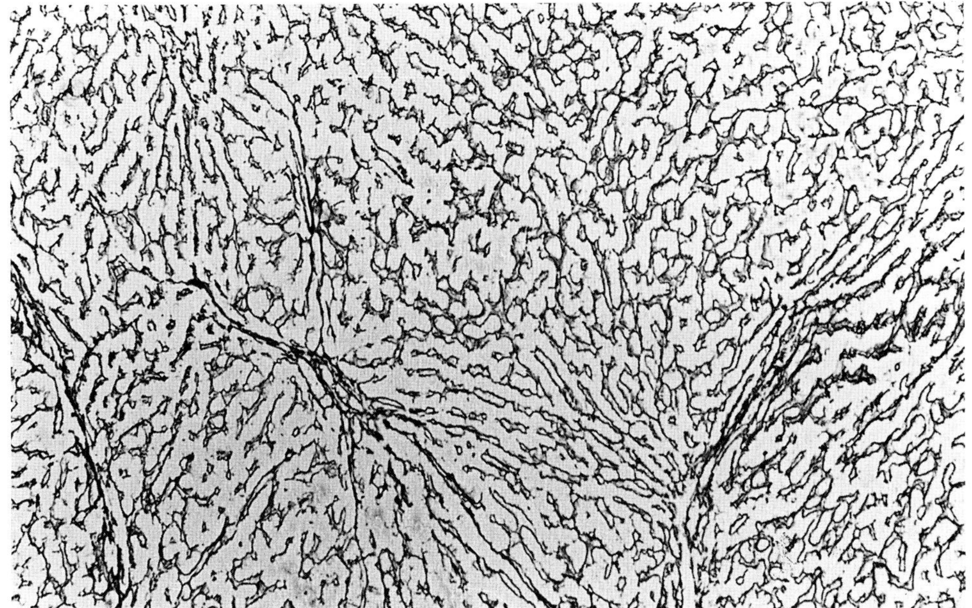

Figure 10.4 *Cirrhosis: distorted reticulin pattern.* The distortion has resulted from abnormal and irregular hepatocyte growth patterns. (Needle biopsy, reticulin).

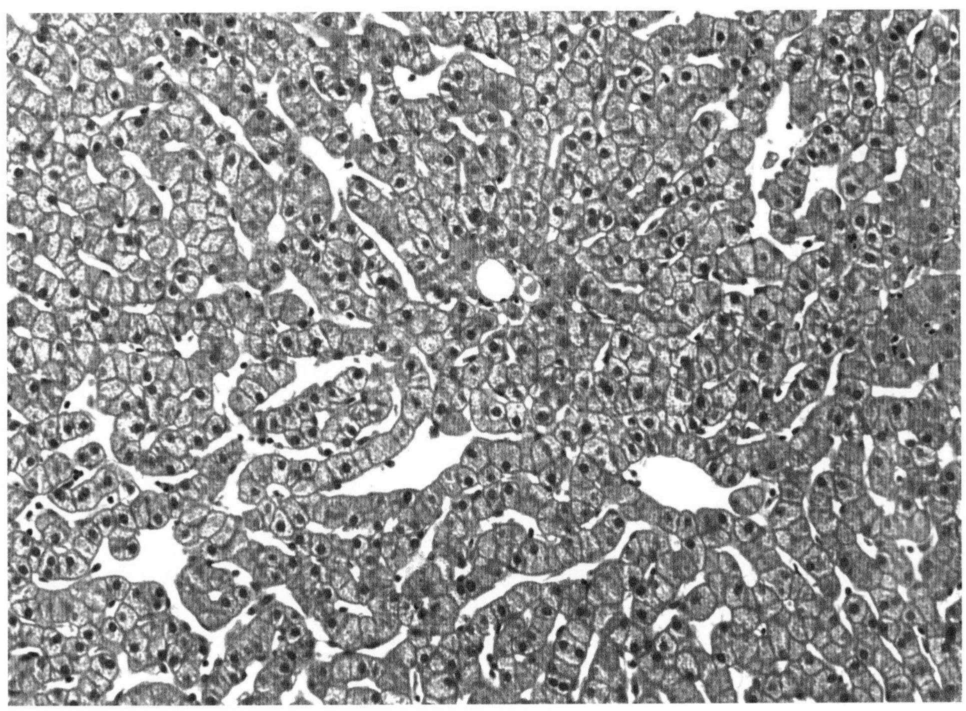

Figure 10.5 *Cirrhosis: abnormal vascular relationships.* Several venous channels are seen near to each other. (Wedge biopsy, H&E).

Hepatocellular changes

In some biopsies from cirrhotic livers, the hepatocytes are normal in appearance and arrangement, so that diagnosis rests on the structural changes discussed above. In others, there are more or less obvious abnormalities of growth.

Regeneration is suggested by thickening of the liver-cell plates (Fig. 10.6). In any liver, an oblique plane of sectioning will cause a few plates to appear more than one cell thick, but widespread double-cell plates are seen when there is active growth. Hepatocytes in hyperplastic areas contain little or no lipofuscin pigment even near terminal venules. Regeneration is not always evident in cirrhosis because it is not a continuous process. Its absence does not therefore exclude the diagnosis. Conversely its presence does not prove cirrhosis, because it is found also in other circumstances, for example after an acute hepatitis and in the pre-cirrhotic stages of chronic biliary diseases.

A very characteristic feature of cirrhosis is the presence of adjacent populations of hepatocytes growing at different rates and having different cell and nuclear characteristics (Fig. 10.7). This **pleomorphism** gives rise to the abnormalities of reticulin pattern already mentioned, notably a tendency for reticulin fibres in the different growth areas to lie in different directions.

In a minority of cirrhotic livers the hepatocytes show structural atypia of a degree sufficient to warrant a label of **dysplasia**, an appearance further discussed in Chapter 11. Two types have been described, large-cell dysplasia[12] and small-cell dysplasia.[13] Because of the unproven status of either type as a precursor of malignant change,[14] some authors prefer to call them large-cell change and small-cell change.[14,15] In the large-cell form, the cells are enlarged and their nuclei hyperchromatic and irregular in shape, with prominent nucleoli (Fig. 10.8). Nuclear-

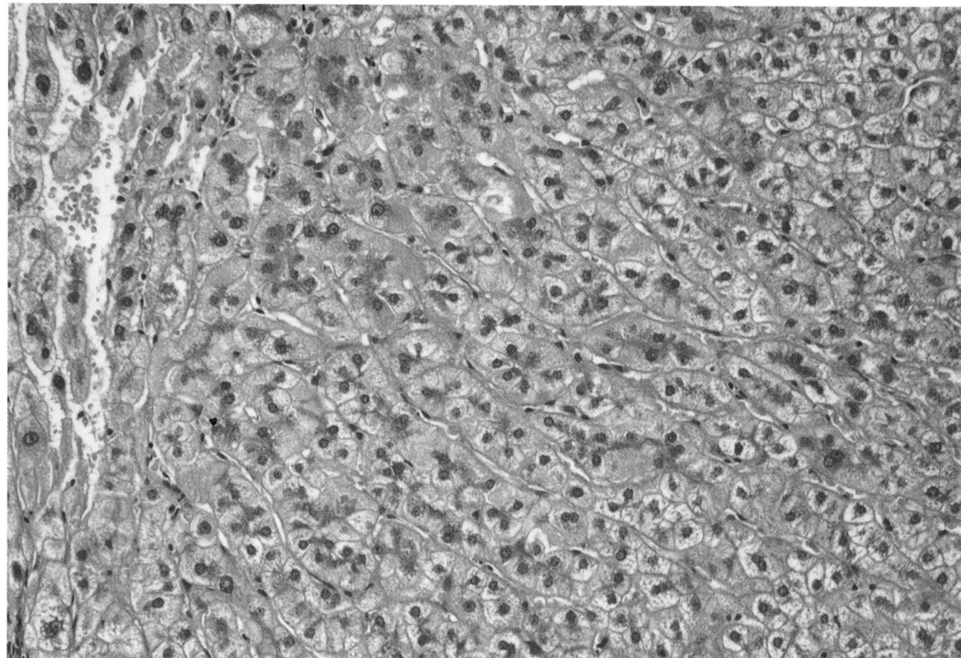

Figure 10.6 *Cirrhosis: hepatocellular regeneration.* Liver-cell plates are two or more cells thick, indicating active growth. (Needle biopsy, H&E).

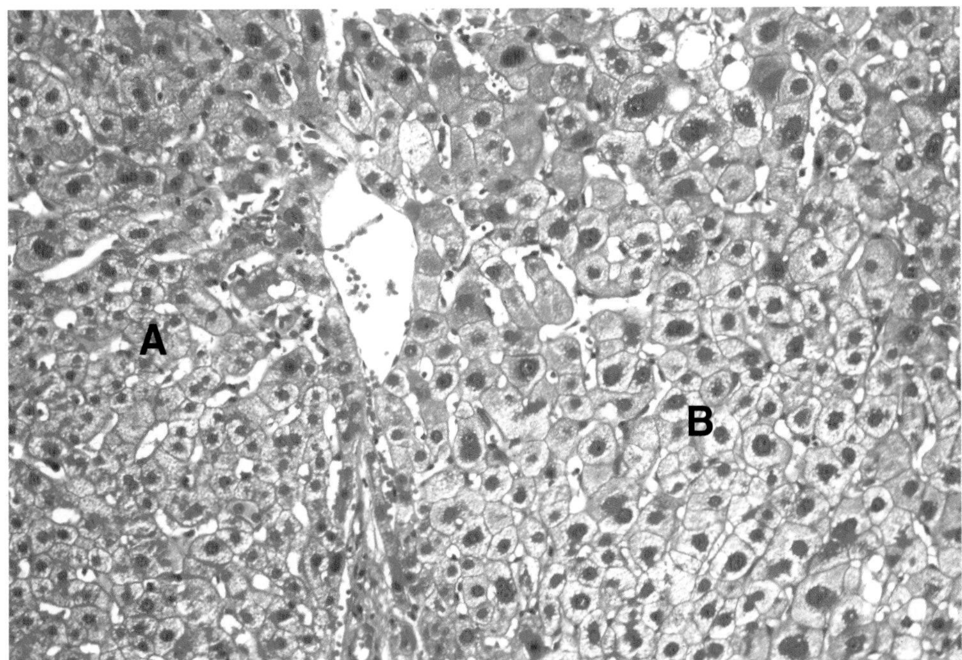

Figure 10.7 *Cirrhosis: different cell populations*. The parenchymal cells in area A are smaller than those in area B which also show a rounded and nodular growth pattern. (Wedge biopsy, H&E).

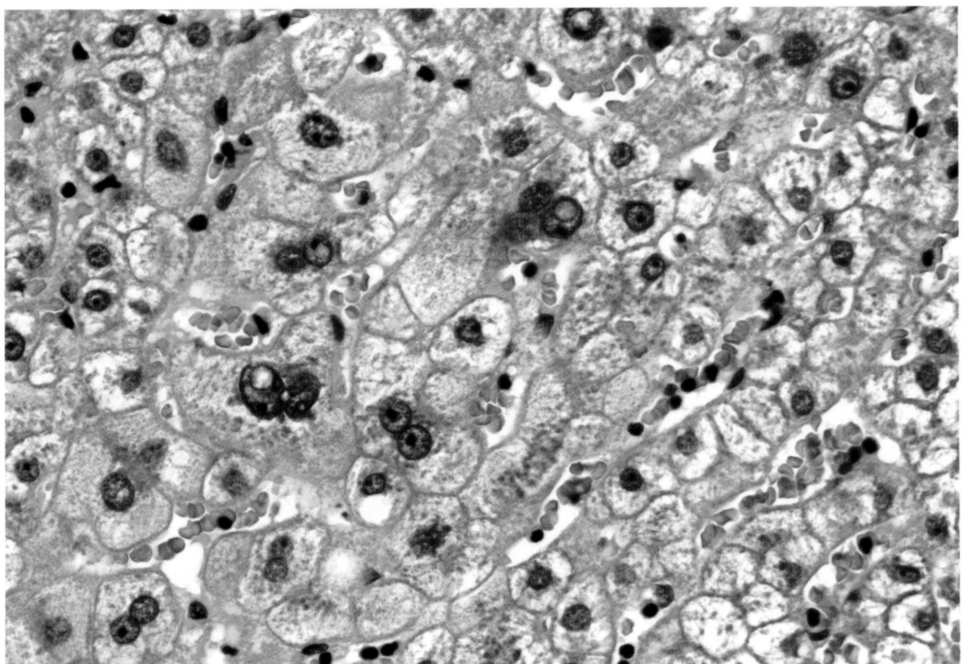

Figure 10.8 *Cirrhosis: large-cell dysplasia (large-cell change)*. The nuclei of the enlarged hepatocytes at centre and left are irregular in shape and vary greatly in size and staining intensity. Several of these cells are multinucleated. Compare with the normal hepatocytes at right and in upper left hand corner. (Wedge biopsy, H&E).

cytoplasmic ratio is normal or only moderately increased.[16] This type of dysplasia was first described in an African population with a high incidence of hepatocellular carcinoma.[12] It is mainly but not exclusively seen in patients with HBV infection. There is evidence of an association with an increased risk of development of this cancer independently of other risk factors.[17,18] The hepatocyte proliferation rate as assessed by expression of silver-stained nuclear organiser regions (AgNOR) was even more strongly predictive of hepatocellular carcinoma in one study.[19] In small-cell dysplasia the nuclear-cytoplasmic ratio is increased but the overall size of the affected cells is less than normal (Fig. 10.9). Zones of dysplastic hepatocytes of either type support a diagnosis of cirrhosis and are regarded by some clinicians as an indication for increased monitoring for hepatocellular carcinoma. A finding of dysplasia of either type should therefore be specifically mentioned in liver biopsy reports.

Differential diagnosis

When there is nodularity and evidence of regeneration but little or no fibrosis, **nodular regenerative hyperplasia** should be considered. In **congenital hepatic fibrosis**, the acinar architecture remains intact and the ductal plate malformation is seen. In **chronic hepatitis** with fibrosis and structural abnormalities, the differential diagnosis is between active cirrhosis and chronic hepatitis which has not yet reached the stage of cirrhosis. This problem cannot always be resolved on the basis of a liver biopsy. Similar doubt may arise in steatohepatitis. The presence of substantial quantities of copper and copper-associated protein in non-cholestatic chronic liver disease supports a diagnosis of cirrhosis.[20] Cirrhotic nodules can usually be distinguished

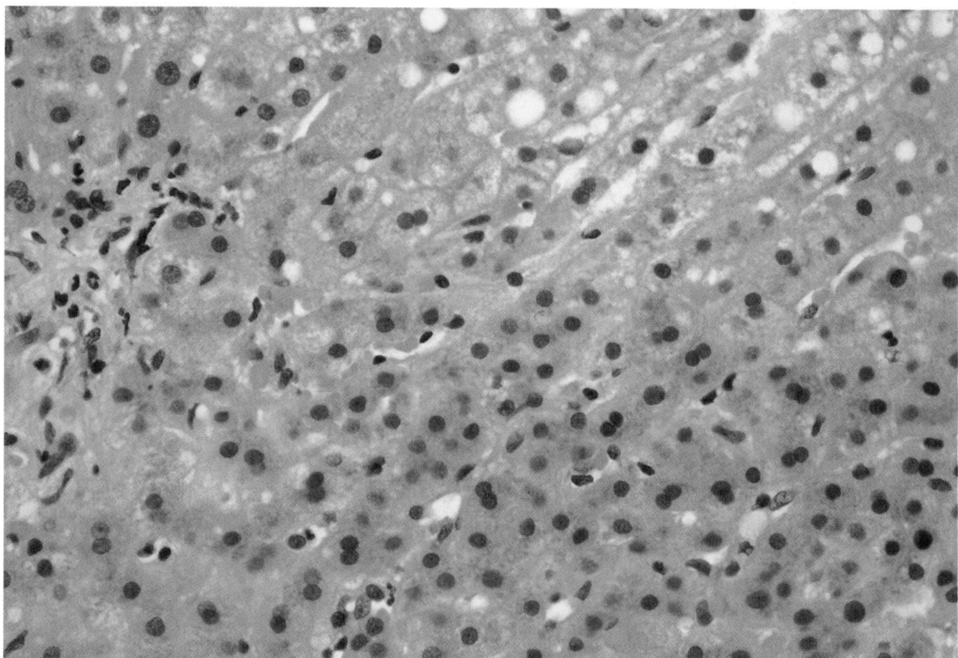

Figure 10.9 *Cirrhosis: small-cell dysplasia (small-cell change).* The hepatocytes below and to the right have normal-sized nuclei, but their overall size is reduced. Nuclear cytoplasmic ratios are therefore increased. (Needle biopsy, H&E).

from well-differentiated **hepatocellular carcinoma**. In the latter, the cell plate architecture is more abnormal, reticulin may be scanty or absent and the cells have malignant cytological characteristics. Also, hepatocellular siderosis is often present secondarily in cirrhosis of varied aetiology (see Ch. 14), but is typically absent in tumour cells of hepatocellular carcinoma.

ASSESSMENT OF CAUSE

Biopsy may help to establish the cause of a cirrhosis. In some of the categories listed in Table 10.3, the histological appearances are diagnostic. The term 'cryptogenic' should only be applied when full clinical and laboratory investigations have been completed and the features listed in Table 10.4 have been assessed. This can be achieved by means of a small range of routine stains. There is evidence to suggest that many examples of cryptogenic cirrhosis result from non-alcoholic steatohepatitis (NASH), not evident histologically at the time of diagnosis.[21] Some cases of cirrhosis are due to mutations in genes for specific cellular keratins.[22]

Table 10.3 Main causes of cirrhosis

Viral hepatitis (B,C,D)
Alcohol abuse
Obesity, insulin resistance/metabolic syndrome
Biliary disease
Metabolic disorders
- Haemochromatosis
- Wilson's disease
- α_1-Antitrypsin deficiency, etc.

Venous outflow obstruction
Drugs and toxins
Autoimmune disease

Table 10.4 Cirrhosis: assessment of cause

Pattern of nodules and fibrosis
Bile ducts
Blood vessels
Steatohepatitis
Evidence of viral infection
Abnormal deposits
- Iron
- Copper, copper-associated protein
- α_1-Antitrypsin globules

Pattern of nodules and fibrosis

Irregularly-shaped nodules suggest the possibility of a biliary cause, especially if there is perinodular oedema, ductular reaction and chronic cholestasis. In a pre-cirrhotic stage of venous outflow obstruction there is regular fibrosis in perivenular regions (acinar zones 3). Sinusoids are dilated. Portal tracts show little or no abnormality or sometimes have changes mimicking biliary tract obstruction.[23] Certain features are indicative of earlier chronic hepatitis that evolved to cirrhosis. Irregular, slender fibrous septa emanating from portal tracts, lymphoplasmacytic infiltrates, lymphoid aggregates or follicles and foci of interface hepatitis should prompt consideration of the several causes of chronic hepatitis.

Confluent fibrosis, which replaces multiple adjacent lobules, is a common feature in several types of cirrhosis, particularly following steatohepatitis and chronic hepatitis of viral or autoimmune aetiology. It is also seen in the less common 'post-hepatitic' cirrhosis, which develops rapidly, within a few months of a severe viral or drug-induced acute hepatitis. Needle biopsy samples in such cases may show entire cores, portions of cores and especially the subcapsular region occupied by fibrous tissue, residual portal tracts and many ductular structures (see Fig. 4.6c), mild chronic inflammatory cell infiltrates, entrapped regenerative liver-cell rosettes and collections of small neo-vessels (see Blood vessels, below).

Bile ducts

Assessment of bile duct numbers in cirrhosis is very important. The number of ducts should approximately equal the number of arteries of similar size and location, but the pathologist must bear in mind that not every portal tract will necessarily contain a bile duct in the plane of section. Definite duct loss almost always indicates primary biliary cirrhosis or primary sclerosing cholangitis. In children or young adults, other ductopenic syndromes should also be considered. Typical bile-duct lesions of primary biliary cirrhosis, with or without granulomas, are still sometimes found at a stage of cirrhosis.

Periductal fibrosis may be very prominent in primary sclerosing cholangitis. Ductular reaction is a non-specific finding, but when severe and focal it often reflects biliary disease. Following extensive hepatocellular damage in cirrhosis, for example after variceal haemorrhage, there is sometimes a very extensive ductular reaction, which can be mistaken for cholangiocarcinoma.

Blood vessels

Occluded, narrowed or recanalised veins suggest that the cirrhosis may be the result of venous outflow block, but are also found in cirrhosis from other causes.[24,25] Portal and hepatic venous thrombosis has indeed been implicated in the progression of cirrhosis in general.[26] Recognition of venous lesions is often difficult without the help of stains for collagen or elastic fibres. Neovascularisation of fibrotic portal tracts, areas of confluent fibrosis and bridging fibrous septa in cirrhosis produces numerous lymphatic and capillary channels, particularly in chronic hepatitis B and C.[27]

Steatohepatitis

This is found in alcohol abusers and in individuals at risk for non-alcoholic fatty liver disease (see Ch. 7), as a manifestation of drug toxicity, or for no obvious underlying reason. In amiodarone toxicity, the fatty change is usually absent. Steatohepatitis must be distinguished from chronic cholestasis, in which there are also swollen hepatocytes containing Mallory bodies.

Evidence of viral infection

Features of chronic hepatitis, particularly interface hepatitis and lymphocytic infiltration, are often but by no means always due to infection with one of the hepatitis viruses. Liver-cell dysplasia also favours a viral cause. Ground-glass hepatocytes, Victoria blue or orcein stains (Fig. 10.10) and immunostains for viral antigens help in the diagnosis of hepatitis B virus infection, but tissue evidence of HBV antigens is not always present or detectable. Lymphoid aggregates or follicles should suggest the possibility of hepatitis C (Fig. 10.11). More than one virus or other causal agent may be responsible for a patient's cirrhosis. Abundant plasma cells raise the possibility of autoimmune hepatitis, but are also sometimes found in viral hepatitis.

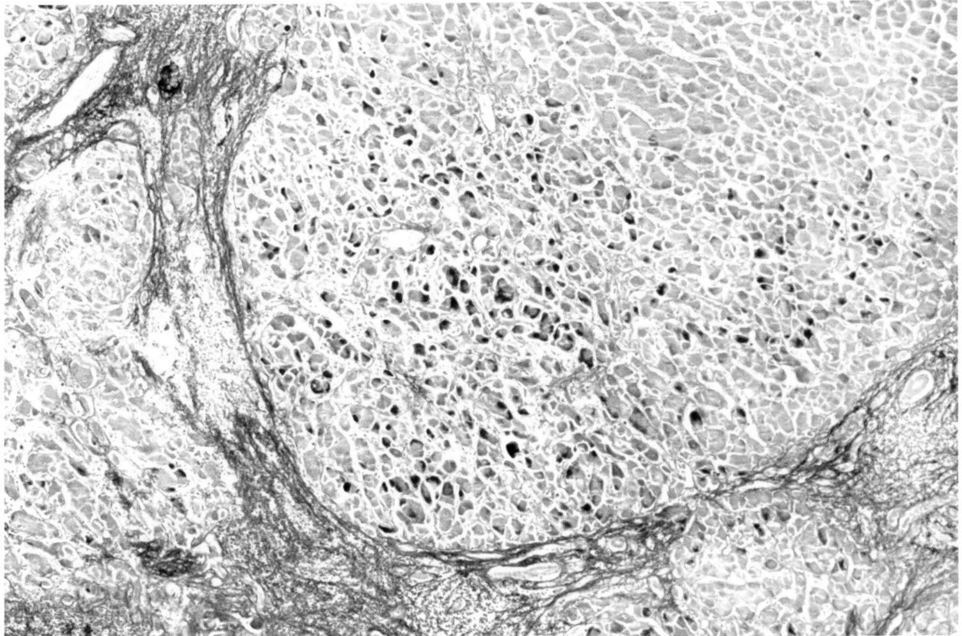

Figure 10.10 *Hepatitis B surface antigen in HBV-related cirrhosis.* Many hepatocytes show positive cytoplasmic staining for HBV surface antigen. This staining method also demonstrates elastic tissue fibres in the fibrous tissue. (Recipient liver from transplantation, Victoria blue).

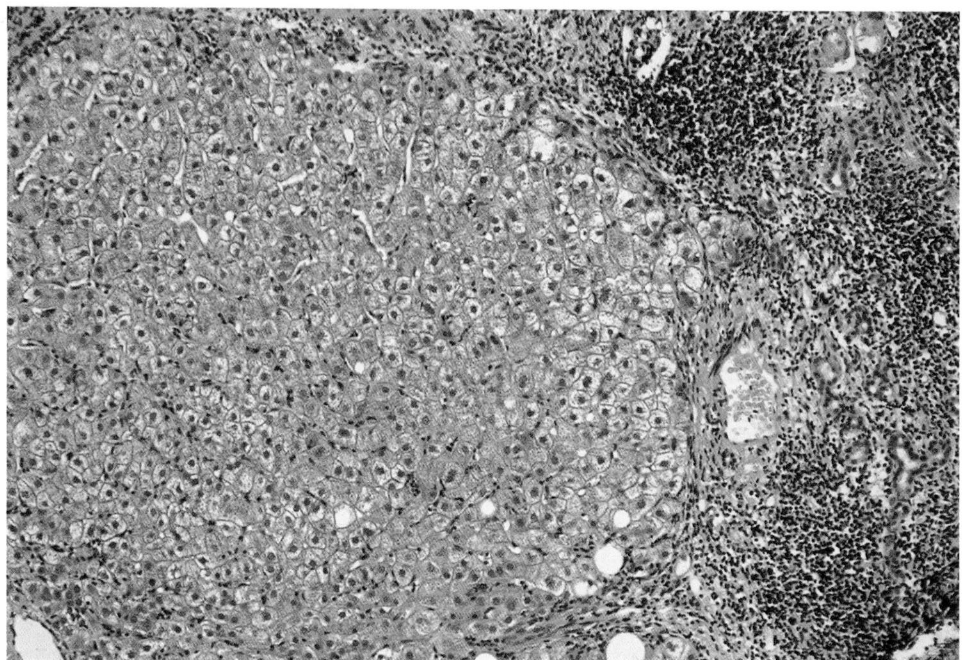

Figure 10.11 *Cirrhosis following hepatitis C virus infection.* Lymphoid aggregates are still visible. (Recipient liver from transplantation, H&E).

Abnormal deposits

Severe siderosis should always raise the possibility of hereditary haemochromatosis, even when another cause is also evident. However, stainable iron often accumulates in cirrhosis from any cause.[28,29] In hereditary haemochromatosis, the nodules are sometimes irregular as in biliary cirrhosis.

Copper and copper-associated protein can often be detected in cirrhosis, whatever its cause.[20] Large amounts at the edges of nodules suggest biliary disease. Staining of entire nodules is seen in Wilson's disease, but other nodules may be negative. In some stages of the disease, the copper is not histochemically demonstrable, so that negative staining does not exclude the diagnosis. Abundant copper and Mallory bodies are also features of Indian childhood cirrhosis and other forms of copper toxicosis.[30,31]

α_1-Antitrypsin bodies should always be looked for in cirrhosis. Immunocytochemical staining is more sensitive than diastase-PAS.

ANATOMICAL TYPE

Because of possible sampling error, the pathologist cannot confidently assess nodule size in the rest of the liver on the basis of a biopsy specimen. This is of little consequence to the patient. Primary classification of cirrhosis by nodule size is no longer appropriate, because aetiology is clinically much more important.

However, nodule size does influence the ease of histological diagnosis. When nodules are of the size order of the lobules from which they are derived, several nodules are usually seen in one biopsy and diagnosis is easy (Figs 10.12, 10.13). When nodules are larger (Fig. 10.14), more subtle diagnostic criteria need to be considered. The most difficult anatomical type to recognise is **incomplete septal cirrhosis**. This is characterised by indistinct nodularity, slender septa, some of which end blindly, poorly-formed small portal tracts and abnormal relationships between portal tracts and efferent venules[32] (Fig. 10.15). There is evidence of hepatocytic hyperplasia, giving rise to crowding of reticulin fibres in adjacent areas. Sinusoidal dilatation is common, while inflammation and necrosis are generally modest or absent. A reticulin preparation is important for diagnosis because the slender septa are easily missed (Figs 10.15, 10.16). The diagnosis is more easily made in wedge biopsies than in needle specimens. A relationship to various forms of non-cirrhotic portal hypertension has been demonstrated,[32–35] but it has also been postulated that incomplete septal cirrhosis can represent a burnt-out form of macronodular cirrhosis.[36] The incomplete septa could reflect resorption of fibrous tissue.

STAGE OF DEVELOPMENT

In some patients, cirrhosis is obvious and appears mature, in the sense that the well-demarcated nodules and dense fibrosis give an impression of long-standing disease.

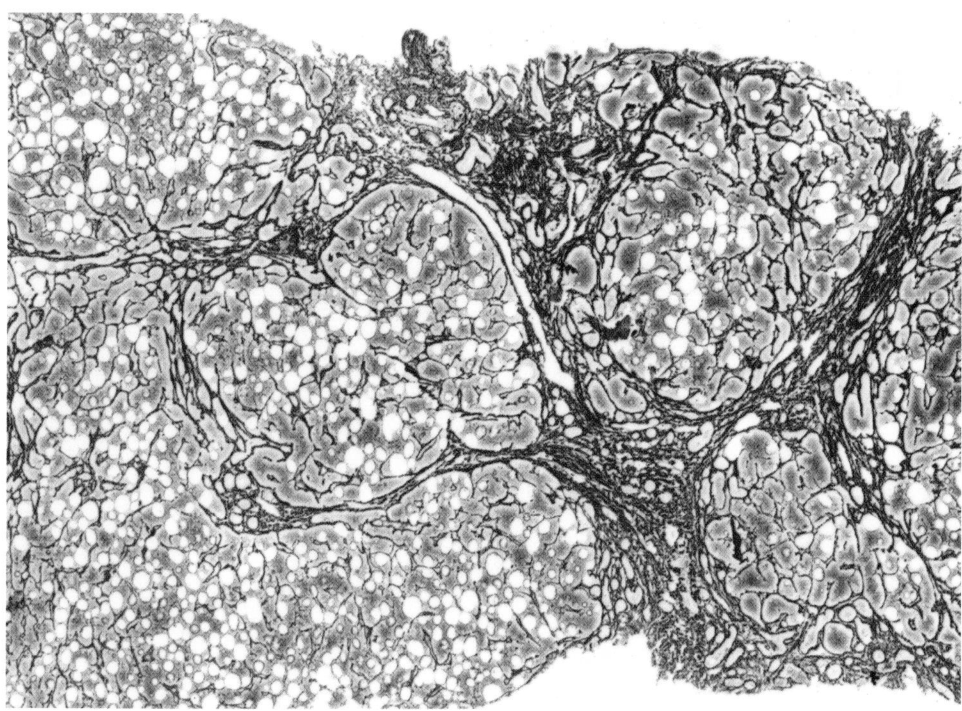

Figure 10.12 *Cirrhosis: micronodular pattern*. Nodules are of lobular size or smaller. (Needle biopsy, reticulin).

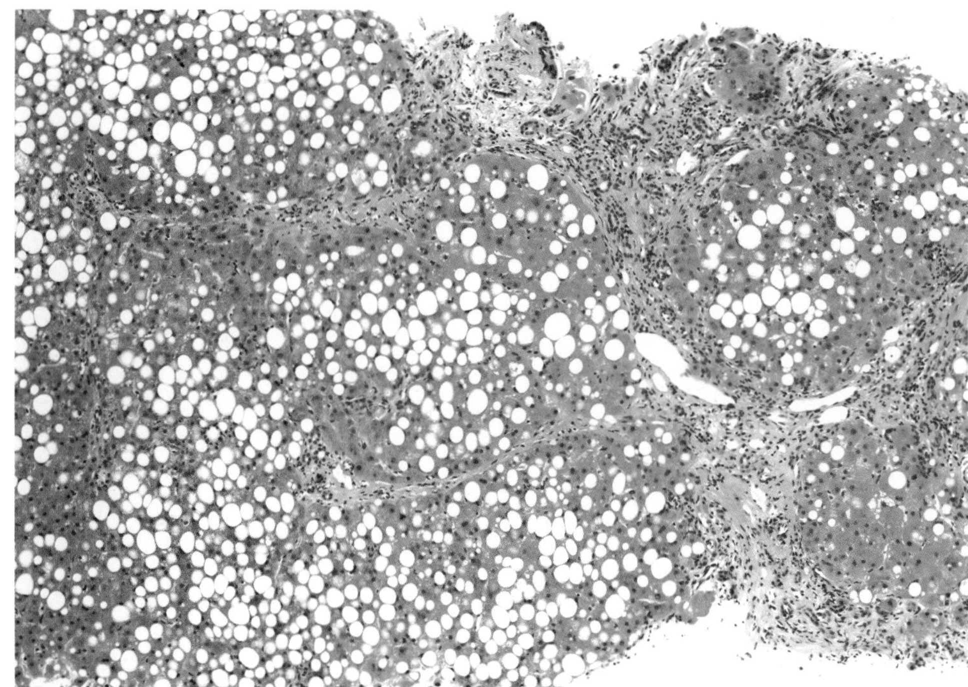

Figure 10.13 *Cirrhosis: micronodular pattern*. Similar field as in Figure 10.12. There is steatosis. (Needle biopsy, H&E).

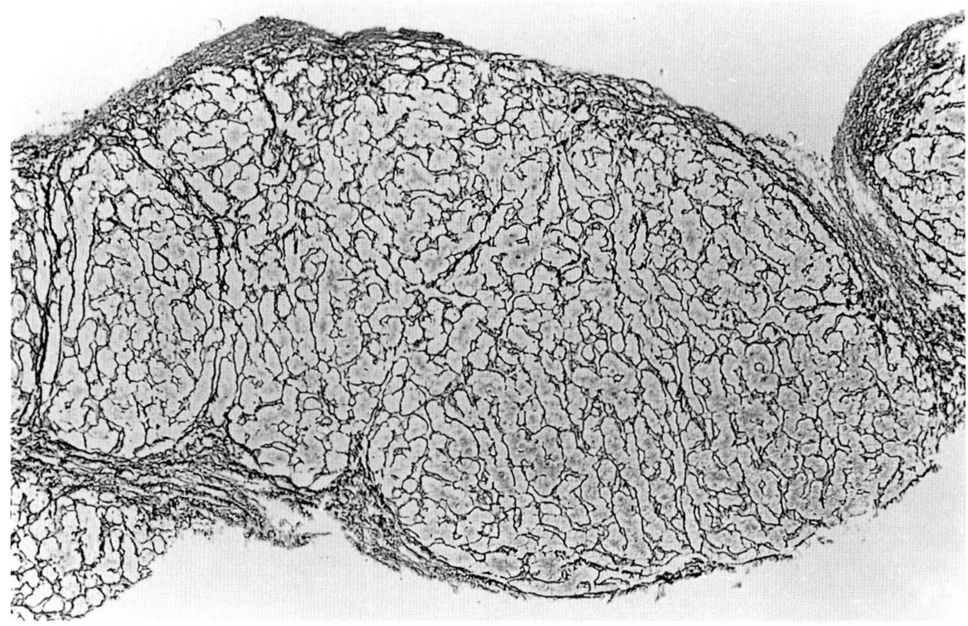

Figure 10.14 *Cirrhosis: macronodular pattern*. Nodules are larger than in Figures 10.12 and 10.13. The magnification is slightly smaller. (Needle biopsy, reticulin).

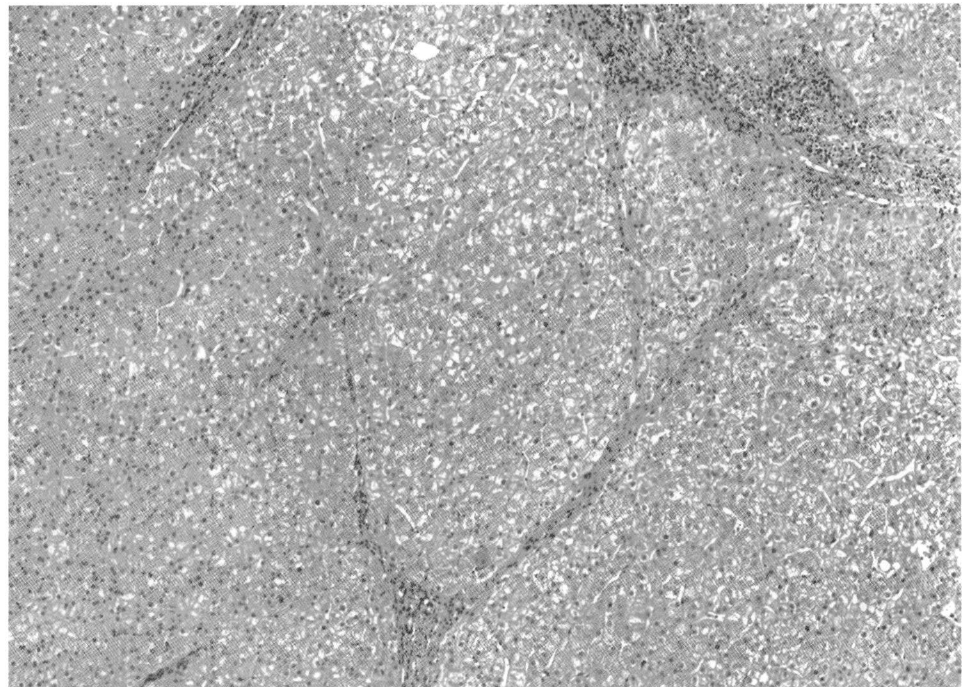

Figure 10.15 *Cirrhosis: incomplete septal pattern*. The parenchyma is nodular but only partially surrounded by fibrous septa. Note the incompleted fibrous septum emerging vertically from the portal tract at bottom. (Wedge biopsy, H&E).

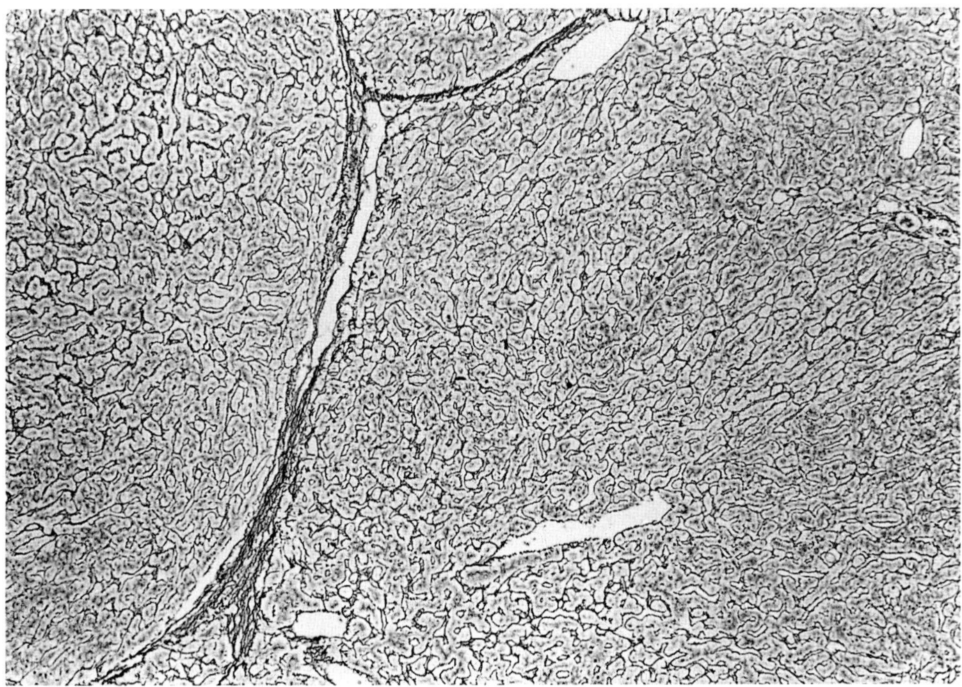

Figure 10.16 *Cirrhosis: incomplete septal pattern*. Slender septa and vessels are present. There is a small portal tract on the right, towards the top of the figure. Wedge biopsy, reticulin.

In others, there is doubt as to whether there is cirrhosis or merely fibrosis. An impression may be gained that cirrhosis is incipient or at an early stage of development (Fig. 10.17). When doubt is unresolved, a report of 'developing cirrhosis' or 'incomplete cirrhosis' is sometimes appropriate. The concept of incomplete cirrhosis is recognised in the staging system of Ishak et al.[37] Once cirrhosis is fully established, reversion to a normal lobular pattern is unlikely. Indeed, reversibility of cirrhosis is a controversial subject[38] and the pathologist should consider this prospect cautiously, taking into account the type of biopsy sample, the underlying disease process and the possibility of sampling error. Diminished fibrosis following therapy does not automatically confer a return to normal liver-cell plate structure and vascular relationships.[2]

Paradoxically, there may be confusion between mild chronic hepatitis and an inactive, well-established cirrhosis. This reflects difficulty in diagnosing some examples of late cirrhosis by needle biopsy, because of a tendency for nodule size to increase with time.

HISTOLOGICAL ACTIVITY

Activity is a convenient term to describe the rate of progression of the cirrhosis. It is usually taken to mean the various forms of liver-cell damage and inflammation typical of chronic viral hepatitis. In cirrhosis following steatohepatitis, however, the severity of the latter should also be taken into account.

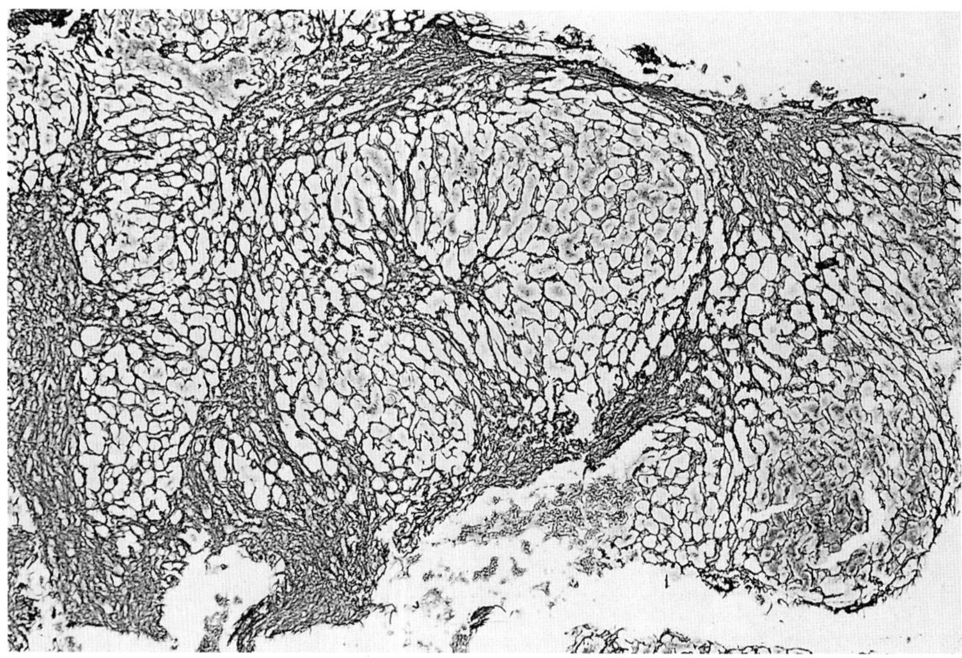

Figure 10.17 *Early (developing) cirrhosis.* There is extensive fibrosis and architectural distortion in this biopsy from an alcohol abuser. Nodules are beginning to form but are not yet clearly defined. Needle biopsy, reticulin.

In an inactive cirrhosis, the interface between septa and nodules is sharply defined (Fig. 10.18). Cellular infiltration is mild and may be confined to the septa. There is little or no focal necrosis or intranodular inflammation. In an active, rapidly progressive cirrhosis however, the interface is blurred by hepatocellular damage and inflammation (Fig. 10.19). Isolated hepatocytes or groups of cells may be seen within the inflamed septa. There is hepatocellular damage and inflammation deep within the nodules.

Histological activity often varies in severity from one part of the liver to another. Comparison of activity in multiple biopsies from an individual patient should therefore be made with caution and with reference to clinical and biochemical data.

COMPLICATIONS

Hypoperfusion leads to coagulative necrosis involving whole nodules or their centres.[31] This is sometimes referred to as **nodular infarction**.

In recent years, advances in imaging and examination of explanted cirrhotic livers after transplantation have led to extensive discussion of the pathology and nomenclature of nodules different in appearance from the rest and usually larger in diameter. The relationship of these nodules to hepatocellular carcinoma has been debated and is further discussed in Chapter 11. An international working party[39] has recommended that the old term adenomatous hyperplasia should no longer be used, and that the nodules should be subdivided into **large regenerative nodules**

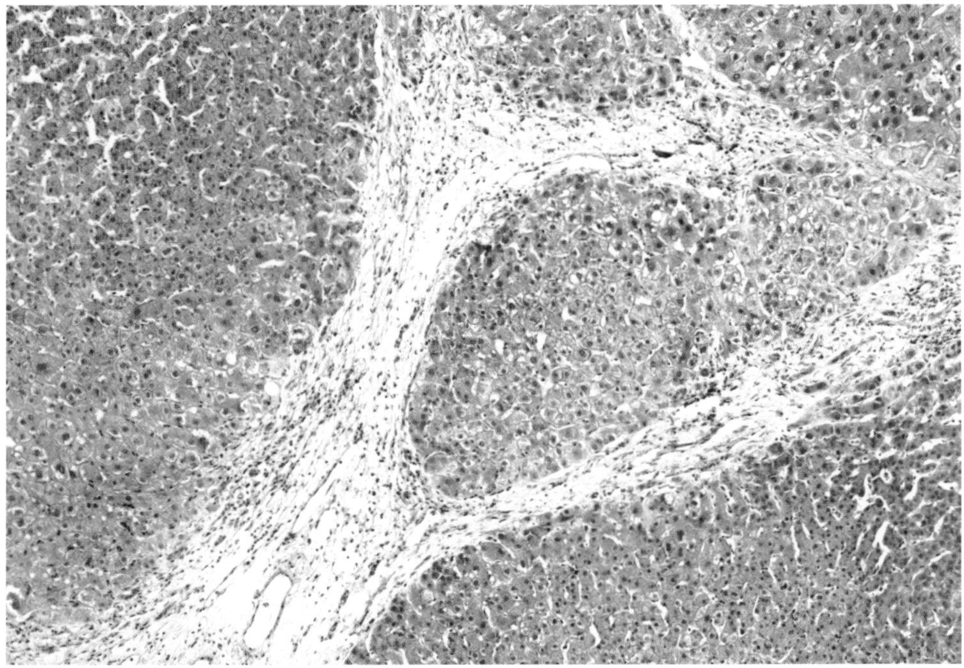

Figure 10.18 *Inactive cirrhosis.* Nodules are sharply outlined and inflammatory cells are scanty. (Wedge biopsy, H&E).

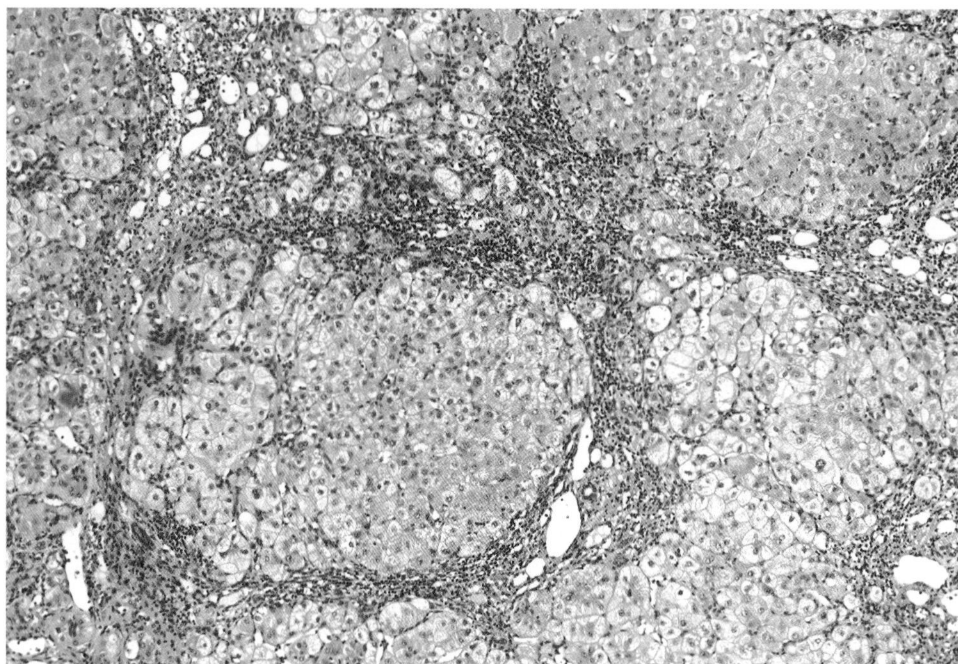

Figure 10.19 *Active cirrhosis.* The outline of the nodule is blurred by interface hepatitis and there is a heavy inflammatory infiltrate. (Wedge biopsy, H&E).

(macroregenerative nodules) and **dysplastic nodules**. The latter are further subclassified as low-grade and high-grade. The dysplastic nodules differ from macroregenerative nodules in their content of dysplastic (atypical) hepatocytes and their more expansile growth pattern. However, the distinction between macroregenerative nodules and low-grade dysplastic nodules is often difficult, as is the distinction between high-grade dysplastic nodules and well-differentiated **hepatocellular carcinoma**, a very important complication of cirrhosis. In addition to the three large nodule types described by the working party, the group also defined **dysplastic foci**, clusters of dysplastic hepatocytes less than 1 mm in diameter. In making a microscopic diagnosis and differentiating between these various, possibly preneoplastic nodules, the pathologist must bear in mind that needle biopsy samples of a nodule may not be representative of the entire nodule and that hepatocellular carcinoma may have arisen in a part not sampled by the needle.

REFERENCES

1 Anthony PP, Ishak KG, Nayak NC, et al. The morphology of cirrhosis: definition, nomenclature, and classification. *Bull World Health Org* 1977; **55**: 521–540.

2 Desmet VJ, Roskams T. Cirrhosis reversal: a duel between dogma and myth. *J Hepatol* 2004; **40**: 860–867.

3 Petz D, Klauck S. Röhl et al. Feasibility of histological grading and staging of chronic viral hepatitis using specimens obtained by thin-needle biopsy. *Virchows Arch* 2003; **442**: 238–244.

4 Colombo M, Ninno E Del, Francis R de, et al. Ultrasound-assisted percutaneous

liver biopsy: superiority of the Tru-Cut over the Menghini needle for diagnosis of cirrhosis. *Gastroenterology* 1988; **95**: 487–489.

5 Bateson MC, Hopwood D, Duguid HL, et al. A comparative trial of liver biopsy needles. *J Clin Pathol* 1980; **33**: 131–133.

6 Littlewood ER, Gilmore IT, Murray-Lyon IM, et al. Comparison of the Trucut and Surecut liver biopsy needles. *J Clin Pathol* 1982; **35**: 761–763.

7 Petrelli M, Scheuer PJ. Variation in subcapsular liver structure and its significance in the interpretation of wedge biopsies. *J Clin Pathol* 1967; **20**: 743–748.

8 Orlando R, Lirussi F, Okolicsanyi L. Laparoscopy and liver biopsy: further evidence that the two procedures improve the diagnosis of liver cirrhosis. A retrospective study of 1,003 consecutive examinations. *J Clin Gastroenterol* 1990; **12**: 47–52.

9 Jalan R, Harrison DJ, Dillon JF, et al. Laparoscopy and histology in the diagnosis of chronic liver disease. *Quart J Med* 1995; **88**: 559–564.

10 Imamura H, Kawasaki S, Bandai Y, et al. Comparison between wedge and needle biopsies for evaluating the degree of cirrhosis. *J Hepatol* 1993; **17**: 215–219.

11 Desmet VJ, Roskams T. Reversal of cirrhosis: evidence-based medicine? *Gastroenterology* 2003; **125**: 629–630.

12 Anthony PP, Vogel CL, Barker LF. Liver cell dysplasia: a premalignant condition. *J Clin Pathol* 1973; **26**: 217–223.

13 Watanabe S, Okita K, Harada T, et al. Morphologic studies of the liver cell dysplasia. *Cancer* 1983; **51**: 2197–2205.

14 Lee RG, Tsamandas AC, Demetris AJ. Large cell change (liver cell dysplasia) and hepatocellular carcinoma in cirrhosis: matched case–control study, pathological analysis, and pathogenetic hypothesis. *Hepatology* 1997; **26**: 1415–1422.

15 Natarajan S, Theise ND, Thung SN, et al. Large-cell change of hepatocytes in cirrhosis may represent a reaction to prolonged cholestasis. *Am J Surg Pathol* 1997; **21**: 312–318.

16 Roncalli M, Borzio M, Tombesi MV, et al. A morphometric study of liver cell dysplasia. *Hum Pathol* 1988; **19**: 471–474.

17 Libbrecht L, Craninx M, Nevens F, et al. Predictive value of liver cell dysplasia for development of hepatocellular carcinoma in patients with non-cirrhotic and cirrhotic chronic viral hepatitis. *Histopathology* 2001; **39**: 66–71.

18 Borzio M, Bruno S, Roncalli M, et al. Liver cell dysplasia is a major risk factor for hepatocellular carcinoma in cirrhosis: a prospective study. *Gastroenterology* 1995; **108**: 812–817.

19 Borzio M, Trerè D, Borzio F, et al. Hepatocyte proliferation rate is a powerful parameter for predicting hepatocellular carcinoma development in liver cirrhosis. *J Clin Pathol: Molecular Pathology* 1998; **51**: 96–101.

20 Guarascio P, Yentis F, Cevikbas U, et al. Value of copper-associated protein in diagnostic assessment of liver biopsy. *J Clin Pathol* 1983; **36**: 18–23.

21 Caldwell SH, Oelsner DH, Iezzoni JC, et al. Cryptogenic cirrhosis: clinical characterization and risk factors for underlying disease. *Hepatology* 1999; **29**: 664–669.

22 Ku N-O, Gish R, Wright TL, et al. Keratin 8 mutations in patients with cryptogenic liver disease. *N Engl J Med* 2001; **344**: 1580–1587.

23 Kakar S, Batts KP, Poterucha JJ, et al. Histologic changes mimicking biliary disease in liver biopsies with venous outflow impairment. *Mod Pathol* 2004; **17**: 874–878.

24 Burt AD, MacSween RN. Hepatic vein lesions in alcoholic liver disease: retrospective biopsy and necropsy study. *J Clin Pathol* 1986; **39**: 63–67.

25 Nakanuma Y, Ohta G, Doishita K. Quantitation and serial section observations of focal venocclusive lesions of hepatic veins in liver cirrhosis. *Virchows Arch (A)* 1985; **405**: 429–438.

26 Wanless IR, Wong F, Blendis LM, et al. Hepatic and portal vein thrombosis in cirrhosis: possible role in development of parenchymal extinction and portal hypertension. *Hepatology* 1995; **21**: 1238–1247.

27 Yamauchi Y, Michitaka K, Onji M. Morphometric analysis of lymphatic and blood vessels in human chronic viral liver diseases. *Am J Pathol* 1998; **153**: 1131–1137.

28 Deugnier Y, Turlin B, Le Quilleuc D, et al. A reappraisal of hepatic siderosis in patients with end-stage cirrhosis: practical implications for the diagnosis of hemochromatosis. *Am J Surg Pathol* 1997; **21**: 669–675.
29 McGuinness PH, Bishop GA, Painter DM, et al. Intrahepatic hepatitis C RNA levels do not correlate with degree of liver injury in patients with chronic hepatitis C. *Hepatology* 1996; **23**: 676–687.
30 Mehrotra R, Pandey RK, Nath P. Hepatic copper in Indian childhood cirrhosis. *Histopathology* 1981; **5**: 659–665.
31 Müller T, Langner C, Fuchsbichler A, et al. Immunohistochemical analysis of Mallory bodies in Wilsonian and non-Wilsonian hepatic copper toxicosis. *Hepatology* 2004; **39**: 963–969.
32 Sciot R, Staessen D, Damme B Van, et al. Incomplete septal cirrhosis: histopathologic aspects. *Histopathology* 1988; **13**: 593–603.
33 Lopez JI. Does incomplete septal cirrhosis link non-cirrhotic nodulations with cirrhosis? *Histopathology* 1989; **15**: 318–320.
34 Bernard P-H, Le Bail B, Cransac M, et al. Progression from idiopathic portal hypertension to incomplete septal cirrhosis with liver failure requiring liver transplantation. *J Hepatol* 2004; **22**: 495–499.
35 Nakanuma Y, Hoso M, Sasaki M, et al. Histopathology of the liver in non-cirrhotic portal hypertension of unknown etiology. *Histopathology* 1996; **28**: 195–204.
36 Nevens F, Staessen D, Sciot R, et al. Clinical aspects of incomplete septal cirrhosis in comparison with macronodular cirrhosis. *Gastroenterology* 1994; **106**: 459–463.
37 Ishak K, Baptista A, Bianchi L, et al. Histological grading and staging of chronic hepatitis. *J Hepatol* 1995; **22**: 696–699.
38 Friedman SL. Liver fibrosis – from bench to bedside. *J Hepatol* 2003; **38**: S38–S53.
39 International Working Party. Terminology of nodular hepatocellular lesions. *Hepatology* 1995; **22**: 983–993.

GENERAL READING

Crawford JM. Liver cirrhosis. In: MacSween RNM, Burt AD, Portmann BC, et al., eds. Pathology of the Liver, 4th edn. Edinburgh: Churchill Livingstone, 2002: 575–620.
Desmet VJ, Roskams T. Cirrhosis reversal: a duel between dogma and myth. *J Hepatol* 2004; **40**: 860–867.

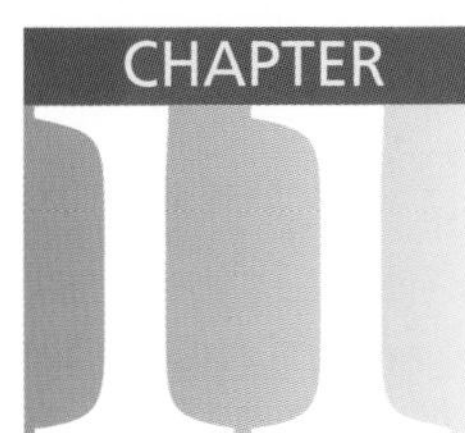

CHAPTER 11

NEOPLASMS AND NODULES

INTRODUCTION

This chapter is intended to provide a working overview of the tumours and tumour-like nodular lesions that the pathologist will encounter with some frequency in everyday practice. The majority of these can be classified according to the putative cells of origin (hepatocytes, bile-duct epithelium and endothelium) from which they arise (Table 11.1) and immunohistochemistry can often be used effectively to distinguish histogenesis. Neoplastic and nodular lesions of adults are covered first, followed by lesions in children and a section on cytopathological diagnosis. The reader is encouraged to consult the references and general reading list for additional details and coverage of some of the rarer tumours.

NEOPLASMS AND NODULES IN ADULTS

Benign lesions

Liver-cell adenoma

Liver-cell adenomas are solitary or occasionally multiple tumours, composed of hepatocytes. Macroscopically they are well defined, but often not encapsulated. The cells of the tumour closely resemble normal hepatocytes (Fig. 11.1). Nuclei are small and regular and mitoses are almost never seen. These features are evident in fine-needle aspiration biopsies.[1] The cells are arranged in normal or thickened trabeculae interspersed with prominent arteries and thin-walled blood vessels. Small liver-cell rosettes (acini) with a central bile-filled or empty lumen may be seen, as in cholestatic liver. In addition to bile, adenomas may contain fat or Dubin-Johnson-like pigment[2], or even show steatohepatitis with Mallory bodies.[3] Non-necrotising granulomas within adenomas have also been described.[4] In adenomas, reticulin is normal or reduced, but extensive loss is in most cases confined to areas of necrosis or haemorrhage. The latter are characteristically found in adenomas in oral contraceptive users and are responsible for pain and for the serious complication of haemoperitoneum. They probably also explain the fibrous scars sometimes found in the lesions. Regular septa, portal tracts and bile ducts are, however, absent; this distinguishes liver-cell adenomas both from non-neoplastic liver and from macroregenerative nodules (large regenerative nodules) in cirrhosis as well as focal

Table 11.1 Classification of liver tumours and nodular lesions

Putative cell of origin	Benign	Malignant
Hepatocyte	Liver-cell adenoma MRN FNH NRH PNT	Hepatocellular carcinoma Fibrolamellar carcinoma Hepatoblastoma
Bile-duct epithelium	Bile-duct adenoma Cystadenoma Adenofibroma	Cholangiocarcinoma Cystadenocarcinoma
Mixed liver-cell and bile-duct cell	Mesenchymal hamartoma	Combined hepatocellular-cholangiocarcinoma
Endothelial cell	Haemangioma Infantile haemangio-endothelioma[a]	Angiosarcoma Epithelioid haemangioendothelioma

MRN, macroregenerative nodule; FNH, focal nodular hyperplasia; NRH, nodular regenerative hyperplasia; PNT, partial nodular transformation.
[a]Some cases may behave more aggressively and are capable of metastasis.

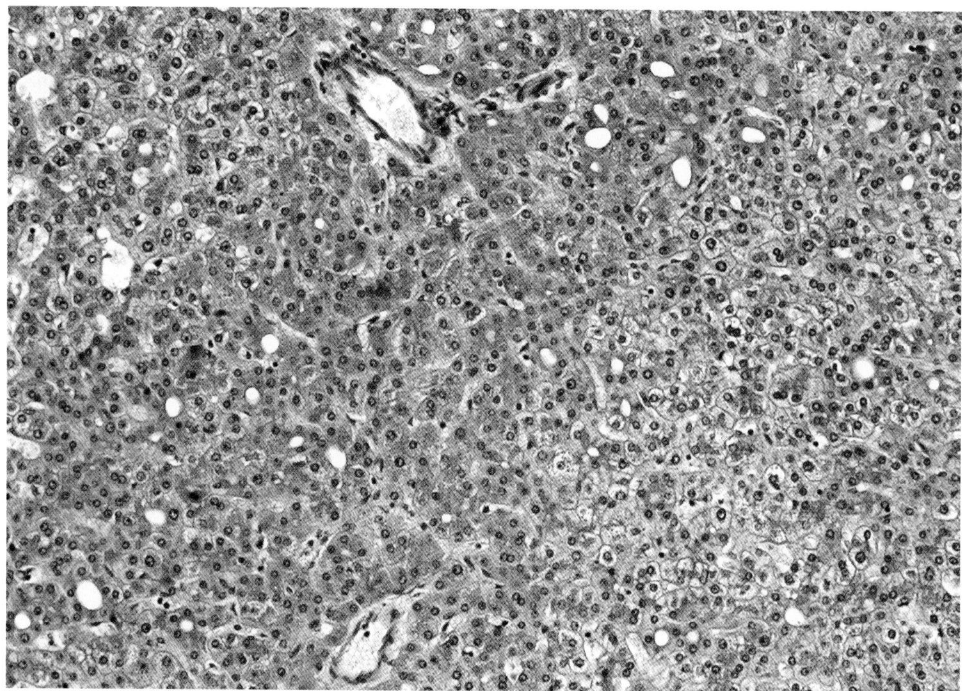

Figure 11.1 *Hepatocellular adenoma*. Liver cells appear normal or contain fat vacuoles. Blood vessels but no portal tracts are seen within the lesion. (Operative specimen, H&E).

nodular hyperplasia (see below). An exception to this rule may occur in patients with multiple adenomas (adenomatosis) where bile ducts can become entrapped within the lesions.[5] The distinction of adenoma from hepatocellular carcinoma is occasionally difficult, but can usually be made confidently on the basis of trabecular pattern, retention of normal amounts of reticulin and appearance of the tumour cells.

Most liver-cell adenomas arise in women of child-bearing age, usually after prolonged use of oral contraceptives.[6] Adenomatosis, in which multiple tumours are seen throughout the liver, is much less common and is found in either sex,[7,8] sometimes in patients taking anabolic/androgenic steroids[9] or in patients without risk factors.[10] Recent data indicate an important role of somatic and germline mutations of hepatocyte nuclear factor (HNF)-1α in the pathogenesis of adenomas and adenomatosis as well as the association with familial cases and diabetes.[11,12] Anabolic/androgenic steroid-related hepatocellular tumours[13] in children or adults sometimes appear malignant histologically but do not necessarily behave in a malignant manner and may therefore be regarded as adenomas rather than carcinomas.[14,15] They may contain areas of peliosis, blood-filled spaces with an incomplete endothelial lining. Liver cell adenomas may also arise in patients with diabetes[16] or type I glycogen storage disease,[17] and in children or young adults (see Neoplasms and nodules in children).

Macroregenerative nodules (large regenerative nodules)

The macroregenerative nodule (MRN) or large regenerative nodule is an unusually large regenerative nodule, which usually develops in cirrhotic liver. Because the MRN is one of several possible settings in which hepatocellular carcinoma may develop, it is covered in greater detail later in this chapter (see Precursors of hepatocellular carcinoma).

Focal nodular hyperplasia (FNH)

This is a fairly common lesion, seen in either sex and at any age. FNH is a reactive, hyperplastic response of polyclonal[18] hepatocytes, fibrous stroma and bile ductules due to a putative pre-existing arterial malformation.[19–22] FNH, unlike liver-cell adenoma, does not appear to be caused by oral contraceptives. Although oral contraceptives may cause an increase in size and vascularity,[23] they do not appear to influence the number or size of these lesions.[24] Bleeding and rupture are rare, as is recurrence after resection.[25] Features of focal nodular hyperplasia and adenoma are only very occasionally seen in the same tumour and the occurrence of the two lesions in the same liver may be coincidental.[26] There may be multiple FNH in the same patient and these individuals often have other lesions, including vascular anomalies (hepatic haemangioma, telangiectasis of the brain, berry aneurysm, dysplastic systemic arteries, portal vein atresia), central nervous system neoplasms (meningioma, astrocytoma)[27,28] and hemihypertrophy.[29]

Macroscopically, the nodules are well demarcated from the normal hepatic parenchyma. They are usually pale and are dissected by fibrous septa into nodules, giving them an appearance very like that of cirrhosis. There may be a prominent central fibrous scar (Fig. 11.2). Histologically, the appearance is also very like that of an inactive cirrhosis. The dense fibrous septa contain large thick-walled and sometimes narrowed arteries, as well as bile duct-like structures probably derived from metaplastic liver-cell plates[30] or from progenitor cells.[21] The telangiectatic form of FNH shows prominent sinusoidal dilatation, abnormal arterioles and ductular structures, but the constituent liver-cell plates often appear thin and atrophic.[31] The presence of bile duct cells in fine-needle aspiration cytology of FNH is helpful in distinguishing this lesion from hepatocellular carcinoma.[32] In fine-needle biopsies obtained under computed tomographic (CT) guidance, the pathologist should be made aware that a mass lesion is being biopsied, since the proliferated bile duct-like

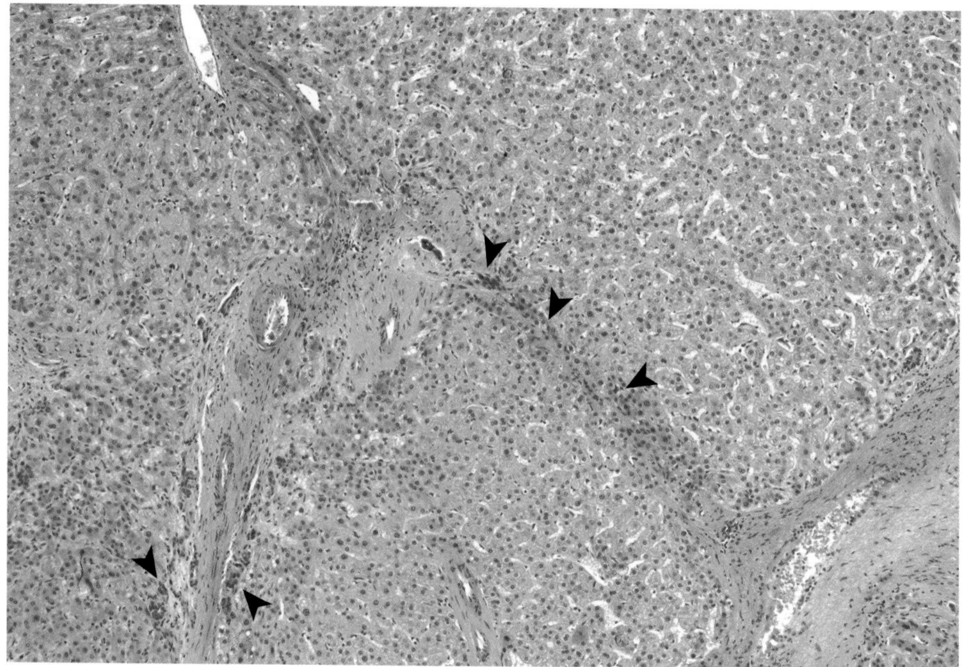

Figure 11.2 *Focal nodular hyperplasia.* Part of a central scar with abnormal arterioles has been sampled. Radiating fibrous septa show small bile duct-like structures at their edges (arrowheads). The parenchyma is nodular. (Operative specimen, H&E).

structures and reactive stroma may otherwise suggest the diagnosis of mechanical bile duct obstruction.

Lesions that grossly resemble FNH are also occasionally seen in Budd-Chiari syndrome.[33] Microscopically, these masses show hyperplastic, regenerative nodules in combination with other features, including central scars and multiple arterial structures. Some vary histologically so as to suggest crossover lesions between large regenerative nodules, FNH and liver-cell adenoma.[34] They appear to result from hyperarterialisation of regions of decreased hepatic venous blood flow.[34,35]

Nodular regenerative hyperplasia (NRH)

In this condition, multiple hyperplastic parenchymal nodules with thickened liver-cell plates are seen, but fibrosis is absent or slight (Fig. 11.3). This distinguishes the lesion from cirrhosis. In some cases, perisinusoidal fibrosis is found in the compressed liver tissue between nodules. Portal tracts may be found at the centres of the nodules but this is not invariable. Diagnosis is often difficult in needle biopsy specimens. The nodularity may be more clearly seen in reticulin preparations (Fig. 11.4). A wedge liver biopsy may be required to establish the diagnosis and to exclude an important differential, incomplete septal cirrhosis (see Ch. 10).

NRH is associated with a wide range of conditions, mainly rheumatic diseases, myeloproliferative disorders and chronic venous congestion.[36–38] Patients with NRH may have received therapeutic drugs, including corticosteroids, anabolic steroids, oral contraceptives, antineoplastics,[39] anticonvulsants and immunosuppressive agents.[36,40,41] NRH has also been associated with the toxic oil syndrome,[42] Behçet's disease,[43] early histologic stages of primary biliary cirrhosis,[44] livers containing

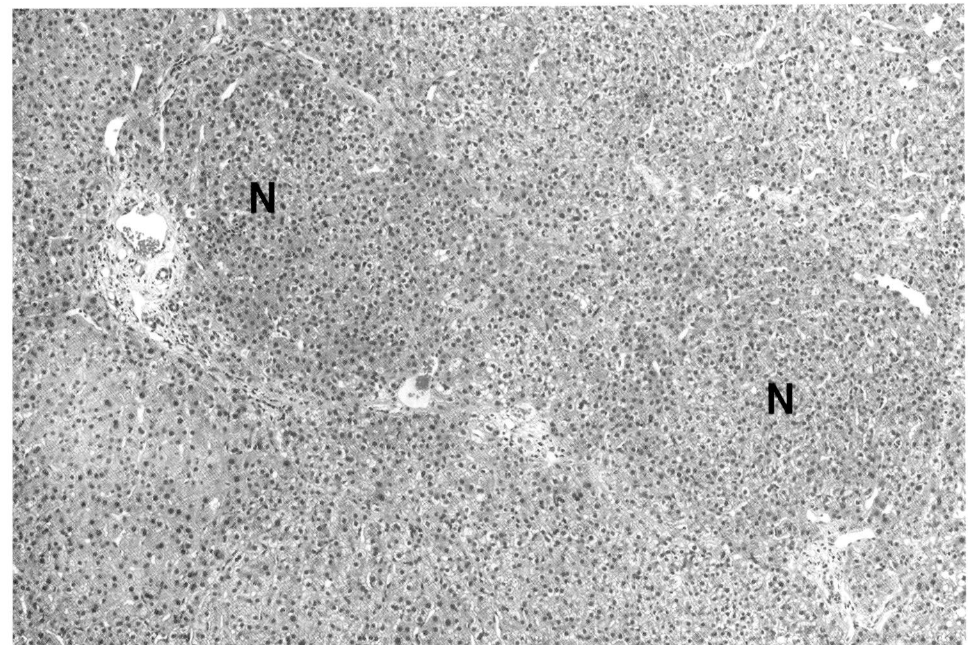

Figure 11.3 *Nodular regenerative hyperplasia*. This abnormal, nodular growth pattern is not accompanied by fibrosis and therefore differs from cirrhosis. The parenchymal nodules (N) are often adjacent to (nodule at left) or surround portal tracts. The intervening liver shows flattened and compressed liver-cell plates and/or sinusoidal dilatation. (Post-mortem liver, H&E).

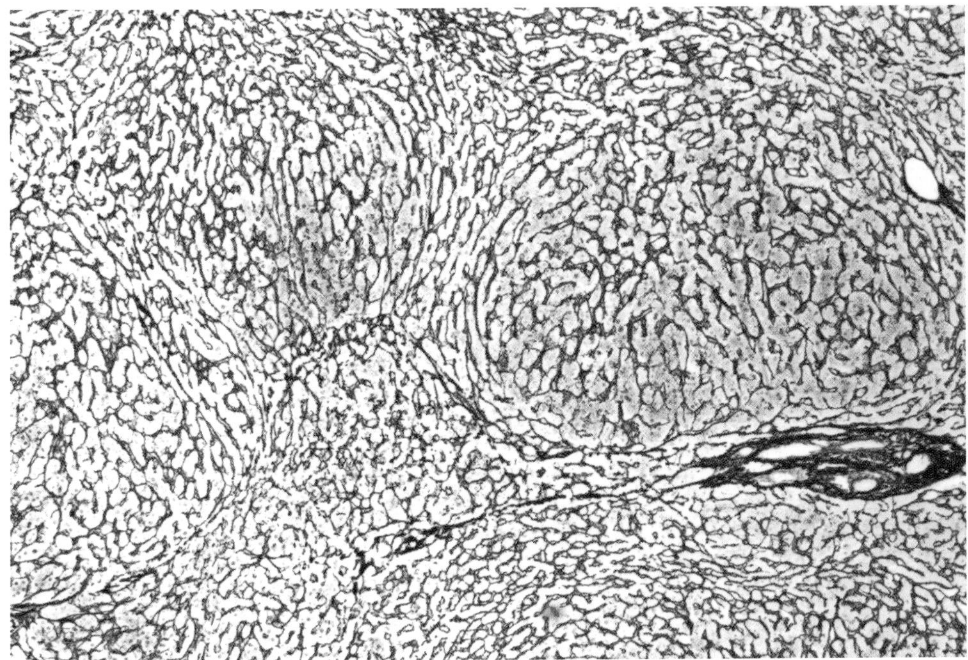

Figure 11.4 *Nodular regenerative hyperplasia*. Reticulin stain of a field similar to that shown in Figure 11.3 highlights the regenerative nodules and the absence of fibrosis. (Post-mortem liver, reticulin).

metastatic neuroendocrine tumours[45] and non-cirrhotic liver in which hepatocellular carcinoma has developed.[46] Some patients with NRH have portal hypertension. Serum alkaline phosphatase and gamma glutamyl transpeptidase may be elevated.[38,44]

Wanless and co-workers have postulated that the basic lesion is portal venous thrombosis, leading to atrophy and compensatory hyperplasia.[47] Arterial lesions, particularly arteriosclerosis of ageing, may also contribute to these changes.[38] Portal venous thrombosis has also been invoked in the pathogenesis of the rare **partial nodular transformation**, in which somewhat larger nodules are found, often localised to the perihilar region.[48,49] Nodular regenerative hyperplasia, focal nodular hyperplasia and partial nodular transformation share the common feature of liver-cell hyperplastic growth in the form of nodules; they have accordingly been grouped under the umbrella heading of 'nodular transformation' by Wanless.[50] The main features of the various non-cirrhotic nodular conditions so far discussed are summarised in Table 11.2.

Bile-duct adenoma

Bile-duct adenomas are small grey-white, usually subcapsular nodules measuring from 1 to 20 mm in diameter,[51] which may represent hamartomatous peribiliary glands rather than a neoplasm.[52] They are more often solitary than multiple. Histologically, they are composed of small well-formed ducts embedded in a stroma of mature fibrous tissue which may contain chronic inflammatory cells, often densely aggregated at the periphery of the lesion[51,53,54] (Fig. 11.5). Their chief importance is that they may be mistaken for metastatic carcinoma, both macroscopically and microscopically. They differ from microhamartomas (von Meyenburg complexes) in that the ducts are smaller and more numerous, are usually not dilated and do not contain bile.[51,55] PAS-positive, diastase-resistant globules of α_1-antitrypsin within the bile-duct epithelium of multiple adenomas were described in a patient with heterozygous α_1-antitrypsin deficiency.[56] The bile-duct adenoma should also be distinguished from the rare **biliary adenofibroma**, a much larger tumour composed of tubulocystic bile-duct structures with apocrine metaplasia and intraluminal bile embedded in fibrous stroma, resembling fibroadenoma of the breast.[57]

Table 11.2 Non-cirrhotic parenchymal nodules

Type Number; involvement of liver	Structure	Portal hypertension
Focal nodular hyperplasia Solitary or few;	Mixed	No
Focal Liver-cell adenoma Solitary or few; rarely many;	Liver cells	No
Focal Nodular regenerative hyperplasia Many; Diffuse	Liver cells	Sometimes
Partial nodular transformation Several; Perihilar	Liver cells, some fibrous tissue	Usually

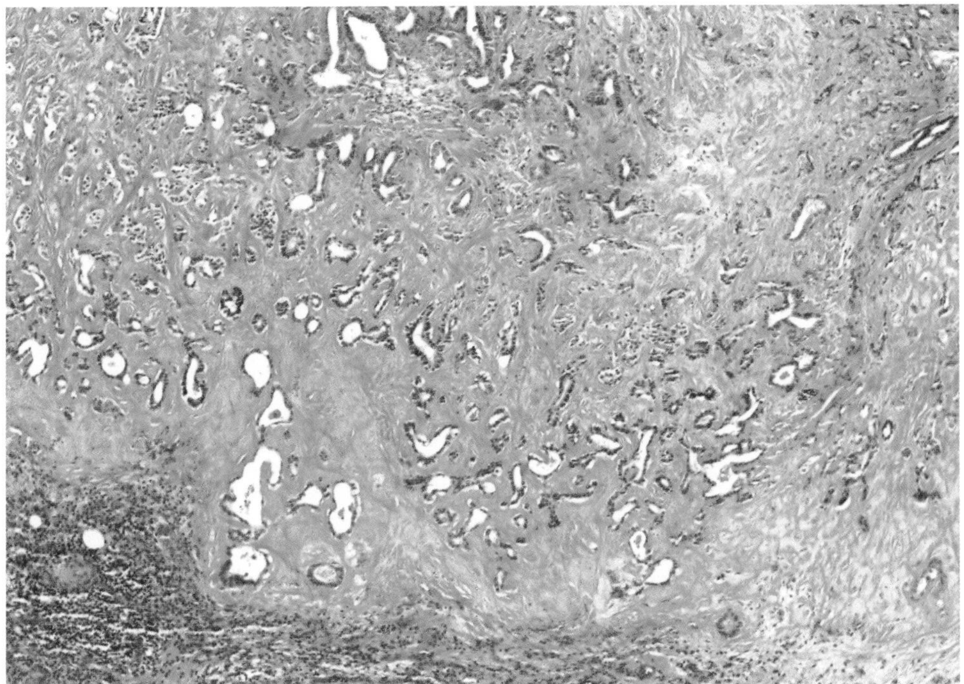

Figure 11.5 *Bile-duct adenoma.* This subcapsular tumour consists of closely packed bile-ducts set in a dense fibrous stroma. A dense collection of lymphocytes is seen at the edge of the lesion (at bottom). (Operative specimen, H&E).

Biliary cystadenoma

This is a multilocular tumour, the cystic spaces of which contain mucoid fluid and are lined by columnar, mucin-secreting epithelium which may form papillary projections. A variant with subepithelial **mesenchymal stroma** containing myofibroblasts occurs in women.[58,59] Malignant change is common.[60]

Haemangioma

The cavernous haemangioma is the most common benign tumour of the liver, found incidentally at autopsy or operation and occasionally seen in biopsy material.[61] A few reach a large and clinically significant size. As in other sites, the lesions are composed of endothelium-lined channels supported by a fibrous stroma (Fig. 11.6). Complications include thrombosis, sclerosis and calcification.[62] Spontaneous rupture is recorded but uncommon. A distinction should be made between cavernous haemangiomas and peliosis; the latter lacks the complete endothelial layer and fibrous trabeculae. **Lymphangioma** of the liver has been reported as part of multiorgan lymphangiomatosis or as a solitary hepatic lesion,[63] but is very rare. The endothelial-lined channels of this neoplasm are empty or contain lymph with occasional leucocytes. It should not be mistaken for mesenchymal hamartoma (see Neoplasms and nodules in children).

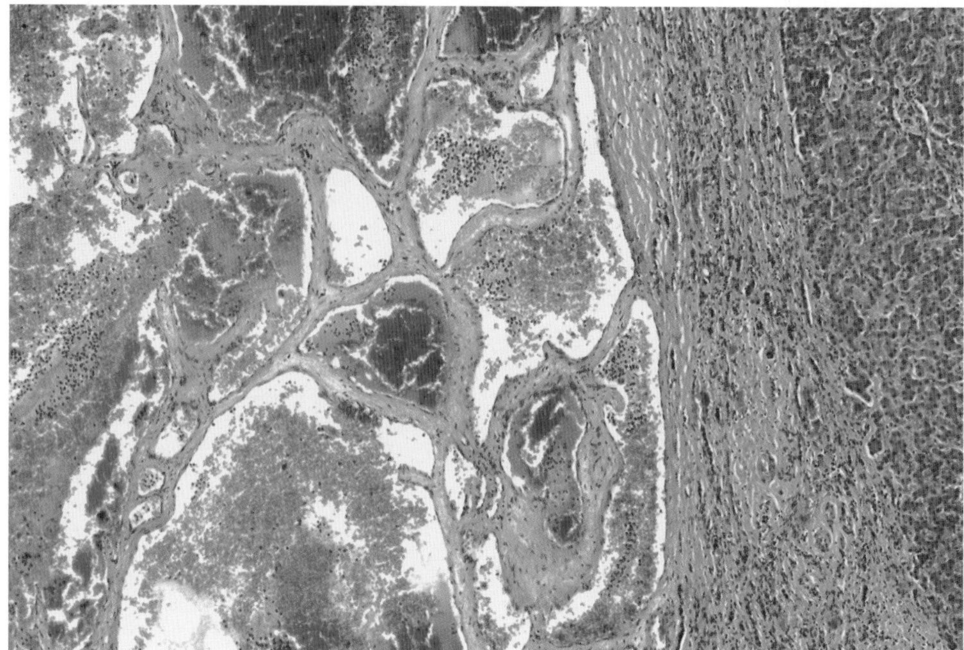

Figure 11.6 *Haemangioma.* Blood-filled spaces are separated by fibrous septa. A thick capsule is seen at right. (Operative specimen, H&E).

Mesenchymal and neural tumours

Connective-tissue elements, adipocytes and smooth muscle of the liver, nerve sheaths of intrahepatic nerves and other mesenchymal cells may give rise to rare tumours, including lipomas, myelolipomas, angiomyelolipomas,[64,65] schwannomas and neurofibromas,[66–68] solitary fibrous tumours[69] and chondromas.[70] **Angiomyolipomas** resemble their more common renal counterparts and contain blood vessels, smooth muscle (myoid cells) and fat.[71] These components allow subcategorisation into mixed, lipomatous, myomatous and angiomatous types, in decreasing order of frequency.[72] Multiple tumours may be present.[73,74] Muscle cells may be partly of epithelioid type, with finely granular eosinophilic cytoplasm and pleomorphic nuclei[75–78] (Fig. 11.7). These may be mistaken for hepatocytes or malignant cells, particularly in cases where the component of fat is minimal. Megakaryocytes and other bone marrow elements are commonly present. Positive HMB-45 immunostaining of the myoid cells is a major diagnostic feature.[72,78] **Pseudolipomas**[79] probably represent separated nodules of peritoneal fat which become embedded in the liver capsule.

Inflammatory pseudotumour

These lesions may be solitary or multiple and usually occur in young, male patients with constitutional symptoms, fever and weight loss. They may sometimes involve structures near the porta hepatis with resultant biliary problems or portal hypertension. The microscopic hallmark of inflammatory pseudotumour is the extensive polyclonal plasma cell infiltrates which are intermixed with lymphocytes, eosinophils, foamy histiocytes and variable degrees of stromal proliferation, including spindle cells in bundles and whorls with associated fibrosis[80] (Fig. 11.8).

and HCC[86,87] and subsequently with a four- to five-fold increased risk of HCC in several studies.[88,89] Affected cells are usually aneuploid[90] and may have attendant chromosomal abnormalities.[91] However, it has been considered merely an effect of cholestasis[92] or a derangement in normal liver-cell polyploidisation[93] and has not been proven to be a direct pathogenetic precursor lesion of HCC. Nevertheless, it is a strong independent risk factor for the development of HCC[94] and thereby identifies patients requiring more diligent surveillance.

Small cell LCD (**small cell change**) is characterised by enlarged, hyperchromatic nuclei within small hepatocytes (increased nuclear-cytoplasmic ratio) arranged in crowded clusters[95] (see Fig 10.9; see also Cytopathological diagnosis; Fig. 11.34). These foci show high cellular proliferation rates,[96] and an overall cytologic resemblance to HCC and may originate from progenitor cells.[94] These features have lent support to small cell dysplasia as a true precursor lesion that is subject to the later cellular events leading to the development of HCC.

Other cellular changes cited as indicators of pre-malignancy include intracytoplasmic Mallory bodies,[97] irregular areas of regeneration showing hepatocyte glycogenosis, oncocytic change (see Ch. 9) or bulging nodularity,[98] iron-negative foci in siderotic macroregenerative nodules[99] and 'iron-free foci' in livers of patients with hereditary haemochromatosis;[100] the latter may show large cell LCD.[100] Clusters of large cell or small cell dysplastic hepatocytes less than 1 mm in diameter have been termed **dysplastic foci** by an international working party.[85]

The **macroregenerative nodule** (**MRN**) is an unusually large regenerative nodule measuring 0.8 cm or more in diameter, which develops in cirrhosis or other chronic liver disease[101] (Fig. 11.9). MRNs are particularly common in macronodular cirrhosis.[102] They may be paler or more bile-stained than the surrounding liver.[85] The

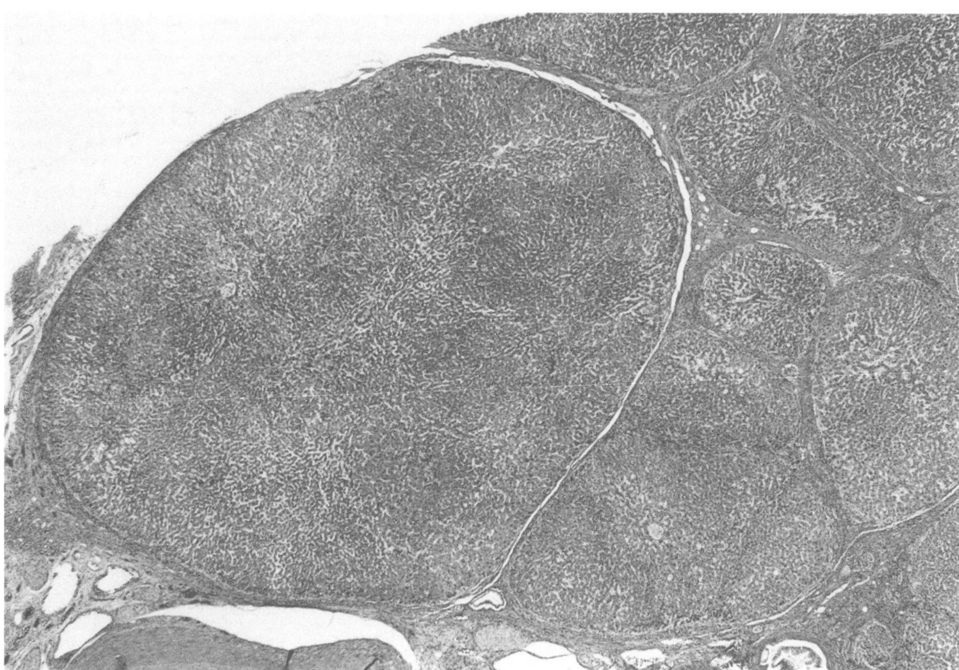

Figure 11.9 *Macroregenerative nodule*. This low magnification view demonstrates the increased size of the nodule at right compared to the cirrhotic nodules at left. (Operative specimen, H&E). (Figure kindly provided by Dr Kamal Ishak, Washington, DC).

cirrhotic liver may harbour several macroregenerative nodules. MRNs may coexist with hepatocellular carcinoma elsewhere in the liver or may contain foci of carcinoma. Cirrhotic explant livers should be carefully examined for these lesions[84,103] and for liver-cell dysplasia.[104]

The MRN histologically shows hyperplastic liver parenchyma arranged in plates 2–3 cells thick, which is typical of cirrhosis. The nodule contains portal tracts and fibrous septa with bile ducts, hepatic arteries and portal vein branches and shows no cellular atypia or disorder in the liver-cell plate arrangement. Steatosis, haemosiderin, bile plugs and Mallory bodies may be present.[101,105] The term 'adenomatous hyperplasia,' a former synonym of MRN, as well as subdivisions into MRN types I and II,[102] are not currently advocated for use.[85]

The **dysplastic nodule (borderline nodule)** shows atypical architectural and/or cytological features that are not acceptable for a benign macroregenerative nodule, but which fall diagnostically short of frank hepatocellular carcinoma.[85,106] Dysplastic nodules may show varying degrees of large and small cell LCD, increased cellularity and foci where the liver cords are less cohesive, focal loss of reticulin fibres or pseudoacini[84,85,103,106] (Fig. 11.10).

The major diagnostic concern is to distinguish MRNs and dysplastic nodules from hepatocellular carcinoma. Certain features seen in these nodules are associated with high risk of progression to carcinoma, including an increased ratio of nuclear density, clear cell change, small cell dysplasia and fatty change.[107] Increased mitotic activity, loss of reticulin fibres, formation of broad trabeculae and an infiltrative margin are helpful evidence of carcinoma.[84,103,108,109] Studies that have demonstrated clonality and loss of heterozygosity[110] and increased cell proliferative indices[111] combined with newer techniques such as spectral karyotype (SKY)[112] and gene

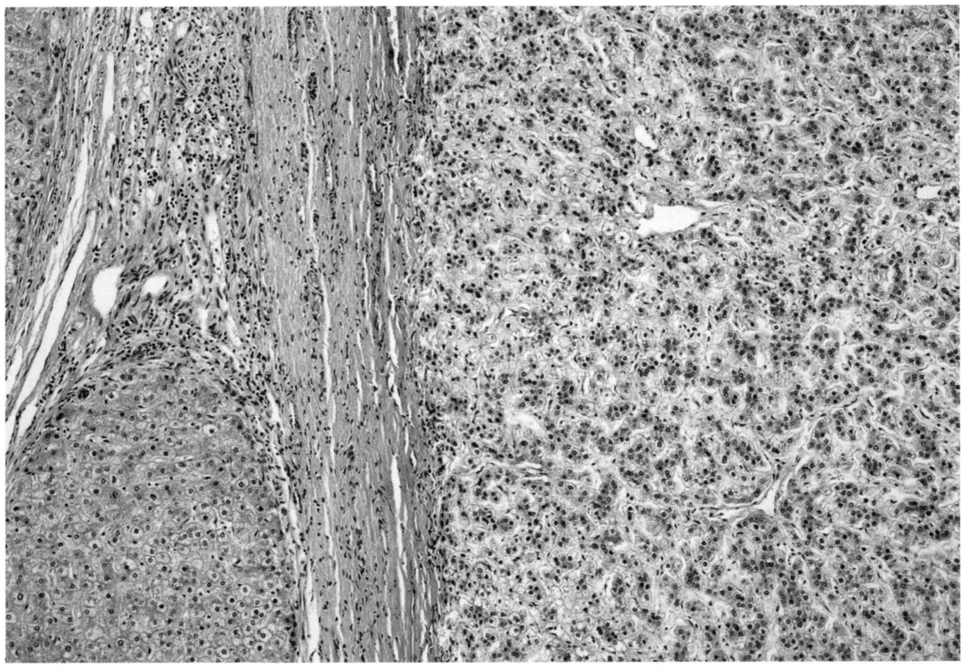

Figure 11.10 *Dysplastic nodule.* The dysplastic nodule at right shows hepatocytes arranged in pseudoacini, with a less cohesive growth pattern centrally. A cirrhotic nodule is present at lower left. The patient had an inactive cirrhosis due to tyrosinaemia. (Explant liver, H&E).

microarray[113] analysis are promising avenues for understanding the key biological and morphological steps in the pathogenesis of HCC.

Hepatocellular carcinoma (HCC)

Hepatocellular carcinoma ranks fifth among malignant tumours worldwide.[87] Epidemiological and other studies of HCC have defined geographical variations in the incidence and prevalence of this tumour, as well as a multifactorial aetiology.[114] Chronic necrosis and inflammation of the liver are important driving forces in the multistep process of hepatocarcinogenesis[115,116] in the context of underlying risk factors such as hepatitis B and C viral infections,[87] iron overload,[117] aflatoxin exposure[118] and the presence of fatty liver disease.[119–121] At the molecular level, identification of genetic changes that control cell cycling and apoptosis,[122] as well as oncogene expression,[123] mutation of tumour suppressor genes such as p53,[124] expression of vascular and cellular growth factors[125–130] and proliferation of hepatic stem cells or their progeny[131,132] comprise a large and growing literature on this subject.

The majority of HCCs develop in cirrhotic liver.[133] The cause of the cirrhosis is usually known, even in many cases labelled as 'cryptogenic' where risk factors for non-alcoholic fatty liver disease (see Ch. 7) become apparent.[120] The non-cirrhotic setting accounts for a substantial number of cases from North America[134] and elsewhere[135] and can be seen in hepatitis B virus carriers[136,137] or suspected occult hepatitis B[135] and in individuals infected with hepatitis C virus.[138] HCC may even develop within ectopic liver.[139] The cirrhosis associated with carcinoma is often macronodular in pattern, except for the micronodular cirrhosis seen in genetic haemochromatosis and chronic hepatitis C. The cirrhosis is usually inactive, although inflammation and necrosis may be seen near the tumour itself. Tumours may be multifocal.[140] Intrahepatic tumour spread is both portal (via portal vein branches) and lobular.[141] Rarely, HCC may spontaneously regress.[87,142,143] Following transplantation, cirrhotic explant livers require careful examination for small carcinomas and precursor lesions which are clinically undetected.[144] Pathology reports on explants or partial resections with HCC should specify the number of lesions and their sizes, as well as the histological grade and evidence of vascular invasion[145] since these factors affect TNM and other prognostic classifications.[146]

The outstanding histological features of hepatocellular carcinoma are the resemblance of the tumour cells to normal hepatocytes and of their arrangement to the trabeculae of normal liver (Fig. 11.11). However, the trabeculae are for the most part thicker and reticulin is often scanty or even absent (Fig. 11.12). This paucireticulin pattern is helpful in fine needle aspiration biopsies (see Cytopathological diagnosis). In exceptional cases where there may be an increase in reticulin, other histological features and/or the clinical behaviour of the tumour must be used as diagnostic criteria of malignancy. Rarely, the trabecular pattern and even bile production is mimicked by primary tumours ('hepatoid carcinomas') of the stomach, ovary and other sites[147] (see Metastatic tumour). Between the tumour trabeculae in HCC there is a network of vascular channels lined by endothelium which is positive with immunostains for CD34,[125,126] factor VIII-related antigen and *Ulex europaeus* lectin.[148] The endothelial lining of these channels is a particularly helpful diagnostic feature in fine needle aspirates (see Cytopathological diagnosis; Fig. 11.36). The absence of portal tracts and a cohesive connective tissue framework in the tumour results in a characteristic fragmentation of needle biopsy specimens with separation of tumour trabeculae that is readily observed at low magnification. Although connective tissue stroma is uncommon except in **fibrolamellar carcinoma**

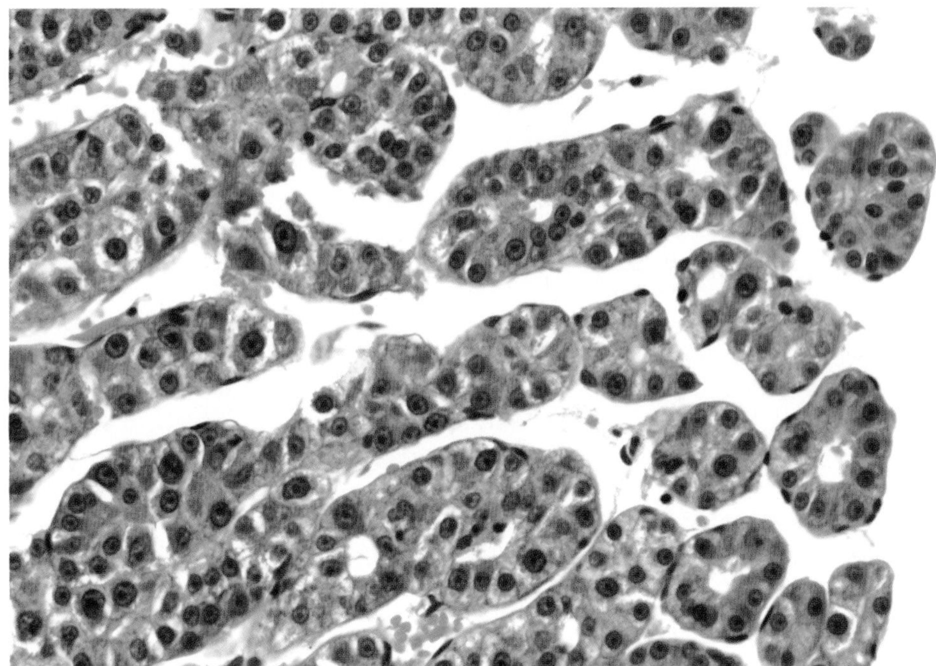

Figure 11.11 *Hepatocellular carcinoma*. Note the trabecular-sinusoidal structure and resemblance of the tumour cells to normal hepatocytes. (Needle biopsy, H&E).

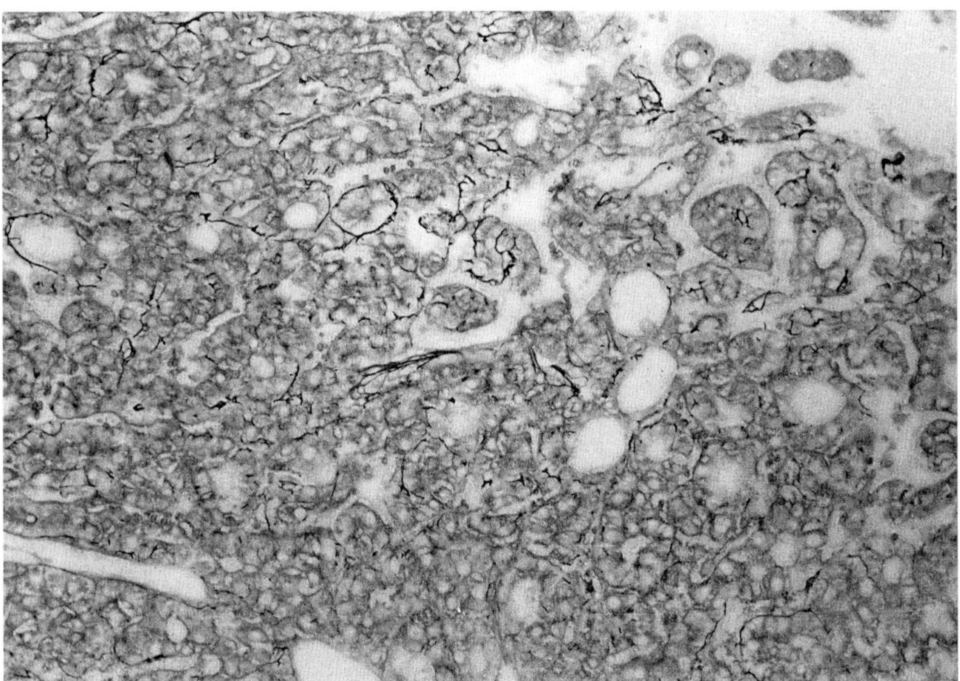

Figure 11.12 *Hepatocellular carcinoma*. Reticulin is scanty in this example. (Needle biopsy, reticulin).

(described below), focal areas of fibrosis may follow tumour necrosis. A form of HCC designated as **sclerosing carcinoma**[149] is often associated with hypercalcaemia; some of these tumours appear to be of bile-duct rather than hepatocellular origin. The **adenoid** (acinar) variant of hepatocellular carcinoma (Fig. 11.13) should not be confused with adenocarcinoma of the biliary tree. Bile-duct carcinomas are usually scirrhous, mucin-secreting tumours, whereas the characteristic secretion of hepatocellular carcinomas is bile, seen in a minority of tumours in spaces homologous with normal bile canaliculi. Mixed or combined tumours designated **hepatocellular-cholangiocarcinoma** are also well described, with special stains and immunohistochemical features representative of both hepatocellular and bile duct epithelial derivation. Stem cell constituents are sometimes present[150] as shown by cytokeratin 7 or 19 positivity (discussed below). Occasionally HCC is infiltrated by T-lymphocytes and shows an improved prognosis.[151]

At a cellular level, variants include giant-cell forms with multinucleated tumour cells (a bad prognostic sign[152]) (Fig. 11.14), spindle-cell or sarcomatoid tumours[153,154] and clear-cell carcinomas. The latter must be distinguished from metastatic renal adenocarcinoma.[155,156] Fine-needle aspiration yields diagnostic material in a high proportion of patients.[157–160] Histologic grading of HCC from 1 to 4 is based on nuclear features, with grade 1 HCC resembling normal hepatocytes and grade 2 showing prominent nucleoli, hyperchromatism and nuclear membrane irregularities.[161] Grades 3 and 4 show progressively greater nuclear pleomorphism, the latter featuring anaplastic and giant tumour cells (Fig. 11.14).

When there is doubt about the hepatocellular origin of a carcinoma, further evidence can sometimes be gained from the characteristics of the tumour cells. In hepatocellular carcinoma, these often contain fat and glycogen and may also contain α_1-antitrypsin globules even in patients without genetic α_1-antitrypsin deficiency.

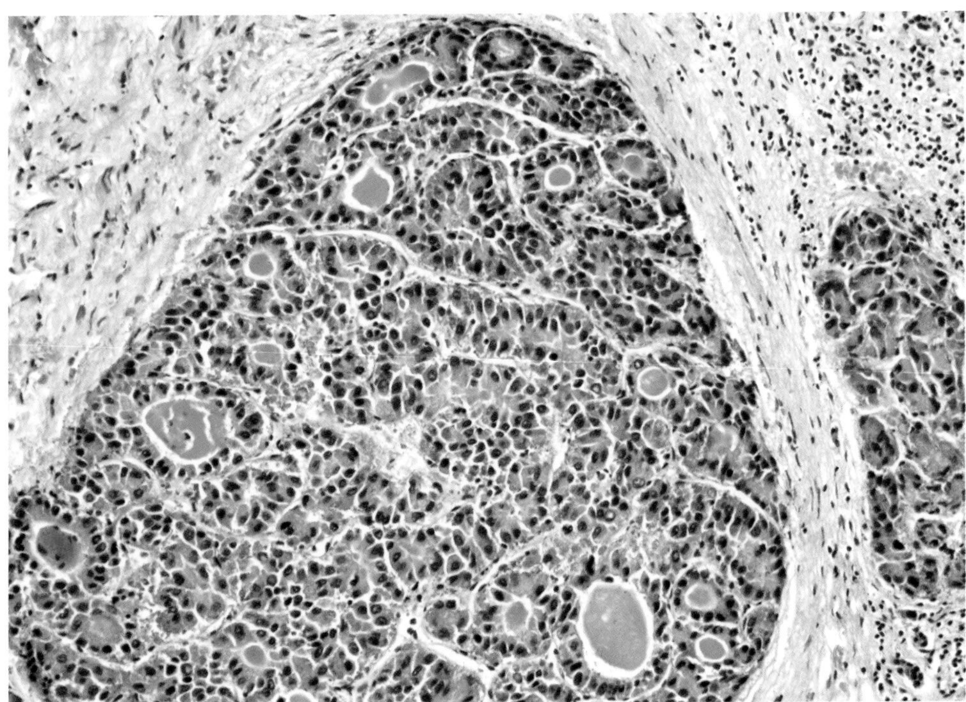

Figure 11.13 *Hepatocellular carcinoma*. Adenoid pattern. Other areas of this tumour showed a more typical trabecular structure. (Post-mortem liver, H&E).

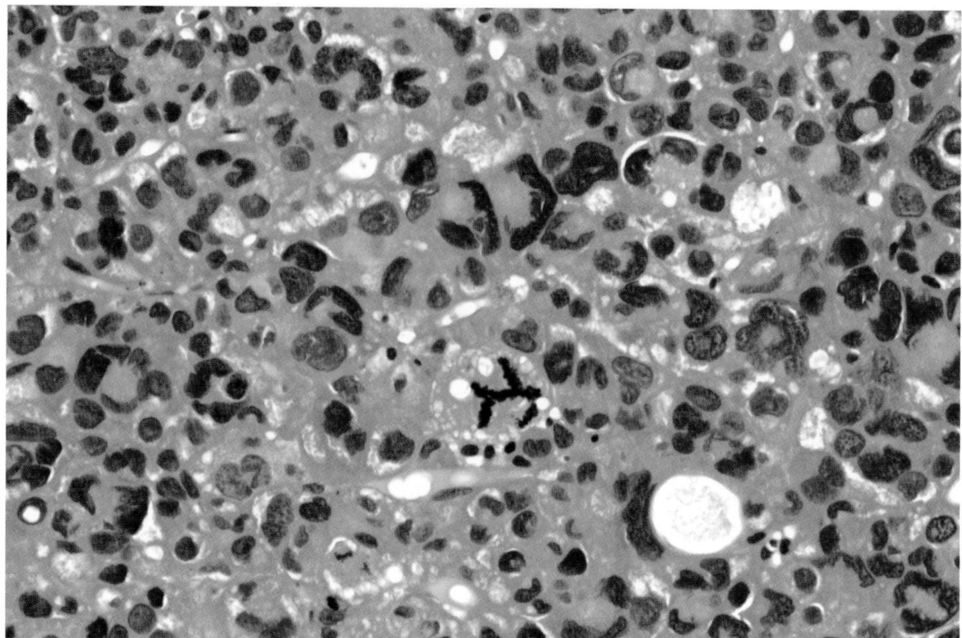

Figure 11.14 *Hepatocellular carcinoma.* This high-grade tumour shows marked anaplasia with giant, multinucleated tumour cells and atypical mitotic figures. (Needle biopsy, H&E).

Mallory bodies are commonly found in the cytoplasm of the tumour cells.[162] Evidence of hepatocellular origin is also provided when immunohistochemical stains of paraffin sections are positive for albumin, fibrinogen, liver-cell cytokeratins (8 and 18), α_1-antitrypsin or α_1-antichymotrypsin.[163–167]

Immunohistochemistry is particularly useful in confirming the diagnosis of HCC (Table 11.4). A good initial approach is to order a panel of four immunostains, including Hep Par 1 (hepatocyte), polyclonal carcinoembryonic antigen (pCEA) and cytokeratins 7 and 20 (CK7 and CK20). Hep Par 1, which stains normal and malignant hepatocytes, is a specific and sensitive marker of HCC, with only rare extrahepatic tumours staining positively.[168] pCEA stains a carbohydrate moiety (biliary glycoprotein) on bile canalicular membranes (serving as an internal control if the biopsy sample includes non-neoplastic liver tissue along with tumour), thereby providing positive staining of apical surfaces or canalicular structures of the HCC cells (Fig. 11.15). Although CD10 also shows similar staining to pCEA, it is far less sensitive.[169] HCC is typically negative for both CK7 and CK20.[170] However, a subset of HCC may stain positively with cytokeratin 7 and/or cytokeratin 19, the latter in particular identifying progenitor cell constituents in the tumour, risk of early postoperative recurrence[171] and a poor prognosis (Professor Tania Roskams, personal communication). The tumour cells are also negative with monoclonal anti-CEA[163] and AE1 cytokeratin.[165] α-Fetoprotein is an unreliable immunostain for HCC,[172] in contrast to hepatoblastoma where most cases stain positively.

Fibrolamellar carcinoma

This tumour usually develops in non-cirrhotic liver in older children and adults and carries a better prognosis (because of its resectability[173]) than typical hepatocellular carcinoma.[174–177] The lesions are solitary or multiple and occasionally resemble focal

Table 11.4 Immunohistochemical stains in the evaluation of hepatic tumours

Tumour	Recommended immunostain(s)
Hepatocellular carcinoma	Hep Par I (hepatocyte)
	polyclonal CEA[a]
	cytokeratin 7/20 pair (–/– staining)[b]
Hepatoblastoma	α-fetoprotein (AFP)
	Hep Par I (hepatocyte)
	polyclonal CEA
Cholangiocarcinoma	cytokeratin 7/19 pair (+/+ staining)
	cytokeratin 7/20 pair (+/+ staining)[b]
Angiomyolipoma	HMB-45
Solitary fibrous tumour	CD34
	Vimentin
Epithelioid haemangioendothelioma	CD34
	CD31
	Factor VIII
Metastatic carcinoma	
Neuroendocrine	chromogranin
	synaptophysin
	neuron-specific enolase
Pancreas	cytokeratin 7/20 pair (+/+ staining)[b]
Colorectal	cytokeratin 7/20 pair (–/+ staining)[b]
Breast	cytokeratin 7/20 pair (+/– staining)[b]
Lung (non-small cell)	cytokeratin 7/20 pair (+/– staining)[b]

[a]Staining is canalicular or apical.
[b]See Chu and Weiss (2002).[170]

nodular hyperplasia macroscopically in having a central fibrous scar.[178] The unique histological features distinguish this tumour from routine hepatocellular carcinoma. Fibrous lamellae arranged in parallel separate groups of large, densely eosinophilic tumour cells,[176,179] which produce transforming growth factor-beta[180] (Fig. 11.16). The eosinophilia is due to the presence of abundant mitochondria.[175,181] Tumour cells commonly contain eosinophilic, diastase-PAS negative globules which stain immunohistochemically for C-reactive protein, fibrinogen and α_1-antitrypsin, as well as cytoplasmic 'pale bodies' which are reactive for fibrinogen.[176] Additional features include bile production (as in other forms of hepatocellular carcinoma), copper and copper-associated protein within tumour cells[182,183] and stainable carcinoembryonic antigen in bile canaliculi.[184] Some fibrolamellar carcinomas have neuroendocrine features[185,186] and in some cases, the tumour shows features of both fibrolamellar and typical hepatocellular carcinoma.[187] Despite isolated reports such as the association of Fanconi anaemia with fibrolamellar carcinoma,[188] the pathogenesis of this tumour is uncertain and risk factors are not apparent.

Bile-duct carcinoma (cholangiocarcinoma)

Carcinoma of the bile ducts can arise anywhere between the papilla of Vater and the smaller branches of the biliary tree within the liver. It is not usually associated with cirrhosis. There are two major anatomic types:[189] one arising either from extrahepatic bile ducts or at the bifurcation of right and left hepatic ducts (the latter perihilar

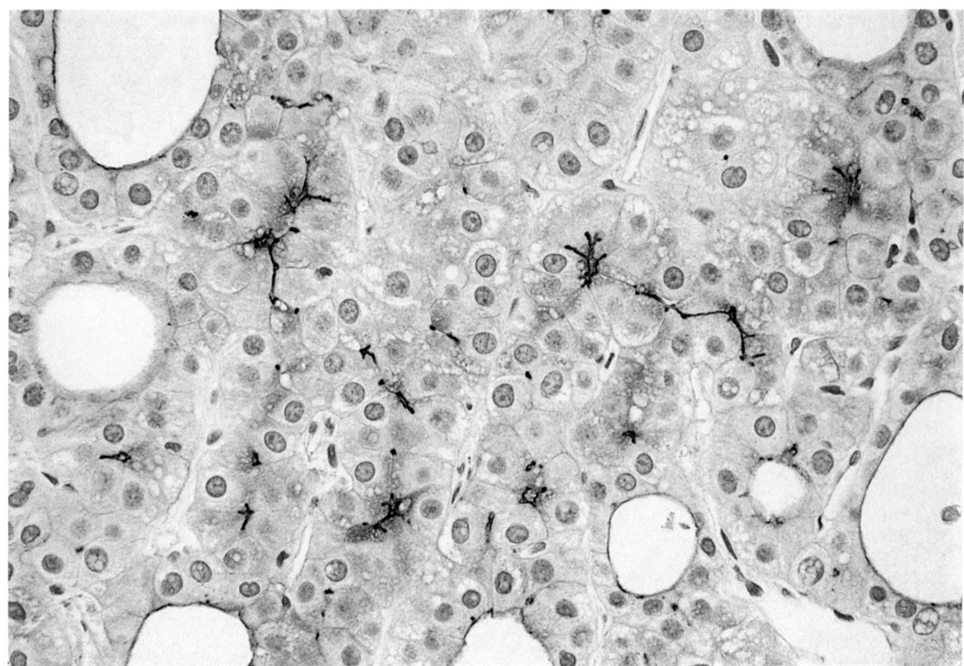

Figure 11.15 Immunohistochemical demonstration of bile canalicular structures in a hepatocellular carcinoma. (The branching spaces are here outlined by the use of polyclonal anti-CEA).

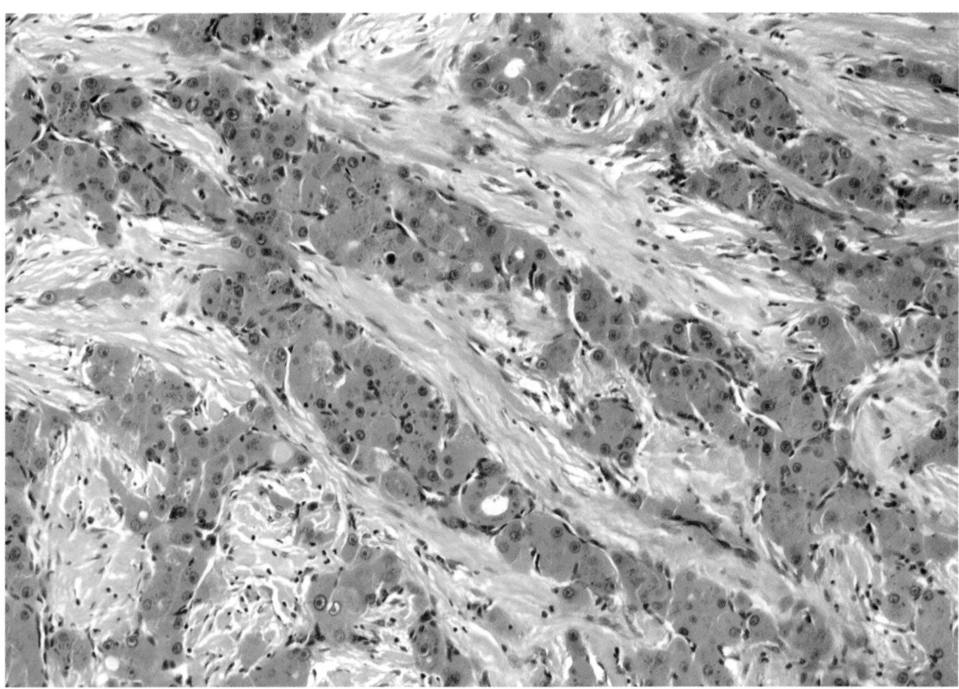

Figure 11.16 *Hepatocellular carcinoma: fibrolamellar type*. Groups of large, eosinophilic tumour cells are surrounded by fibrous septa in parallel arrays. (Needle biopsy, H&E).

cholangiocarcinoma sometimes referred to as a **Klatskin tumour**[190]) and a second type presenting as an intrahepatic mass.[191] Carcinoma of the hepatic ducts is an important cause of biliary obstruction, which may be missed at laparotomy unless the intrahepatic bile ducts are explored or visualised. The most commonly known predisposing factors to bile-duct cancer are infestation with oriental flukes, primary sclerosing cholangitis[192] and congenital cystic lesions of the biliary tree.[193] Of these, Caroli's disease and choledochal cysts are important precursors, but carcinoma may also arise in von Meyenburg complexes (bile-duct microhamartomas)[194] and in congenital hepatic fibrosis.[195] Development of carcinoma in bile duct adenoma is also reported.[196] In Japan, hepatitis C virus infection has been suggested as a risk factor[197] and intrahepatic cholangiocarcinoma is a known consequence of hepatolithiasis.[198] Investigations at the molecular level indicate pathogenetic roles for K-*ras* and *p53* mutations, increased expression of receptor tyrosine kinase c-erB-2 and c-met and expression of human telomerase reverse transcriptase (hTERT).[189]

Microscopically, bile-duct carcinomas are mucin-secreting adenocarcinomas with a reactive, desmoplastic fibrous stroma (Fig. 11.17). A fairly uniform gland size (medium to small) is often maintained within these tumours, in comparison to the wide size variations seen in glands of metastatic pancreatic carcinoma. The tumour cells are cuboidal or columnar and may assume a papillary pattern. Adenosquamous, squamous, mucinous,[199] clear cell[200] and anaplastic histologic types are less common.[201] Intra- and perineural invasion are common. The presence of free stromal mucin, small groups and isolated tumour cells in fibrous stroma and the concurrence of apparently normal epithelium and abnormal tumour cells within a duct-like structure all help to distinguish cholangiocarcinoma from metastatic tumour.[202] Cholangiocarcinoma must be distinguished from the acinar type of hepatocellular carcinoma, a distinction usually made with confidence on the basis of

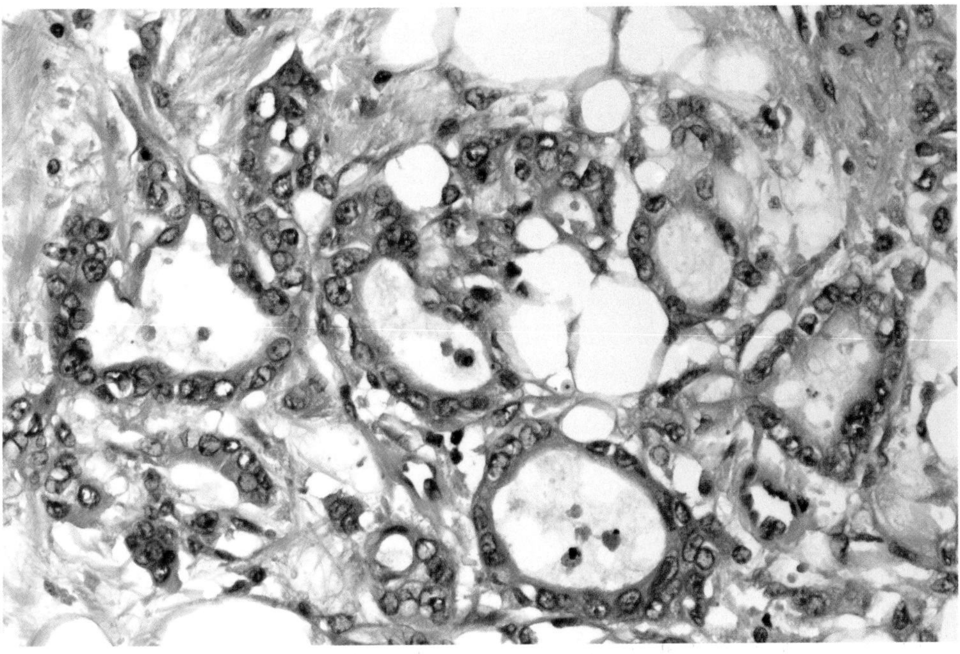

Figure 11.17 *Bile-duct carcinoma.* There are islands of adenocarcinoma in the connective tissue. The appearances are different from those of the hepatocellular carcinoma of adenoid pattern shown in Fig. 11.13. (Operative specimen, H&E).

mucin or bile secretion respectively. In difficult cases positive staining for epithelial membrane antigen,[203] tissue polypeptide antigen,[204] biliary cytokeratins[164] (7 and 19), Lewis(x) and Lewis(y) blood group-related antigens,[205] and α-amylase[206] helps to exclude hepatocellular carcinoma. In the uncommon tumour which shows combined hepatocellular-cholangiocarcinoma, cytokeratins 7 and 19 and epithelial membrane antigen immunostaining is positive in the cholangiocellular component.[207,208] Other rare mixed tumours show sarcomatoid[209] or fibrolamellar regions.[210] The differential diagnosis of bile-duct cancer includes epithelioid haemangioendothelioma. Bile-duct tumours are very occasionally of neuroendocrine type, with characteristic neurosecretory granules in their cytoplasm.

Cystadenocarcinomas are rare malignant tumours which sometimes develop from benign cystadenomas.[58,60] Although these have been considered distinct from the more aggressive carcinomas arising from pre-existing congenital cystic lesions,[211] occasional tumours with features of cystadenocarcinoma develop in fibropolycystic disease.[212]

Angiosarcoma

This uncommon, highly malignant tumour forms multiple or, less often, solitary haemorrhagic masses. Predisposing factors include treatment with arsenic,[213] injection of the radioactive contrast medium Thorotrast[214–216] and industrial exposure to vinyl chloride.[217] Other postulated factors include copper-containing vineyard sprays,[218] steroid hormones,[219–221] phenelzine[222] and urethane.[223] Positive staining of tumour cells for factor VIII-related antigen and other endothelial markers is evidence of their endothelial origin.[224,225] Their growth is characteristically along sinusoids and around surviving, hyperplastic hepatocytes (Fig. 11.18). The presence of the latter may lead to confusion with hepatocellular carcinoma, with which angiosarcoma, however, occasionally coexists. Infiltration of sinusoids beyond the main tumour mass makes the outlines of the tumour indistinct. Both cavernous and solid areas may be present. Other features include islands of haemopoietic cells and areas of thrombosis and infarction.

The non-neoplastic liver tissue is usually not cirrhotic, but may show fibrosis and other changes attributable to the predisposing factors listed above, including deposits of refractile Thorotrast granules in macrophages. Features seen irrespective of the cause include focal dilatation of sinusoids, hyperplasia of hepatocytes, sinusoid-lining cells and perisinusoidal cells and increased perisinusoidal reticulin.[226] These changes may precede the development of the tumour.[227]

Epithelioid haemangioendothelioma

This endothelial tumour of soft tissues or the lung (intravascular bronchioloalveolar tumour) may uncommonly present as a primary liver tumour. In the liver, it is seen in patients from the second to eighth decades of life, with women more commonly affected.[228–230] Its prognosis varies very widely, some patients surviving for decades while others die within months of diagnosis.[231] Histologically, it may be confused with adenocarcinoma or with veno-occlusive disease. Its causes are unknown, but a relationship to oral contraceptive use has been postulated.[232]

The lesion consists of proliferated endothelial cells with pleomorphic nuclei, arranged in clusters or singly, some of them with rounded lumens (Fig. 11.19). The lumens may be mistaken for lipid or for mucin droplets in a signet-ring cell adenocarcinoma. Two types of tumour cells have been described,[228,230] dendritic and

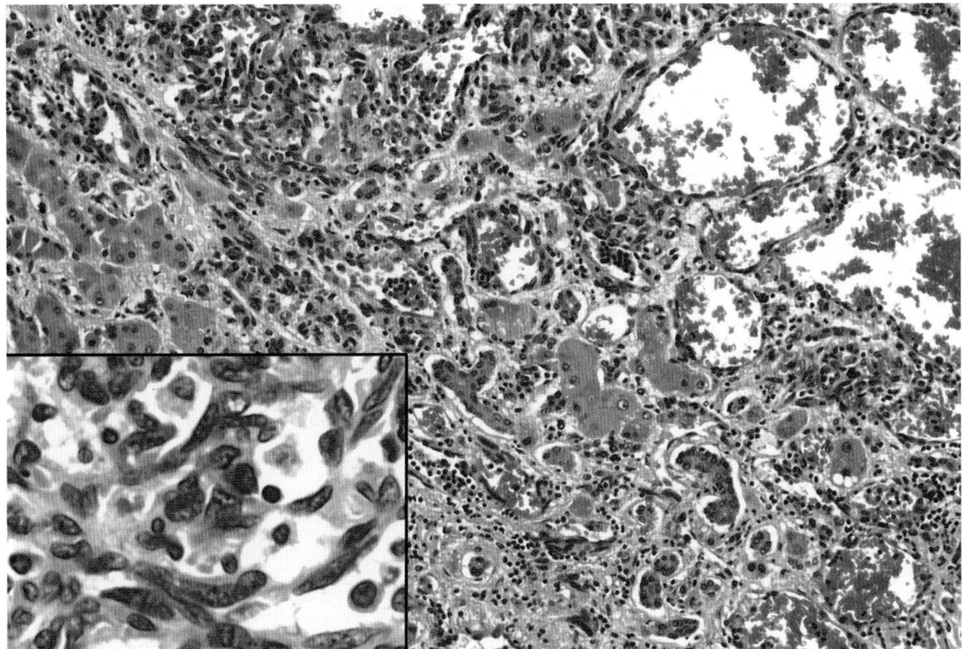

Figure 11.18 *Angiosarcoma*. Elongated tumour cells surround islands of hepatocytes (centre) in this highly vascular tumour. *Inset*: Pleomorphic endothelial cells line the vascular spaces. (Operative specimen, H&E).

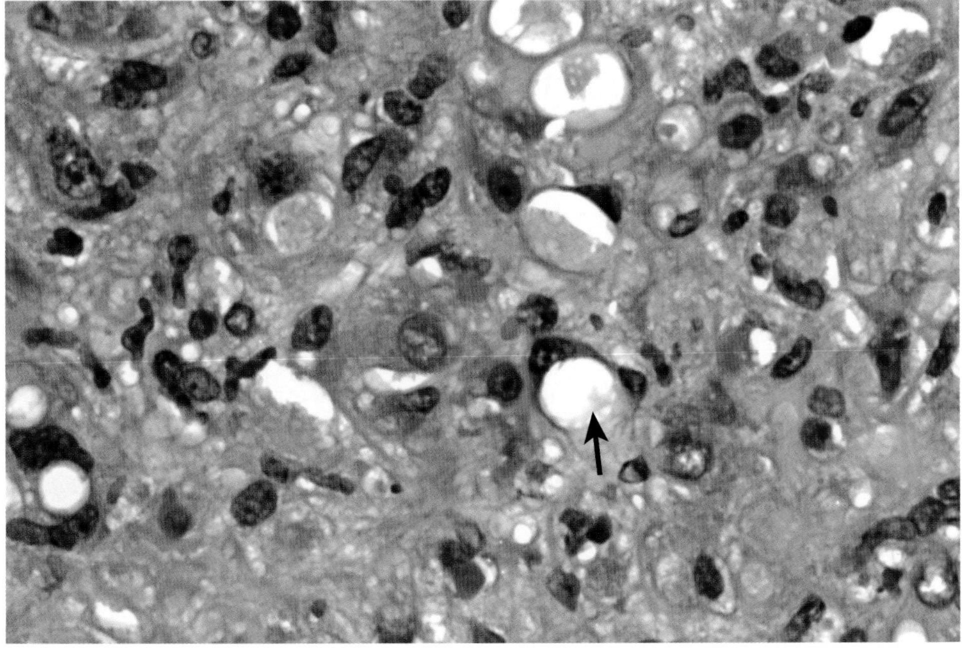

Figure 11.19 *Epithelioid haemangioendothelioma*. Individual tumour cells and small groups are set in a dense fibrous stroma. Some of the tumour cells have formed vascular lumens (arrow). (Operative specimen, H&E).

epithelioid, the latter giving rise to the adenocarcinoma-like appearance. The tumour cells should be positive on immunostaining for one or more endothelial markers (CD34, CD31, factor VIII[230]). CD34 immunostaining is more sensitive than factor VIII.[233] Further evidence of vascular differentiation is seen ultrastructurally where Weibel-Palade bodies in tumour cells and a tumour tissue component of pericytes have been noted.[234] High cellularity is a predictor of unfavourable prognosis, whereas nuclear pleomorphism and mitotic count are not.[230]

Vascular occlusion by dense fibrous tissue containing tumour cells, a characteristic feature, is seen in both portal and hepatic vein branches. This is best seen with connective tissue stains. The problem of confusion with veno-occlusive disease or even steatohepatitis is compounded by the fact that the tumour sometimes has a zonal distribution, affecting perivenular regions of each lobule in a more or less regular fashion (Fig. 11.20).

EXTRAHEPATIC MALIGNANCY AND THE LIVER

Patients with extrahepatic tumour may have biochemical evidence of hepatic dysfunction in the absence of liver metastases, particularly when the tumour is a renal adenocarcinoma. Liver biopsies in such patients have shown Kupffer-cell proliferation, hepatocellular swelling, focal necrosis, fatty change and mild

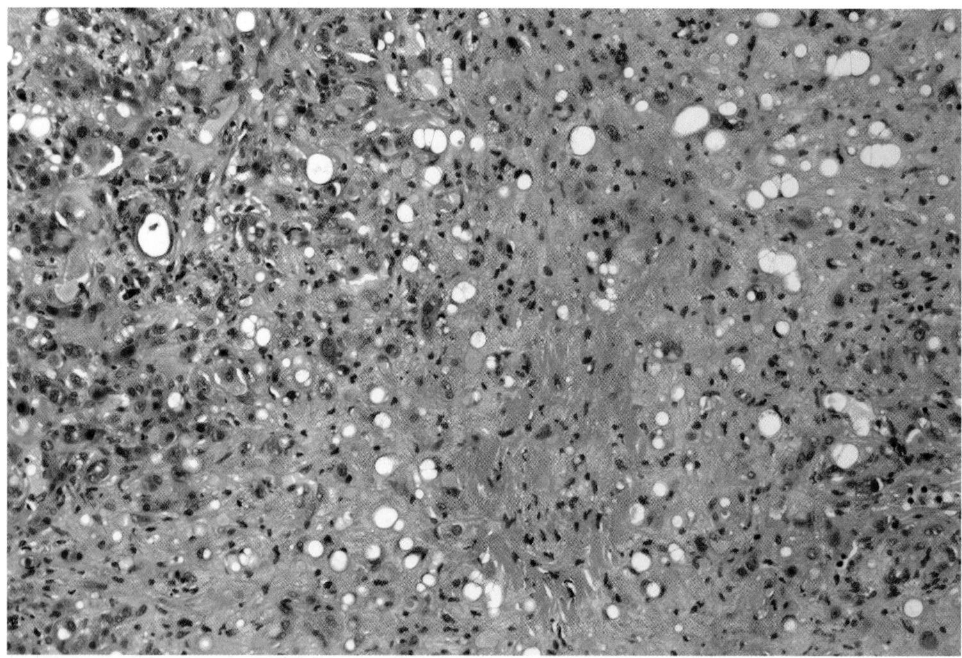

Figure 11.20 *Epithelioid haemangioendothelioma.* In this example the tumour has a zonal distribution, mimicking the fibrosis of venous outflow obstruction. The tumour stroma is predominantly seen in the perivenular and mid-zonal regions, while surviving periportal hepatocytes and ductular reaction are evident at left and at lower right. (Operative specimen, H&E).

inflammation.[235,236] Granulomas are occasionally found and there may be cholestasis, especially in Hodgkin's disease (see below).

Metastatic tumour

Blind percutaneous needle biopsy may reveal metastatic tumour, but the yield of correct diagnoses is increased if the needle is guided by means of an imaging method. Multiple punctures may be needed to sample the tumour. Guided fine-needle aspiration is a helpful diagnostic procedure[237,238] and cytological examination of aspiration fluid and touch preparations of biopsy specimens increase the yield of positive results.[239] Step sections of biopsy specimens should be examined if tumour is suspected clinically but initial sections are negative. The primary site of a tumour can sometimes be determined histologically. Some metastases, notably from renal adenocarcinoma, can mimic hepatocellular carcinoma and metastatic tumour may invade liver-cell plates, giving a false impression of primary carcinoma arising within them (Fig. 11.21). Primary extrahepatic carcinomas of the stomach, sex cord-stromal tumours of the ovary and other sites[147] may closely resemble HCC in both their primary sites and in metastatic foci. These 'hepatoid carcinomas' may produce bile or be positive with polyclonal CEA or α-fetoprotein immunostains.

Biopsy specimens from the vicinity of a metastasis typically show portal oedema, ductular reaction and infiltration by neutrophils, as well as focal sinusoidal dilatation[240] (see Fig. 1.5). The ductular structures sometimes have abnormal

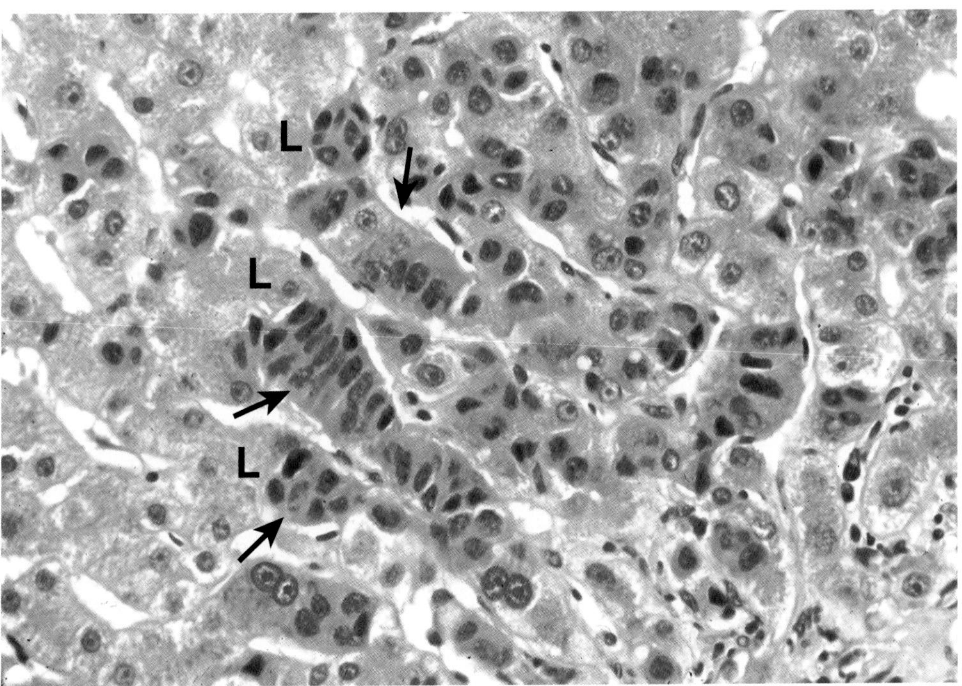

Figure 11.21 *Metastatic tumour*. Cells of a carcinoid tumour (arrows) have invaded liver cell plates (L), giving a false impression of origin from the latter. (Needle biopsy, H&E).

epithelium with atypical, hyperchromatic nuclei. The portal changes are reminiscent of those seen in biliary obstruction.

Lymphomas and leukaemias

Hodgkin's disease

Liver biopsy plays an important part in staging; wedge biopsies are more likely than multiple needle biopsies to reveal deposits and either may be positive, in spite of normal macroscopic appearances of the liver at laparotomy.[241] Negative biopsy does not rule out liver involvement. Hepatic involvement by Hodgkin's disease is usually associated with splenic involvement.[242] Step sections of initially negative small biopsies should be examined because the infiltrates of Hodgkin's disease are unevenly distributed and may be sparse. Correct diagnosis of an infiltrate may be difficult because Reed-Sternberg cells are often very scanty, so that the correct diagnosis must be suspected on the basis of other features. These include an abnormal population of cells with deeply-stained angular nuclei or vesicular nuclei with prominent nucleoli (Fig. 11.22), irregular infiltration beyond portal tracts with destruction of hepatocytes and abundant reticulin fibres. There is a variable component of reactive lymphoid cells, eosinophils and histiocytes. The differential diagnosis of Hodgkin's disease in the liver includes reactive infiltrates and other lymphomas, especially of the T-cell type.

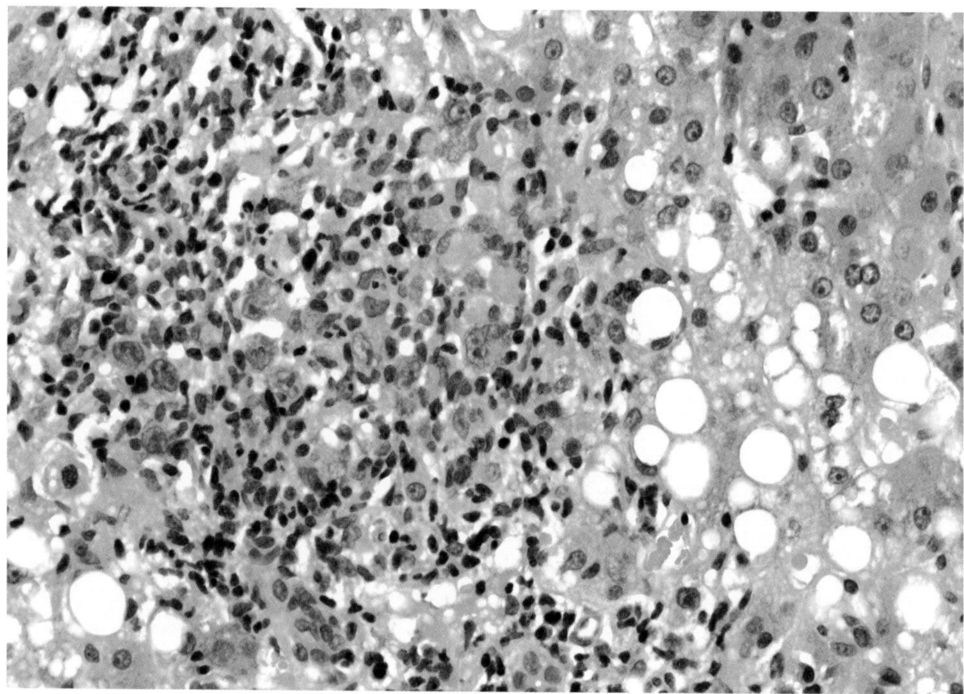

Figure 11.22 *Hodgkin's disease*. The portal infiltrate is composed of a variety of cells, including large tumour cells with angular, hyperchromatic nuclei. (Needle biopsy, H&E).

features as in adults.[280] Hepatosplenomegaly and portal hypertension may be present and in some patients there is a history of prior chemotherapy or anticonvulsant medication.

Mesenchymal hamartoma

This is an uncommon lesion of infancy and childhood, rarely seen in older subjects. Loose, oedematous connective tissue rich in blood vessels contains lymphangioma-like cystic spaces, bile ducts and hepatocytes (Fig. 11.24).[281,282] Haemopoietic cells are often present. The edge of the lesion is irregular, gradually merging with adjacent normal liver. In adults the bile duct elements may be difficult to find and the collagenous stroma is densely hyalinised.[283] An undifferentiated embryonal sarcoma arising in mesenchymal hamartoma has been reported.[284]

Infantile haemangioendothelioma

This solitary or multicentric tumour is composed of capillary-like vascular channels lined by plump endothelium (Fig. 11.25) which with time undergo progressive maturation, scarring and eventual involution.[65,285,286] Central portions of the tumour

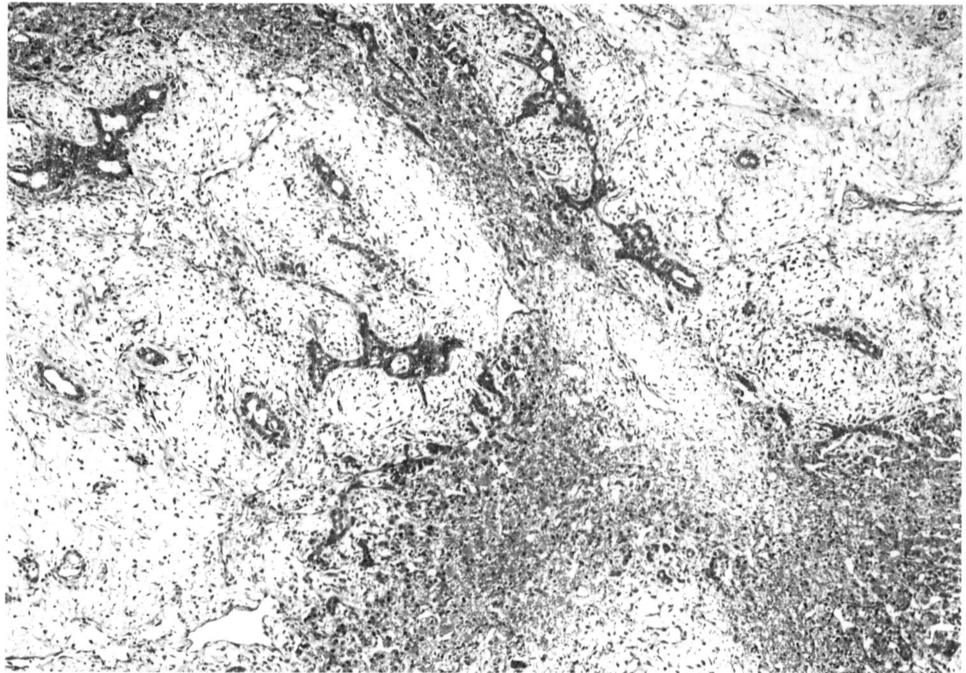

Figure 11.24 *Mesenchymal hamartoma*. Loose connective tissue (left and right) containing bile ducts and blood vessels is separated by intervening hepatocellular parenchyma. (Operative specimen, H&E).

may show increased fibrous stroma and thrombosis and dystrophic calcification are sometimes present. The margin of the tumour often merges into adjacent liver parenchyma. Dehner and Ishak[285] described Type I tumours with cytologically bland endothelium and Type II tumours capable of aggressive behaviour and metastasis, with atypical, hyperchromatic endothelium and intravascular budding. The latter are now considered angiosarcomas.[286a] Most cases present in the first 6 months of life with hepatomegaly, abdominal mass or diffuse abdominal enlargement.[65,285,287] There may be high-output cardiac failure due to shunting through the tumour, liver failure or tumour rupture. The possibility that some of these tumours will pursue a malignant course should be kept in mind in evaluating the histopathology of individual cases.

Malignant lesions

Hepatoblastoma

Hepatoblastoma is the most common liver tumour in childhood,[288] usually presenting under 2 years of age. The prognosis depends on surgical resectability and histologic type. These tumours are usually solitary and histologically classified as **epithelial, mixed epithelial-mesenchymal** and **anaplastic (undifferentiated)** types.[289–292]

The epithelial type consists of fetal or embryonal liver cells, or both. Fetal cells somewhat resemble adult hepatocytes in appearance, but are smaller (Fig. 11.26). The fat and glycogen content in some fetal cells gives them a pale appearance,

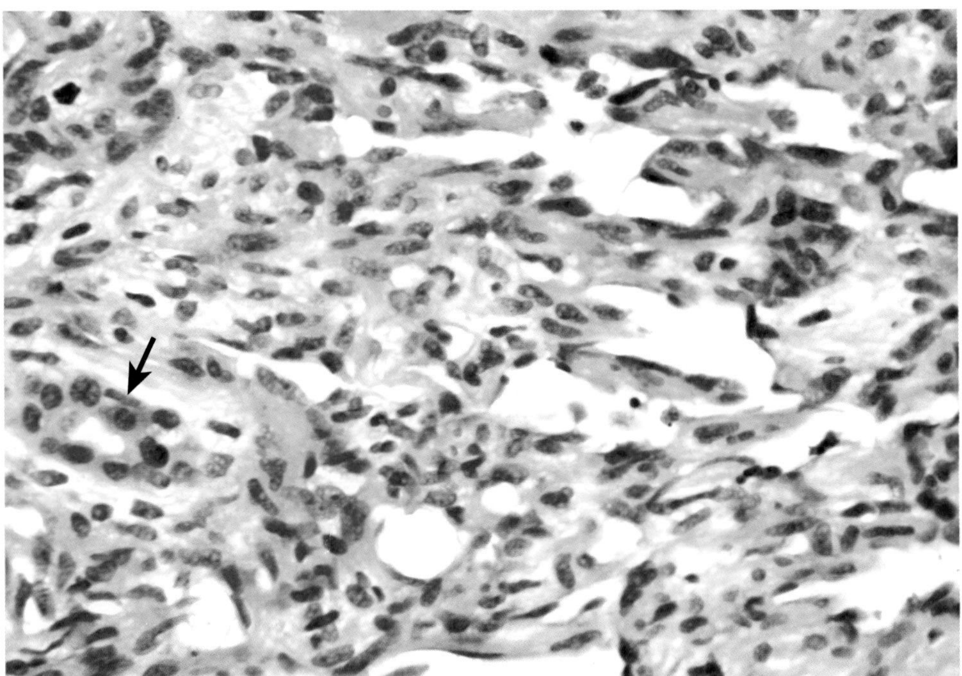

Figure 11.25 *Infantile haemangioendothelioma*. The tumour is composed of vascular channels lined by plump endothelium. Entrapped bile ducts are often present (arrow). (Operative specimen, H&E).

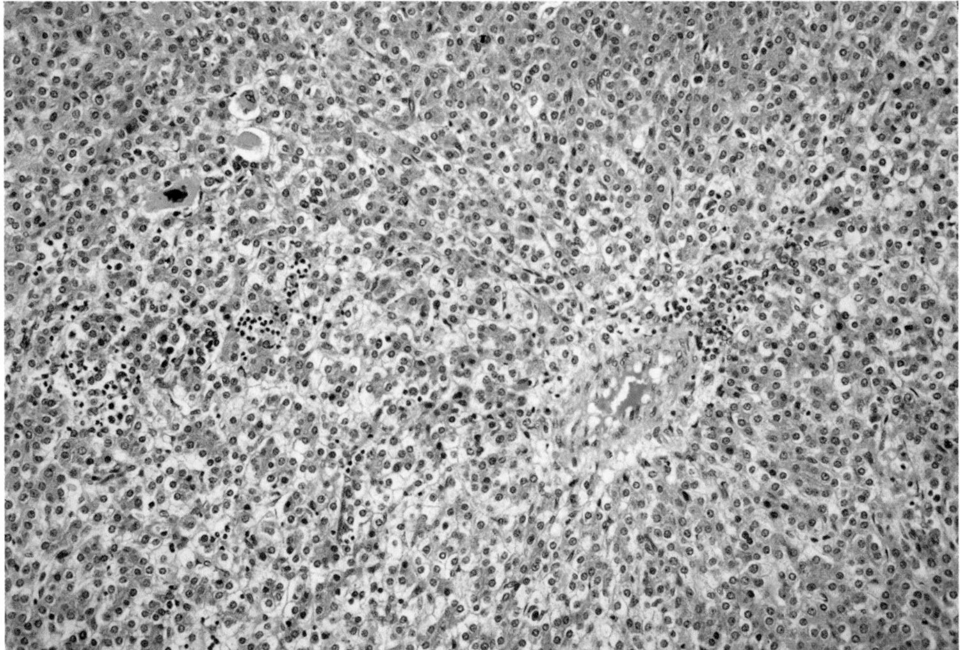

Figure 11.26 *Hepatoblastoma, fetal epithelial type.* The tumour grows in cords of small hepatocytes with a 'light and dark' herringbone pattern due to the admixed clear (glycogenated) and eosinophilic liver cells. Foci of extramedullary haemopoiesis, including several megakaryocytes and clusters of erythrocyte precursors, are seen at upper left. (Operative specimen, H&E).

thereby rendering a 'light-and-dark' pattern to fetal areas at low magnification. These areas are also characterised by foci of extramedullary haemopoiesis and an absence of mitoses. By histologic pattern, the purely fetal type has the best prognosis.[293] Embryonal cells have less cytoplasm, higher nuclear:cytoplasmic ratios, higher cell proliferative indices,[294] poorly defined cellular margins and mitotic activity (Fig. 11.27). They may form rosettes, acini or tubules. Squamous differentiation may be present in epithelial hepatoblastomas. The anaplastic type shows sheets of cells resembling neuroblastoma cells with little cytoplasm, hyperchromatic nuclei and no mitoses. Gonzalez-Crussi et al.[295] described a **'macrotrabecular'** pattern reminiscent of hepatocellular carcinoma but containing fetal or embryonal cells. Anaplastic and macrotrabecular variants have the worst prognosis.[289] Mixed epithelial-mesenchymal hepatoblastomas contain mesenchymal elements such as osteoid and cartilage in addition to epithelium. Staining for α-fetoprotein is common in hepatoblastoma and depending on the type of histologic differentiation immunohistochemistry may also be positive for α_1-antitrypsin, cytokeratins, vimentin and carcinoembryonic antigen.[296]

Sarcoma and lymphoma

Undifferentiated sarcomas with a poor prognosis occasionally develop in the liver in children.[297] Epithelium trapped within the tumour may give rise to confusion. Light microscopic and ultrastructural features suggest malignant fibrous histiocytoma[298,299] or myoblastic differentiation.[299] Immunohistochemical results are

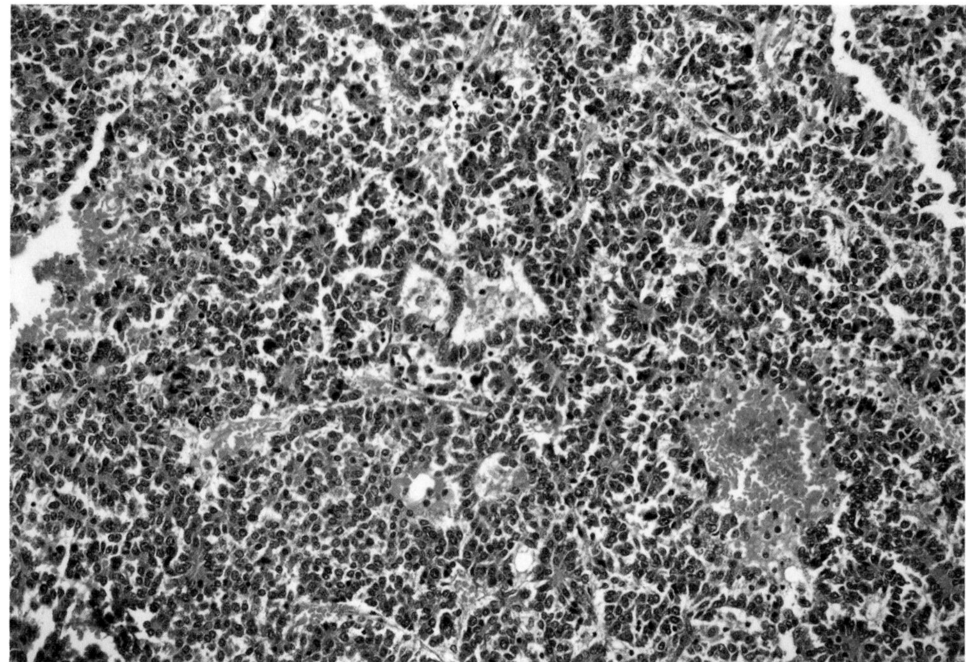

Figure 11.27 *Hepatoblastoma, embryonal epithelial type.* Tumour cells grow in tubules and show an increased nuclear:cytoplasmic ratio. Darkly stained mitotic figures can be identified in some cells. (Operative specimen, H&E).

inconsistent, with reports of staining for histiocytic markers, desmin, vimentin and even cytokeratin.[299,300] Another form of sarcoma, arising in the biliary tract, is the **embryonal rhabdomyosarcoma** or **sarcoma botryoides**.[293] Mixed stromal-epithelial tumors **(nested stromal epithelial tumours)** with calcifaction or ossification have uncertain malignant potential but usually show indolent behavior.[300a,300b] Exceptionally rare **primary non-Hodgkin's lymphoma** in the liver has been reported in childhood.[301]

Hepatocellular carcinoma

This resembles the adult type histologically, but cirrhosis is usually absent.[293] Predisposing causes include tyrosinaemia and type I glycogenosis. The fibrolamellar type of carcinoma has been described in older children, with better prognosis than hepatocellular carcinoma in general.[175]

CYTOPATHOLOGICAL DIAGNOSIS

Fine needle aspiration biopsy (FNAB) is often used to investigate hepatic masses, particularly in patients with cirrhosis where HCC is suspected.[302] This technique may demonstrate lesional tissue as well as components of normal or non-neoplastic liver. In the latter regard, the interpreter must be familiar with the cytologic appearances of normal liver, cirrhosis or dysplasia, which are discussed below.

Normal or reactive liver

Aspirates from non-neoplastic liver will contain **normal** or **reactive hepatocytes**, which are present as single cells, clusters or two-dimensional monolayer sheets (Fig. 11.28). Normal hepatocytes may be arranged in trabeculae, but these should consist of three cells or less, without enveloping endothelium (Fig. 11.29). Individual hepatocytes are polygonal cells with well-defined borders and centrally placed, round nuclei, which often have conspicuous nucleoli and occasionally show intranuclear cytoplasmic pseudoinclusions (vesicular inclusions). The latter may also be seen in hepatocellular carcinoma (HCC) and are therefore not diagnostic. The nuclei of benign hepatocytes may vary considerably in size (not shape) and this is a helpful diagnostic sign which contrasts with the more monomorphic nuclei seen in HCC.[303] The appearance of pigment in the liver varies according to the staining method used.[303,304] The presence of lipofuscin in hepatocytes is indicative of a benign process.

Benign aspirates may also contain **bile duct epithelium**, which is usually not present in specimens from liver cell adenoma and HCC.[305] Bile duct epithelial cells are smaller than hepatocytes, are arranged in monolayers with a 'honeycomb' glandular pattern (Fig. 11.30) and have eccentrically located nuclei in a pale, non-granular cytoplasm. The nuclei have fine chromatin and no prominent nucleoli. Aspirates may also contain sheets of benign **mesothelium** derived from the peritoneum (Fig. 11.31).

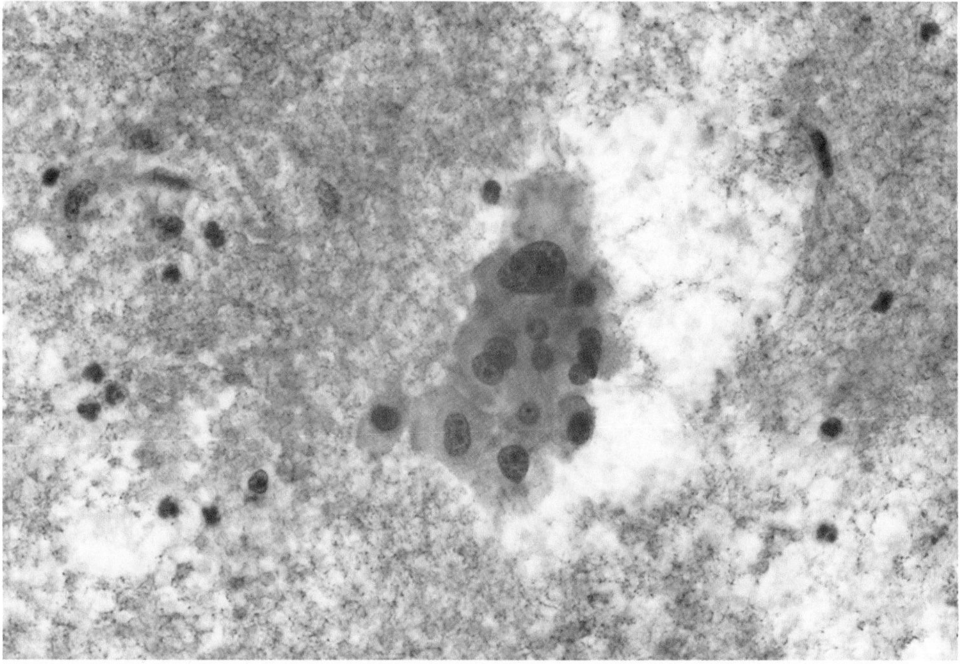

Figure 11.28 *Normal hepatocytes.* A cluster of normal liver cells includes several binucleated hepatocytes and an enlarged, polyploid cell at top. Prominent nucleoli are visible. (Papanicolaou).

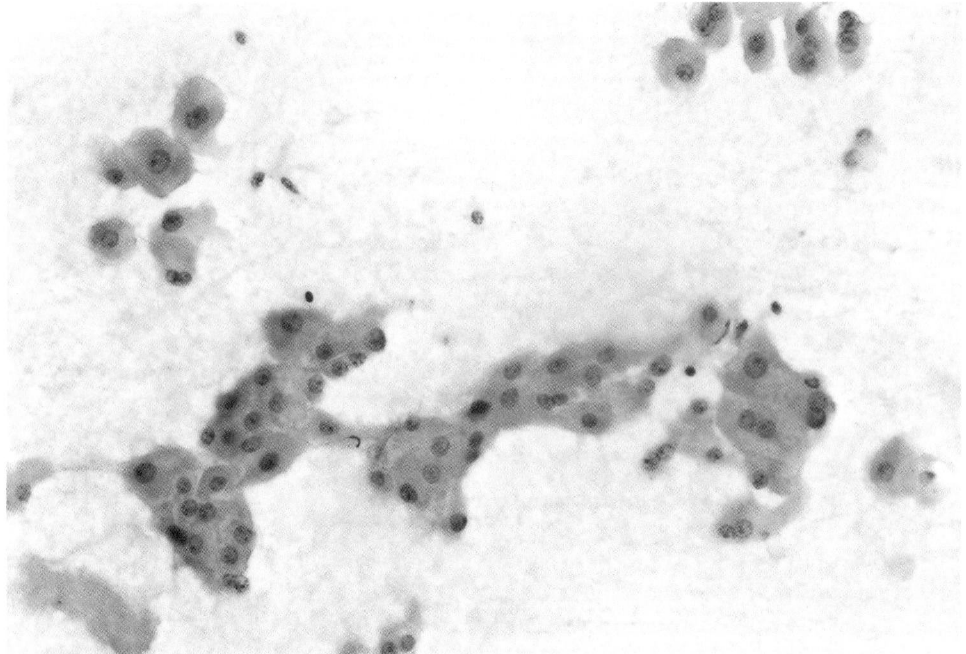

Figure 11.29 *Normal hepatocyte trabeculae*. Normal trabeculae of hepatocytes on aspirate contain up to two or three cells. (Papanicolaou).

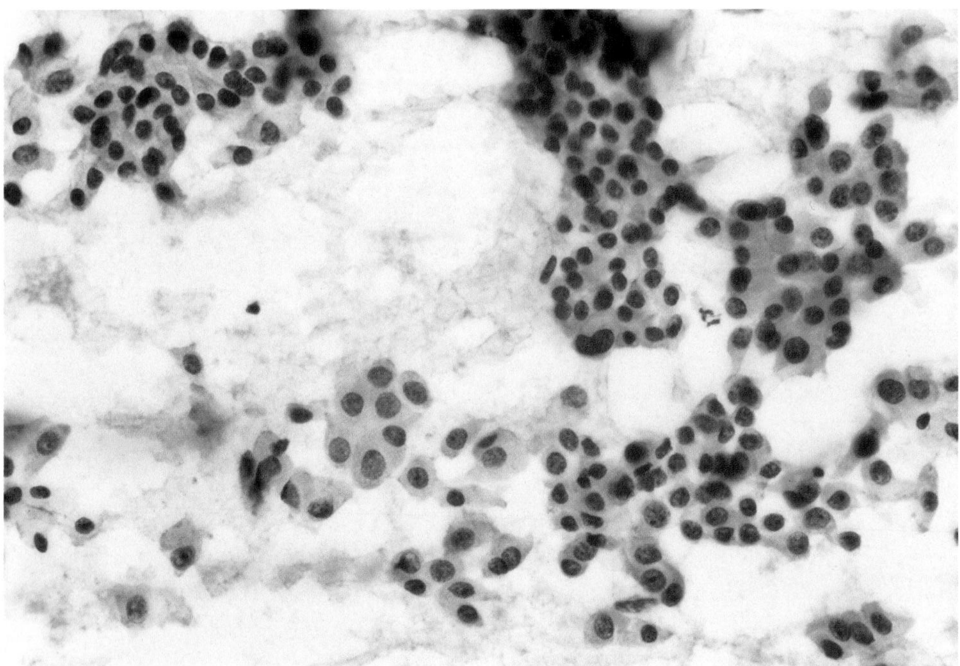

Figure 11.30 *Bile duct epithelium*. Clusters of bile duct epithelial cells are distinguishable from the group of hepatocytes near the centre by their smaller size and round, nondescript nuclei. Microglandular structures are also focally present. (Papanicolaou).

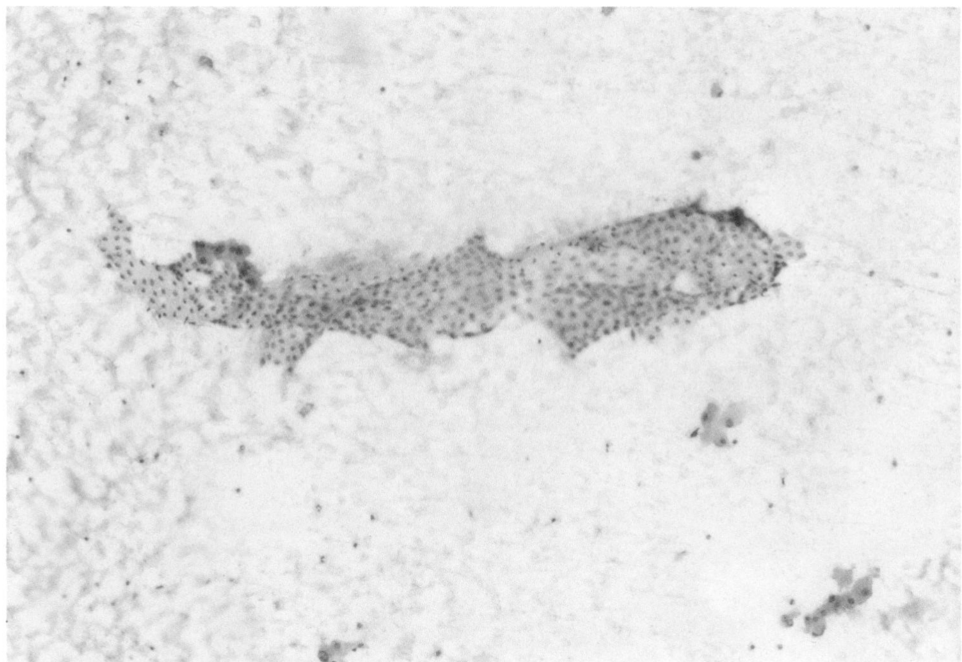

Figure 11.31 *Mesothelium.* A sheet of mesothelial cells from the peritoneum shows a characteristic clear 'window' at right. (Papanicolaou).

Cirrhosis and liver-cell dysplasia

Aspirates from cirrhotic liver may contain portions of connective tissue and fibroblasts (Fig. 11.32), bile duct epithelium, reactive hepatocytes arranged in clusters with jagged edges (rather than smooth-edged trabeculae as in HCC) and mixed chronic inflammatory cells (mostly lymphocytes). A definitive diagnosis of cirrhosis based only on FNAB is usually not possible.[306]

Large-cell and small-cell dysplasia can also be identified on FNAB. The type and degree of nuclear atypia distinguish dysplastic hepatocytes from normal or reactive liver cells. In large-cell dysplasia, nuclei are enlarged, hyperchromatic and pleomorphic, with one or more prominent nucleoli (Fig. 11.33). Coarse nuclear chromatin and pseudoinclusions of invaginated cytoplasm are often present. The presence of cellular enlargement with ample cytoplasm maintains a relatively normal nuclear:cytoplasmic ratio. In small-cell dysplasia this ratio is increased because the atypical nuclei are found in cells that are smaller than normal hepatocytes (Fig. 11.34). The aspirated cell clusters in which dysplastic hepatocytes may be found are accompanied by normal or reactive hepatocytes with heterogeneous nuclear features and cell sizes, an important distinction from aspirates of hepatocellular carcinoma, which typically show a relatively monomorphous population of hepatocytes.[307]

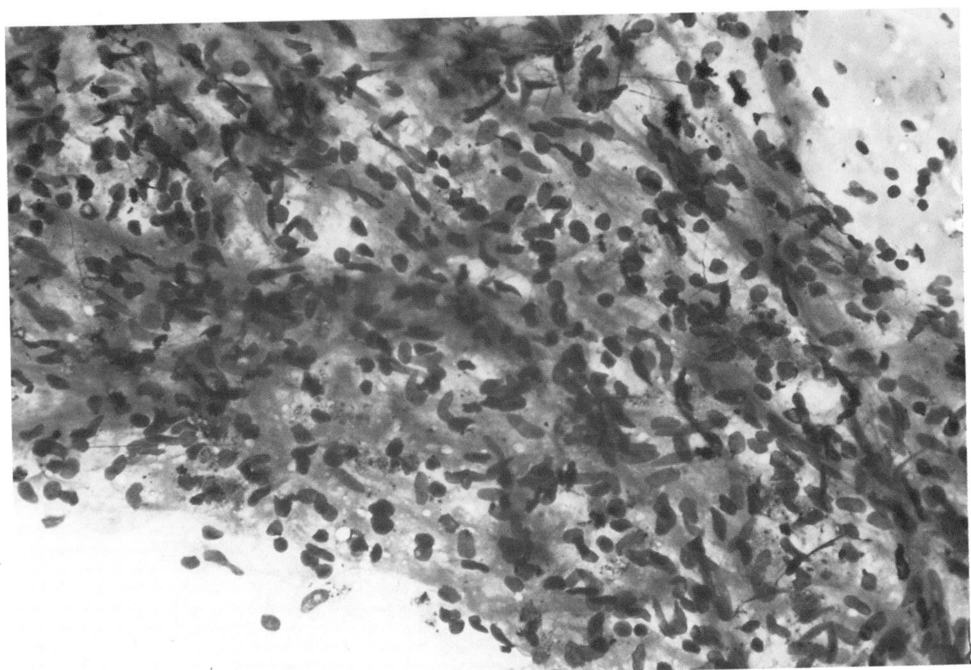

Figure 11.32 *Cirrhosis*. The aspirate includes interweaving spindled fibroblasts, stroma and the round nuclei of lymphocytes. (Diff-Quick).

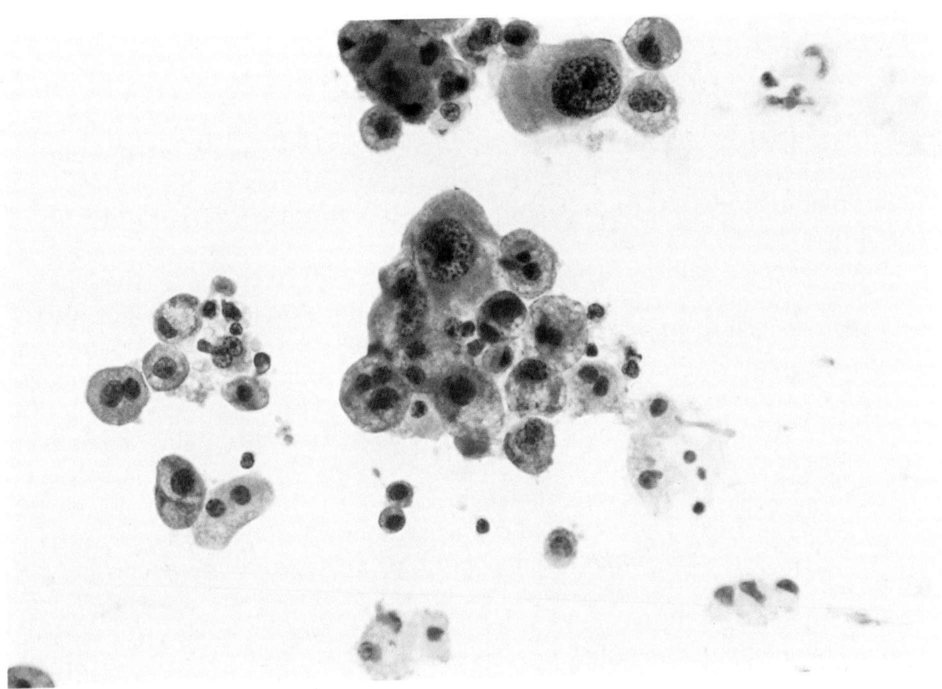

Figure 11.33 *Large-cell dysplasia*. Two groups of hepatocytes (top and centre) contain large dysplastic cells intermixed with smaller reactive hepatocytes. The dysplastic cells have hyperchromatic nuclei, coarse chromatin and prominent nucleoli. Normal hepatocytes are seen at left and at bottom. (Papanicolaou). (Illustration kindly provided by Dr Alastair Deery, London).

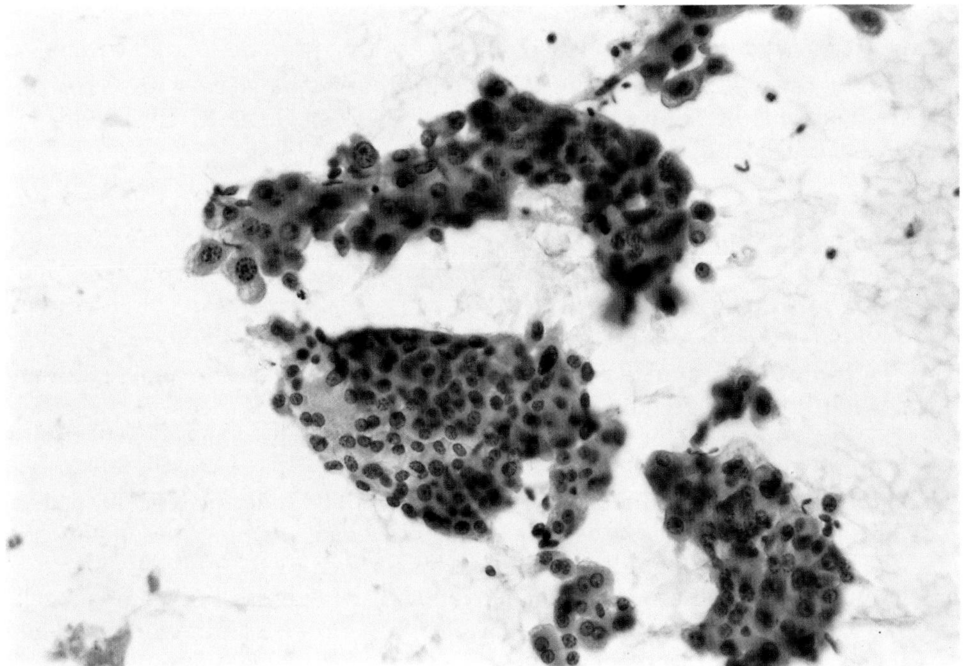

Figure 11.34 *Small-cell dysplasia.* The cluster of small hepatocytes slightly below centre shows hyperchromatic atypical nuclei. (Papanicolaou). (Illustration kindly provided by Dr Alastair Deery, London).

Liver-cell adenoma

The cytological diagnosis rendered from the FNAB smear of liver-cell adenoma is typically 'compatible with' this tumour since the specimen usually shows single hepatocytes or clusters which resemble benign, normal liver cells.[305] Bile duct epithelium and connective tissue should be absent, in contrast to focal nodular hyperplasia.

Focal nodular hyperplasia (FNH)

Establishing the cytologic diagnosis of FNH is based on finding one or more of the several cellular elements comprising this lesion (hepatocytes, fibrous tissue, bile-duct epithelium) within the smear. The presence of bile-duct epithelium in duct-like structures or clusters effectively rules out liver cell adenoma and HCC. The bile-duct epithelium may show nuclear variation and conspicuous nucleoli.[308] Fibrous tissue and bile-duct epithelium are not always present in the aspirate, but the bland appearance of the hepatocytes, with small, round nuclei lacking prominent nucleoli, implies a benign lesion. The hepatocytes are arranged in clusters with irregular or jagged edges without traversing or peripheral endothelium.

Haemangioma

Aspirates of haemangiomas are bloody and numerous red blood cells are seen on the smear. Fragments of fibrous tissue[309] and/or single or clustered spindle-shaped endothelial cells may also be present (Fig. 11.35).

Hepatocellular carcinoma (HCC)

The low power appearance of smears from HCC provides several important diagnostic features, especially the rounded edges of tumour cells in clusters or trabeculae (in contrast to the ragged edges of normal or reactive hepatocyte clusters) and endothelial cells which traverse clusters of tumour cells as well as wrap around the periphery of clusters or trabeculae (Figs 11.36, 11.37). The paucireticulin pattern of HCC is helpful in fine needle aspiration biopsies where low power examination of glass slides shows a finely granular smear (in contrast to the preserved cores or larger tissue fragments seen with benign liver diseases and masses).[310] Tumour cells are polygonal with central nuclei that may have either coarse or fine chromatin and prominent nucleoli or macronucleoli (Fig. 11.38). There is usually less variability in the features of HCC cells on smear than in normal or reactive hepatocytes. Atypical naked nuclei[311] (exceptionally large and irregular nuclei without visible cytoplasm) are also an important diagnostic feature (Fig. 11.39). A stepwise logistic regression study showed that the three features which best differentiate HCC from normal or

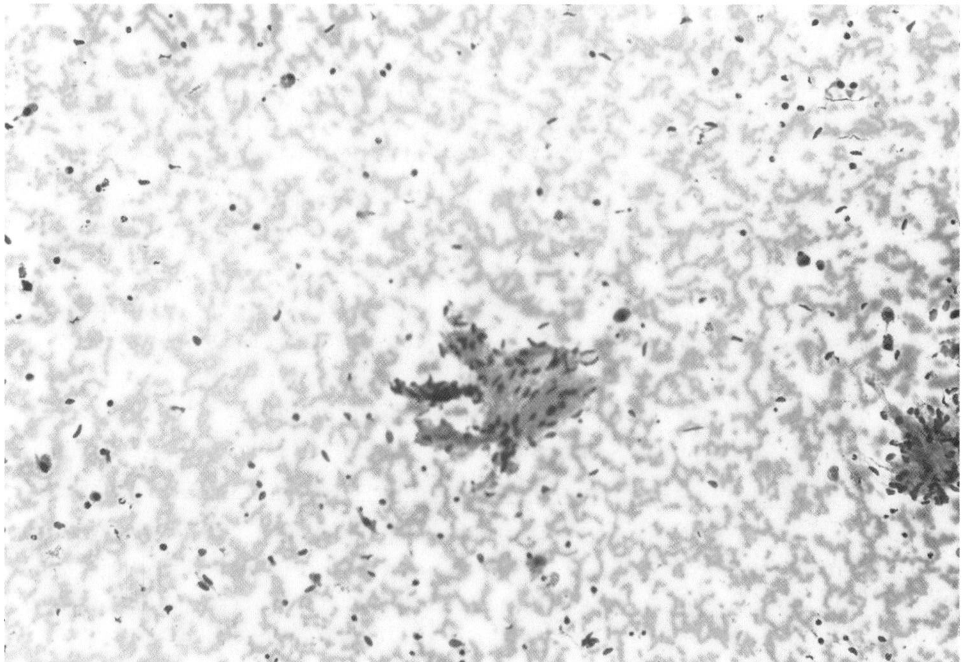

Figure 11.35 *Haemangioma.* A focus of stromal cells is present with an extensive background of red blood cells. Scattered spindle-shaped endothelial or fibroblast nuclei are seen amidst the erythrocytes. (Papanicolaou).

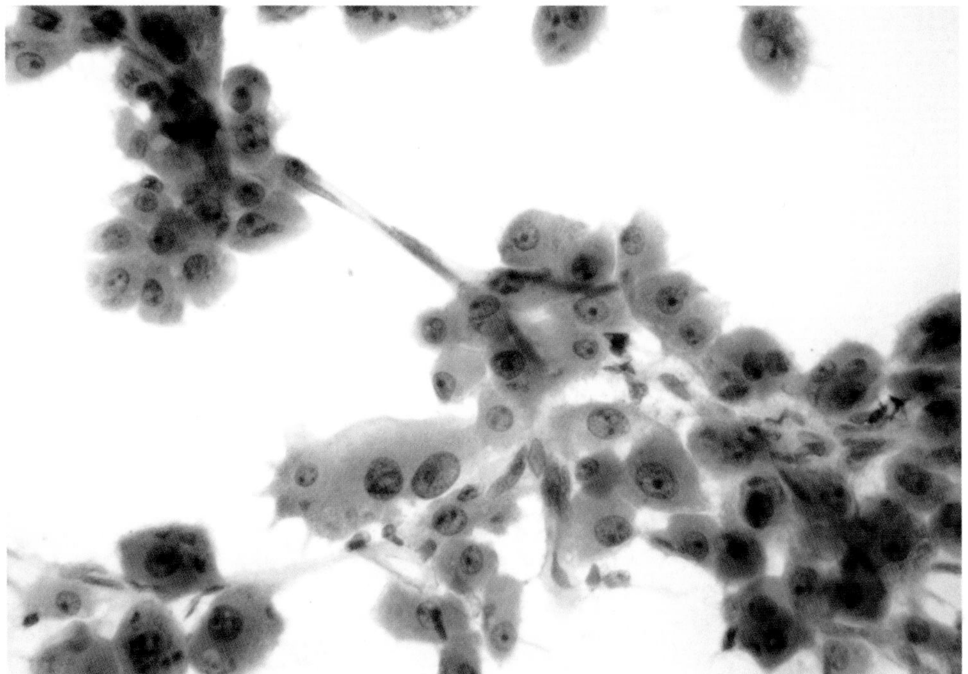

Figure 11.36 *Hepatocellular carcinoma*. Malignant hepatocytes in clusters are traversed by slender strings of endothelium. (Papanicolaou).

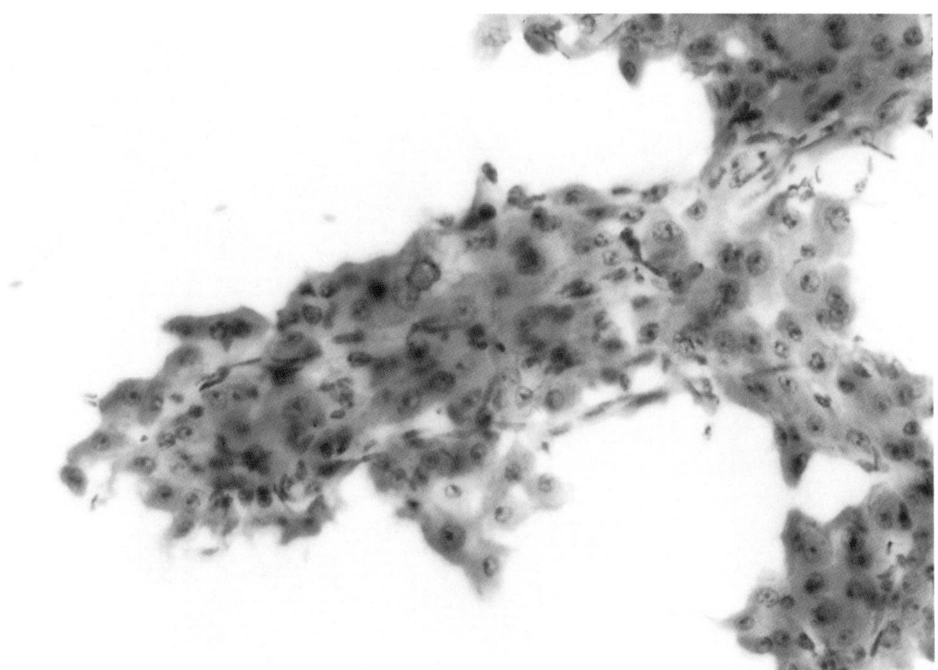

Figure 11.37 *Hepatocellular carcinoma*. Flattened endothelium is seen peripherally at the edge of a trabecula of hepatocellular carcinoma. (Papanicolaou).

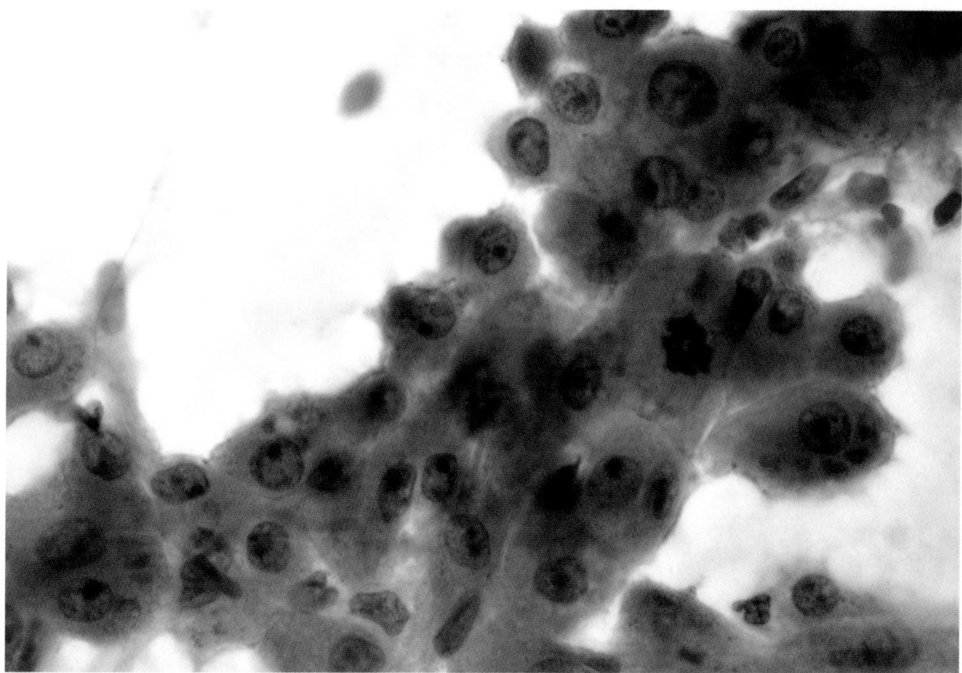

Figure 11.38 *Hepatocellular carcinoma*. Malignant hepatocytes have fairly uniform nuclei, which are centrally or peripherally located. Prominent nucleoli are seen throughout and a mitotic figure is present at right centre. (Papanicolaou).

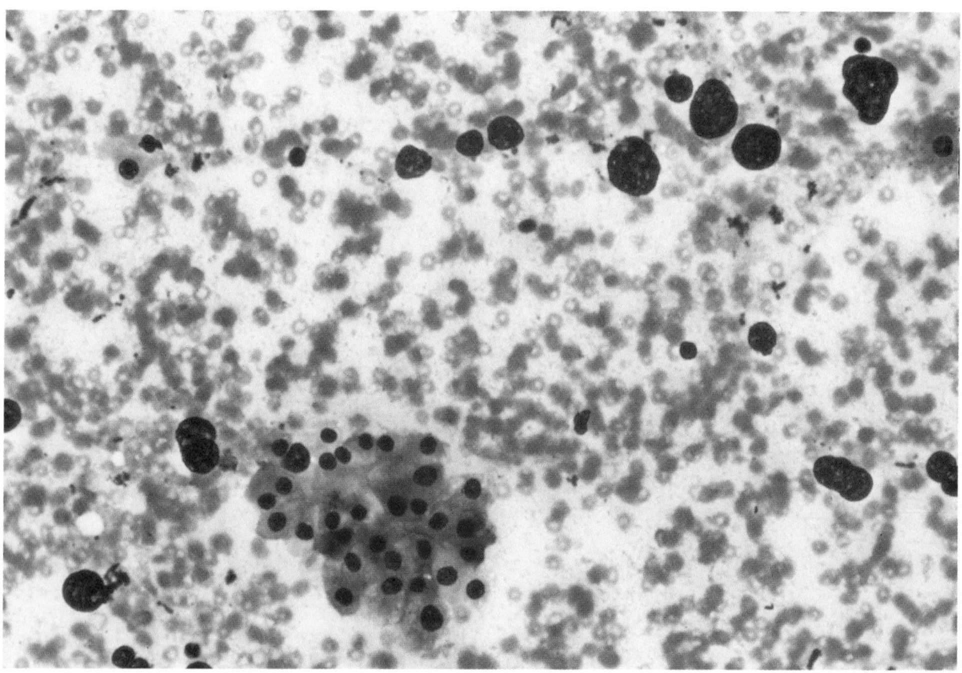

Figure 11.39 *Hepatocellular carcinoma*. A cluster of malignant hepatocytes is present along with 'naked nuclei'. (Diff-Quick).

reactive liver are: increased nucleus-to-cytoplasm ratio; a trabecular pattern of tumour cells enclosed by endothelium; and atypical naked nuclei.[303,312] Table 11.5 summarises some of the major FNAB cytologic features of HCC. The presence of bile within or between tumour cells is indicative of their hepatocellular origin, but bile may only be seen in half the cases[313] and can also be present in smears from non-neoplastic liver.

Variants of HCC which may be present include acinar, clear cell and fibrolamellar carcinoma. As with typical HCC, the presence of peripheral endothelial wrapping or traversal of endothelium across tumour cell clusters favours HCC. When **clear cells** are identified, there are also usually non-clear cell HCC cells present which help distinguish the tumour from renal, adrenal and ovarian neoplasms.[314] **Fibrolamellar carcinoma** can be diagnosed if the smear includes fibrous tissue or fibroblasts and the distinctive polygonal cells with granular, eosinophilic cytoplasm[315] (Fig. 11.40). The tumour cells of fibrolamellar carcinoma are often dispersed or dyshesive, in comparison to the cell clusters and trabeculae of typical HCC.[316]

When metastatic carcinoma must be differentiated from HCC on FNAB, the cytopathologist should bear in mind that nearly all hepatocellular carcinomas will have two or three of the following key diagnostic criteria:[303] polygonal cells with centrally placed nuclei; malignant cells traversed by sinusoidal capillaries; and bile.

Hepatoblastoma

The **epithelial type** of hepatoblastoma cytologically resembles HCC and on smear shows cohesive nests, sheets or trabeculae of malignant hepatocytes (Fig. 11.41). The tumour cells have hyperchromatic nuclei which may overlap and show prominent nucleoli. Fetal and embryonal subtypes are difficult to distinguish on FNAB alone.[317] There may be extramedullary haemopoiesis, formation of acini and naked tumour cell nuclei.[317,318] The **mesenchymal type** of hepatoblastoma, or the mixed epithelial-mesenchymal variant, may be represented by spindle cells in the smear.

Cholangiocarcinoma

Aspirate smears from cholangiocarcinoma demonstrate three-dimensional clusters of atypical cells with a small amount of cytoplasm and nuclei with granular

Table 11.5 Major FNAB features of hepatocellular carcinoma

Polygonal cells with central or paracentral nuclei
Relative homogeneity of tumour cells
High nuclear:cytoplasmic ratio
Cell nests and trabeculae with smooth edges
Traversing and/or peripheral endothelium
Atypical naked nuclei

FNAB, fine needle aspiration biopsy.

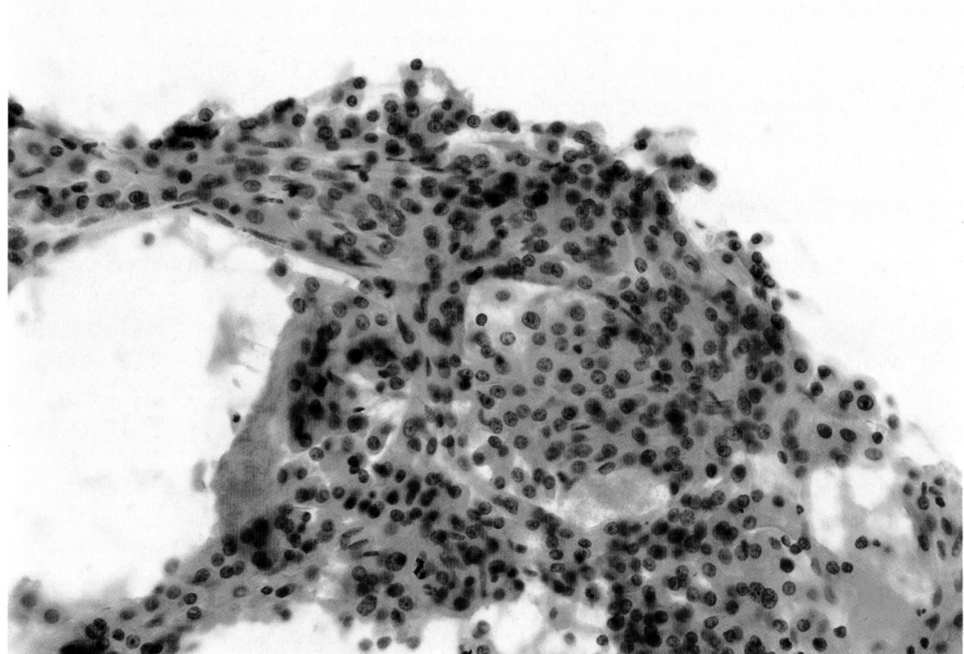

Figure 11.40 *Fibrolamellar carcinoma*. The malignant hepatocytes in this aspirate have ample granular cytoplasm and prominent nucleoli. (Papanicolaou). (Illustration kindly provided by Dr Alastair Deery, London).

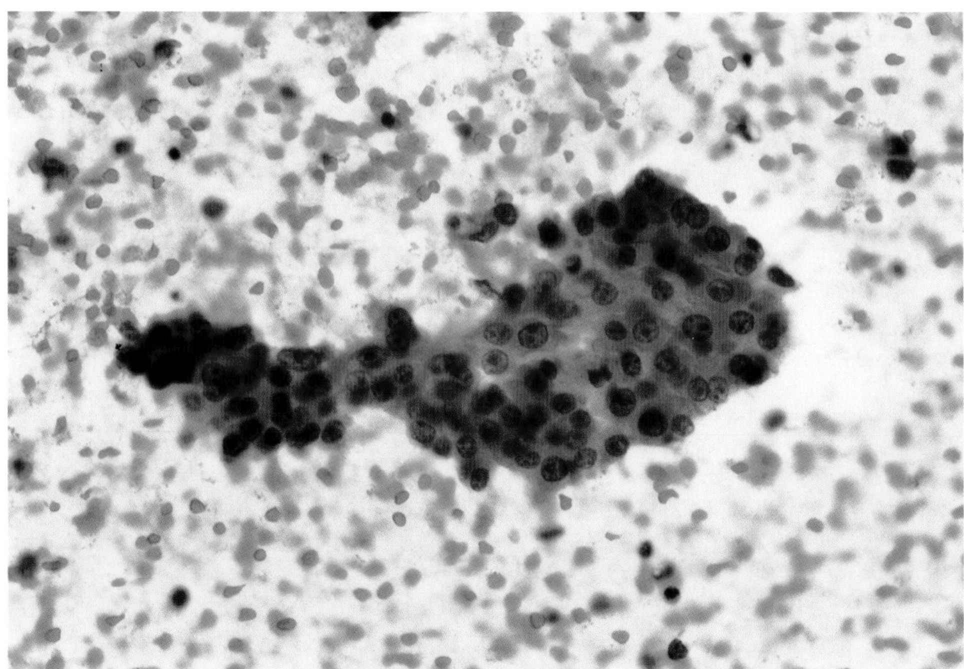

Figure 11.41 *Hepatoblastoma*. The cell cluster is packed with malignant epithelium. Nuclear features resemble those seen in hepatocellular carcinoma. (Papanicolaou).

chromatin and one or more prominent nucleoli. Tumour cells may also be arranged in acini and cannot be readily distinguished on routine stains from metastatic pancreatic or other adenocarcinomas.[315]

Angiosarcoma

The smear of this tumour is typically bloody and features a necrotic background with dyshesive, pleomorphic spindle cells. Factor VIII and CD34 immunostains are diagnostically helpful.[319]

Lymphoma

Lymphoid proliferations in the liver, including lymphoma and post-transplant lymphoproliferative disease,[320] can be diagnosed on FNAB according to cytologic criteria used for aspirates from extrahepatic sites. Smears show dispersed single, monomorphous lymphoid cells with 'blue blobs' of stripped cytoplasm (lymphoglandular bodies[321]) in the background (Fig. 11.42). Blue blobs may also be present in smears containing non-neoplastic lymphocytes.

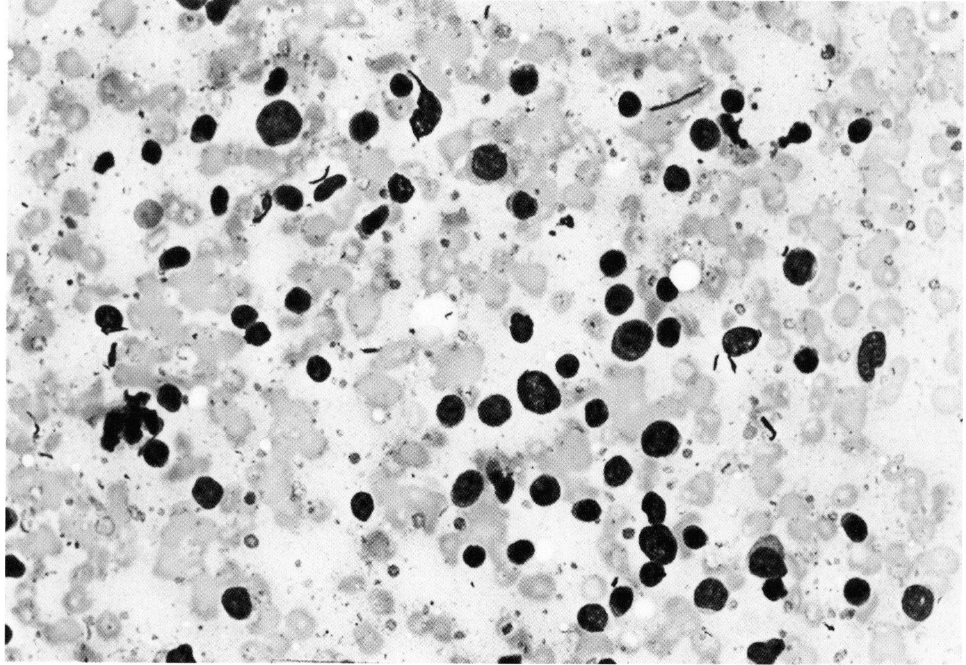

Figure 11.42 *Lymphoma.* Dissociated malignant lymphoid cells are present with a background of smaller 'blue blobs' (lymphoglandular bodies). (Diff-Quick).

Metastatic tumours

Adenocarcinoma from the colon and pancreas on aspirate smears presents as cell clusters with round or oval vesicular nuclei, prominent nucleoli and delicate cytoplasm. The presence of columnar cells with cigar-shaped, palisaded nuclei and apical cytoplasm or vacuoles (goblet cells) is characteristic of **colon carcinoma** (Fig. 11.43). The cytologic features of **breast carcinoma** include the tendency to smear as dyshesive cell groups or single cells with eccentric nuclei and cone-shaped cytoplasm. Relative uniformity of cell size and shape, prominent small nucleoli and the absence of marked atypia are seen in infiltrating duct carcinoma. Lobular carcinoma may show single file lines of cells with nuclear moulding. **Neuroendocrine carcinomas** on smear feature organoid nests (carcinoid tumours) or loose groups or sheets (islet cell carcinoma). The coarse 'salt and pepper' chromatin pattern is characteristic of these neoplasms, with islet cell carcinomas often showing more nuclear pleomorphism with prominent nucleoli than carcinoid tumours (Fig. 11.44). **Malignant melanoma** often metastasises to the liver and may be confused with hepatocellular carcinoma on FNAB because of features in common, including eosinophilic macronucleoli, nuclear pseudoinclusions, polygonal cell shape and cohesive cell groups. However, in contrast to HCC, aspirates of melanoma are more likely to show single, dyshesive cells with eccentric nuclei and intracellular melanin pigment (Fig. 11.45). If cell grouping is present, it is unlikely to be accompanied by the traversing or peripheral endothelium seen in HCC. Immunostains for HMB-45 and S-100 should be undertaken if melanoma is a possible diagnosis, particularly if pigment is absent.

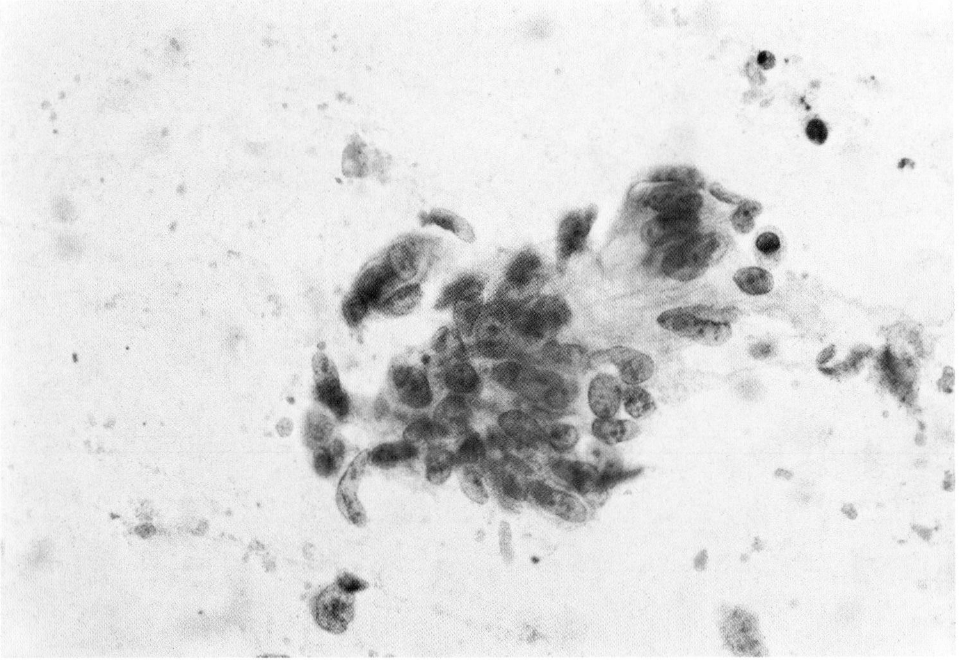

Figure 11.43 *Metastatic colonic adenocarcinoma.* Several rows of columnar cells are present and the cluster at upper right contains a goblet cell with a large cytoplasmic vacuole. (Papanicolaou).

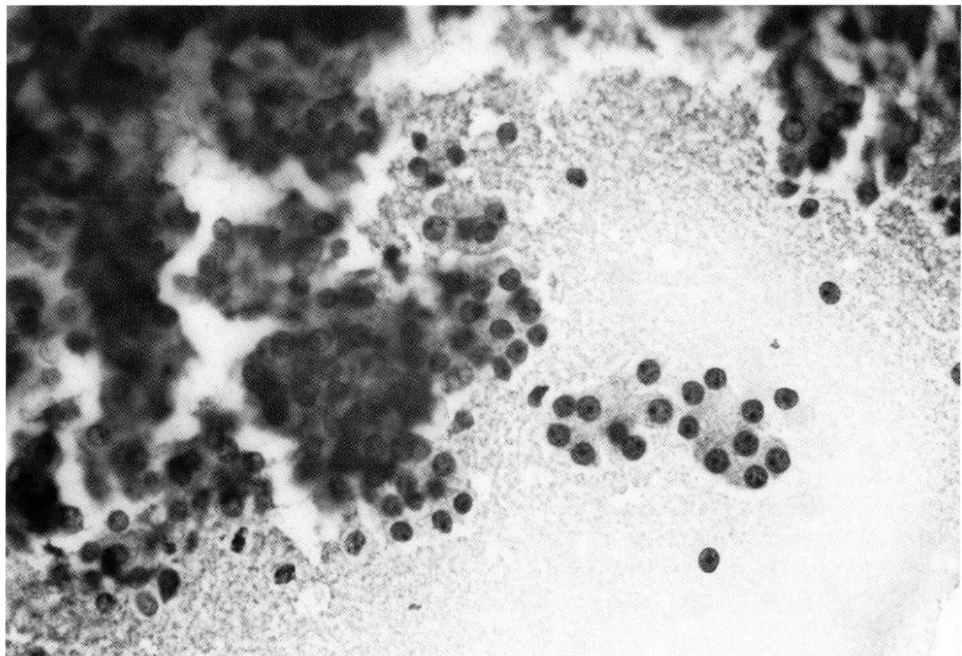

Figure 11.44 *Metastatic neuroendocrine carcinoma*. Clusters of fairly homogeneous small cells with regular nuclei and substantial cytoplasm are seen. The patient had a pancreatic islet cell carcinoma. Thick trabecular structures are seen at left. (Diff-Quick).

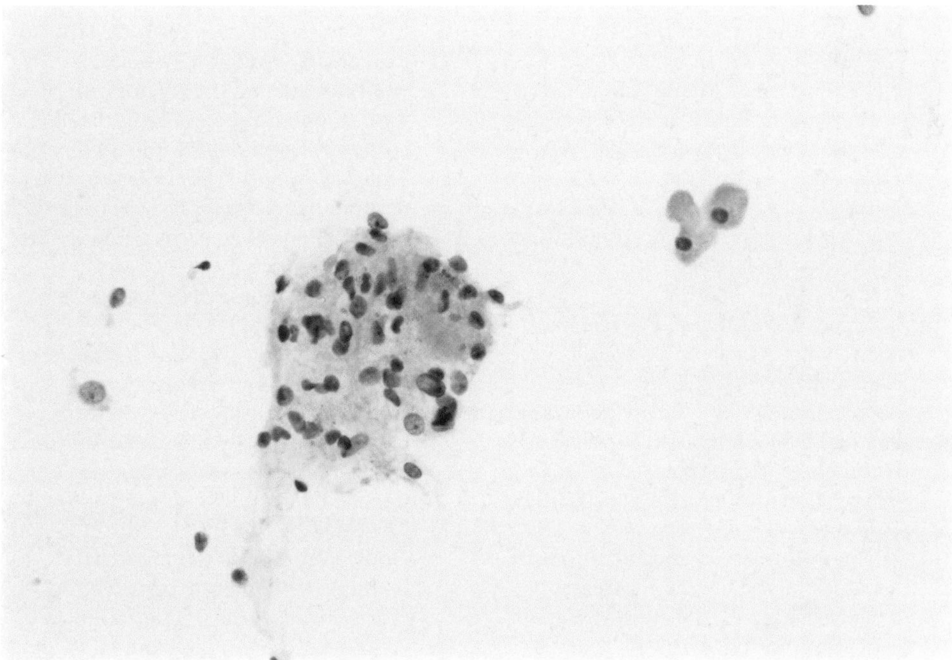

Figure 11.45 *Metastatic uveal melanoma*. A cluster of melanoma cells with intracellular melanin pigment is present. Several normal hepatocytes are seen at upper right. (Papanicolaou). (Illustration kindly provided by Dr Alastair Deery, London).

REFERENCES

1 Tao L-C. Oral contraceptive-associated liver cell adenoma and hepatocellular carcinoma. Cytomorphology and mechanism of malignant transformation. *Cancer* 1991; **68**: 341–347.

2 Hasan N, Coutts M, Portmann B. Pigmented liver cell adenoma in two male patients. *Am J Surg Pathol* 2000; **24**: 1429–1432.

3 Heffelfinger S, Irani DR, Finegold MJ. "Alcoholic hepatitis" in a hepatic adenoma. *Hum Pathol* 1987; **18**: 751–754.

4 Le Bail B, Jouhanole H, Deugnier Y, et al. Liver adenomatosis with granulomas in two patients on long-term oral contraceptives. *Am J Surg Pathol* 1992; **16**: 982–987.

5 Lepreux S, Laurent C, Blanc JF, et al. The identification of small nodules in liver adenomatosis. *J Hepatol* 2003; **39**: 77–85.

6 Rooks JB, Ory HW, Ishak KG, et al. Epidemiology of hepatocellular adenoma. The role of oral contraceptive use. *JAMA* 1979; **242**: 644–648.

7 Lui AF, Hiratzka LF, Hirose FM. Multiple adenomas of the liver. *Cancer* 1980; **45**: 1001–1004.

8 Flejou JF, Barge J, Menu Y, et al. Liver adenomatosis. Entity distinct liver adenoma? *Gastroenterology* 1985; **89**: 1132–1138.

9 Kahn H, Manzarbeitia C, Theise N, et al. Danazol-induced hepatocellular adenomas. *Arch Pathol Lab Med* 1991; **115**: 1054–1057.

10 Gokhale R, Whitington PR. Hepatic adenomatosis in an adolescent. *J Ped Gastroenterol Nutr* 1996; **23**: 482–486.

11 Bacq Y, Jacquemin E, Balabaud C, et al. Familial liver adenomatosis associated with hepatocyte nuclear factor 1α? inactivation. *Gastroenterology* 2003; **125**: 1470–1475.

12 Zucman-Rossi J. Genetic alterations in hepatocellular adenomas: recent findings and new challenges. *J Hepatol* 2004; **40**: 1036–1039.

13 Soe KL, Soe M, Gluud C. Liver pathology associated with the use of anabolic-androgenic steroids. *Liver* 1992; **12**: 73–79.

14 Letter APP. hepatoma associated with androgenic steroids. *Lancet* 1975; **1**: 685–686.

15 Chandra RS, Kapur SP, Kelleher J Jr., et al. Benign hepatocellular tumors in the young. A clinicopathologic spectrum. *Arch Pathol Lab Med* 1984; **108**: 168–171.

16 Foster JH, Donohue TA, Berman MM. Familial liver-cell adenomas and diabetes mellitus. *N Engl J Med* 1978; **299**: 239–241.

17 Coire CI, Qizilbash AH, Castelli MF. Hepatic adenomata in type Ia glycogen storage disease. *Arch Pathol Lab Med* 1987; **111**: 166–169.

18 Paradis V, Laurent A, Flejou J-F, et al. Evidence for the polyclonal nature of focal nodular hyperplasia of the liver by the study of X-chromosome inactivation. *Hepatology* 1997; **26**: 891–895.

19 Wanless IR, Mawdsley C, Adams R. On the pathogenesis of focal nodular hyperplasia of the liver. *Hepatology* 1985; **5**: 1194–1200.

20 Fukukura Y, Nakashima O, Kusaba A, et al. Angioarchitecture and blood circulation in focal nodular hyperplasia of the liver. *J Hepatol* 1998; **29**: 470–475.

21 Roskams T, Vos R De, Desmet V. 'Undifferentiated progenitor cells' in focal nodular hyperplasia of the liver. *Histopathology* 1996; **28**: 291–299.

22 Scoazec J-Y, Flejou J-F, D'Errico A, et al. Focal nodular hyperplasia of the liver: composition of the extracellular matrix and expression of cell–cell and cell–matrix adhesion molecules. *Hum Pathol* 1995; **26**: 1114–1125.

23 Nime F, Pickren JW, Vana J, et al. The histology of liver tumors in oral contraceptive users observed during a national survey by the American College of Surgeons Commission on Cancer. *Cancer* 1979; **44**: 1481–1489.

24 Mathieu D, Kobeiter H, Maison P, et al. Oral contraceptive use and focal nodular hyperplasia of the liver. *Gastroenterology* 2000; **118**: 560–564.

25 Sadowski DC, Lee SS, Wanless IR, et al. Progressive type of focal nodular hyperplasia characterized by multiple tumors and recurrence. *Hepatology* 1995; **21**: 970–975.

26 Friedman LS, Gang DL, Hedberg SE, et al. Simultaneous occurrence of hepatic adenoma and focal nodular hyperplasia: report of a case and review of the literature. *Hepatology* 1984; **4**: 536–540.
27 Wanless IR, Albrecht S, Bilbao J, et al. Multiple focal nodular hyperplasia of the liver associated with vascular malformations of various organs and neoplasia of the brain: a new syndrome. *Mod Pathol* 1989; **2**: 456–462.
28 Portmann B, Stewart S, Higenbottam TW, et al. Nodular transformation of the liver associated with portal and pulmonary arterial hypertension. *Gastroenterology* 1993; **104**: 616–621.
29 Haber M, Reuben A, Burrell M, et al. Multiple focal nodular hyperplasia of the liver associated with hemihypertrophy and vascular malformations. *Gastroenterology* 1995; **108**: 1256–1262.
30 Butron Vila MM, Haot J, Desmet VJ. Cholestatic features in focal nodular hyperplasia of the liver. *Liver* 1984; **4**: 387–395.
31 Lepreux S, Laurent C, Le Bail B, et al. Multiple telangiectatic focal nodular hyperplasia: vascular abnormalities. *Virchows Arch* 2003; **442**: 226–230.
32 Ruschenburg I, Droese M. Fine needle aspiration cytology of focal nodular hyperplasia of the liver. *Acta Cytol* 1989; **33**: 857–860.
33 Schilling MK, Zimmermann A, Redaelli C, et al. Liver nodules resembling focal nodular hyperplasia after hepatic venous thrombosis. *J Hepatol* 2000; **33**: 673–676.
34 Ibarrola C, Castellano VM, Colina F. Focal hyperplastic hepatocellular nodules in hepatic venous outflow obstruction: a clinicopathological study of four patients and 24 nodules. *Histopathology* 2004; **44**: 172–179.
35 Wanless IR. Epithelioid hemangioendothelioma, multiple focal nodular hyperplasias and cavernous hemangiomas of the liver. *Arch Pathol Lab Med* 2000; **124**: 1105–1107.
36 Stromeyer FW, Ishak KG. Nodular transformation (nodular 'regenerative' hyperplasia) of the liver. A clinicopathologic study of 30 cases. *Hum Pathol* 1981; **12**: 60–71.
37 Thorne C, Urowitz MB, Wanless I, et al. Liver disease in Felty's syndrome. *Am J Med* 1982; **73**: 35–40.
38 Wanless IR. Micronodular transformation (nodular regenerative hyperplasia) of the liver: a report of 64 cases among 2,500 autopsies and a new classification of benign hepatocellular nodules. *Hepatology* 1990; **11**: 787–797.
39 Dubinsky MC, Vasiliauskas EA, Singh H, et al. 6-Thioguanine can cause serious liver injury in inflammatory bowel disease patients. *Gastroenterology* 2003; **125**: 298–303.
40 Paradinas FJ, Bull TB, Westaby D, et al. Hyperplasia and prolapse of hepatocytes into hepatic veins during longterm methyltestosterone therapy: possible relationships of these changes to the development of peliosis hepatis and liver tumours. *Histopathology* 1977; **1**: 225–246.
41 Baker BL, Axiotis C, Hurwitz ES, et al. Nodular regenerative hyperplasia of the liver in idiopathic hypereosinophilic syndrome. *J Clin Gastroenterol* 1991; **13**: 452–456.
42 Solis-Herruzo JA, Vidal JV, Colina F, et al. Nodular regenerative hyperplasia of the liver associated with the toxic oil syndrome: report of five cases. *Hepatology* 1986; **6**: 687–693.
43 Bloxham CA, Henderson DC, Hampson J, et al. Nodular regenerative hyperplasia of the liver in Behçet's disease. *Histopathology* 1992; **20**: 452–454.
44 Colina F, Pinedo F, Solís A, et al. Nodular regenerative hyperplasia of the liver in early histological stages of primary biliary cirrhosis. *Gastroenterology* 1992; **102**: 1319–1324.
45 Minato H, Nakanuma Y. Nodular regenerative hyperplasia of the liver associated with metastases of pancreatic endocrine tumour: report of two autopsy cases. *Virchows Arch [A]* 1992; **421**: 171–174.
46 Kobayashi S, Saito K, Nakanuma Y. Nodular regenerative hyperplasia of the liver in hepatocellular carcinoma. *J Clin Gastroenterol* 1993; **16**: 155–159.
47 Wanless IR, Godwin TA, Allen F, et al. Nodular regenerative hyperplasia of the liver in hematologic disorders: a possible response to obliterative portal

venopathy. A morphometric study of nine cases with an hypothesis on the pathogenesis. *Medicine* 1980; **59**: 367–379.

48 Wanless IR, Lentz JS, Roberts EA. Partial nodular transformation of liver in an adult with persistent ductus venosus. Review with hypothesis on pathogenesis. *Arch Pathol Lab Med* 1985; **109**: 427–432.

49 Terayama N, Terada T, Hoso M, et al. Partial nodular transformation of the liver with portal vein thrombosis. *J Clin Gastroenterol* 1995; **20**: 71–76.

50 Wanless IR. Vascular disorders. In: MacSween RNM, Anthony PP, Scheuer PJ, et al., eds. Pathology of the Liver, 3rd edn. Edinburgh: Churchill Livingstone, 1994: Ch. 14: 535–562.

51 Allaire GS, Rabin L, Ishak KG, et al. Bile duct adenoma. A study of 152 cases. *Am J Surg Pathol* 1988; **12**: 708–715.

52 Bhathal PS, Hughes NR, Goodman ZD. The so-called bile duct adenoma is a peribiliary gland hamartoma. *Am J Surg Pathol* 1996; **20**: 858–864.

53 Cho C, Rullis I, Rogers LS. Bile duct adenomas as liver nodules. *Arch Surg* 1978; **113**: 272–274.

54 Gold JH, Guzman IJ, Rosai J. Benign tumors of the liver. Pathologic examination of 45 cases. *Am J Clin Pathol* 1978; **70**: 6–17.

55 Govindarajan S, Peters RL. The bile duct adenoma. A lesion distinct from Meyenburg complex. *Arch Pathol Lab Med* 1984; **108**: 922–924.

56 Scheele PM, Bonar MJ, Zumwalt R, et al. Bile duct adenomas in heterozygous (MZ) deficiency of α1-protease inhibitor. *Arch Pathol Lab Med* 1988; **112**: 945–947.

57 Varnholt H, Vauthey J-N, Dal Cin P, et al. Biliary adenofibroma. A rare neoplasm of bile duct origin with an indolent behavior. *Am J Surg Pathol* 2003; **27**: 693–698.

58 Wheeler DA, Edmondson HA. Cystadenoma with mesenchymal stroma (CMS) in the liver and bile ducts. A clinicopathologic study of 17 cases, 4 with malignant change. *Cancer* 1985; **56**: 1434–1445.

59 Gourley WK, Kumar D, Bouton MS, et al. Cystadenoma and cystadenocarcinoma with mesenchymal stroma of the liver. Immunohistochemical analysis. *Arch Pathol Lab Med* 1992; **116**: 1047–1050.

60 Ishak KG, Willis GW, Cummins SD, et al. Biliary cystadenoma and cystadenocarcinoma: report of 14 cases and review of the literature. [Review]. *Cancer* 1977; **39**: 322–338.

61 Tung GA, Cronan JJ. Percutaneous needle biopsy of hepatic cavernous hemangioma. *J Clin Gastroenterol* 1993; **16**: 117–122.

62 Berry CL. Solitary 'necrotic nodule' of the liver: a probable pathogenesis. *J Clin Pathol* 1985; **38**: 1278–1280.

63 Steenbergen W Van, Joosten E, Marchal G, et al. Hepatic lymphangiomatosis. Report of a case and review of the literature. *Gastroenterology* 1985; **88**: 1968–1972.

64 Peters WM, Dixon MF, Williams NS. Angiomyolipoma of the liver. *Histopathology* 1983; **7**: 99–106.

65 Goodman ZD. Benign tumors of the liver. In: Okuda K, Ishak KG, eds. Neoplasms of the Liver, 1st edn. Tokyo: Springer-Verlag, 1990: 105.

66 Hytiroglou P, Linton P, Klion F, et al. Benign schwannoma of the liver. *Arch Pathol Lab Med* 1993; **117**: 216–218.

67 Lederman SM, Martin EC, Laffey KT, et al. Hepatic neurofibromatosis, malignant schwannoma and angiosarcoma in von Recklinghausen's disease. *Gastroenterology* 1989; **92**: 234–239.

68 Andreu V, Elizalde I, Mallafré C, et al. Plexiform neurofibromatosis and angiosarcoma of the liver in Von Recklinghausen disease. *Am J Gastroenterol* 1997; **92**: 1229–1230.

69 Moran CA, Ishak KG, Goodman ZD. Solitary fibrous tumor of the liver: a clinicopathologic and immunohistochemical study of nine cases. *Ann Diagn Pathol* 1998; **2**: 19–24.

70 Fried RH, Wardzala A, Willson RA, et al. Benign cartilaginous tumor (chondroma) of the liver. *Gastroenterology* 1992; **103**: 678–680.

71 Nonomura A, Mizukami Y, Isobe M, et al. Smallest angiomyolipoma of the liver in the oldest patient. *Liver* 1993; **13**: 51–53.

72 Tsui WMS, Colombari R, Portmann BC, et al. Hepatic angiomyolipoma. A

clinicopathologic study of 30 cases and delineation of unusual morphologic variants. *Am J Surg Pathol* 1999; **23**: 34–48.

73 Nonomura A, Mizukami Y, Kadoya M, et al. Multiple angiomyolipoma of the liver. *J Clin Gastroenterol* 1995; **20**: 248–251.

74 Kyokane T, Akita Y, Katayama M, et al. Multiple angiomyolipomas of the liver (case report). *Hepato Gastroenterol* 1995; **42**: 510–515.

75 Pounder DJ. Hepatic angiomyolipoma. *Am J Surg Pathol* 1982; **6**: 677–681.

76 Goodman ZD, Ishak KG. Angiomyolipomas of the liver. *Am J Surg Pathol* 1984; **8**: 745–750.

77 Hoffman AL, Emre S, Verham RP, et al. Hepatic angiomyolipoma: two case reports of caudate-based lesions and review of the literature. *Liver Transplant Surg* 1997; **3**: 46–53.

78 Terris B, Fléjou J-F, Picot R, et al. Hepatic angiomyolipoma. A report of four cases with immunohistochemical and DNA-flow cytometric studies. *Arch Pathol Lab Med* 1996; **120**: 68–72.

79 Karhunen PJ. Hepatic pseudolipoma. *J Clin Pathol* 1985; **38**: 877–879.

80 Shek TWH, Ng IOL, Chan KW. Inflammatory pseudotumor of the liver. Report of four cases and review of the literature. *Am J Surg Pathol* 1993; **17**: 231–238.

81 Lawrence B, Perez-Atayde A, Hibbard MK, et al. TPM3-ALK and TPM4-ALK oncogenes in inflammatory myofibroblastic tumors. *Am J Pathol* 2000; **157**: 377–384.

82 Cessna MH, Zhou H, Sanger WG, et al. Expression of ALK1 and p80 in inflammatory myofibroblastic tumor and its mesenchymal mimics: a study of 135 cases. *Mod Pathol* 2002; **15**: 931–938.

83 Shek TWH, Ho FCS, Ng GOL, et al. Follicular dendritic cell tumor of the liver. Evidence for an Epstein–Barr virus-related clonal proliferation of follicular dendritic cells. *Am J Surg Pathol* 1996; **20**: 313–324.

84 Ferrell LD, Crawford JM, Dhillon AP, et al. Proposal for standardized criteria for the diagnosis of benign, borderline and malignant hepatocellular lesions arising in chronic advanced liver disease. *Am J Surg Pathol* 1993; **17**: 1113–1123.

85 International Working Party. Terminology of nodular hepatocellular lesions. *Hepatology* 1995; **22**: 983–993.

86 Anthony PP, Vogel CL, Barker LF. Liver cell dysplasia: a premalignant condition. *J Clin Pathol* 1973; **26**: 217–223.

87 Anthony PP. Hepatocellular carcinoma: an overview. *Histopathology* 2001; **39**: 109–118.

88 Borzio M, Bruno S, Roncalli M, et al. Liver cell dysplasia is a major risk factor for hepatocellular carcinoma in cirrhosis: a prospective study. *Gastroenterology* 1995; **108**: 812–817.

89 Ganne-Carrié N, Chastang C, Chapel F, et al. Predictive score for the development of hepatocellular carcinoma and additional value of liver large cell dysplasia in Western patients with cirrhosis. *Hepatology* 1996; **23**: 1112–1118.

90 Thomas RM, Berman JJ, Yetter RA, et al. Liver cell dysplasia: a DNA aneuploid lesion with distinct morphologic features. *Hum Pathol* 1992; **23**: 496–503.

91 Terris B, Ingster O, Rubbia L, et al. Interphase cytogenetic analysis reveals numerical chromosome aberrations in large liver cell dysplasia. *J Hepatol* 1997; **27**: 313–319.

92 Natarajan S, Theise ND, Thung SN, et al. Large-cell change of hepatocytes in cirrhosis may represent a reaction to prolonged cholestasis. *Am J Surg Pathol* 1997; **21**: 312–318.

93 Lee RG, Tsamandas AC, Demetris AJ. Large cell change (liver cell dysplasia) and hepatocellular carcinoma in cirrhosis: matched case–control study, pathological analysis and pathogenetic hypothesis. *Hepatology* 1997; **26**: 1415–1422.

94 Libbrecht L, Craninx M, Nevens F, et al. Predictive value of liver cell dysplasia for development of hepatocellular carcinoma in patients with non-cirrhotic and cirrhotic chronic viral hepatitis. *Histopathology* 2001; **39**: 66–71.

95 Watanabe S, Okita K, Harada T, et al. Morphologic studies of the liver cell dysplasia. *Cancer* 1983; **51**: 2197–2205.

96 Adachi E, Hashimoto H, Tsuneyoshi M. Proliferating cell nuclear antigen in hepatocellular carcinoma and small cell liver dysplasia. *Cancer* 1993; **72**: 2902–2909.

97 Terada T, Hoso M, Nakanuma Y. Mallory body clustering in adenomatous hyperplasia in human cirrhotic livers. *Hum Pathol* 1989; **20**: 886–890.

98 Ueno Y, Moriyama M, Uchida T, et al. Irregular regeneration of hepatocytes is an important factor in the hepatocarcinogenesis of liver disease. *Hepatology* 2001; **33**: 357–362.

99 Terada T, Nakanuma Y. Iron-negative foci in siderotic macroregenerative nodules in human cirrhotic liver. *Arch Pathol Lab Med* 1989; **113**: 916–920.

100 Deugnier YM, Charalambous P, Le Quilleuc D, et al. Preneoplastic significance of hepatic iron-free foci in genetic hemochromatosis: a study of 185 patients. *Hepatology* 1993; **18**: 1363–1369.

101 Nakanuma Y, Terada T, Ueda K, et al. Adenomatous hyperplasia of the liver as a precancerous lesion. *Liver* 1993; **13**: 1–9.

102 Furuya K, Nakamura M, Yamamoto Y, et al. Macroregenerative nodule of the liver. A clinicopathologic study of 345 autopsy cases of chronic liver disease. *Cancer* 1988; **61**: 99–105.

103 Terada T, Ueda K, Nakanuma Y. Histopathological and morphometric analysis of atypical adenomatous hyperplasia of human cirrhotic livers. *Virchows Arch [A]* 1993; **422**: 381–388.

104 Le Bail B, Bernard P-H, Carles J, et al. Prevalence of liver cell dysplasia and association with HCC in a series of 100 cirrhotic liver explants. *J Hepatol* 1997; **27**: 835–842.

105 Ferrell LD. Hepatocellular nodules in the cirrhotic liver: diagnostic features and proposed nomenclature. In: Ferrell LD, ed. Diagnostic Problems in Liver Pathology. Philadelphia, PA: Hanley & Belfus, 1994: 105.

106 Gastaldi M, Massacrier A, Planells R, et al. Detection by in situ hybridization of hepatitis C virus positive and negative RNA strands using digoxigenin-labeled cRNA probes in human liver cells. *J Hepatol* 1995; **23**: 509–518.

107 Terasaki S, Kaneko S, Kobayashi K, et al. Histological features predicting malignant transformation of nonmalignant hepatocellular nodules: a prospective study. *Gastroenterology* 1998; **115**: 1216–1222.

108 Theise ND, Schwartz M, Miller C, et al. Macroregenerative nodules and hepatocellular carcinoma in forty-four sequential adults liver explants with cirrhosis. *Hepatology* 1992; **16**: 949–955.

109 Eguchi A, Nakashima O, Okudaira S, et al. Adenomatous hyperplasia in the vicinity of small hepatocellular carcinoma. *Hepatology* 1992; **15**: 843–848.

110 Aihara T, Noguchi S, Sasaki Y, et al. Clonal analysis of precancerous lesion of hepatocellular carcinoma. *Gastroenterology* 1996; **111**: 455–461.

111 Donato MF, Arosio E, Ninno E Del, et al. High rates of hepatocellular carcinoma in cirrhotic patients with high liver cell proliferative activity. *Hepatology* 2001; **34**: 523–528.

112 Wong N, Lai P, Pang E, et al. A comprehensive karyotypic study on human hepatocellular carcinoma by spectral karyotyping. *Hepatology* 2000; **32**: 1060–1068.

113 Shirota Y, Kaneko S, Honda M, et al. Identification of differentially expressed genes in hepatocellular carcinoma with cDNA microarrays. *Hepatology* 2001; **33**: 832–840.

114 Di Bisceglie AM, Carithers RL, Gores GJ. Hepatocellular carcinoma. *Hepatology* 1998; **28**: 1161–1165.

115 Schirmacher P, Rogler CE, Dienes HP. Current pathogenetic and molecular concepts in viral liver carcinogenesis. *Virchows Arch [B]* 1993; **63**: 71–89.

116 Popper H, Thung SN, McMahon BJ, et al. Evolution of hepatocellular carcinoma associated with chronic hepatitis B virus infection in Alaskan Eskimos. *Arch Pathol Lab Med* 1988; **112**: 498–504.

117 Mandishona E, MacPhail AP, Gordeuk VR, et al. Dietary iron overload as a risk factor for hepatocellular carcinoma in black Africans. *Hepatology* 1998; **27**: 1563–1566.

118 Sun Z, Lu P, Gail MH, et al. Increased risk of hepatocellular carcinoma in male hepatitis B surface antigen

carriers with chronic hepatitis who have detectable urinary aflatoxin metabolite M1. *Hepatology* 1999; **30**: 379–383.

119 Nair S, Mason A, Eason J, et al. Is obesity an independent risk factor for hepatocellular carcinoma in cirrhosis? *Hepatology* 2002; **36**: 150–155.

120 Marrero JA, Fontana RJ, Su GL, et al. NAFLD may be a common underlying liver disease in patients with hepatocellular carcinoma in the United States. *Hepatology* 2002; **36**: 1349–1354.

121 Shimada M, Hashimoto E, Taniai M, et al. Hepatocellular carcinoma in patients with non-alcoholic steatohepatitis. *J Hepatol* 2002; **37**: 154–160.

122 Paradis V, Bièche I, Dargère D, et al. Molecular profiling of hepatocellular carcinomas (HCC) using a large-scale real-time RT-PCR approach. Determination of a molecular diagnostic index. *Am J Pathol* 2003; **163**: 733–741.

123 Chen Q, Seol D-W, Carr B, et al. Co-expression and regulation of Met and Ron proto-oncogenes in human hepatocellular carcinoma tissues and cell lines. *Hepatology* 1997; **26**: 59–66.

124 Tannapfel A, Wittekind C. Genes involved in hepatocellular carcinoma: deregulation in cell cycling and apoptosis. *Virchows Arch* 2002; **44**: 345–352.

125 Park YN, Yang C-P, Fernandez GJ, et al. Neoangiogenesis and sinusoidal 'capillarization' in dysplastic nodules of the liver. *Am J Surg Pathol* 1998; **22**: 656–662.

126 Kimura H, Nakajima T, Kagawa K, et al. Angiogenesis in hepatocellular carcinoma as evaluated by CD34 immunohistochemistry. *Liver* 1998; **18**: 14–19.

127 El-Assal ON, Yamanoi A, Soda Y, et al. Clinical significance of microvessel density and vascular endothelial growth factor expression in hepatocellular carcinoma and surrounding liver: possible involvement of vascular endothelial growth factor in the angiogenesis of cirrhotic liver. *Hepatology* 1998; **27**: 1554–1562.

128 Yamaguchi R, Yano H, Iemura A, et al. Expression of vascular endothelial growth factor in human hepatocellular carcinoma. *Hepatology* 1998; **28**: 68–77.

129 Torimura T, Sata M, Ueno T, et al. Increased expression of vascular endothelial growth factor is associated with tumor progression in hepatocellular carcinoma. *Hum Pathol* 1998; **29**: 986–991.

130 Nehrbass D, Klimek F, Bannasch P. Overexpression of insulin receptor substrate-1 emerges early in hepatocarcinogenesis and elicits preneoplastic hepatic glycogenosis. *Am J Pathol* 1998; **152**: 341–345.

131 Hsia CC, Evarts RP, Nakatsukasa H, et al. Occurrence of oval-type cells in hepatitis B virus-associated human hepatocarcinogenesis. *Hepatology* 1992; **16**: 1327–1333.

132 Desmet V, Vos R De. Ultrastructural characteristics of novel epithelial cell types identified in human pathologic liver specimens with chronic ductular reaction. *Am J Pathol* 1992; **140**: 1441–1450.

133 Anthony PP. Tumours and tumour-like lesions of the liver and biliary tract. In: MacSween RNM, Anthony PP, Scheuer PJ, et al., eds. Pathology of the Liver, 3rd edn. Edinburgh: Churchill Livingstone, 1994: 16.

134 Nzeako UC, Goodman ZD, Ishak KG. Hepatocellular carcinoma in cirrhotic and noncirrhotic livers. A clinico-histopathologic study of 804 North American patients. *Am J Clin Pathol* 1996; **105**: 65–75.

135 Bralet M-P, Régimbeau J-M, Pineau P, et al. Hepatocellular carcinoma occurring in nonfibrotic liver: epidemiologic and histopathologic analysis of 80 French cases. *Hepatology* 2000; **32**: 200–204.

136 Shikata T, Yamazaki S, Uzawa T. Hepatocellular carcinoma and chronic persistent hepatitis. *Acta Pathol Jap* 1977; **27**: 297–304.

137 Tabarin A, Bioulac-Sage P, Boussarie L, et al. Hepatocellular carcinoma developed on noncirrhotic livers. *Arch Pathol Lab Med* 1987; **111**: 174–180.

138 El-Refaie A, Savage K, Bhattacharya S, et al. HCV-associated hepatocellular carcinoma without cirrhosis. *J Hepatol* 1996; **24**: 277–285.

139 Le Bail B, Carles J, Saric J, et al. Ectopic liver and hepatocarcinogenesis. *Hepatology* 1999; **30**: 585–586.
140 Miyagawa S, Kawasaki S, Makuuchi M. Comparison of the characteristics of hepatocellular carcinoma between hepatitis B and C viral infection: tumor multicentricity in cirrhotic liver with hepatitis C. *Hepatology* 1996; **24**: 307–310.
141 Kondo Y, Wada K. Intrahepatic metastasis of hepatocellular carcinoma: a histopathologic study. *Hum Pathol* 1991; **22**: 125–130.
142 Halteren HK van, Salemans JMJI, Peters H, et al. Spontaneous regression of hepatocellular carcinoma. *J Hepatol* 1997; **27**: 211–215.
143 Kaczynski J, Hansson G, Remotti H, et al. Spontaneous regression of hepatocellular carcinoma. *Histopathology* 1998; **32**: 147–150.
144 Libbrecht L, Bielen D, Verslype C, et al. Focal lesions in cirrhotic explant livers: pathological evaluation and accuracy of pretransplantation imaging examinations. *Liver Transplant* 2002; **8**: 749–761.
145 Lauwers GY, Terris B, Balis UJ, et al. Prognostic histologic indicators of curatively resected hepatocellular carcinomas. *Am J Surg Pathol* 2002; **26**: 25–34.
146 Cillo U, Bassanello M, Vitale A, et al. The critical issue of hepatocellular carcinoma prognostic classification: which is the best tool available? *J Hepatol* 2004; **40**: 124–131.
147 Lopez-Beltran A, Luque RJ, Quintero A, et al. Hepatoid adenocarcinoma of the urinary bladder. *Virchows Arch* 2003; **442**: 381–387.
148 Dhillon AP, Colombari R, Savage K, et al. An immunohistochemical study of the blood vessels within primary hepatocellular tumours. *Liver* 1992; **12**: 311–318.
149 Omata M, Peters RL, Tatter D. Sclerosing hepatic carcinoma: relationship to hypercalcemia. *Liver* 1981; **1**: 33–49.
150 Theise ND, Yao JL, Harada K, et al. Hepatic 'stem cell' malignancies in adults: four cases. *Histopathology* 2003; **43**: 263–271.
151 Wada Y, Nakashima O, Kutami R, et al. Clinicopathological study on hepatocellular carcinoma with lymphocytic infiltration. *Hepatology* 1998; **27**: 407–414.
152 Nzeako UC, Goodman ZD, Ishak KG. Comparison of tumor pathology with duration of survival of North American patients with hepatocellular carcinoma. *Cancer* 1995; **76**: 579–588.
153 Kakizoe S, Kojiro M, Nakashima T. Hepatocellular carcinoma with sarcomatous change. *Cancer* 1987; **59**: 310–316.
154 Haratake J, Horie A. An immunohistochemical study of sarcomatoid liver carcinomas. *Cancer* 1991; **68**: 93–97.
155 Buchanan TF, Jr., Huvos AG. Clear-cell carcinoma of the liver. A clinicopathologic study of 13 patients. *Am J Clin Pathol* 1974; **61**: 529–539.
156 Wu PC, Lai CL, Lam KC, et al. Clear cell carcinoma of liver. An ultrastructural study. *Cancer* 1983; **52**: 504–507.
157 Ajdukiewicz A, Crowden A, Hudson E, et al. Liver aspiration in the diagnosis of hepatocellular carcinoma in the Gambia. *J Clin Pathol* 1985; **38**: 185–192.
158 Noguchi S, Yamamoto R, Tatsuta M, et al. Cell features and patterns in fine-needle aspirates of hepatocellular carcinoma. *Cancer* 1986; **58**: 321–328.
159 Pedio G, Landolt U, Zöbeli L, et al. Fine needle aspiration of the liver. Significance of hepatocytic naked nuclei in the diagnosis of hepatocellular carcinoma. *Acta Cytol* 1988; **32**: 437–442.
160 Bottles K, Cohen MB, Holly EA, et al. A step-wise logistic regression analysis of hepatocellular carcinoma. An aspiration biopsy study. *Cancer* 1988; **62**: 558–563.
161 Ishak KG, Goodman ZD, Stocker JT. Tumors of the Liver and Intrahepatic Bile Ducts. Washington, DC: Armed Forces Institute of Pathology, 2001: 199–230.
162 Nakanuma Y, Ohta G. Expression of Mallory bodies in hepatocellular carcinoma in man and its significance. *Cancer* 1986; **57**: 81–86.
163 Hurlimann J, Gardiol D. Immunohistochemistry in the differential diagnosis of liver

carcinomas. *Am J Surg Pathol* 1991; **15**: 280–288.

164 Eyken P Van, Sciot R, Paterson A, et al. Cytokeratin expression in hepatocellular carcinoma: an immunohistochemical study. *Hum Pathol* 1988; **19**: 562–568.

165 Lai Y-S, Thung SN, Gerber MA, et al. Expression of cytokeratins in normal and diseased livers and in primary liver carcinomas. *Arch Pathol Lab Med* 1989; **113**: 134–138.

166 Thung SN, Gerber MA, Sarno E, et al. Distribution of five antigens in hepatocellular carcinoma. *Lab Invest* 1979; **41**: 101–105.

167 Ordonez NG, Manning JT Jr. Comparison of alpha-1-antitrypsin and alpha-1-antichymotrypsin in hepatocellular carcinoma: an immunoperoxidase study. *Am J Gastroenterol* 1984; **79**: 959–963.

168 Fan Z, Rijn M van de, Montgomery K, et al. Hep Par 1 antibody stain for the differential diagnosis of hepatocellular carcinoma: 676 tumors tested using tissue microarrays and conventional tissue sections. *Mod Pathol* 2003; **16**: 137–144.

169 Morrison C, Marsh W, Frankel WL. A comparison of CD10 to pCEA, MOC-31 and hepatocyte for the distinction of malignant tumors in the liver. *Mod Pathol* 2002; **15**: 1279–1287.

170 Chu PG, Weiss LM. Keratin expression in human tissues and neoplasms. *Histopathology* 2002; **40**: 403–439.

171 Uenishi T, Kubo S, Yamamoto T, et al. Cytokeratin 19 expression in hepatocellular carcinoma predicts early postoperative recurrence. *Cancer Sci* 2003; **94**: 851–857.

172 Lau SK, Prakash S, Geller SA, Alsabeh R. Comparative immunohistochemical profile of hepatocellular carcinoma, cholangiocarcinoma and metastatic adenocarcinoma. *Hum Pathol* 2002; **33**: 1175–1181.

173 Nagorney DM, Adson MA, Weiland LH, et al. Fibrolamellar hepatoma. *Am J Surg* 1985; **149**: 113–119.

174 Berman MM, Libbey NP, Foster JH. Hepatocellular carcinoma. Polygonal cell type with fibrous stroma – an atypical variant with a favorable prognosis. *Cancer* 1980; **46**: 1448–1455.

175 Craig JR, Peters RL, Edmondson HA, et al. Fibrolamellar carcinoma of the liver: a tumor of adolescents and young adults with distinctive clinico-pathologic features. *Cancer* 1980; **46**: 372–379.

176 Berman MA, Burnham JA, Sheahan DG. Fibrolamellar carcinoma of the liver: an immunohistochemical study of nineteen cases and a review of the literature. *Hum Pathol* 1988; **19**: 784–794.

177 El-Serag HB, Davila JA. Is fibrolamellar carcinoma different from hepatocellular carcinoma? A US population-based study. *Hepatology* 2004; **39**: 798–803.

178 Vecchio FM, Fabiano A, Ghirlanda G, et al. Fibrolamellar carcinoma of the liver: the malignant counterpart of focal nodular hyperplasia with oncocytic change. *Am J Clin Pathol* 1984; **81**: 521–526.

179 Vecchio FM. Fibrolamellar carcinoma of the liver: a distinct entity within the hepatocellular tumors. A review. *Appl Pathol* 1988; **6**: 139–148.

180 Orsatti G, Hytiroglou P, Thung SN, et al. Lamellar fibrosis in the fibrolamellar variant of hepatocellular carcinoma: a role for transforming growth factor beta. *Liver* 1997; **17**: 152–156.

181 Farhi DC, Shikes RH, Silverberg SG. Ultrastructure of fibrolamellar oncocytic hepatoma. *Cancer* 1982; **50**: 702–709.

182 Lefkowitch JH, Muschel R, Price JB, et al. Copper and copper-binding protein in fibrolamellar liver cell carcinoma. *Cancer* 1983; **51**: 97–100.

183 Vecchio FM, Federico F, Dina MA. Copper and hepatocellular carcinoma. *Digestion* 1986; **35**: 109–114.

184 Teitelbaum DH, Tuttle S, Carey LC, et al. Fibrolamellar carcinoma of the liver. Review of three cases and the presentation of a characteristic set of tumor markers defining this tumor. *Ann Surg* 1985; **202**: 36–41.

185 Payne CM, Nagle RB, Paplanus SH, et al. Fibrolamellar carcinoma of liver: a primary malignant oncocytic carcinoid? *Ultrastruc Pathol* 1986; **10**: 539–552.

186 Subramony C, Herrera GA, Lockard V. Neuroendocrine differentiation in hepatic neoplasms: report of four cases. *Surg Pathol* 1993; **5**: 17–33.

187 Okano A, Hajiro K, Takakuwa H, et al.

Fibrolamellar carcinoma of the liver with a mixture of ordinary hepatocellular carcinoma: a case report. *Am J Gastroenterol* 1998; **93**: 1144–1145.

188 LeBrun DP, Silver MM, Freedman MH, et al. Fibrolamellar carcinoma of the liver in a patient with Fanconi anemia. *Hum Pathol* 1991; **22**: 396–398.

189 Gores GJ. Cholangiocarcinoma. Current concept and insights. *Hepatology* 2003; **37**: 961–969.

190 Klatskin G. Adenocarcinoma of the hepatic duct at its bifurcation within the porta hepatis. An unusual tumor with distinctive clinical and pathological features. *Am J Med* 1965; **38**: 241–256.

191 Schlinkert RT, Nagorney DM, Heerden JA Van, et al. Intrahepatic cholangiocarcinoma: clinical aspects, pathology and treatment. *HPB Surg* 1992; **5**: 95–102.

192 Case records of the Massachusetts General Hospital. Case 29-1987. *N Engl J Med* 1987; **317**: 153–160.

193 Bloustein PA. Association of carcinoma with congenital cystic conditions of the liver and bile ducts. *Am J Gastroenterol* 1977; **67**: 40–46.

194 Burns CD, Kuhns JG, Wieman J. Cholangiocarcinoma in association with multiple biliary microhamartomas. *Arch Pathol Lab Med* 1990; **114**: 1287–1289.

195 Yamato T, Sasaki M, Hoso M, et al. Intrahepatic cholangiocarcinoma arising in congenital hepatic fibrosis: report of an autopsy case. *J Hepatol* 1998; **28**: 717–722.

196 Hasebe T, Sakamoto M, Mukai K, et al. Cholangiocarcinoma arising in bile duct adenoma with focal area of bile duct hamartoma. *Virchows Arch* 1995; **426**: 209–213.

197 Kobayashi M, Ikeda K, Saitoh S, et al. Incidence of primary cholangiocellular carcinoma of the liver in Japanese patients with hepatitis C virus-related cirrhosis. *Cancer* 2000; **88**: 2471–2477.

198 Lau GKK, Davis GL, Wu SPC, et al. Hepatic expression of hepatitis C virus RNA in chronic hepatitis C: a study by in situ reverse-transcription polymerase chain reaction. *Hepatology* 1996; **23**: 1318–1323.

199 Chow LTC, Ahuja AT, Kwong KH, et al. Mucinous cholangiocarcinoma: an unusual complication of hepatolithiasis and recurrent pyogenic cholangitis. *Histopathology* 1997; **30**: 491–494.

200 Tihan T, Blumgart L, Klimstra DS. Clear cell papillary carcinoma of the liver: an unusual variant of peripheral cholangiocarcinoma. *Hum Pathol* 1998; **29**: 196–200.

201 Nakajima T, Knodo Y, Miyazaki M, et al. A histopathologic study of 102 cases of intrahepatic cholangiocarcinoma: histologic classification and modes of spreading. *Hum Pathol* 1988; **19**: 1228–1234.

202 Weinbren K, Mutum SS. Pathological aspects of cholangiocarcinoma. *J Pathol* 1983; **139**: 217–238.

203 Bonetti F, Chilosi M, Pisa R, et al. Epithelial membrane antigen expression in cholangiocarcinoma. An useful immunohistochemical tool for differential diagnosis with hepatocarcinoma. *Virchows Arch A Pathol Anat Histopathol* 1983; **401**: 307–313.

204 Pastolero GC, Wakabayashi T, Oka T, et al. Tissue polypeptide antigen – a marker antigen differentiating cholangiolar tumors from other hepatic tumors. *Am J Clin Pathol* 1987; **87**: 168–173.

205 Jovanovic R, Jagirdar J, Thung SN, et al. Blood-group-related antigen Lewis-X and Lewis-Y in the differential diagnosis of cholangiocarcinoma and hepatocellular carcinoma. *Arch Pathol Lab Med* 1989; **113**: 139–142.

206 Terada T, Nakanuma Y. An immunohistochemical survey of amylase isoenzymes in cholangiocarcinoma and hepatocellular carcinoma. *Arch Pathol Lab Med* 1993; **117**: 160–162.

207 Maeda T, Adachi E, Kajiyama K, et al. Combined hepatocellular and cholangiocarcinoma: proposed criteria according to cytokeratin expression and analysis of clinicopathologic features. *Hum Pathol* 1995; **26**: 956–964.

208 Haratake J, Hashimoto H. An immunohistochemical analysis of 13 cases with combined hepatocellular and cholangiocellular carcinoma. *Liver* 1995; **15**: 9–15.

209 Papotti M, Sambataro D, Marchesa P, et al. A combined hepatocellular/

cholangiocellular carcinoma with sarcomatoid features. *Liver* 1997; **17**: 47–52.

210 Goodman ZD, Ishak KG, Langloss JM, et al. Combined hepatocellular-cholangiocarcinoma. A histologic and immunohistochemical study. *Cancer* 1985; **55**: 124–135.

211 Azizah N, Paradinas FJ. Cholangiocarcinoma coexisting with developmental liver cysts: a distinct entity different from liver cystadenocarcinoma. *Histopathology* 1980; **4**: 391–400.

212 Theise ND, Miller F, Worman HJ, et al. Biliary cystadenocarcinoma arising in a liver with fibropolycystic disease. *Arch Pathol Lab Med* 1993; **117**: 163–165.

213 Lander JJ, Stanley RJ, Sumner HW, et al. Angiosarcoma of the liver associated with Fowler's solution (potassium arsenite). *Gastroenterology* 1975; **68**: 1582–1586.

214 Horta JS. Late effects of thorotrast on the liver and spleen and their efferent lymph nodes. *Ann N Y Acad Sci* 1967; **145**: 676–699.

215 Visfeldt J, Poulsen H. On the histopathology of liver and liver tumours in thorium- dioxide patients. *Acta Pathol Microbiol Scand A* 1972; **80**: 97–108.

216 Winberg CD, Ranchod M. Thorotrast induced hepatic cholangiocarcinoma and angiosarcoma. *Hum Pathol* 1979; **10**: 108–112.

217 Thomas LB, Popper H, Berk PD, et al. Vinyl-chloride-induced liver disease. From idiopathic portal hypertension (Banti's syndrome) to angiosarcomas. *N Engl J Med* 1975; **292**: 17–22.

218 Pimentel JC, Menezes AP. Liver disease in vineyard sprayers. *Gastroenterology* 1977; **72**: 275–283.

219 Hoch-Ligeti C. Angiosarcoma of the liver associated with diethylstilbestrol. *JAMA* 1978; **240**: 1510–1511.

220 Falk H, Thomas LB, Popper H, et al. Hepatic angiosarcoma associated with androgenic-anabolic steroids. *Lancet* 1979; **2**: 1120–1123.

221 Monroe PS, Riddell RH, Siegler M et al. Hepatic angiosarcoma. Possible relationship to long-term oral contraceptive ingestion. *JAMA* 1981; **246**: 64–65.

222 Daneshmend TK, Scott GL, Bradfield JW. Angiosarcoma of liver associated with phenelzine. *Br Med J* 1979; **1**: 1679–1679.

223 Cadranel JF, Legendre C, Desaint B, et al. Liver disease from surreptitious administration of urethane. *J Clin Gastroenterol* 1993; **17**: 52–56.

224 Fortwengler HP Jr., Jones D, Espinosa E et al. Evidence for endothelial cell origin of vinyl chloride-induced hepatic angiosarcoma. *Gastroenterology* 1981; **80**: 1415–1419.

225 Manning JT Jr., Ordonez NG, Barton JH. Endothelial cell origin of thorium oxide-induced angiosarcoma of liver. *Arch Pathol Lab Med* 1983; **107**: 456–458.

226 Popper H, Thomas LB, Telles NC, et al. Development of hepatic angiosarcoma in man induced by vinyl chloride, thorotrast and arsenic. Comparison with cases of unknown etiology. *Am J Pathol* 1978; **92**: 349–369.

227 Tamburro CH, Makk L, Popper H. Early hepatic histologic alterations among chemical (vinyl monomer) workers. *Hepatology* 1984; **4**: 413–418.

228 Ishak KG, Sesterhenn IA, Goodman ZD, et al. Epithelioid hemangioendothelioma of the liver: a clinicopathologic and follow-up study of 32 cases. *Hum Pathol* 1984; **15**: 839–852.

229 Ishak KG. Malignant mesenchymal tumors of the liver. In: Okuda K, Ishak KG, eds. Neoplasms of the Liver, 1st edn. Tokyo: Springer-Verlag, 1987: 159.

230 Makhlouf HR, Ishak KG, Goodman ZD. Epithelioid hemangioendothelioma of the liver. A clinicopathologic study of 137 cases. *Cancer* 1999; **85**: 562–582.

231 Ekfors TO, Joensuu K, Toivio I, et al. Fatal epithelioid haemangio-endothelioma presenting in the lung and liver. *Virchows Arch A Pathol Anat Histopathol* 1986; **410**: 9–16.

232 Dean PJ, Haggitt RC, O'Hara CJ. Malignant epithelioid hemangioendothelioma of the liver in young women. Relationship to oral contraceptive use. *Am J Surg Pathol* 1985; **9**: 695–704.

233 Demetris AJ, Minervini M, Raikow RB, et al. Hepatic epithelioid hemangioendothelioma. Biological questions based on pattern of recurrence in an allograft and tumor

immunophenotype. *Am J Surg Pathol* 1997; **21**: 263–270.

234 Scoazec J-Y, Degott C, Reynes M, et al. Epithelioid hemangioendothelioma of the liver: an ultrastructural study. *Hum Pathol* 1989; **20**: 673–681.

235 Utz DC, Warren MM, Gregg JA, et al. Reversible hepatic dysfunction associated with hypernephroma. *Mayo Clin Proc* 1970; **45**: 161–169.

236 Strickland RC, Schenker S. The nephrogenic hepatic dysfunction syndrome: a review. [Review]. *Am J Dig Dis* 1977; **22**: 49–55.

237 Tao LC, Donat EE, Ho CS, et al. Percutaneous fine-needle aspiration biopsy of the liver. Cytodiagnosis of hepatic cancer. *Acta Cytol* 1979; **23**: 287–291.

238 Axe SR, Erozan YS, Ermatinger SV. Fine-needle aspiration of the liver. A comparison of smear and rinse preparations in the detection of cancer. *Am J Clin Pathol* 1986; **86**: 281–285.

239 Atterbury CE, Enriquez RE, Desuto-Nagy GI, et al. Comparison of the histologic and cytologic diagnosis of liver biopsies in hepatic cancer. *Gastroenterology* 1979; **76**: 1352–1357.

240 Gerber MA, Thung SN, Bodenheimer HC Jr., et al. Characteristic histologic triad in liver adjacent to metastatic neoplasm. *Liver* 1986; **6**: 85–88.

241 Glees JP, Thomas M, Redding WH, et al. Liver biopsy at lymphoma laparotomy [letter]. *Lancet* 1978; **1**: 210–211.

242 Kim H, Dorfman RF, Rosenberg SA. Pathology of malignant lymphomas of the liver: application in staging. In: Popper H, Schaffner F, eds. Progress in Liver Diseases, Vol. V, 1st edn. New York: Grune & Stratton, 1976: 683.

243 Leslie KO, Colby TV. Hepatic parenchymal lymphoid aggregates in Hodgkin's disease. *Hum Pathol* 1984; **15**: 808–809.

244 Abt AB, Kirschner RH, Belliveau RE, et al. Hepatic pathology associated with Hodgkin's disease. *Cancer* 1974; **33**: 1564–1571.

245 Bruguera M, Caballero T, Carreras E, et al. Hepatic sinusoidal dilatation in Hodgkin's disease. *Liver* 1987; **7**: 76–80.

246 Perera DR, Greene ML, Fenster LF. Cholestasis associated with extrabiliary Hodgkin's disease. Report of three cases and review of four others. *Gastroenterology* 1974; **67**: 680–685.

247 Hubscher SG, Lumley MA, Elias E. Vanishing bile duct syndrome: a possible mechanism for intrahepatic cholestasis in Hodgkin's lymphoma. *Hepatology* 1993; **17**: 70–77.

248 Lefkowitch JH, Falkow S, Whitlock RT. Hepatic Hodgkin's disease simulating cholestatic hepatitis with liver failure. *Arch Pathol Lab Med* 1985; **109**: 424–426.

249 Wolf-Peeters C De. Liver involvement in lymphomas. *Ann Diagn Pathol* 1998; **2**: 363–369.

250 Trudel M, Aramendi T, Caplan S. Large-cell lymphoma presenting with hepatic sinusoidal infiltration. *Arch Pathol Lab Med* 1991; **115**: 821–824.

251 Dubois A, Dauzat M, Pignodel C, et al. Portal hypertension in lympho-proliferative and myeloproliferative disorders: hemodynamic and histological correlations. *Hepatology* 1993; **17**: 246–250.

252 Saló J, Nomdedeu B, Bruguera M, et al. Acute liver failure due to non-Hodgkin's lymphoma. *Am J Gastroenterol* 1993; **88**: 774–776.

253 Verdi CJ, Grogan TM, Protell R, et al. Liver biopsy immunotyping to characterize lymphoid malignancies. *Hepatology* 1986; **6**: 6–13.

254 Freeman C, Berg JW, Cutler SJ. Occurrence and prognosis of extranodal lymphomas. *Cancer* 1972; **29**: 252–260.

255 Zafrani ES, Gaulard P. Primary lymphoma of the liver. *Liver* 1993; **13**: 57–61.

256 Stemmer S, Geffen DB, Goldstein J, et al. Primary small noncleaved cell lymphoma of the liver. *J Clin Gastroenterol* 1993; **16**: 65–69.

257 Maes M, Depardieu C, Dargent J-L, et al. Primary low-grade B-cell lymphoma of MALT-type occurring in the liver: a study of two cases. *J Hepatol* 1997; **27**: 922–927.

258 Isaacson PG, Banks PM, Best PV, et al. Primary low-grade hepatic B-cell lymphoma of mucosa-associated lymphoid tissue (MALT)-type. *Am J Surg Pathol* 1995; **19**: 571–575.

259 Scoazec J-Y, Degott C, Brousse N, et al. Non-Hodgkin's lymphoma presenting

as a primary tumor of the liver: presentation, diagnosis and outcome in eight patients. *Hepatology* 1991; **13**: 870–875.

260 Kim JH, Kim HY, Kang I, et al. A case of primary hepatic lymphoma with hepatitis C liver cirrhosis. *Am J Gastroenterol* 2000; **95**: 2377–2380.

261 Rasul I, Shepherd FA, Kamel-Reid S, et al. Detection of occult low-grade B-cell non-Hodgkin's lymphoma in patient's with chronic hepatitis C infection and mixed cryoglobulinemia. *Hepatology* 1999; **29**: 543–547.

262 Ohshima K, Haraoka S, Harada N, et al. Hepatosplenic γδ T-cell lymphoma: relation to Epstein-Barr virus and activated cytotoxic molecules. *Histopathology* 2000; **36**: 127–135.

263 Suarez F, Wlodarski I, Rigal-Huguet F, et al. Hepatosplenic αβ T-cell lymphoma. An unusual case with clinical, histologic and cytogenetic features of γδ hepatosplenic T-cell lymphoma. *Am J Surg Pathol* 2000; **24**: 1027–1032.

264 Thomas FB, Clausen KP, Greenberger NJ. Liver disease in multiple myeloma. *Arch Intern Med* 1973; **132**: 195–202.

265 Weichhold W, Labouyrie E, Merlio JP et al. Primary extramedullary plasmacytoma of the liver. A case report. *Am J Surg Pathol* 1995; **19**: 1197–1202.

266 Brooks AP. Portal hypertension in Waldenstrom's macroglobulinaemia. *Br Med J* 1976; **1**: 689–690.

267 Lévy S, Capron D, Joly J-P, et al. Hepatic nodules as single organ involvement in an adult with Langerhans cell granulomatosis. *J Clin Gastroenterol* 1998; **26**: 69–73.

268 Foschini MP, Milandri GL, Dina RE, et al. Benign regressing histiocytosis of the liver. *Histopathology* 1995; **26**: 363–366.

269 Kaplan KJ, Goodman ZD, Ishak KG. Liver involvement in Langerhans' cell histiocytosis: a study of nine cases. *Mod Pathol* 1999; **12**: 370–378.

270 Yam LT, Chan CH, Li CY. Hepatic involvement in systemic mast cell disease. *Am J Med* 1986; **80**: 819–826.

271 Scheimberg IB, Pollock DJ, Collins PW, et al. Pathology of the liver in leukaemia and lymphoma. A study of 110 autopsies. *Histopathology* 1995; **26**: 311–321.

272 Schwartz JB, Shamsuddin AM. The effects of leukemic infiltrates in various organs in chronic lymphocytic leukemia. *Hum Pathol* 1981; **12**: 432–440.

273 Roquet ML, Zafrani ES, Farcet JP, et al. Histopathological lesions of the liver in hairy cell leukemia: a report of 14 cases. *Hepatology* 1985; **5**: 496–500.

274 Yam LT, Janckila AJ, Chan CH, et al. Hepatic involvement in hairy cell leukemia. *Cancer* 1983; **51**: 1497–1504.

275 Zafrani ES, Degos F, Guigui B, et al. The hepatic sinusoid in hairy cell leukemia: an ultrastructural study of 12 cases. *Hum Pathol* 1987; **18**: 801–807.

276 Grouls V, Stiens R. Hepatic involvement in hairy cell leukemia: diagnosis by tartrate-resistant acid phosphatase enzyme histochemistry on formalin fixed and paraffin-embedded liver biopsy specimens. Pathology. *Res Pract* 1984; **178**: 332–334.

277 Wheeler DA, Edmondson HA, Reynolds TB. Spontaneous liver cell adenoma in children. *Am J Clin Pathol* 1986; **85**: 6–12.

278 Resnick MB, Kozakewich HPW, Perez-Atayde AR. Hepatic adenoma in the pediatric age group. Clinicopathological observations and assessment of cell proliferative activity. *Am J Surg Pathol* 1995; **19**: 1181–1190.

279 Janes CH, McGill DB, Ludwig J, et al. Liver cell adenoma at the age of 3 years and transplantation 19 years later after development of carcinoma: a case report. *Hepatology* 1993; **17**: 583–585.

280 Moran CA, Mullick FG, Ishak KG. Nodular regenerative hyperplasia of the liver in children. *Am J Surg Pathol* 1991; **15**: 449–454.

281 Srouji MN, Chatten J, Schulman WM, et al. Mesenchymal hamartoma of the liver in infants. [Review]. *Cancer* 1978; **42**: 2483–2489.

282 Stocker JT, Ishak KG. Mesenchymal hamartoma of the liver: report of 30 cases and review of the literature. *Ped Pathol* 1983; **1**: 245–267.

283 Cook JR, Pfeifer JD, Dehner LP. Mesenchymal hamartoma of the liver in the adult: association with distinct clinical features and histological changes. *Hum Pathol* 2002; **33**: 893–898.

284 Lauwers GY, Grant LD, Donnelly WH, et al. Hepatic undifferentiated (embryonal) sarcoma arising in a mesenchymal hamartoma. *Am J Surg Pathol* 1997; **21**: 1248–1254.

285 Dehner LP, Ishak KG. Vascular tumors of the liver in infants and children. A study of 30 cases and review of the literature. *Arch Pathol* 1971; **92**: 101–111.

286 Selby DM, Stocker JT, Waclawiw MA, et al. Infantile hemangioendothelioma of the liver. *Hepatology* 1994; **20**: 39–45.

286a Dimashkieh HH, M. JQ, Wyatt-Ashmead J, Collins MH. Pediatric hepatic angiosarcoma: case report and review of the literature. *Pediatr Dev Pathol* 2004; **7**: 527–532.

287 Dachman AH, Lichtenstein JE, Friedman AC, et al. Infantile hemangioendothelioma of the liver: a radiologic-pathologic-clinical correlation. *AJR* 1983; **140**: 1091–1096.

288 Darbari A, Sabin KM, Shapiro CN, et al. Epidemiology of primary hepatic malignancies in U.S. children. *Hepatology* 2003; **38**: 560–566.

289 Stocker JT, Ishak KG. Hepatoblastoma. In: Okuda K, Ishak KG, eds. Neoplasms of the Liver, 1st edn. Tokyo: Springer-Verlag, 1987: 127.

290 Ishak KG, Glunz PR. Hepatoblastoma and hepatocarcinoma in infancy and childhood. Report of 47 cases. *Cancer* 1967; **20**: 396–422.

291 Lack EE, Neave C. Vawter GF. Hepatoblastoma. A clinical and pathologic study of 54 cases. *Am J Surg Pathol* 1982; **6**: 693–705.

292 Kasai M, Watanabe I. Histologic classification of liver cell carcinoma in infancy and childhood and its clinical evaluation. *Cancer* 1970; **25**: 551–563.

293 Weinberg AG, Finegold MJ. Primary hepatic tumors of childhood. [Review]. *Hum Pathol* 1983; **14**: 512–537.

294 Rugge M, Sonego F, Pollice L, et al. Hepatoblastoma: DNA nuclear content, proliferative indices and pathology. *Liver* 1998; **18**: 128–133.

295 Gonzalez-Crussi F, Upton MP, Maurer HS. Hepatoblastoma. Attempt at characterization of histologic subtypes. *Am J Surg Pathol* 1982; **6**: 599–612.

296 Abenoza P, Manivel JC, Wick MR, et al. Hepatoblastoma: an immunohistochemical and ultrastructural study. *Hum Pathol* 1987; **18**: 1025–1035.

297 Stocker JT, Ishak KG. Undifferentiated (embryonal) sarcoma of the liver: report of 31 cases. *Cancer* 1978; **42**: 336–348.

298 Keating S, Taylor GP. Undifferentiated (embryonal) sarcoma of the liver: ultrastructural and immunohistochemical similarities with malignant fibrous histiocytoma. *Hum Pathol* 1985; **16**: 693–699.

299 Aoyama C, Hachitanda Y, Sato JK, et al. Undifferentiated (embryonal) sarcoma of the liver. A tumor of uncertain histogenesis showing divergent differentiation. *Am J Surg Pathol* 1991; **15**: 615–624.

300 Lack EE, Schloo BL, Azumi N, et al. Undifferentiated (embryonal) sarcoma of the liver. Clinical and pathologic study of 16 cases with emphasis on immunohistochemical features. *Am J Surg Pathol* 1991; **15**: 1–16.

300a Heerema-McKenney A, Leuschner I, Smith N et al. Nested stromal epithelial tumor of the liver. Six cases of a distinctive pediatric neoplasm with frequent calcifications and association with Cushing syndrome. *Am J Surg Pathol* 2005; **29**: 10–20.

300b Hill DA, Swanson PE, Anderson K et al. Desmoplastic nested spindle cell tumor of liver. Report of four cases of a proposed newentity. *Am J Surg Pathol* 2005; **29**:1–9.

301 Mills AE. Undifferentiated primary hepatic non-Hodgkin's lymphoma in childhood. *Am J Surg Pathol* 1988; **12**: 721–726.

302 Caturelli E, Solmi L, Anti M, et al. Ultrasound guided fine needle biopsy of early hepatocellular carcinoma complicating liver cirrhosis: a multicentre study. *Gut* 2004; **53**: 1356–1362.

303 Bottles K, Cohen MB. An approach to fine-needle aspiration biopsy diagnosis of hepatic masses. *Diagn Cytopathol* 1991; **7**: 204–210.

304 Frias-Hidvegi D. Guides to Clinical Aspiration Biopsy. Liver and Pancreas. New York & Tokyo: Igaku-Shoin, 1988: 27–42.

305 Suen KC. Diagnosis of primary hepatic neoplasms by fine needle aspiration cytology. *Diagn Cytopathol* 1986; **2**: 99–109.

306 Perry MD, Johnson WW. Needle biopsy of the liver for the diagnosis of

nonneoplastic liver disease. *Acta Cytol* 1985; **29**: 385–390.

307 Tao L-C. Are oral contraceptive-associated liver cell adenomas premalignant? *Acta Cytol* 1992; **36**: 338–344.

308 Ruschenberg I, Droese M. Fine needle aspiration cytology of focal nodular hyperplasia of the liver. *Acta Cytol* 1989; **33**: 857–860.

309 Taavitsainen M, Airaksinin T, Kreula J, et al. Fine-needle aspiration biopsy of liver hemangioma. *Acta Radiol* 1990; **31**: 69–71.

310 Yang GCH, Yang G-Y, Tao L-C. Distinguishing well-differentiated hepatocellular carcinoma from benign liver by the physical features of fine-needle aspirates. *Mod Pathol* 2004; **17**: 798–802.

311 Pedio G, Landolt U, Zobeli L, et al. Fine needle aspiration of the liver. Significance of hepatocytic naked nuclei in the diagnosis of hepatocellular carcinoma. *Acta Cytol* 1988; **32**: 437–442.

312 Cohen MB, Haber MM, Holly EA, et al. Cytologic criteria to distinguish hepatocellular carcinoma from non-neoplastic liver. *Am J Clin Pathol* 1990; **93**: 444.

313 Wee A, Nilsson B, Chan-Wilde C, et al. Fine needle aspiration biopsy of hepatocellular carcinoma: some unusual features. *Acta Cytol* 1991; **35**: 661–670.

314 Donat EE, Anderson V, Tao L-C. Cytodiagnosis of clear cell hepatocellular carcinoma. A case report. *Acta Cytol* 1991; **35**: 671–675.

315 Nguyen G-K. Fine-needle aspiration biopsy cytology of hepatic tumors in adults. *Pathol Annu* 1986; **21**: 321–349.

316 Davenport RD. Cytologic diagnosis of fibrolamellar carcinoma of the liver by fine-needle aspiration. *Diagn Cytopathol* 1990; **6**: 275–279.

317 Wakely PEJ, Silverman JF, Geisinger KR, et al. Fine needle aspiration cytology of hepatoblastoma. *Mod Pathol* 1990; **3**: 688–693.

318 Dekmezian R, Sneigi N, Papok S, et al. Fine needle aspiration cytology of pediatric patients with primary hepatic tumors. *Diagn Cytopathol* 1988; **4**: 162–168.

319 Saleh HA, Tao LC. Hepatic angiosarcoma: aspiration biopsy cytology and immunocytochemical contribution. *Diagn Cytopathol* 1998; **18**: 208–211.

320 Siddiqui MT, Reddy VB, Castelli MJ, et al. Role of fine-needle aspiration in clinical management of transplant patients. *Diagn Cytopathol* 1997; **17**: 429–435.

321 Flanders E, Kornstein M, Wakely P, et al. Lymphoglandular bodies in fine-needle aspiration cytology smears. *Am J Clin Pathol* 1993; **99**: 566–569.

GENERAL READING

Okuda K, Ishak KG (eds). Neoplasms of the Liver. Tokyo: Springer-Verlag, 1987.

Anthony PP. Tumours and tumour-like lesions of the liver and biliary tract: aetiology, epidemiology and pathology. In: MacSween RNM, Anthony PP, Scheuer PJ, et al., eds. Pathology of the Liver, 4th edn. Edinburgh: Churchill Livingstone, 2002: 711–776.

Bannasch P, Schröder CH. Tumours and tumour-like lesions of the liver and biliary tract: pathogenesis of primary liver tumours. In: MacSween RNM, Anthony PP, Scheuer PJ, et al., eds. Pathology of the Liver, 4th edn. Edinburgh: Churchill Livingstone, 2002: 777–825.

Anthony PP. Hepatocellular carcinoma: an overview. *Histopathology* 2001; **39**: 109–118.

Gores GJ. Cholangiocarcinoma: current concepts and insights. *Hepatology* 2003; **37**: 961–969.

Pitman MB, Szyfelbein WM. Fine Needle Aspiration Biopsy of the Liver. Pitman MB, Szyfelbein WM, eds. A Color Atlas. Boston: Butterworth-Heinemann, 1994.

DeMay RM. Practical Principles of Cytopathology. Chicago: ASCP Press, 1999: 307–320.

Tao L-C. Liver and pancreas. In: Bibbo M, ed. Comprehensive Cytopathology, 2nd edn. Philadelphia: WB Saunders, 1997: 827–864.

CHAPTER 12

VASCULAR DISORDERS

THE HEPATIC ARTERIES

The effects of occlusion of hepatic artery branches are unpredictable because of the liver's double blood supply and variable collateral flow. Potential effects of thrombotic or other occlusion include infarction and ischaemic damage to the biliary tree leading to stricture formation, cholangitis or duct rupture.[1–3] The branches of the hepatic artery are sometimes involved in **polyarteritis nodosa**,[2,4] the arteritis of **systemic lupus erythematosus**,[5] **Schönlein-Henoch purpura**[3] and **giant cell arteritis**.[6] In the latter, the liver may contain granulomas of classical[7] or fibrin-ring type.[8] The arterial lesions of these systemic diseases are not often seen in needle biopsies of the liver. Vasculitis affecting small intrahepatic vessels is sometimes a manifestation of infection or neoplasia.

In some older subjects, especially those with systemic hypertension, small arteries and arterioles in portal tracts appear thickened and hyaline. **Amyloidosis** can give rise to thickening of arterial walls in the absence of sinusoidal deposits.

The arteriovenous malformations and telangiectases of **hereditary haemorrhagic telangiectasia** are sometimes found in the liver, with or without surrounding fibrosis. The presentation is either as portal hypertension (accompanied by hepatic encephalopathy and nodular regeneration[9,10]), biliary disease (sometimes resembling primary sclerosing cholangitis or Caroli's disease) or cardiac failure due to arteriovenous shunting.[11] Patients with liver involvement may have raised serum alkaline phosphatase levels without jaundice ('anicteric cholestasis'), attributed to abnormal blood supply to the biliary tree.[12] Severely damaged medium-sized bile ducts are occasionally seen histologically.

Infarcts of the liver result from arteritis, aneurysms, thrombosis, embolism or surgical ligation. They may complicate pregnancy or liver transplantation. Infarction can also follow occlusion of portal-vein branches[13] and may even be found in the absence of demonstrable vascular obstruction. The pathological features are as in other organs: there are well-defined zones of coagulative necrosis with congested and inflamed borders (Fig. 12.1). Portal tracts may survive within the infarcted areas. Coagulative necrosis of the centres of cirrhotic nodules following hypoperfusion is sometimes called nodular infarction.

Shock, heart failure and heat-stroke

Severe hypoperfusion of the hepatic parenchyma leads to necrosis, usually in perivenular regions (acinar zone 3) but also, additionally or alternatively, in

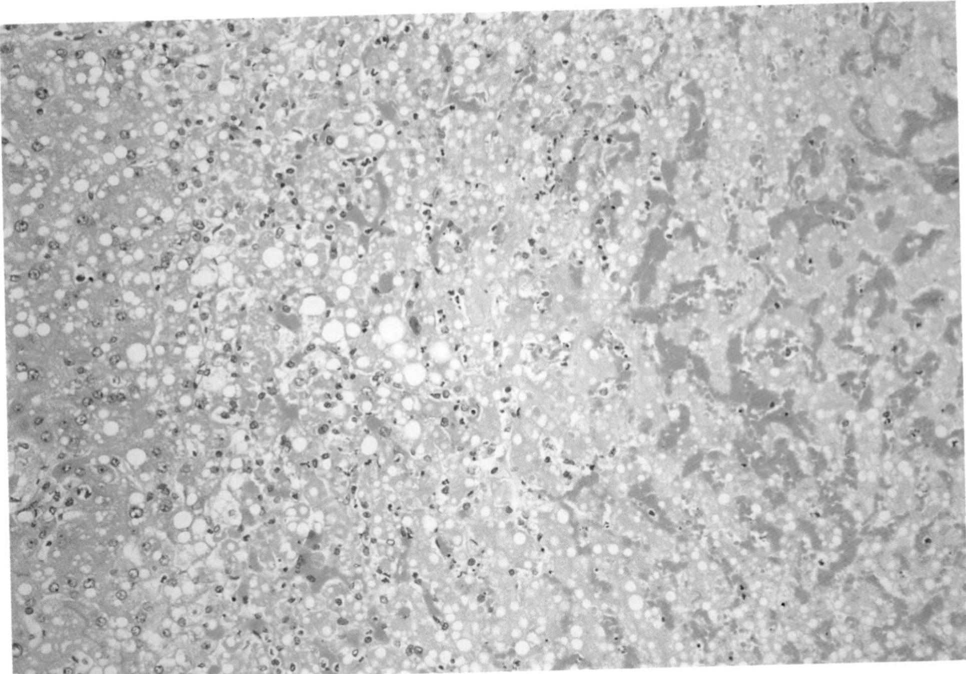

Figure 12.1 *Infarct*. The dead parenchyma to the right is intensely congested. Surviving liver tissue (left) is fatty. (Post-mortem liver, H&E).

mid-zonal regions (zone 2).[14] Portal tracts and the periportal parenchyma typically remain normal. In contrast to the necrosis of acute hepatitis there is usually little or no inflammation, but in some patients neutrophils and mononuclear cells accumulate in limited numbers.[15] Affected areas may be congested and contain large, ceroid-laden macrophages. There may be cholestasis and evidence of regenerative hyperplasia in the surviving parenchyma. The reticulin network shows regular condensation in the necrotic areas. Similar changes are seen in patients with heat-stroke (Fig. 12.2). There may be steatosis in the surviving parenchyma. Inflammation ranges from absent in mild cases[16] to severe when the damage is extensive.[17] Systemic candidiasis is a complication.

One of the most important causes of this type of necrosis is heart failure with consequent hypoperfusion of the liver. The term ischaemic hepatitis is commonly used for the viral hepatitis-like clinical picture which may ensue.[18] Congestive heart failure leads to sinusoidal dilatation (see Venous congestion and outflow obstruction, below).

THE PORTAL VEINS

Thrombosis of the main portal veins may result from infection (local or in the portal venous drainage area), cirrhosis,[19] liver transplantation, disorders of coagulation and venous outflow obstruction.[20] Invasion by hepatocellular carcinoma is a common cause. In some patients no reason for the thrombosis can be discovered, but an underlying thrombophilic condition should always be excluded.[19] In the acute phase

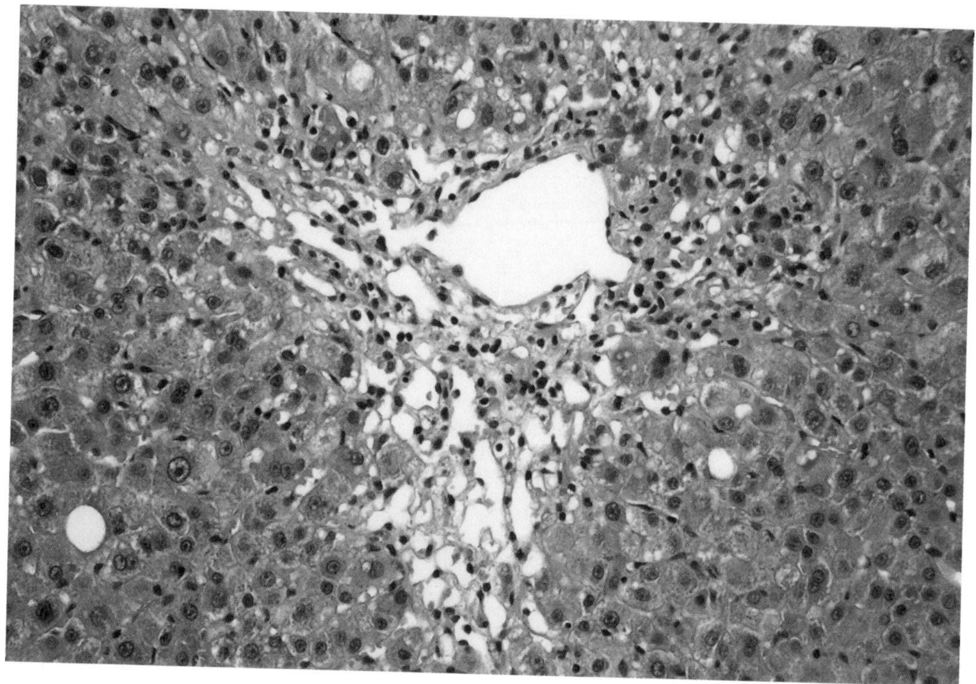

Figure 12.2 *Heat-stroke*. There has been confluent necrosis in acinar zone 3. (Section kindly provided by Professor Helmut Denk). (Needle biopsy, H&E).

of pylephlebitis, septic thrombi may be seen in portal-vein branches in portal tracts (Fig. 12.3).

Possible results of portal vein thrombosis include diffuse or focal parenchymal atrophy, increase in the number of apoptotic hepatocytes,[21] parenchymal nodularity (see Nodular regenerative hyperplasia) and a mild degree of portal fibrosis. Focal atrophy, also known as Zahn's infarction, is often found at the margins of tumour nodules. Occasionally portal venous obstruction leads to true infarction of the hepatic parenchyma.[13] In many patients with thrombosis of the main portal veins the liver remains histologically normal.

Portal hypertension

Portal hypertension is most often the result of cirrhosis. Other causes include schistosomiasis, alcohol-related liver disease, non-alcoholic steatohepatitis, congenital hepatic fibrosis, the tropical splenomegaly syndrome, hepatic venous outflow obstruction and portal venous thrombosis. The latter probably contributes to portal hypertension in polycythaemia and other haematological diseases.[22] In lymphoproliferative and myeloproliferative disorders, the portal infiltration may be a further pathogenetic factor.[23] The anatomical subdivision of portal hypertension into pre-hepatic, intrahepatic and post-hepatic forms should be considered in conjunction with specific structural alterations in classifying the individual case.[24]

There remains a somewhat ill-defined group of patients with portal hypertension not attributable to cirrhosis or to the other causes mentioned above

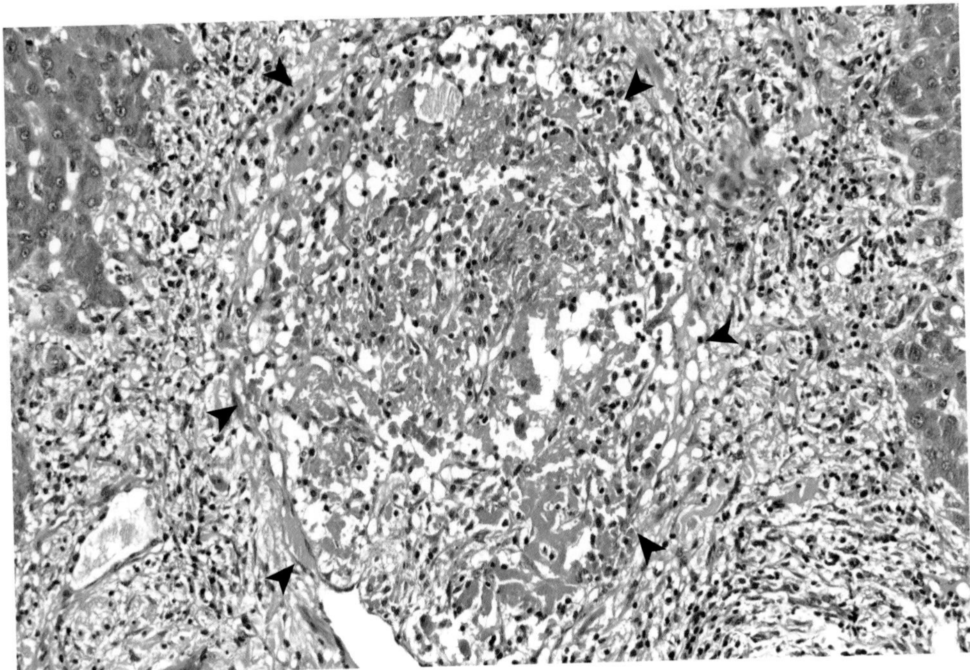

Figure 12.3 *Pylephlebitis*. Thrombus with inflammatory cells, outlined by arrowheads, fills a portal-vein branch. The surrounding portal tract is also inflamed. (Wedge biopsy, H&E).

(**non-cirrhotic portal hypertension**). In a few cases, the condition is attributable to a toxin or toxins such as arsenic,[25] vinyl chloride[26,27] or cytotoxic drugs,[28] but in the majority no cause can be found. Several different labels have been used to describe aspects of this group (**hepatoportal sclerosis, non-cirrhotic portal fibrosis, idiopathic portal hypertension**). The term **obliterative portal venopathy** indicates that there may be demonstrable thrombosis or narrowing of portal-vein branches, but this is not always the case and it is not clear whether the portal venous narrowing or occlusion is primary or secondary.

Needle liver biopsies from patients with non-cirrhotic portal hypertension are often normal or show only non-specific changes. Abnormalities are more likely to be seen in operative wedge biopsies. Portal-vein branches are sometimes thickened and narrowed, unusually inconspicuous or replaced by multiple small, thin-walled channels. Their overall area is reduced, while portal tract lymphatics increase in number.[29] Dilated venules appear to herniate into the adjacent parenchyma[30,31] (Fig. 12.4). There may be portal fibrosis and enlargement, with or without inflammatory-cell infiltration (Fig. 12.5). Slender fibrous septa extending from the portal tracts give an appearance indistinguishable from incomplete septal cirrhosis.[32] These septa sometimes connect with bridge-like zones of necrosis.[30] There may be randomly distributed thin-walled vessels in the lobules ('megasinusoids') and sclerosis or dilatation of efferent veins.[30]

Diffuse or localized nodular hyperplasia of the parenchyma is commonly seen in these patients. There is thus overlap between hepatoportal sclerosis, nodular regenerative hyperplasia, incomplete septal cirrhosis[32,33] and, rarely, partial nodular transformation.[34] Nodular regenerative hyperplasia, however, is also found in the absence of clinically evident portal hypertension.

In patients exposed to vinyl chloride monomer and other carcinogens there may be, in addition to the above features, perisinusoidal fibrosis and an increase in the

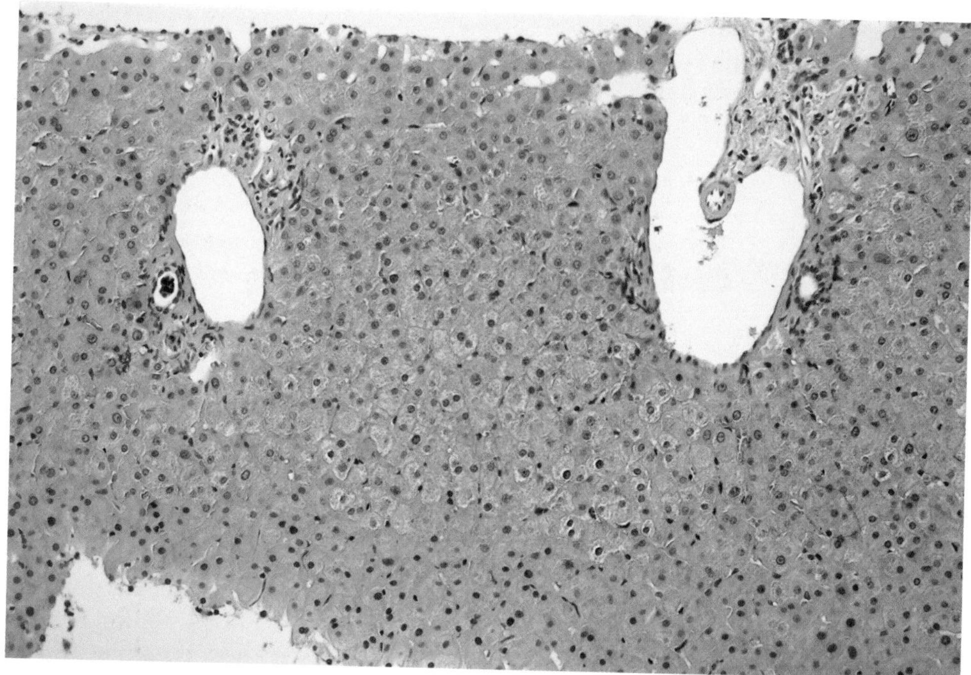

Figure 12.4 *Non-cirrhotic portal hypertension*. The portal-vein branches in the two portal tracts are widely dilated and appear to have herniated into the parenchyma. (Section kindly provided by Professor Helmut Denk). (Needle biopsy, H&E).

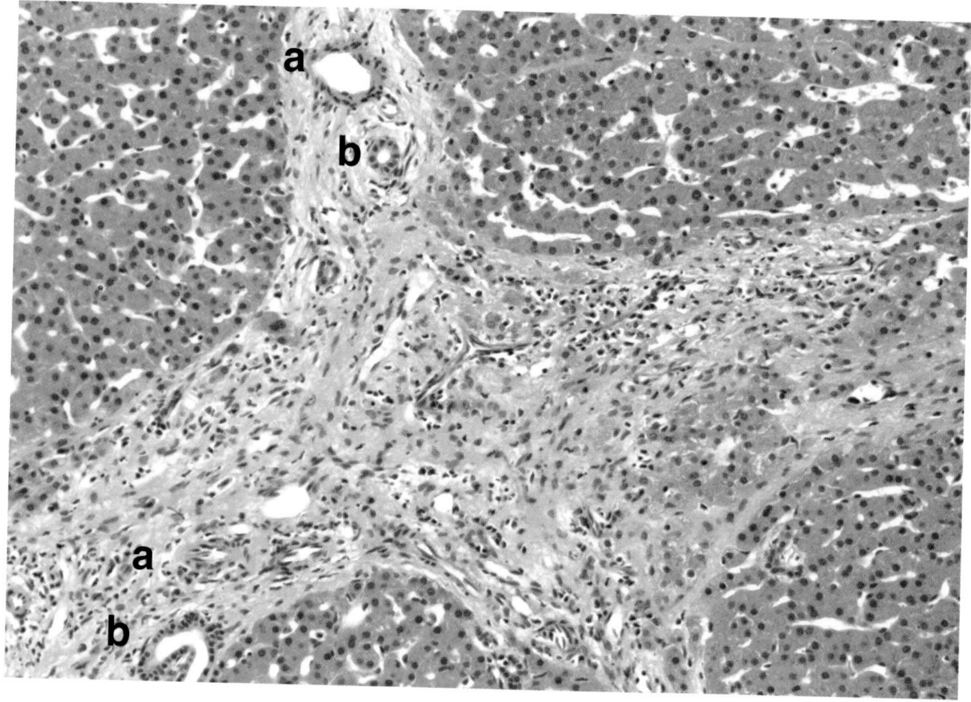

Figure 12.5 *Non-cirrhotic portal hypertension*. An enlarged, sclerotic portal tract contains (a) arteries and (b) bile ducts, but portal vein branches are inconspicuous. (Wedge biopsy, H&E).

number and size of sinusoidal cells.[26,27] Perisinusoidal fibrosis may also contribute to the portal hypertension which develops in some patients after renal transplantation.[35] Prolonged drug therapy has been suggested as a possible mechanism.

THE HEPATIC SINUSOIDS

The width of the sinusoids in liver biopsy specimens is very variable. It is influenced not only by the state of the patient's circulation at the time of biopsy, but also by fixation and tissue processing. Slight variations in width are therefore of doubtful significance.

The amount of connective tissue in sinusoidal walls should also be assessed critically, since its appearance varies with section thickness. A definite increase in fibres is characteristic of chronic venous outflow obstruction and of steatohepatitis. In the former the pattern of fibrosis is usually linear (peri- or parasinusoidal fibrosis), while in steatohepatitis the fibrosis surrounds hepatocytes (pericellular fibrosis). Other causes and associations, some of them already mentioned above, include congenital syphilis, vinyl chloride toxicity, heroin addiction,[36] hypervitaminosis A,[37] diabetes,[38] renal transplantation, myeloid metaplasia[39] and thrombocytopenic purpura.[40] Endothelial cells lining the hepatic sinusoids sometimes contain iron-rich granules of uncertain significance, especially in viral hepatitis[41] and alcoholic liver disease. Immunoglobulin-containing eosinophilic granules have been reported, particularly in chronic hepatitis[42,43] (see Fig. 9.10).

Definite and regular **dilatation** of the sinusoidal network is associated with several conditions, the most important being venous outflow obstruction (see below). It has been reported in patients with tumours or granulomas even when these did not involve the liver,[44] in Crohn's disease,[45] in patients with anti-cardiolipin antibodies and features of the antiphospholipid syndrome,[46] haemophagocytic syndrome[47] and in heroin addicts.[48] Sinusoidal dilatation and congestion in the absence of venous outflow obstruction may also be seen with portal vein thrombosis and congenital absence, rheumatoid arthritis, Still disease and in wedge biopsies taken during abdominal surgery.[49] Dilatation of periportal and mid-zonal sinusoids has been described in a small number of patients taking oral contraceptives[50,51] (Fig. 12.6). In some patients with renal cell carcinoma there is focal dilatation of mid-zonal sinusoids.[52]

Peliosis hepatis

The borderline between regular diffuse dilatation and the focal dilatation known as peliosis hepatis is not always sharp.[52,53] In peliosis, blood-filled cysts are found in the parenchyma (Fig. 12.7), ranging in size from less than one to several millimetres in diameter. The endothelial lining is usually incomplete.[54] Peliosis is found in association with many different conditions and circumstances including wasting diseases, asphyxia,[55] neoplasia,[56] liver and renal transplantation,[57,58] drug therapy[59,60] and bacterial infection.[61] The lesion is often discovered incidentally, but rupture leading to haemoperitoneum has been reported.[61,62] Bacillary peliosis hepatis is a

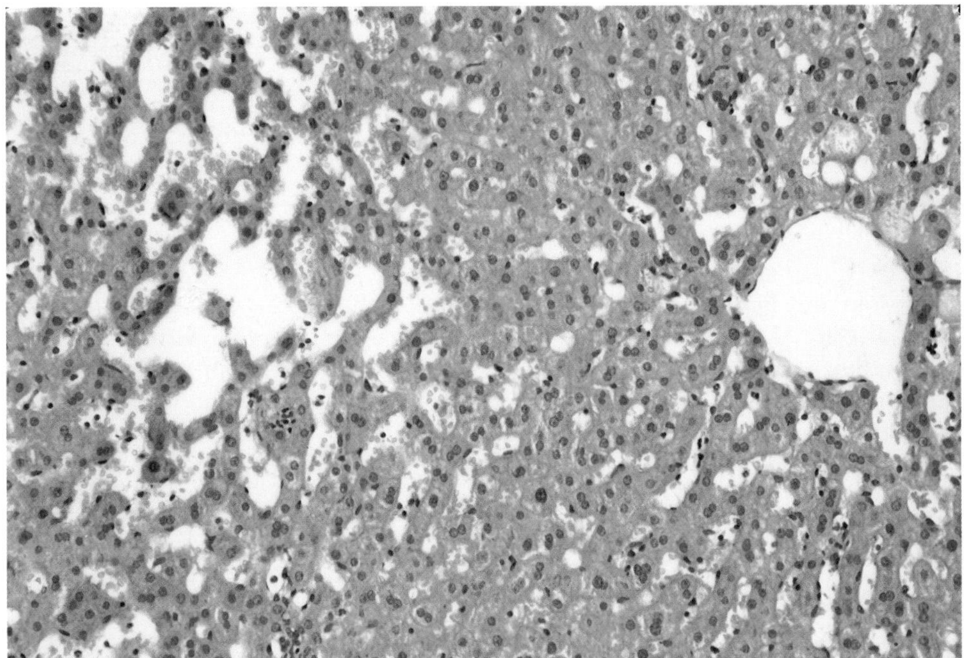

Figure 12.6 *Sinusoidal dilatation.* Dilated periportal and mid-zonal sinusoids are seen to the left and a terminal hepatic venule to the right. The dilatation was attributed to an oral contraceptive steroid. (Section kindly provided by Professor Hemming Poulsen). (Needle biopsy, H&E).

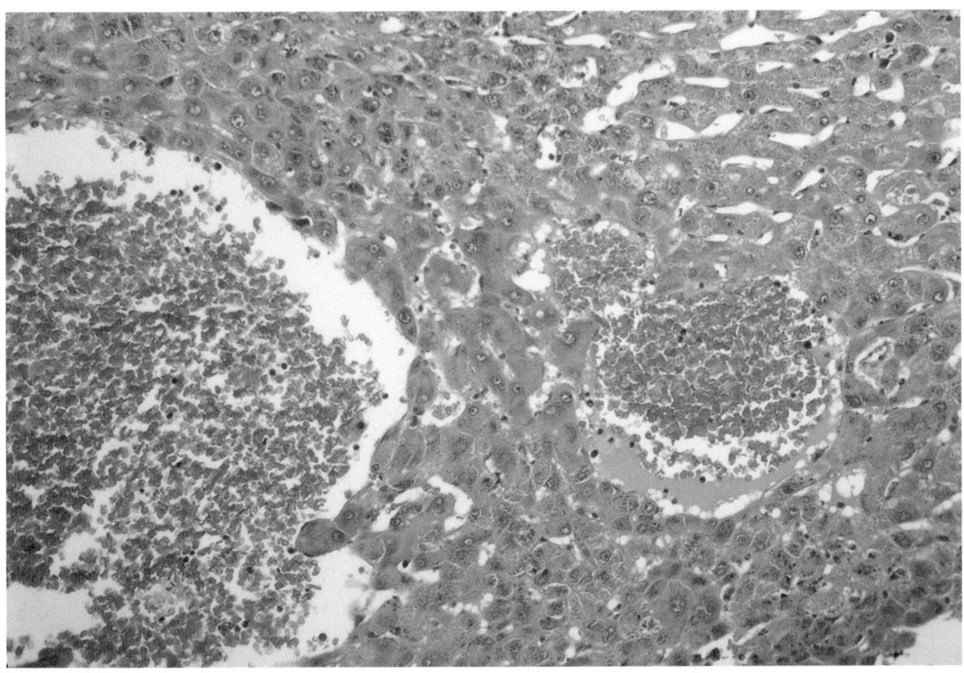

Figure 12.7 *Peliosis.* There are blood-filled spaces within the parenchyma. (Needle biopsy, H&E).

different lesion, and is attributed to the bacteria which cause cutaneous bacillary angiomatosis in patients with AIDS. Their presence in silver preparations distinguishes the condition from simple peliosis.

Disseminated intravascular coagulation

This commonly involves the liver.[63] Sinusoids and small portal vessels contain fibrin thrombi (Fig. 12.8), but the fibrin is often difficult to identify with certainty in conventional sections. Similar changes are seen in eclampsia, in association with periportal necrosis and acute inflammation. In congestive cardiac failure thrombi may form in the sinusoids.[64]

Sickle-cell disease

In most patients with sickle-cell disease clumps of sickled erythrocytes are found in dilated sinusoids[65] (Fig. 12.9). Lesions of peliosis may develop and there is often some degree of perisinusoidal fibrosis. There is erythrophagocytosis, and hypertrophied Kupffer cells and hepatocytes contain iron. Hepatocytes may show atrophy and ischaemic necrosis[66] as well as evidence of regeneration. The degree of sickling seen does not correlate with biochemical or clinical evidence of liver

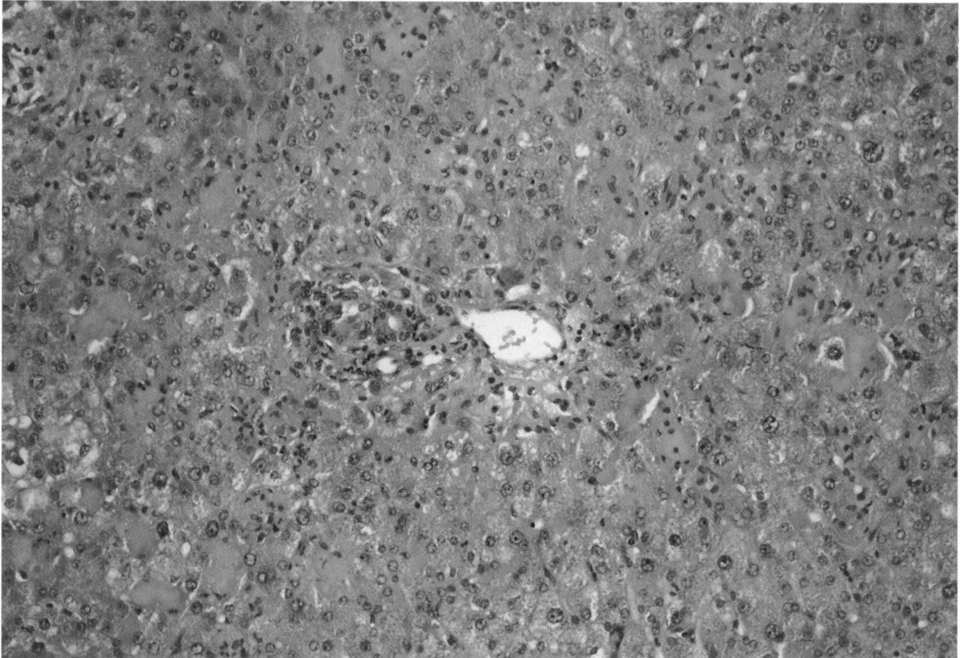

Figure 12.8 *Disseminated intravascular coagulation.* Periportal sinusoids are filled with fibrin and neutrophils. (Needle biopsy, H&E).

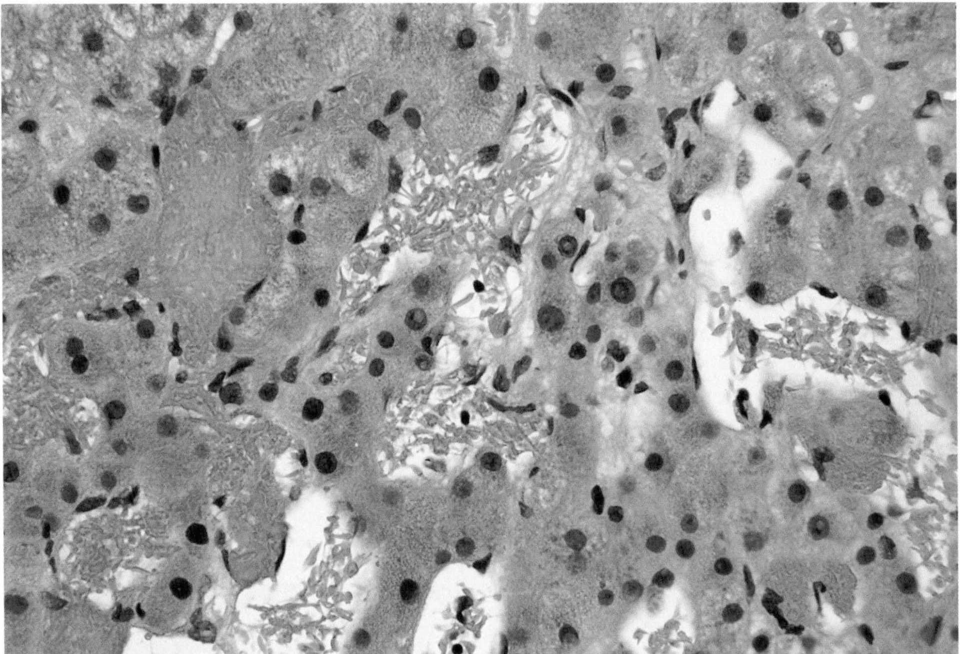

Figure 12.9 *Sickle-cell disease.* Clumped and sickled erythrocytes are seen in distended sinusoids. (Needle biopsy, H&E).

damage, and some hepatic manifestations in patients with sickle-cell disease are thought to be the result of complications such as transfusion-related hepatitis,[67] siderosis, cholelithiasis and venous outflow obstruction. Cirrhosis occasionally develops, possibly as a consequence of viral hepatitis.

VENOUS CONGESTION AND OUTFLOW OBSTRUCTION

Interference with the venous outflow of the liver results from a multitude of causes ranging from congestive cardiac failure to occlusion of the smallest tributaries of the hepatic veins within the liver. Space-occupying lesions such as tumours may cause localized obstruction affecting only parts of the liver. The term **Budd-Chiari syndrome** is often used to describe the clinical findings when the inferior vena cava or main hepatic veins are obstructed, and is sometimes extended to obstruction at the level of the heart. Ludwig and colleagues[68] argue convincingly that classification should be based on the nature and location of the obstruction, and that the label Budd-Chiari syndrome should be used sparingly and only until the cause of the obstruction is known. Indeed, the pathologist faced with a severely congested liver biopsy is often unsure about the level and nature of the block. Use of the term **venous outflow obstruction** is then appropriate.

Congestive cardiac failure

The terminal hepatic venules and adjacent sinusoids show variable combinations of dilatation and congestion in patients with congestive failure.[69] The degree of dilatation or congestion can vary from lobule to lobule in a given tissue section. As already noted, the congestion may be accompanied by hepatocellular necrosis if there is also a significant element of hypoperfusion (Fig. 12.10), as in the combination of right- and left-sided heart failure. Sinusoidal and venous thrombosis may also contribute to hepatocellular damage.[64] Blood may infiltrate the liver-cell plates.[70] Canalicular cholestasis is sometimes seen, and must be distinguished from the commonly found ceroid pigment in Kupffer cells. Inflammation is typically mild or absent, and portal tracts usually remain normal. Periportal necrosis occurs rarely.[69] There may be regenerative hyperplasia of hepatocytes; chronic venous congestion is one cause of nodular regenerative hyperplasia and, very rarely, cirrhosis.[69] Perivenular and perisinusoidal fibrosis ('cardiac sclerosis') reflects prior episodes of failure.[15,69] In some patients, hepatocytes contain PAS-positive globules which probably represent phagosomes containing imbibed plasma proteins.[71] The globules are usually located in or near the congested areas. They can be distinguished from the globules of α_1-antitrypsin deficiency by their location and if necessary by immunochemical staining.

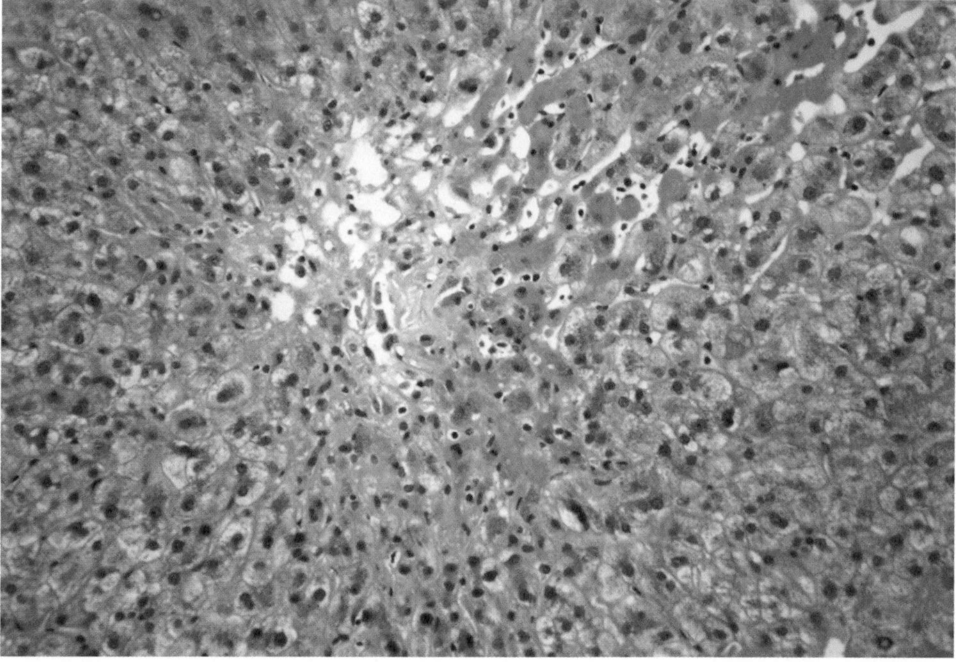

Figure 12.10 *Venous congestion.* Perivenular sinusoids are dilated. The pale zone of necrosis indicates an element of hypoperfusion. Kupffer cells in and around this area are loaded with brown ceroid pigment. (Needle biopsy, H&E).

Obstruction to large veins

Obstruction of the inferior vena cava or the main hepatic veins typically causes severe congestion. The many causes include thrombosis related to myeloproliferative disorders,[72] predisposing coagulopathies[73] and other haematological diseases. Disorders characterized by vasculitis, such as Behçet's disease, may be complicated by either venous outflow obstruction[74,75] or portal vein obstruction.[76] An association of outflow obstruction with the use of oral contraceptives lacks conclusive proof.[77] Fibrous webs may represent a late consequence of thrombosis,[78,79] but there is some evidence to support an alternative, non-thrombotic pathogenesis.[80] Occasionally the obstruction results from administration of anti-tumour drugs[81] or infection.[82] In some patients no cause can be discovered. While in Western countries primary hepatic vein thrombosis is commoner than obliterative disease of the inferior vena cava ('obliterative cavopathy'), the reverse is true in the developing world.[83] Caval obstruction is often complicated by hepatocellular carcinoma.

In the acute stages, much of the parenchyma may be replaced by blood. Sinusoids at the border between the haemorrhagic zones and the surviving parenchyma are dilated and empty (Fig. 12.11). Small efferent veins may be narrowed or blocked, depending on the cause of the obstruction (see discussion of veno-occlusive disease, below). Portal vein branches may also be thrombosed.[84] In acute or chronic venous outflow obstruction it is common to find normal-appearing portal tracts, but there may also be portal features that mimic biliary tract disease, including a ductular reaction, inflammation and portal and/or periportal fibrosis, typically unassociated with cholestasis.[85] Eventually the haemorrhage and congestion lead to fibrosis or even cirrhosis (Fig. 12.12). The pattern of cirrhosis

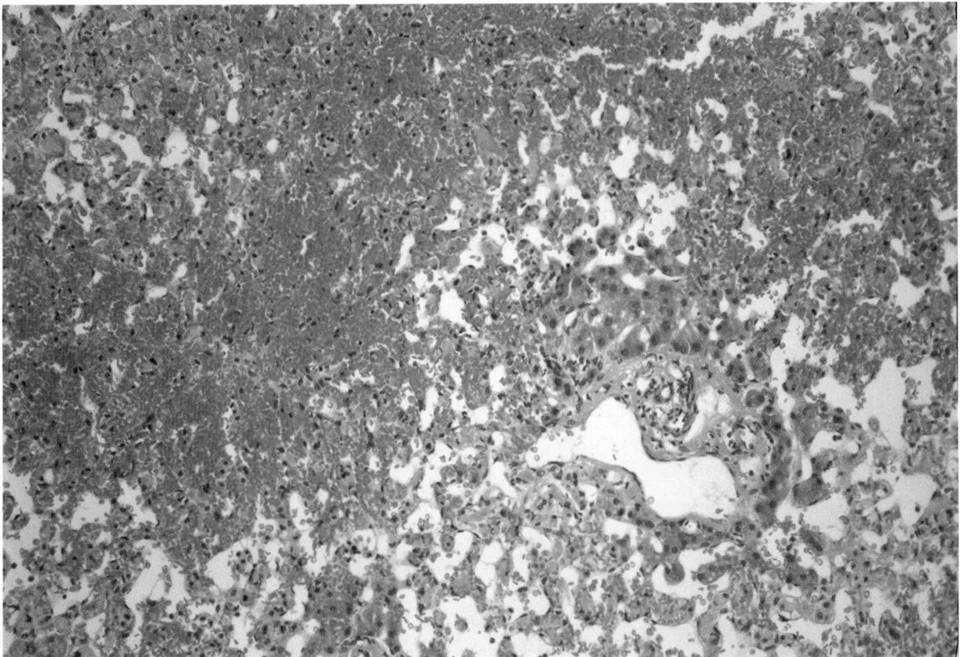

Figure 12.11 *Acute venous outflow obstruction*. In this example, due to obstruction of major veins (Budd-Chiari syndrome), much of the parenchyma has been replaced by blood. A few hepatocytes have survived around the portal tract (below right). (Wedge biopsy, H&E).

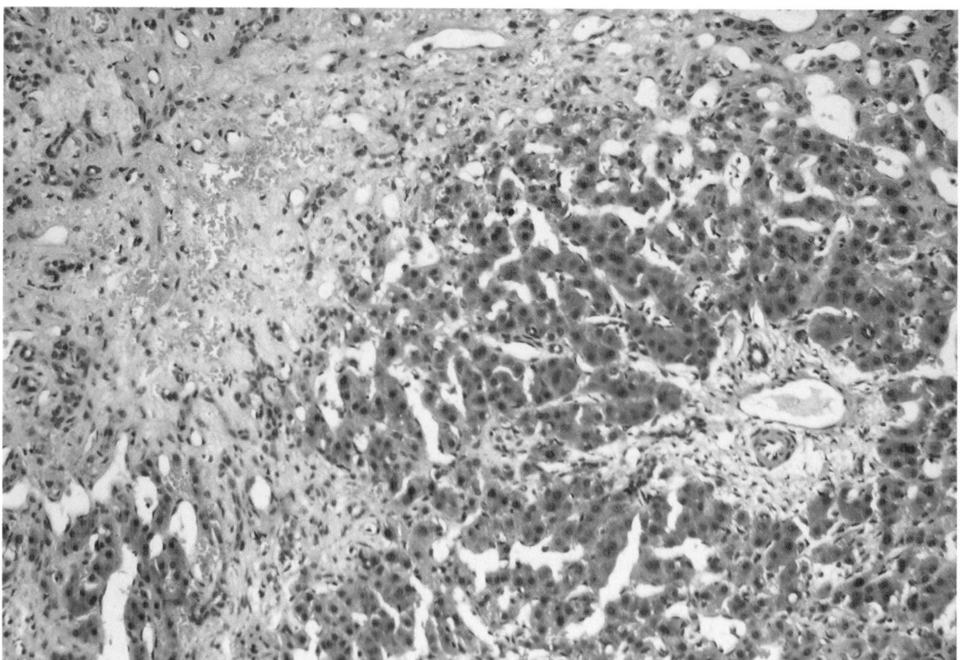

Figure 12.12 *Chronic venous outflow obstruction.* Late in the disease fibrous tissue has been laid down in the congested areas, top left. Surviving parenchyma shows 'reversed lobulation' around a portal tract. (Needle biopsy, H&E).

following venous outflow obstruction is influenced by the presence or absence of concomitant portal venous thrombosis; this is associated with extensive portal-central-portal bridging and with presence of portal tracts within the fibrous septa.[20] In some cases parenchymal nodularity is due to nodular regenerative hyperplasia rather than true cirrhosis, and isolated nodules resembling focal nodular hyperplasia can develop as a result of locally increased arterial blood flow.[84]

Fibrosis is often difficult to distinguish from simple acute condensation of pre-existing reticulin and collagen. Stains for elastic fibres are then sometimes helpful, as in the distinction between bridging necrosis and fibrosis. Two further diagnostic problems should be noted. First, blocked veins may be missed in haematoxylin and eosin-stained sections so that a collagen stain should be examined if venous outflow obstruction is suspected. Thin-walled bypass channels should not be mistaken for patent veins. Second, the obstruction may not affect all the hepatic veins, so that parts of the liver escape serious congestion. As a result, biopsy samples may show considerable regional variability which can lead to diagnostic confusion. It follows that a near-normal liver biopsy does not exclude a diagnosis of venous outflow obstruction.

Veno-occlusive disease (VOD)

In VOD, the smallest tributaries of the hepatic veins, the terminal hepatic venules and sublobular veins, are occluded by fibrous tissue (Fig. 12.13). The venous lesions can thus be detected in needle biopsies. There is often associated fibrosis of

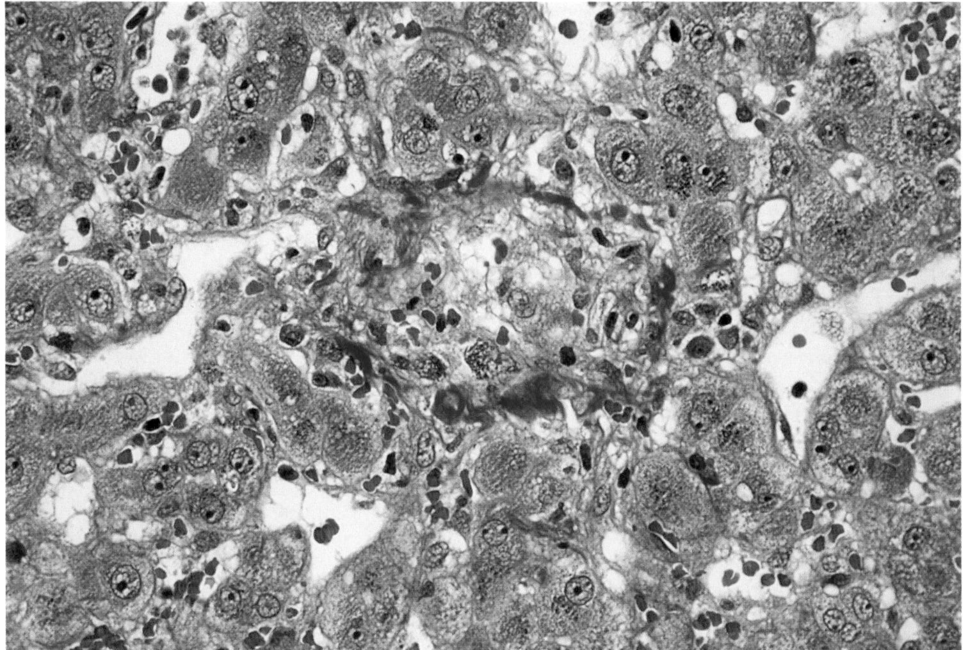

Figure 12.13 *Veno-occlusive disease (VOD).* A terminal hepatic venule has been occluded by recently-formed collagen and cells, following liver transplantation. (Section kindly provided by Professor A P Dhillon). (Needle biopsy, Chromotrope aniline blue).

sinusoidal walls (perisinusoidal fibrosis), probably mediated by hepatic stellate cells.[86] Apart from these lesions, the changes are as for obstruction of large veins. As already noted, the borderline between obstruction to large and small veins is not sharp, since both may be affected by thrombosis, for example in patients with coagulation disorders. Furthermore, thrombosis of large or medium-sized hepatic veins may lead to fibrous intimal thickening of smaller vessels. Rarely, an exuberant form of fibrous obliteration involves veins of all calibres and has been shown to recur after liver transplantation.[87]

As in the case of obstruction to larger veins, there are many causes of VOD. The classical cause, ingestion of pyrrolizidine alkaloids, remains a hazard.[88] Sinusoidal endothelium in general is also susceptible to similar toxic injury, suggesting the term **sinusoidal obstruction syndrome** as an alternative to VOD.[89] Venous occlusion is increasingly seen following bone-marrow, renal or liver transplantation.[86,90–92] Other associations and causes are irradiation of the liver,[93] AIDS,[94] heroin addiction,[36] primary vascular disease,[95] Hodgkin's disease,[96] drug therapy[60,97] and arsenic poisoning.[98] Epithelioid haemangioendothelioma of the liver can mimic VOD because of the characteristic vascular occlusions produced by tumour invasion, and can also give rise to clinical and histological features of the Budd-Chiari syndrome.[99] Finally, careful examination of connective tissue stains may reveal occluded veins in the livers of patients with alcohol-related liver disease[100] and indeed in cirrhosis from any cause.[101]

REFERENCES

1 Valente JF, Alonso MH, Weber FL, et al. Late hepatic artery thrombosis in liver allograft recipients is associated with intrahepatic biliary necrosis. *Transplantation* 1996; **61**: 61–65.

2 Goritsas CP, Repanti M, Papadaki E, et al. Intrahepatic bile duct injury and nodular regenerative hyperplasia of the liver in a patient with polyarteritis nodosa. *J Hepatol* 1997; **26**: 727–730.

3 Viola S, Meyer M, Fabre M, et al. Ischemic necrosis of bile ducts complicating Schönlein-Henoch purpura. *Gastroenterology* 1999; **117**: 211–214.

4 Parangi S, Oz MC, Blume RS, et al. Hepatobiliary complications of polyarteritis nodosa. *Arch Surg* 1991; **126**: 909–912.

5 Matsumoto T, Yoshimine T, Shimouchi K, et al. The liver in systemic lupus erythematosus: pathologic analysis of 52 cases and review of Japanese autopsy registry data. *Hum Pathol* 1992; **23**: 1151–1158.

6 Rousselet M-C, Kettani S, Rohmer V, et al. A case of temporal arteritis with intrahepatic arterial involvement. *Path Res Pr* 1989; **185**: 329–331.

7 Heneghan MA, Feeley KM, DeFaoite N, et al. Granulomatous liver disease and giant-cell arteritis. *Dig Dis Sci* 1998; **43**: 2164–2167.

8 Bayser L De, Roblot P, Ramassamy A, et al. Hepatic fibrin-ring granulomas in giant cell arteritis. *Gastroenterology* 1993; **105**: 272–273.

9 Martini GA. The liver in hereditary haemorrhagic telangiectasia: an inborn error of vascular structure with multiple manifestations: a reappraisal. *Gut* 1978; **19**: 531–537.

10 Wanless IR, Gryfe A. Nodular transformation of the liver in hereditary hemorrhagic telangiectasia. *Arch Pathol Lab Med* 1986; **110**: 331–335.

11 Larson AM. Liver disease in hereditary hemorrhagic telangiectasia. *J Clin Gastroenterol* 2003; **36**: 149–158.

12 Bernard G, Mion F, Henry L, et al. Hepatic involvement in hereditary hemorrhagic telangiectasia: clinical, radiological, and hemodynamic studies of 11 cases. *Gastroenterology* 1993; **105**: 482–487.

13 Saegusa M, Takano Y, Okudaira M. Human hepatic infarction: histopathological and postmortem angiological studies. *Liver* 1993; **13**: 239–245.

14 Monte SM de la, Arcidi JM, Moore GW, et al. Midzonal necrosis as a pattern of hepatocellular injury after shock. *Gastroenterology* 1984; **86**: 627–631.

15 Lefkowitch JH, Mendez L. Morphologic features of hepatic injury in cardiac disease and shock. *J Hepatol* 1986; **2**: 313–327.

16 Sort P, Mas A, Salmeron JM, et al. Recurrent liver involvement in heatstroke. *Liver* 1996; **16**: 334–337.

17 Hassanein T, Perper JA, Tepperman L, et al. Liver failure occurring as a component of exertional heatstroke. *Gastroenterology* 1991; **100**: 1442–1447.

18 Gitlin N, Serio KM. Ischemic hepatitis: widening horizons. *Am J Gastroenterol* 1992; **87**: 831–836.

19 Amitrano L, Guardascione MA, Brancaccio V, et al. Risk factors and clinical presentation of portal vein thrombosis in patients with liver cirrhosis. *J Hepatol* 2004; **40**: 736–741.

20 Tanaka M, Wanless IR. Pathology of the liver in Budd-Chiari syndrome: portal vein thrombosis and the histogenesis of veno-centric cirrhosis, veno-portal cirrhosis, and large regenerative nodules. *Hepatology* 1998; **27**: 488–496.

21 Shimamatsu K, Wanless IR. Role of ischemia in causing apoptosis, atrophy, and nodular hyperplasia in human liver. *Hepatology* 1997; **26**: 343–350.

22 Wanless IR, Peterson P, Das A, et al. Hepatic vascular disease and portal hypertension in polycythemia vera and agnogenic myeloid metaplasia: a clinicopathological study of 145 patients examined at autopsy. *Hepatology* 1990; **12**: 1166–1174.

23 Dubois A, Dauzat M, Pignodel C, et al. Portal hypertension in lymphoproliferative and myeloproliferative disorders: hemodynamic and histological correlations. *Hepatology* 1993; **17**: 246–250.

24 Roskams T, Baptista A, Bianchi L, et al. Histopathology of portal hypertension: a practical guideline. *Histopathology* 2003; **42**: 2–13.

25 Nevens F, Fevery J, Steenbergen W Van, et al. Arsenic and non-cirrhotic portal hypertension. A report of eight cases. *J Hepatol* 1990; **11**: 80–85.

26 Thomas LB, Popper H, Berk PD, et al. Vinyl-chloride-induced liver disease. From idiopathic portal hypertension (Banti's syndrome) to angiosarcomas. *N Engl J Med* 1975; **292**: 17–22.

27 Popper H, Thomas LB, Telles NC, et al. Development of hepatic angiosarcoma in man induced by vinyl chloride, thorotrast, and arsenic. Comparison with cases of unknown etiology. *Am J Pathol* 1978; **92**: 349–369.

28 Shepherd P, Harrison DJ. Idiopathic portal hypertension associated with cytotoxic drugs. *J Clin Pathol* 2004; **43**: 206–210.

29 Oikawa H, Masuda T, Sato S-I, et al. Changes in lymph vessels and portal veins in the portal tract of patients with idiopathic portal hypertension: a morphometric study. *Hepatology* 1998; **27**: 1607–1610.

30 Ludwig J, Hashimoto E, Obata H, et al. Idiopathic portal hypertension: a histopathological study of 26 Japanese cases. *Histopathology* 1993; **22**: 227–234.

31 Ohbu M, Okudaira M, Watanabe K, et al. Histopathological study of intrahepatic aberrant vessels in cases of noncirrhotic portal hypertension. *Hepatology* 1994; **20**: 302–308.

32 Nakanuma Y, Hoso M, Sasaki M, et al. Histopathology of the liver in non-cirrhotic portal hypertension of unknown etiology. *Histopathology* 1996; **28**: 195–204.

33 Bernard P-H, Le Bail B, Cransac M, et al. Progression from idiopathic portal hypertension to incomplete septal cirrhosis with liver failure requiring liver transplantation. *J Hepatol* 2004; **22**: 495–499.

34 Ibarrola C, Colina F. Clinicopathological features of nine cases of non-cirrhotic portal hypertension: current definitions and criteria are inadequate. *Histopathology* 2003; **42**: 251–264.

35 Nataf C, Feldmann G, Lebrec D, et al. Idiopathic portal hypertension (perisinusoidal fibrosis) after renal transplantation. *Gut* 1979; **20**: 531–537.

36 Trigueiro de Araújo MS, Gerard F, Chossegros P et al. Vascular hepatotoxicity related to heroin addiction. *Virchows Arch (A)* 1990; **417**: 497–503.

37 Bioulac-Sage P, Quinton A, Saric J, et al. Chance discovery of hepatic fibrosis in patient with asymptomatic hypervitaminosis A. *Arch Pathol Lab Med* 1988; **112**: 505–509.

38 Latry P, Bioulac-Sage P, Echinard E, et al. Perisinusoidal fibrosis and basement membrane-like material in the livers of diabetic patients. *Hum Pathol* 1987; **18**: 775–780.

39 Degott C, Capron J, Bettan L, et al. Myeloid metaplasia, perisinusoidal fibrosis, and nodular regenerative hyperplasia of the liver. *Liver* 1985; **5**: 276–281.

40 Lafon ME, Bioulac-Sage P, Grimaud JA, et al. Perisinusoidal fibrosis of the liver in patients with thrombocytopenic purpura. *Virchows Arch (A)* 1987; **411**: 553–559.

41 Bardadin KA, Scheuer PJ. Endothelial cell changes in acute hepatitis. A light and electron microscopic study. *J Pathol* 1984; **144**: 213–220.

42 Iwamura S, Enzan H, Saibara T, et al. Appearance of sinusoidal inclusion-containing endothelial cells in liver disease. *Hepatology* 1994; **20**: 604–610.

43 Iwamura S, Enzan H, Saibara T, et al. Hepatic sinusoidal endothelial cells can store and metabolize serum immunoglobulin. *Hepatology* 1995; **22**: 1456–1461.

44 Bruguera M, Aranguibel F, Ros E, et al. Incidence and clinical significance of sinusoidal dilatation in liver biopsies. *Gastroenterology* 1978; **75**: 474–478.

45 Capron JP, Lemay JL, Gontier MF, et al. Hepatic sinusoidal dilatation in Crohn's disease. *Scand J Gastroenterol* 1979; **14**: 987–992.

46 Saadoun D, Cazals-Hatem D, Denninger M-H, et al. Association of idiopathic hepatic sinusoidal dilatation with the immunological features of the antiphospholipid syndrome. *Gut* 2004; **53**: 1516–1519.

47 Kerguenec C de, Hillaire S, Molinié V, et al. Hepatic manifestations of

hemophagocytic syndrome: a study of 30 cases. *Am J Gastroenterol* 2001; **96**: 852–857.
48 Trigueiro de Araújo MS, Gerard F, Chossegros P et al. Lack of hepatocyte involvement in the genesis of the sinusoidal dilatation related to heroin addiction: a morphometric study. *Virchows Arch (A)* 1992; **420**: 149–153.
49 Kakar S, Kamath PS, Burgart LJ. Sinusoidal dilatation and congestion in liver biopsy. Is it always due to venous outflow impairment? *Arch Pathol Lab Med* 2004; **128**: 901–904.
50 Winkler K, Poulsen H. Liver disease with periportal sinusoidal dilatation. A possible complication to contraceptive steroids. *Scand J Gastroenterol* 1975; **10**: 699–704.
51 Winkler K, Christoffersen P. A reappraisal of Poulsen's disease (hepatic zone 1 sinusoidal dilatation). *APMIS* 1991 **(Suppl 23)**: 86–90.
52 Aoyagi T, Mori I, Ueyama Y, et al. Sinusoidal dilatation of the liver as a paraneoplastic manifestation of renal cell carcinoma. *Hum Pathol* 1989; **20**: 1193–1197.
53 Oligny LL, Lough J. Hepatic sinusoidal ectasia. *Hum Pathol* 1992; **23**: 953–956.
54 Wold LE, Ludwig J. Peliosis hepatis: two morphologic variants? *Hum Pathol* 1981; **12**: 388–389.
55 Selby DM, Stocker JT. Focal peliosis hepatis, a sequela of asphyxial death? *Ped Pathol Lab Med* 1995; **15**: 589–596.
56 Fine KD, Solano M, Polter DE, et al. Malignant histiocytosis in a patient presenting with hepatic dysfunction and peliosis hepatis. *Am J Gastroenterol* 1995; **90**: 485–488.
57 Degott C, Rueff B, Kreis H, et al. Peliosis hepatis in recipients of renal transplants. *Gut* 1978; **19**: 748–753.
58 Scheuer PJ, Schachter LA, Mathur S, et al. Peliosis hepatis after liver transplantation. *J Clin Pathol* 1990; **43**: 1036–1037.
59 Soe KL, Soe M, Gluud C. Liver pathology associated with the use of anabolic-androgenic steroids. *Liver* 1992; **12**: 73–79.
60 Modzelewski JRJ, Daeschner C, Joshi VV, et al. Veno-occlusive disease of the liver induced by low-dose cyclophosphamide. *Mod Pathol* 1994; **7**: 967–972.
61 Jacquemin E, Pariente D, Fabre M, et al. Peliosis hepatis with initial presentation as acute hepatic failure and intraperitoneal hemorrhage in children. *J Hepatol* 1999; **30**: 1146–1150.
62 Takiff H, Brems JJ, Pockros PJ, et al. Focal hemorrhagic necrosis of the liver. A rare cause of hemoperitoneum. *Dig Dis Sci* 1992; **37**: 1910–1914.
63 Shimamura K, Oka K, Nakazawa M, et al. Distribution patterns of microthrombi in disseminated intravascular coagulation. *Arch Pathol Lab Med* 1983; **107**: 543–547.
64 Wanless IR, Liu JJ, Butany J. Role of thrombosis in the pathogenesis of congestive hepatic fibrosis (cardiac cirrhosis). *Hepatology* 1995; **21**: 1232–1237.
65 Banerjee S, Owen C, Chopra S. Sickle cell hepatopathy. *Hepatology* 2001; **33**: 1021–1028.
66 Charlotte F, Bachir D, Nénert M, et al. Vascular lesions of the liver in sickle cell disease. A clinicopathological study in 26 living patients. *Arch Pathol Lab Med* 1995; **119**: 46–52.
67 Comer GM, Ozick LA, Sachdev RK, et al. Transfusion-related chronic liver disease in sickle cell anemia. *Am J Gastroenterol* 1991; **86**: 1232–1234.
68 Ludwig J, Hashimoto E, McGill DB, et al. Classification of hepatic venous outflow obstruction: ambiguous terminology of the Budd-Chiari syndrome. *Mayo Clin Proc* 1990; **65**: 51–55.
69 Myers RP, Cerini R, Sayegh R, et al. Cardiac hepatopathy: clinical, hemodynamic, and histologic characteristics and correlations. *Hepatology* 2003; **37**: 393–400.
70 Kanel GC, Ucci AA, Kaplan MM, et al. A distinctive perivenular hepatic lesion associated with heart failure. *Am J Clin Pathol* 1980; **73**: 235–239.
71 Klatt EC, Koss MN, Young TS, et al. Hepatic hyaline globules associated with passive congestion. *Arch Pathol Lab Med* 1988; **112**: 510–513.
72 Boughton BJ. Hepatic and portal vein thrombosis. Closely associated with chronic myeloproliferative disorders. *Br Med J* 1991; **302**: 192–193.
73 Valla D-C. The diagnosis and management of the Budd-Chiari syndrome: consensus and controversies. *Hepatology* 2003; **38**: 793–803.

74 Bismuth E, Hadengue A, Hammel P, et al. Hepatic vein thrombosis in Behçet's disease. *Hepatology* 1990; **11**: 969–974.
75 Bayraktar Y, Balkanci F, Bayraktar M, et al. Budd-Chiari syndrome: a common complication of Behçet's disease. *Am J Gastroenterol* 1997; **92**: 858–862.
76 Bayraktar Y, Balkanci F, Kansu E, et al. Cavernous transformation of the portal vein: a common manifestation of Behçet's syndrome. *Am J Gastroenterol* 1995; **90**: 1476–1479.
77 Maddrey WC. Hepatic vein thrombosis (Budd-Chiari syndrome): possible association with the use of oral contraceptives. *Semin Liver Dis* 1987; **7**: 32–39.
78 Blanshard C, Dodge G, Pasi J, et al. Membranous obstruction of the inferior vena cava in a patient with factor V Leiden: evidence for a post-thrombotic aetiology. *J Hepatol* 1997; **26**: 731–735.
79 Valla D, Hadengue A, el Younsi M, et al. Hepatic venous outflow block caused by short-length hepatic vein stenoses. *Hepatology* 1997; **25**: 814–819.
80 Riemens SC, Haagsma EB, Kok T, et al. Familial occurrence of membranous obstruction of the inferior vena cava: arguments in favor of a congenital etiology. *J Hepatol* 1995; **22**: 404–409.
81 Greenstone MA, Dowd PM, Mikhailidis DP, et al. Hepatic vascular lesions associated with dacarbazine treatment. *Br Med J Clin Res* 1981; **282**: 1744–1745.
82 Vallaeys JH, Praet MM, Roels HJ, et al. The Budd-Chiari syndrome caused by a zygomycete. A new pathogenesis of hepatic vein thrombosis. *Arch Pathol Lab Med* 1989; **113**: 1171–1174.
83 Okuda K, Kage M, Shrestha SM. Proposal of a new nomenclature for Budd-Chiari syndrome: hepatic vein thrombosis versus thrombosis of the inferior vena cava at its hepatic portion. *Hepatology* 1998; **28**: 1191–1198.
84 Cazals-Hatem D, Vilgrain V, Genin P, et al. Arterial and portal circulation and parenchymal changes in Budd-Chiari syndrome: a study in 17 explanted livers. *Hepatology* 2003; **37**: 510–519.
85 Gouysse G, Couvelard A, Frachon S, et al. Relationship between vascular development and vascular differentiation during liver organogenesis in humans. *J Hepatol* 2002; **37**: 730–740.
86 Sato Y, Asada Y, Hara S, et al. Hepatic stellate cells (Ito cells) in veno-occlusive disease of the liver after allogeneic bone marrow transplantation. *Histopathology* 1999; **34**: 66–70.
87 Fiel MI, Schiano TD, Klion FM, et al. Recurring fibro-obliterative venopathy in liver allografts. *Am J Surg Pathol* 1999; **23**: 734–737.
88 Chojkier M. Hepatic sinusoidal-obstruction syndrome: toxicity of pyrrolizidine alkaloids. *J Hepatol* 2003; **39**: 437–446.
89 DeLeve LD, Shulman HM, McDonald GB. Toxic injury to hepatic sinusoids: sinusoidal obstruction syndrome (veno-occlusive disease). *Semin Liver Dis* 2002; **22**: 27–42.
90 Katzka DA, Saul SH, Jorkasky D, et al. Azathioprine and hepatic venoocclusive disease in renal transplant patients. *Gastroenterology* 1986; **90**: 446–454.
91 Shulman HM, Fisher LB, Schoch HG et al. Venoocclusive disease of the liver after marrow transplantation: histological correlates of clinical signs and symptoms. *Hepatology* 1994; **19**: 1171–1180.
92 Dhillon AP, Burroughs AK, Hudson M, et al. Hepatic venular stenosis after orthotopic liver transplantation. *Hepatology* 1994; **19**: 106–111.
93 Lawrence TS, Robertson JM, Anscher MS, et al. Hepatic toxicity resulting from cancer treatment. *Int J Radiat Oncol Biol Phys* 1995; **31**: 1237–1248.
94 Buckley JA, Hutchins GM. Association of hepatic veno-occlusive disease with the acquired immunodeficiency syndrome. *Mod Pathol* 1995; **8**: 398–401.
95 Ito N, Kimura A, Nishikawa M, et al. Veno-occlusive disease of the liver in a patient with allergic granulomatous angiitis. *Am J Gastroenterol* 1988; **83**: 316–319.
96 Lohse AW, Dienes HP, Wolfel T, et al. Veno-occlusive disease of the liver in Hodgkin's disease prior to and resolution following chemotherapy. *J Hepatol* 1995; **22**: 378.
97 Nakhleh RE, Wesen C, Snover DC, et al. Venoocclusive lesions of the central veins and portal vein radicles secondary to intraarterial 5-fluoro-2′-deoxyuridine infusion. *Hum Pathol* 1989; **20**: 1218–1220.
98 Labadie H, Stoessel P, Callard P, et al. Hepatic venoocclusive disease and

perisinusoidal fibrosis secondary to arsenic poisoning. *Gastroenterology* 1990; **99**: 1140–1143.

99 Walsh MM, Hytiroglou P, Thung SN, et al. Epithelioid hemangioendothelioma of the liver mimicking Budd-Chiari syndrome. *Arch Pathol Lab Med* 1998; **122**: 846–848.

100 Burt AD, MacSween RN. Hepatic vein lesions in alcoholic liver disease: retrospective biopsy and necropsy study. *J Clin Pathol* 1986; **39**: 63–67.

101 Nakanuma Y, Ohta G, Doishita K. Quantitation and serial section observations of focal venocclusive lesions of hepatic veins in liver cirrhosis. *Virchows Arch (A)* 1985; **405**: 429–438.

GENERAL READING

Wanless IR. Vascular disorders. In: MacSween RNM, Burt AD, Portmann BC, et al., eds. Pathology of the Liver, 4th edn. Edinburgh: Churchill Livingstone, 2002: 539–574.

Roskams T, Baptista A, Bianchi L, et al. Histopathology of portal hypertension: a practical guideline. *Histopathology* 2003; **42**: 2–13.

Okudaira M, Ohbu M, Okuda K. Idiopathic portal hypertension and its pathology. *Semin Liver Dis* 2002; **22**: 59–72.

Cazals-Hatem D, Vilgrain V, Genin P, et al. Arterial and portal circulation and parenchymal changes in Budd-Chiari syndrome: a study in 17 explanted livers. *Hepatology* 2003; **37**: 510–519.

DeLeve LD, Shulman HM, McDonald GB. Toxic injury to hepatic sinusoids: sinusoidal obstruction syndrome (veno-occlusive disease). *Semin Liver Dis* 2002; **22**: 27–42.

CHAPTER 13

CHILDHOOD LIVER DISEASE AND METABOLIC DISORDERS

INTRODUCTION

Paediatric liver biopsies present a unique set of diagnostic problems for the pathologist, many of which become clinically apparent in the first few months of life as neonatal cholestasis.[1] Among the important disorders one must consider in evaluating neonatal liver biopsies are extrahepatic biliary atresia, paucity of intrahepatic bile ducts (syndromatic and non-syndromatic types), metabolic diseases, viral hepatitis and the hepatic effects of parenteral nutrition (Table 13.1). Common to many of these conditions are the histological features of cholestasis and giant-cell hepatitis (formation of multinucleated hepatocytes). Because these features are not specifically diagnostic of any one neonatal liver disease, the pathologist must be acquainted with other biopsy changes by which to establish or suggest the diagnosis. In many instances, assays of metabolic enzymes and products in serum and liver tissue take diagnostic precedence over routine histopathological interpretation. Electron microscopy may be required to assess the structure of organelles or storage material in hepatocytes or Kupffer cells, particularly when lysosomal storage disorders are being considered. Consultation with investigators dealing with mitochondriopathies,[2] mutations of bile salt transport proteins[3] and expression of proteins involved in blood vessel and bile duct morphogenesis (e.g. Jagged proteins and Notch receptors) should be considered if special studies are

Table 13.1 Liver biopsy interpretation in neonatal cholestasis

Aetiology	Histological features
Extrahepatic biliary atresia	Ductular reaction; ductular cholestasis; portal and periportal fibrosis
Paucity of intrahepatic bile ducts	Loss of interlobular bile ducts (bile duct:hepatic artery ratio <1)
Neonatal hepatitis	Portal and lobular mononuclear cell inflammation; apoptotic bodies
Metabolic disorders	Steatosis; fibrosis or cirrhosis; storage product in liver cells or Kupffer cells (see specific disorder)
Parenteral nutrition	Ductular reaction; portal fibrosis or cirrhosis

Many of the conditions shown in Table 13.1 are associated with histological cholestasis and formation of giant multinucleated hepatocytes, in addition to the diagnostic features listed.

needed to determine the cause of neonatal cholestasis. Childhood liver tumours are discussed in Chapter 11.

DIAGNOSTIC APPROACH TO THE NEONATAL LIVER BIOPSY

Histopathological examination of neonatal liver biopsies may benefit from a systematic checklist of questions by which the major diagnostic concerns in neonatal liver disease can be evaluated. A simplified, stepwise set of seven questions can be asked:

1. *Is the acinar structure normal for age?* As described in Chapter 3, the hepatic plates are two cells thick until 5 or 6 years of age and should not be misconstrued as a pathologic change. As with adult biopsies, the presence of fibrosis, nodularity or cirrhosis should be noted early in the biopsy evaluation and correlated with other histological features, which may define the aetiology.
2. *Are cholestasis and giant cells present?* As indicated above, neither of these is diagnostically specific. If present, the next interpretive steps should be examination of portal tracts for evidence of biliary tract obstruction (atresia, etc.) and of portal tracts and parenchyma for evidence of hepatitis.
3. *Are histological changes of hepatitis present?* Mononuclear cell infiltrates within lobules and portal tracts associated with liver-cell degeneration should be sought when considering cytomegalovirus, Epstein-Barr virus, rubella or hepatitis virus infections.
4. *Are the interlobular bile ducts normal?* This question has three major ramifications. Abundance of bile ducts usually signifies some form of biliary obstruction, such as extrahepatic atresia or choledochal cyst. Paucity of bile ducts (ductopenia, vanishing bile duct syndrome) may be due to developmental, metabolic, or infectious causes. Last, malformations of bile ducts comprise a spectrum of problems related to abnormal remodelling of the embryonic bile duct plate (fibropolycystic diseases).
5. *Does the biopsy specimen contain iron or copper?* Although rare, neonatal haemochromatosis[4] and Indian childhood cirrhosis (copper toxicosis in young children) are serious liver diseases with high mortality rates that must be excluded. In the older child and adolescent, Wilson's disease (Ch. 14) must not be overlooked. It should be noted, however, that fetal and neonatal liver contains much higher copper levels compared to adults, with an irregular tissue distribution.[5] Mild siderosis is also within the spectrum of normal findings in the fetal and neonatal liver.[6]
6. *Has the biopsy specimen been studied by diastase-PAS or immunoperoxidase staining to exclude α_1-antitrypsin deficiency?* The expression of α_1-antitrypsin deficiency is variable, and biopsies may not show diagnostic staining of retained enzyme within liver cells prior to 13 to 15 weeks of age. This condition should be histologically excluded whenever possible.
7. *Are storage cells present?* Abnormal storage products in liver cells or Kupffer cells may be seen in various metabolic diseases which cause hepatomegaly and failure to thrive. These should be sought on routine haematoxylin and eosin as well as special stains.

Inflammation and hepatocellular damage in the neonatal period may result from infections and from inborn errors of metabolism. The former include type B hepatitis, cytomegalovirus infection and rubella among others, the latter α_1-antitrypsin deficiency, galactosaemia and bile acid synthetic defects.[7] Disorders at the ultrastructural or molecular level may also need to be considered, such as neonatal hepatitis due to depletion of mitochondrial DNA.[8] A diagnosis of neonatal hepatitis is therefore a signal for further investigation. The histological picture is broadly similar whatever the cause. There is a variable degree of hepatocellular swelling and multinucleation, cholestasis and portal inflammation. Lobular inflammation may be mild. Liver-cell necrosis and swelling result in collapse and distortion of the reticulin framework (Fig. 13.1). Fibrosis is sometimes already well developed, as in neonatal haemochromatosis (Ch. 14) or the severe perinatal liver disease which may rarely be seen in Down syndrome.[9] Giant multinucleated hepatocytes are commonly seen, whatever the cause of the hepatitis (Fig. 13.2). The outcome of neonatal giant-cell hepatitis is resolution, liver failure, cirrhosis or a chronic cholestatic course. The variety of different outcomes is well illustrated in α_1-antitrypsin deficiency.[10]

From a histological point of view, the main differential diagnosis of neonatal hepatitis is extrahepatic biliary obstruction, which may require surgical treatment. Giant multinucleated hepatocytes and an altered reticulin structure are more prominent in hepatitis than in biliary obstruction while cholestasis is usually more severe in atresia and there is typically a ductular reaction.

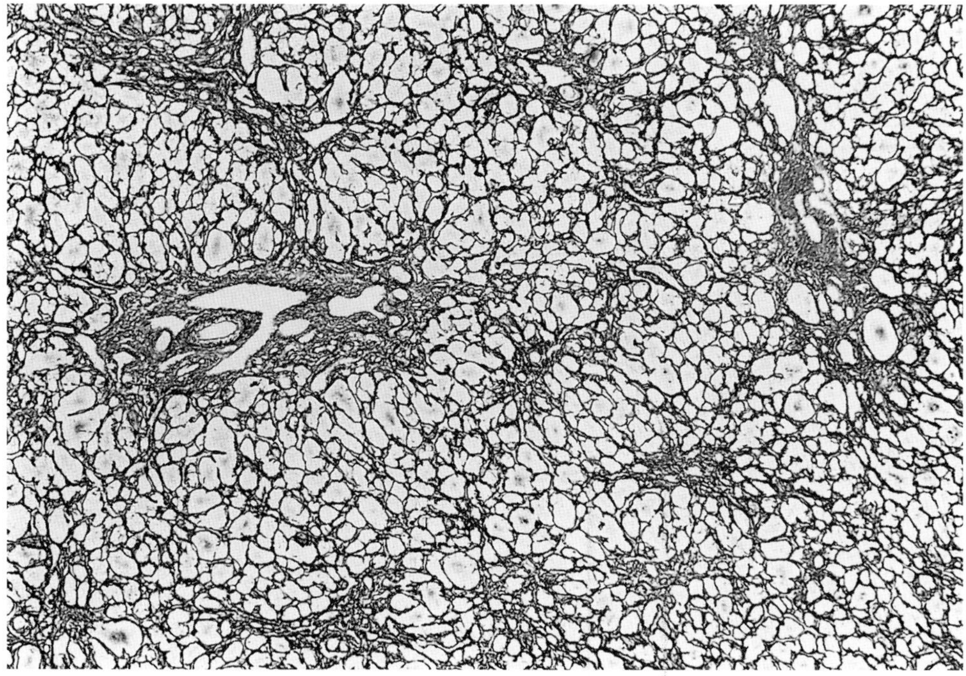

Figure 13.1 *Neonatal (giant-cell) hepatitis*. Fibrosis extends from portal tracts into the lobules and architecture is distorted. (Wedge biopsy, reticulin).

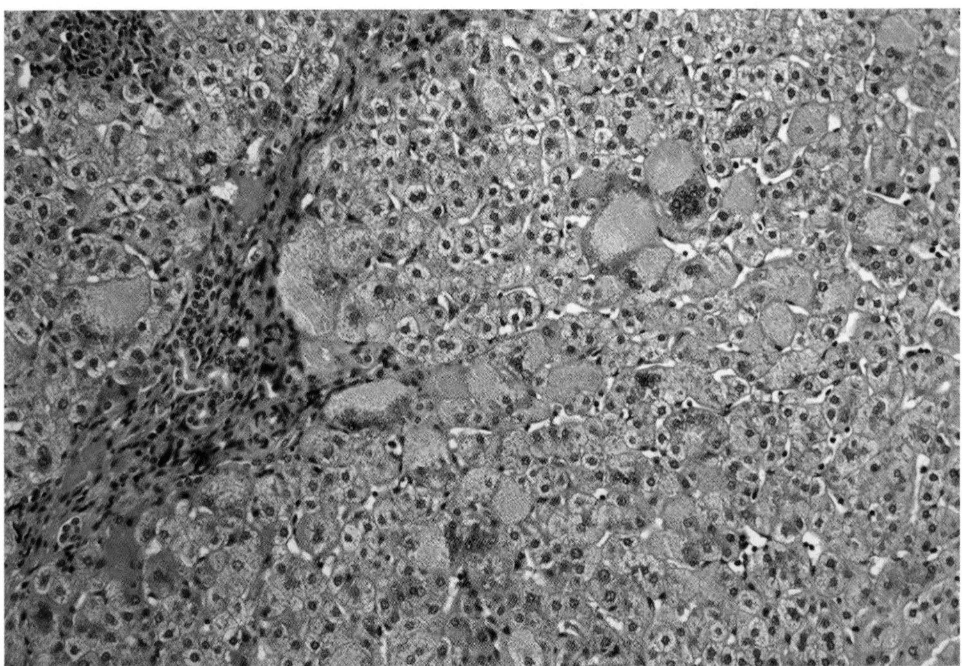

Figure 13.2 *Neonatal (giant-cell) hepatitis.* The parenchyma consists of multinucleated giant liver cells and the portal tract shown is infiltrated by lymphocytes. (Wedge biopsy, H&E).

EXTRAHEPATIC BILIARY ATRESIA

This condition results from inflammation and destruction of all or part of the extrahepatic bile duct system *in utero* or in the perinatal period.[11] Pathologic studies of atretic bile duct segments[12–14] show chronic inflammation and obliterative fibrosis, sometimes with a few remaining bile-duct cells[15] seen on routine stains or cytokeratin immunostaining. Satisfactory bile drainage and an improved outcome after the Kasai portoenterostomy[16] have sometimes been associated with identification of bile ducts with lumens of 150 μm or greater at the proximal resection margin.[13] Optimal surgical results are obtained if the Kasai procedure (hepatic portoenterostomy) is performed within the first 8 weeks of life.[17] Many patients, nevertheless, later require liver transplantation.[18]

The trigger for the destructive process in extrahepatic atresia is unknown, but considerations have included viral infections (reovirus type 3, rotavirus), exposure to toxins, abnormal remodelling of the embryonic bile duct plate and disorders of Jagged protein-Notch receptor signalling.[11] DNA microarray studies suggest a gene profile of abnormal cell signalling and transcription regulation.[19] There may be associated congenital abnormalities, including polysplenia[20] and intrahepatic biliary cysts[21] in approximately 20% of cases with more severe and earlier disease (the 'embryonic' form of biliary atresia). In contrast, the majority of patients have the 'perinatal' form without such anomalies. Expression of various regulatory genes appears to differentiate the two types.[22] The process of biliary atresia is a dynamic one, which may also involve the intrahepatic bile ducts,[23,24] even after Kasai surgery.[25]

Liver biopsy shows cholestasis and portal tract changes resembling those of large bile-duct obstruction in the adult. Portal tracts are enlarged by oedema, a striking ductular reaction and infiltrating neutrophils with fewer chronic inflammatory cells (Fig. 13.3). Native interlobular bile ducts are usually intact and can be identified near hepatic arterioles. Bile-containing portal macrophages are often also present. Ductular structures may contain inspissated bile ('ductular cholestasis') and occasionally resemble the embryonic bile duct plate described by Jørgensen[26] (Figs 13.4, 13.5). A prominent ductular reaction is the major histological point of distinction from neonatal hepatitis.[27] There is panlobular cholestasis with accentuation in zone 3. Giant cells are common, but not as numerous or as striking as in neonatal hepatitis. The degree of portal fibrosis[28] depends on the duration of the obstruction and the age at diagnosis. The overall lobular architecture remains intact except in patients diagnosed late in the disease who may then show secondary biliary cirrhosis (see Fig. 5.11). The differential diagnosis includes biliary obstruction by a choledochal cyst, chronic injury associated with parenteral nutrition (see Parenteral nutrition) and various inborn errors of metabolism.

PAUCITY OF INTRAHEPATIC BILE DUCTS IN CHILDHOOD

Two varieties of intrahepatic bile duct paucity (formerly called intrahepatic biliary atresia) are recognised in childhood, syndromatic and nonsyndromatic.[29] In syndromatic paucity[30,31] (Alagille's syndrome, arteriohepatic dysplasia), loss of small intrahepatic bile ducts is associated with abnormal facies, vertebral anomalies and various other malformations. The pathogenesis is linked to mutations in the *Jagged*

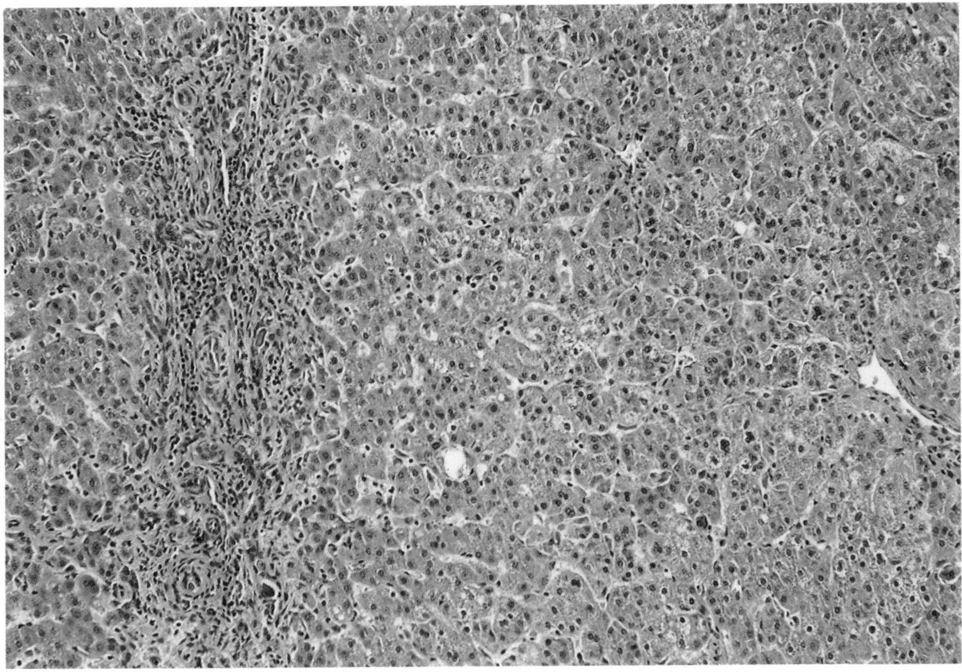

Figure 13.3 *Extrahepatic biliary atresia.* An expanded, inflamed portal tract at left contains many proliferated bile ducts, some of which are filled with inspissated bile. There is also panlobular cholestasis. (Wedge biopsy, H&E).

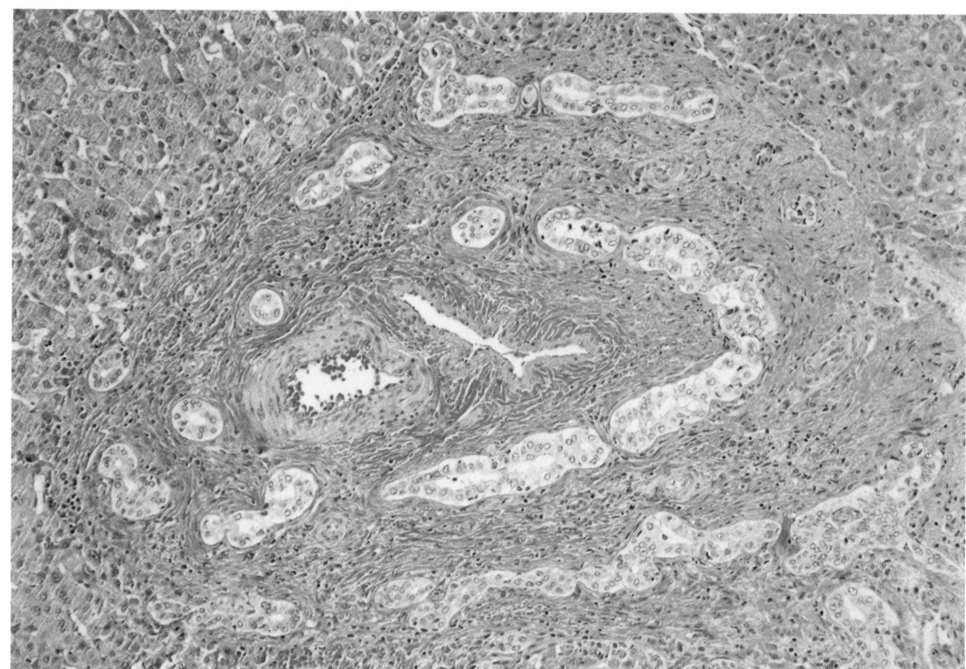

Figure 13.4 *Extrahepatic biliary atresia with bile duct plate-like structures*. The proliferating bile duct structures in this case resemble the embryonic bile duct plate. (Wedge biopsy, H&E).

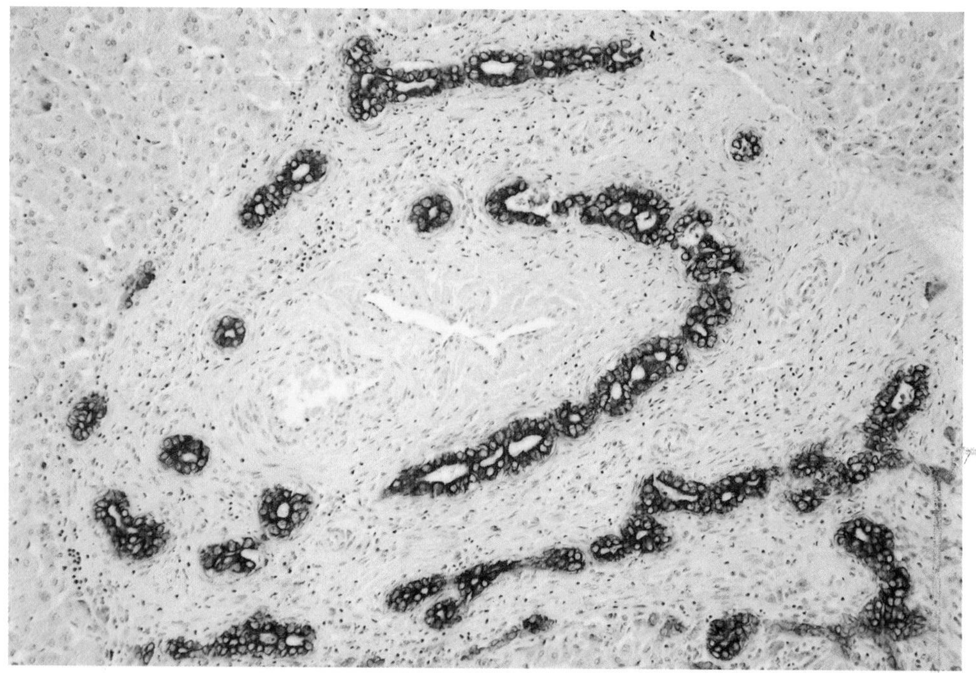

Figure 13.5 *Extrahepatic biliary atresia with bile duct plate-like structures*. The field shown in Figure 13.4 stained with antibodies to cytokeratins highlights the circumferential portal bile duct structures resembling the embryonic bile duct plate. (Wedge biopsy, specific immunoperoxidase).

1 gene, which produce a structurally abnormal ligand for binding to the Notch 1 receptor, which is involved in cell–cell interactions in differentiation and the development of intrahepatic bile ducts.[32] Increased mortality in these patients is linked to the presence of intracardiac congenital heart disease.[33] In non-syndromatic paucity, duct loss is not associated with facial or other anomalies. In some patients, it may be related to a definable cause such as α_1-antitrypsin deficiency or cytomegalovirus infection,[34] while in others there is no detectable aetiological factor. The exact time of onset of bile duct injury is difficult to establish accurately and probably varies from case to case. Some patients have active destruction of ducts in the first few weeks of life[31] and later stabilise, potentially with few symptoms or only mild chronic cholestasis, into young adulthood. In others, cirrhosis and liver failure may develop within months or many years later.[35] It has been speculated that there may be a small subgroup of patients with non-syndromatic paucity in which cholestatic disease first presents in adulthood[35] ('idiopathic adulthood ductopenia').[36]

Histologically, in both forms of intrahepatic duct paucity there is canalicular cholestasis and chronic periportal cholestasis. Portal tracts show a variable degree of fibrosis, and small bile ducts are scanty or absent[37] (Fig. 13.6). Step sections and cytokeratin 7 or 19 immunostaining may be needed for thorough assessment of duct numbers which, as in primary biliary cirrhosis, should approximately correspond to the number of arteries of similar size. A ductular reaction is usually not a prominent feature, in contrast to extrahepatic biliary atresia. Inflammation is often slight or even absent but lymphoid aggregates may be seen in the place of bile ducts (Fig. 13.7). Secondary biliary cirrhosis develops in some patients.[35,38] α_1-Antitrypsin deficiency should be looked for in all patients with paucity of ducts. Duct paucity has also been described in association with Langerhans' cell histiocytosis.[39,40] As primary

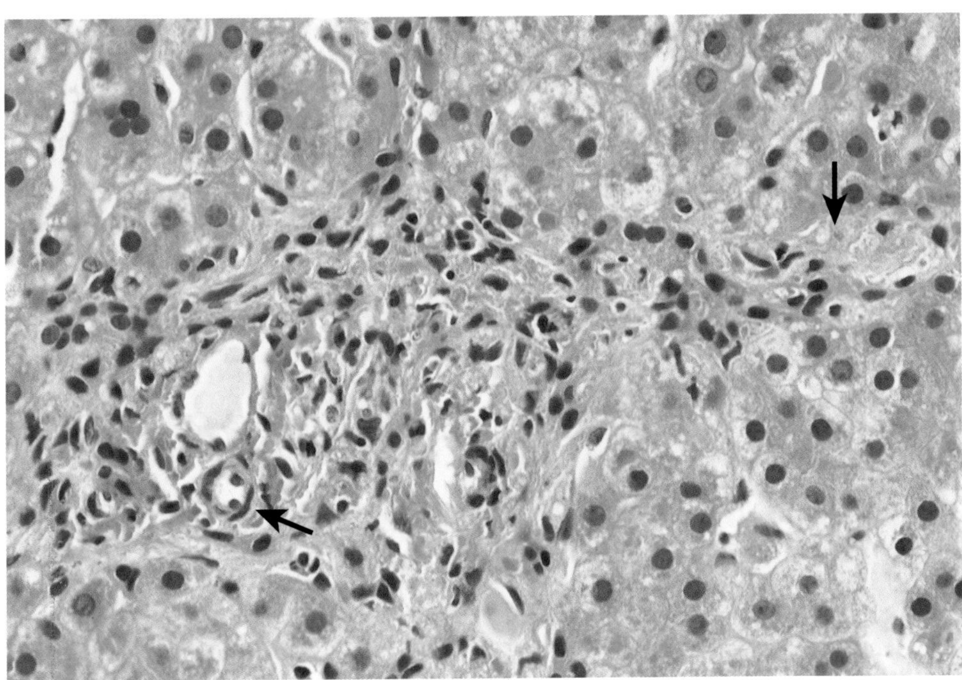

Figure 13.6 *Paucity of bile ducts in childhood.* The portal tract shows an artery (left arrow) but no corresponding bile duct of similar calibre. There is periportal cholestasis (right arrow). (Needle biopsy, H&E).

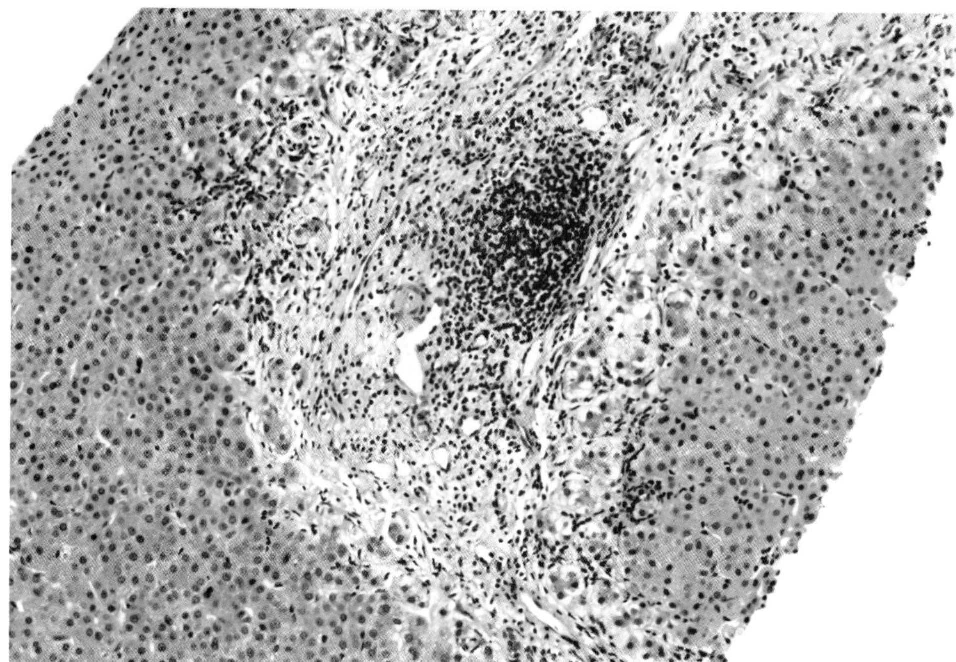

Figure 13.7 *Paucity of bile ducts in childhood.* A lymphoid aggregate is present at the former site of the bile duct. (Needle biopsy, H&E).

sclerosing cholangitis can also present in childhood,[41] it should be considered in the differential diagnosis.

FIBROPOLYCYSTIC DISEASES

This term covers a number of congenital abnormalities involving bile ducts, many of them related to an abnormal remodelling of the embryonic 'bile duct plate'.[42–45] They include congenital hepatic fibrosis, Caroli's disease (congenital dilatation of the intrahepatic bile ducts), microhamartoma (von Meyenburg complex), choledochal cyst and both infantile and adult forms of polycystic disease. The first four of these carry an increased risk of carcinoma of the biliary tree.[46–49] The bile duct plate, first seen at approximately 8 weeks of gestation, is a layer of primitive small cells encircling the portal tract mesenchyme (see Figs 13.4, 13.5). Progressive involution of most of these cells, with acquisition of strong cytokeratin 7 and 19 positivity in those remaining, is the process by which mature interlobular bile ducts of the portal tracts are formed.[43] Persistence of portions of the ductal plate and abnormal remodelling (the 'ductal plate malformation' described by Jørgensen[26]) lead to ectatic and irregularly shaped bile ducts set in dense fibrous stroma, the basic histopathological feature common to all fibropolycystic diseases.

Congenital hepatic fibrosis

This recessively inherited condition presents as hepatomegaly or the effects of portal hypertension, usually in childhood but occasionally in adults.[50] Some cases have been associated with phosphomannose isomerase deficiency in which the resultant hypoglycosylation may affect remodelling of the bile duct plate.[51] The liver is enlarged and very hard. Islands of normal liver parenchyma with unaltered vascular relationships are separated by broad and narrow septa of dense, mature fibrous tissue containing elongated or cystic spaces lined by regular biliary epithelium (Fig. 13.8). These represent cross-sections of the hollow structures comprising the ductal plate malformation. Two separate sets of duct-like structures can often be identified, one lying centrally in the septa, the other near the parenchyma. The lumens may contain inspissated bile. Portal vein branches are small and inconspicuous in some cases. There is usually no cholestasis, necrosis, inflammation or hepatocellular regeneration. In older patients with congenital hepatic fibrosis, the abnormal duct-like structures may be less apparent because of atrophy.

Congenital hepatic fibrosis must be differentiated from cirrhosis, in which there is nodular regeneration and often inflammation and necrosis, and in which the abnormal biliary channels are not seen. The shape of the parenchymal islands in congenital hepatic fibrosis is very similar to that seen in secondary biliary cirrhosis (see Fig. 5.11). In this condition the septa contain irregular, newly proliferated bile ducts rather than congenitally abnormal plates, the connective tissue of the septa is loose and inflamed, and there may be cholestatic features. Histological cholangitis, other types of inflammation or cholestasis in a liver with the characteristic features of congenital hepatic fibrosis should raise the possibility of coexisting Caroli's disease. The combination comprises Caroli's syndrome.

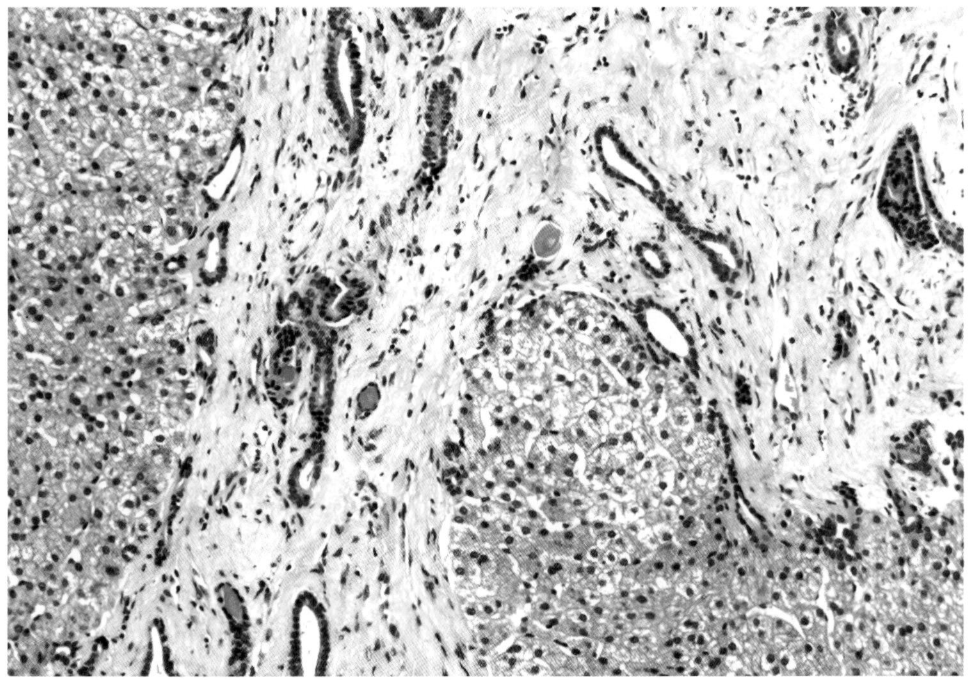

Figure 13.8 *Congenital hepatic fibrosis*. Normal parenchyma is surrounded by fibrous septa containing many epithelium-lined structures of biliary origin. (Needle biopsy, H&E).

Caroli's disease (congenital dilatation of the intrahepatic bile ducts)

This cystic malformation can affect different parts of the intrahepatic biliary tree, and is seen alone or in combination with other congenital abnormalities, notably congenital hepatic fibrosis.[52] Because the cysts communicate with the rest of the biliary tree, there is a risk of ascending bacterial infection. Liver biopsy then shows the changes of cholangitis, with or without associated congenital hepatic fibrosis. The lesion of Caroli's disease must be distinguished from the acquired cholangiectases sometimes found in primary sclerosing cholangitis.[53]

Microhamartoma

Microhamartomas (von Meyenburg complexes) are rounded nodules closely related to portal tracts, containing multiple biliary channels lined by regular epithelium and set in a stroma of dense fibrous tissue (Fig. 13.9). They may be grossly visible on the liver surface as 1 to 2 mm white nodules. The lumens of the biliary structures sometimes contain inspissated bile. Serial sectioning shows that they are interconnected.[54] Microhamartomas are usually found incidentally, and do not normally give rise to symptoms or abnormalities of liver function. They are often multiple, in which case they may very occasionally be associated with portal

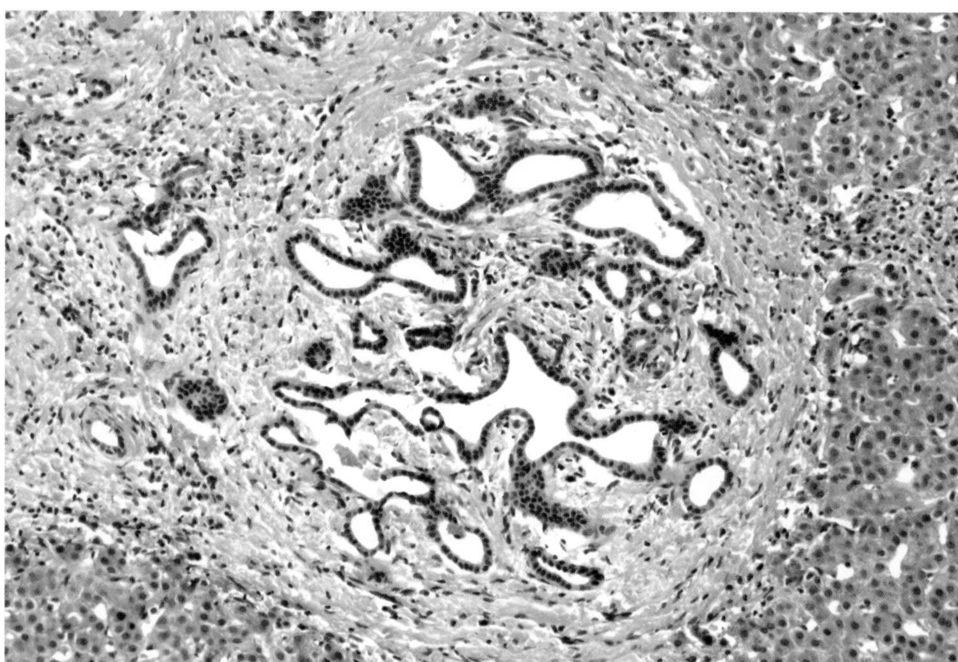

Figure 13.9 *Microhamartoma.* A cluster of duct-like structures is seen in a portal tract. Note resemblance to congenital hepatic fibrosis, shown in Figure 13.8. (Wedge biopsy, H&E).

hypertension; distinction from congenital hepatic fibrosis is then difficult. If a small nodule on the liver surface is seen during surgery, frozen section may occasionally be requested in order to exclude metastatic carcinoma. The irregularly dilated duct structures, inspissated bile and circumscription seen in microhamartomas are helpful in making this distinction.

Polycystic disease

The infantile type of polycystic disease is regularly associated with renal involvement.[43,55] Portal tracts contain multiple cystic channels set in a fibrous stroma. In the adult type the cysts are lined by epithelium of biliary type (Fig. 13.10) but are not connected with the rest of the biliary tree. Solitary congenital cysts are histologically similar. The cuboidal or flattened epithelial lining helps distinguish these cysts from **ciliated hepatic foregut cysts** which are lined by ciliated cells and mucin-secreting goblet cells.[56] The presence of microhamartomas and features of Caroli's disease in individuals with polycystic disease favours a continuum in the expression of fibropolycystic disease.[57–59] The genomic basis of autosomal dominant polycystic liver disease has been elucidated.[59a]

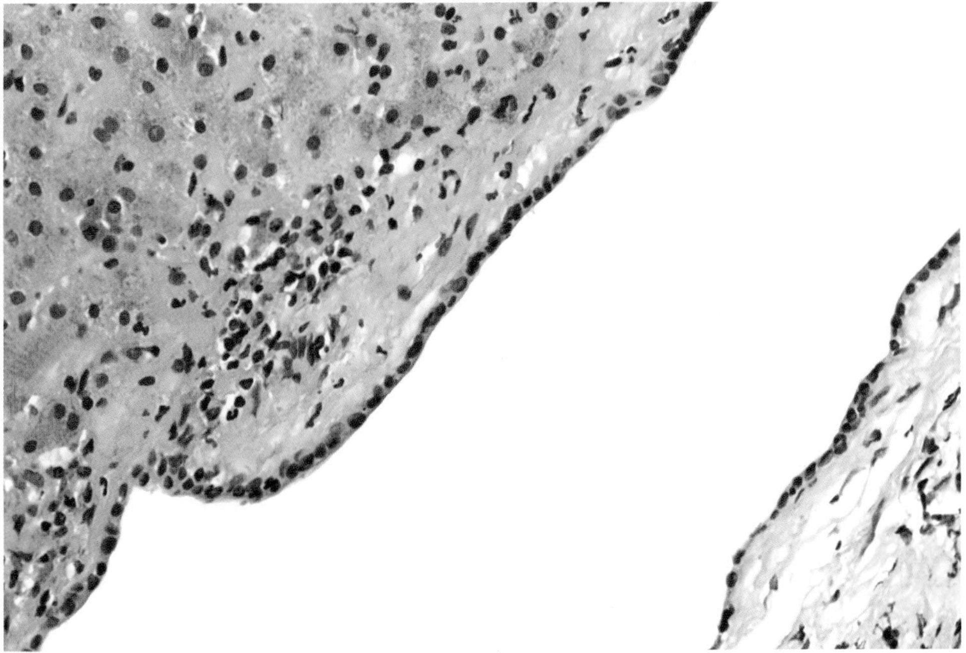

Figure 13.10 *Cystic liver.* A cyst (centre) is lined by a single layer of low cuboidal epithelium. (Wedge biopsy, H&E).

Cystic fibrosis

In this inherited disease in which abnormally viscous exocrine secretions are present in the pancreas, salivary glands, alimentary tract and lungs, the prevalence of liver disease is variable and in part age-dependent.[60–62] Sub-clinical liver disease may be significant.[61] Jaundice in the neonatal period has been attributed to bile-duct obstruction by abnormally viscous bile and to gastrointestinal obstruction by meconium. Intercurrent hepatitis may also be responsible. Steatosis is common, although not always related to malnutrition.[63] Paucity of intrahepatic bile ducts in cystic fibrosis has also been reported.[64] In a proportion of older children, a characteristic lesion of intrahepatic bile ducts is found.[65] Dense plugs of PAS-positive material are seen within dilated, proliferated ducts (Fig. 13.11). Bile-duct cells may undergo degeneration and necrosis.[63] There is surrounding fibrosis[66] and a variable degree of inflammatory infiltration, which may be associated with abnormal intrahepatic ducts on cholangiography.[61] Eventually the fibrous areas may join, separating parenchymal islands. The term **focal biliary fibrosis** expresses the uneven involvement of the intrahepatic bile ducts in this process, with parts of the liver remaining unaffected. In some patients the disease evolves to secondary biliary cirrhosis.[65]

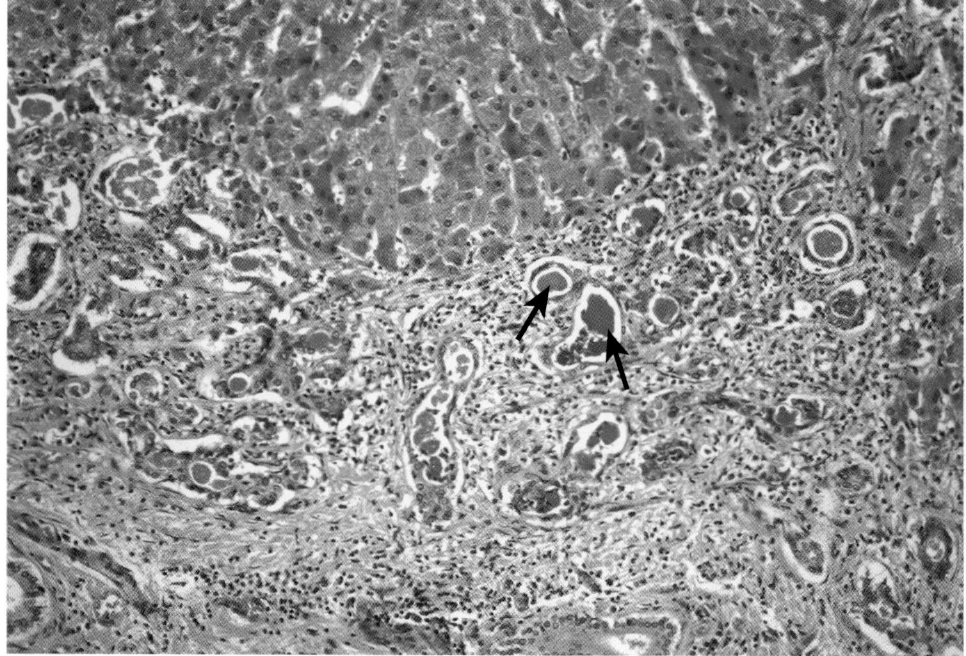

Figure 13.11 *Cystic fibrosis*. Proliferated bile ducts in an enlarged, fibrosed portal tract contain dense inspissated material (arrows). (Post-mortem liver, H&E).

Storage disorders: general remarks

Inherited metabolic defects leading to the abnormal accumulation of lipids, proteins and carbohydrates in the liver are many and varied; for a full description of the morphological changes, recent reviews should be consulted.[67–69] Ishak[67] helpfully discusses the differential diagnosis of individual histological features. Liver biopsy is sometimes useful in diagnosis, though by no means always decisive. The following points are offered as practical suggestions for occasions when biopsy is contemplated in children suspected of having storage disorders.

1. Storage disorders can involve hepatocytes (e.g. glycogenoses, α_1-antitrypsin deficiency), macrophages (e.g. Gaucher's disease), or both (e.g. Niemann-Pick disease, mucopolysaccharidoses,[70] cholesterol ester storage disease). When Kupffer cells are involved, they may swell to the size of hepatocytes and their involvement may not at first be apparent; the use of stains other than haematoxylin and eosin, especially PAS and trichrome stains, then usually makes the Kupffer cell involvement obvious.
2. Suspicion of a possible storage disorder is one of the few indications for electron microscopy of part of the biopsy specimen as a diagnostic procedure, because characteristic ultrastructural appearances sometimes enable a correct diagnosis to be established quickly.[71] Even when the changes are not diagnostic, they can direct attention to a particular group of diseases, and suggest the next line of investigation. Arrangements for electron microscopy should be made beforehand, so that part of the specimen can be put into the correct fixative without delay. In centres without facilities for electron microscopy, part of the specimen should still be correctly fixed and possibly embedded and sent to a referral centre later if light microscopic findings warrant this.
3. Arrangements should also be made to freeze part of the specimen and to store it in liquid nitrogen for possible biochemical analysis and histochemical staining of frozen sections. Speed is essential to avoid loss of enzyme activity. Again, a specialist centre may need to be consulted, because few centres or pathologists have the necessary expertise to investigate the rarer metabolic diseases.

Many inherited metabolic diseases affect the liver and several may lead to cirrhosis[67] (glycogenosis type III, IV and VI, galactosaemia, tyrosinaemia type I, α_1-antitrypsin deficiency, Wilson's disease, hereditary haemochromatosis). Liver transplantation may be indicated in some patients.[18,72,73] The discussion in this chapter will be limited primarily to the disorders mentioned under point 1 above. Haemochromatosis and Wilson's disease are described in Chapter 14.

Glycogen storage diseases (glycogenoses)

Most forms of glycogen storage disease involve the liver.[74] In type I glycogenosis (von Gierke's disease) fat and glycogen accumulate in the cytoplasm of hepatocytes. These appear swollen, pale-staining and sometimes vacuolated with haematoxylin and eosin, and have centrally placed nuclei (Fig. 13.12). Mallory bodies may be found in the cytoplasm.[75] The abundant glycogen displaces the organelles of affected cells to the periphery, giving them a plant cell-like appearance. Some liver-cell nuclei also contain glycogen. Sinusoids are compressed. The overall appearance has been described as a uniform mosaic pattern.[74] Slender periportal fibrous scars often

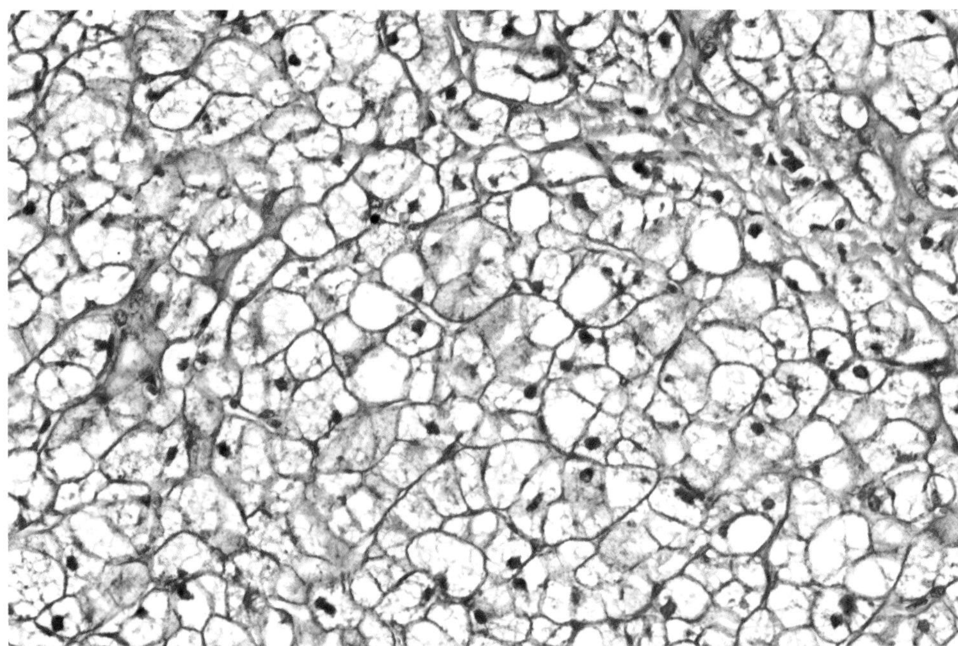

Figure 13.12 *Glycogenosis*. In this example of type I glycogen storage disease, hepatocytes are swollen and resemble plant cells. (Wedge biopsy, H&E).

develop. Liver-cell adenomas[76,77] or even, rarely, carcinomas[78] may develop. Rapid fixation in buffered formal saline usually enables abundant glycogen to be demonstrated in hepatocytes in paraffin sections, but it should be noted that the diagnosis does not rest only on the demonstration of glycogen, which is plentiful in normal liver. Features closely resembling type I glycogenosis can be seen in poorly controlled diabetics in **Mauriac syndrome** (see Ch. 7).

In type II glycogenosis (Pompe's disease), the highly soluble storage material is contained in enlarged lysosomes, visible as vacuoles in hepatocytes and Kupffer cells by light microscopy. Many other tissues are involved. Type III glycogenosis has been subdivided into several biochemical subtypes. Histological appearances are like those of type I, but fat is less abundant and there may be fibrosis or cirrhosis.[79] Type IV (amylopectinosis) is characterised by abnormal glycogen in the form of well-defined cytoplasmic inclusions in hepatocytes.[80] The glycogen is only incompletely removed by diastase digestion. The inclusions have a ground-glass appearance and must be distinguished from hepatitis B virus surface antigen and other similar cytoplasmic inclusions.[81] In other types of glycogenosis there is often much variation in the degree of hepatocellular swelling in different areas, in contrast to the regular distribution of the changes in type I.[74]

α_1-Antitrypsin deficiency

Individuals with decreased levels of the serum protease inhibitor α_1-antitrypsin (α_1-antitrypsin deficiency) may present with liver disease as neonates (neonatal cholestasis), in adolescence or in adulthood, even beyond 60 years of age.[82–84] There are at least 75 different alleles of the α_1-antitrypsin (AAT) gene, two of which determine an individual's phenotype. The most common phenotype, PiMM, is associated with normal serum levels of AAT. Individuals with heterozygous (PiMZ) and homozygous deficiency (PiZZ) have moderately and profoundly reduced serum levels of AAT respectively. The accumulation of characteristic PAS-positive, diastase-resistant globules in the hepatocytes of AAT-deficient individuals (Fig. 13.13) is based on a structural change in the glycoprotein which is encoded by the mutant Z gene.[85] An amino acid substitution (lysine for glutamic acid at position 342) results in abnormal folding and polymerization[85a] of the protein with failure of both its secretion from the endoplasmic reticulum[85] and its subsequent degradation. In this regard AAT deficiency is conceptually similar to Alzheimer's and Parkinson's diseases where inclusions result from conformational disorders of serine proteases ('serpinopathies').[86]

The globules of AAT which accumulate range from less than 1 μm to 10 μm or more in diameter. They are mainly found in periportal hepatocytes, a similar distribution to the much smaller granules of copper-associated protein and haemosiderin, from which they need to be distinguished. In doubtful cases, immunohistochemical staining enables AAT to be identified with certainty (Fig. 13.14). Moreover, immunohistochemical staining is more sensitive than diastase-PAS positivity, and is helpful when diastase-PAS positive globules are scanty or unevenly distributed. Conversely, immunohistochemically positive material is found in some patients without the genetic deficiency, usually with a panlobular or perivenular rather than a periportal distribution[87,88] and particularly in livers with sinusoidal congestion and hypoxia.[89] From a practical point of view, it is wise to regard the presence of diastase-resistant PAS-positive globules in periportal liver cells as evidence for α_1-antitrypsin deficiency until proved otherwise.[90]

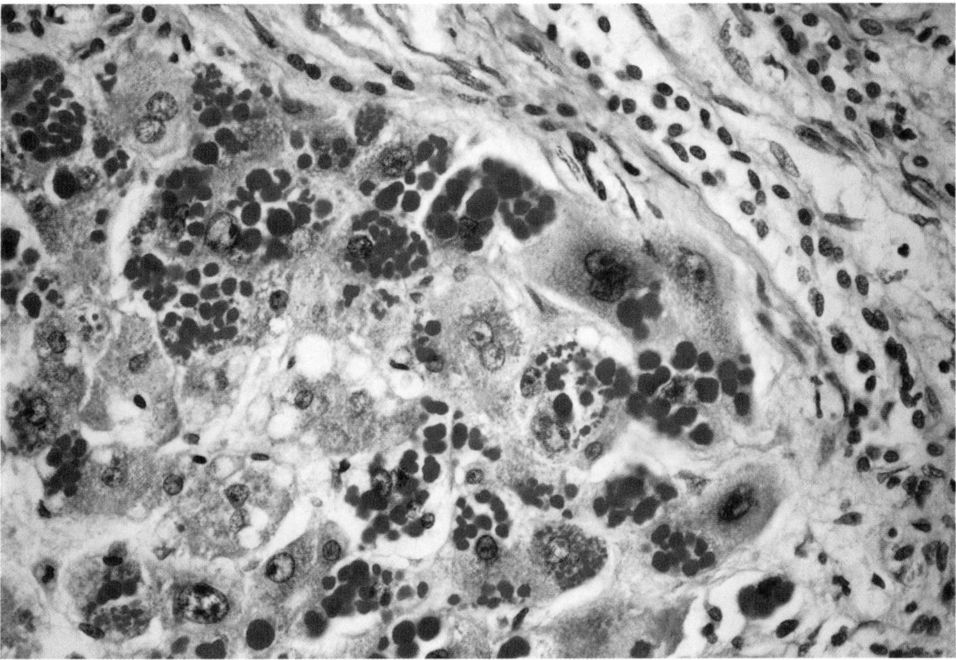

Figure 13.13 α_1-*Antitrypsin deficiency*. Hepatocytes near a fibrous septum contain many magenta globules of different sizes. (Post-mortem liver, diastase-PAS).

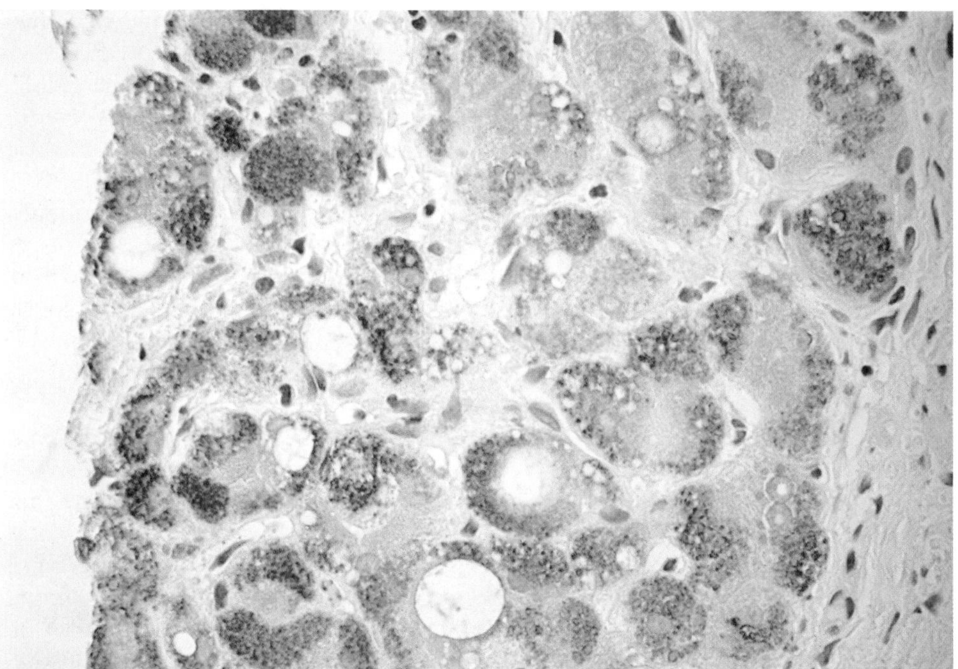

Figure 13.14 α_1-*Antitrypsin deficiency*. Periportal hepatocytes contain numerous globules of α_1-antitrypsin, stained brown by the immunoperoxidase method. Each globule typically is stained around the perimeter, with a central unstained region. (Needle biopsy, specific immunoperoxidase).

Intracellular AAT globules have been vividly demonstrated in a transgenic mouse model of the disease.[91]

Some children with homozygous AAT deficiency develop neonatal cholestasis. Histological changes include a ductular reaction and fibrosis, but the typical globules may not be seen until the age of three or four months.[92] The subsequent course varies; many children improve, while others develop a chronic cholestatic syndrome with paucity of bile ducts or cirrhosis.[10,84,93] Cirrhosis in children with AAT deficiency often has 'biliary' features, such as a ductular reaction and partial preservation of lobular architecture.

Adults carrying two Z alleles present with pulmonary emphysema or liver disease, but may also be symptom-free and healthy. Liver biopsy may show little apart from the PAS-positive globules, or varying degrees of fibrosis. Cirrhosis may have developed, and is either inactive or shows features of chronic hepatitis. An increased prevalence of hepatitis B and C viral infections in AAT deficiency may contribute to this picture.[94] The characteristic globules are found predominantly in periportal or periseptal hepatocytes. They are seen most easily in sections stained with diastase-PAS, phosphotungstic acid haematoxylin or specific immunoperoxidase, but are also seen in trichrome preparations and, when large and abundant, are faintly visible with haematoxylin and eosin. Similar globules are seen in some hepatocellular carcinomas in patients with or without the Z allele.[95,96] Furthermore, an increased risk of hepatocellular carcinoma has been reported in male patients with AAT deficiency.[97] Chronic hepatitis, cirrhosis, large cell liver-cell dysplasia and hepatocellular carcinoma may also be seen in heterozygous (PiMZ) AAT deficiency[98] and in individuals with other allelic variants such as Mmalton.[99–101]

Brief mention should be made of several other endoplasmic reticulum inclusions found in hepatocytes in patients who may have chronic hepatitis or cirrhosis. Diastase-PAS-negative periportal granules of α_1-antichymotrypsin can be identified by specific immunohistochemical staining in **partial α_1-antichymotrypsin deficiency**.[102,103] In **fibrinogen storage disease** there are diastase-PAS-negative intracellular pale inclusions resembling ground-glass hepatocytes.[102]

Gaucher's disease (glycosyl ceramide lipidosis)

Cerebrosides accumulate in Kupffer cells and portal macrophages, which are enlarged, moderately diastase-PAS positive, and have a finely striated appearance (Fig. 13.15). The affected cells compress hepatocytes and sinusoids and may give rise to portal hypertension. Pericellular fibrosis is a common finding.[104]

Niemann-Pick disease (sphingomyelin lipidosis)

There are several variants of this disorder, and the clinical features range from severe and fatal neurological disease in infancy to symptomless hepatosplenomegaly in adults. The typical morphological feature of Niemann-Pick disease is the accumulation of sphingomyelin in both hepatocytes and macrophages. The latter are

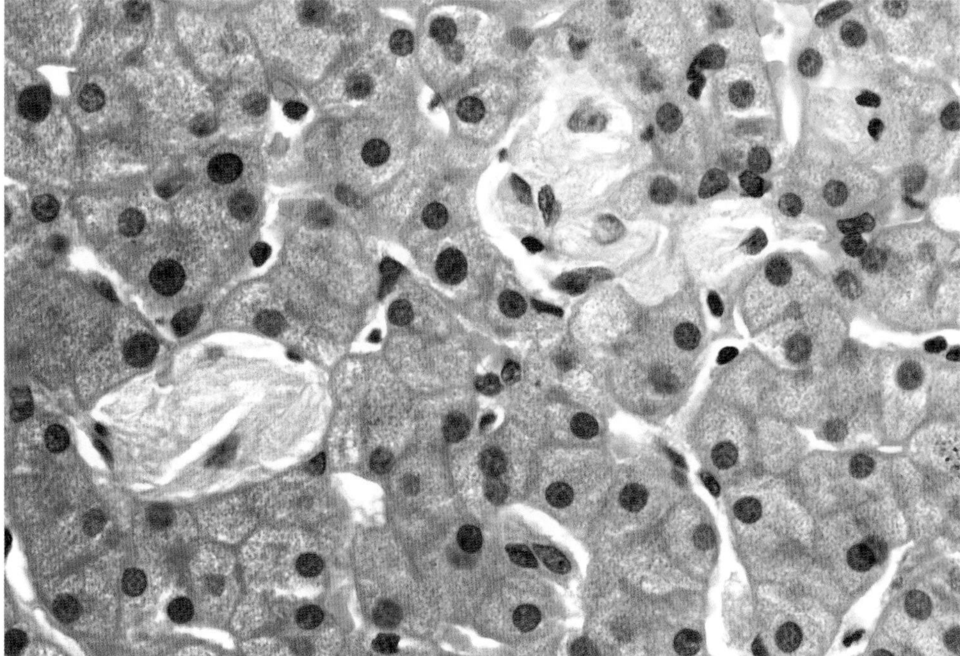

Figure 13.15 *Gaucher's disease.* Pale-staining, striated Kupffer cells containing stored lipid are present within sinusoids. (Wedge biopsy, H&E).

greatly swollen, foamy and diastase-PAS positive to a variable extent. They can readily be distinguished from glycogen-rich liver cells in sections stained by the PAS method (Fig. 13.16). In addition to sphingomyelin, portal phagocytes, especially in the adult form, may also contain a brown lipofuscin-like pigment; these, as well as similar cells in bone marrow, stain a sea-blue colour by the Giemsa method. Niemann-Pick disease is thus one cause of the so-called sea-blue histiocyte syndrome.[105] Type B Niemann-Pick disease may progress to cirrhosis.[73,106]

Wolman's disease and cholesterol ester storage disease

In these apparently related conditions, the first a severe and usually fatal disease of infants, the second a milder disease of older children, cholesterol esters accumulate in hepatocytes and macrophages.[107,108] Hepatocytes also contain much triglyceride. The diagnosis may be suspected from the bright orange colour of the liver biopsy core. By light microscopy hepatocytes appear fat-laden and macrophages are enlarged and foamy. Crystalline deposits may be seen within affected cells, particularly in frozen sections. The excess lipid is birefringent. Other features which may be found include ductular proliferation, pericellular fibrosis and even cirrhosis.[108]

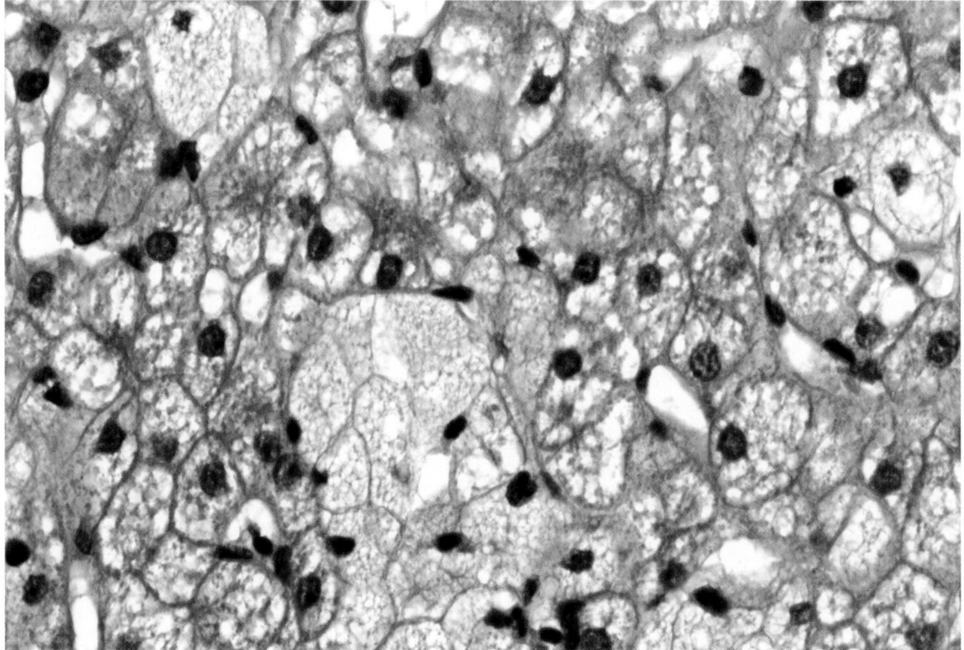

Figure 13.16 *Niemann-Pick disease.* The darker cells are glycogen-rich PAS-positive hepatocytes. Between them are large, pale-staining Kupffer cells (K) filled with lipid. (Wedge biopsy, PAS).

Galactosaemia

Severe fatty change appears early in children with an inherited deficiency of galactose-1-phosphate uridyl transferase. Ductular reaction and cholestasis may also be present. Within a few weeks, liver-cell plates become transformed into tubular, duct-like structures (cholestatic rosettes) which dominate the histological picture, and there is siderosis and extramedullary haemopoiesis. Fibrosis and cirrhosis then develop. Institution of a galactose-free diet may result in substantial histological improvement.[109]

Histologically, the differential diagnosis includes **hereditary fructose intolerance**, in which the changes are somewhat similar but less severe. Also similar but more severe are the histological changes of **tyrosinaemia**. In this condition adenoma-like nodules are often seen, containing much fat.[67,68] Siderosis is also prominent. Hepatocellular carcinoma can develop, particularly in children over the age of 2 years, and liver transplantation is an important therapeutic option to forestall this event.[110]

Disorders of ureagenesis

Deficiencies in enzymes of the urea cycle, including ornithine transcarbamylase (OTC) and carbamyl-phosphate synthase (CPS), may produce fatal hyperammon-aemia in children and rarely in adults.[111] In these disorders, the liver shows microvesicular steatosis which may be accompanied by aggregates of clear hepatocytes (**focal glycogenosis**[112]) (Fig. 13.17). These glycogen-enriched regions stain brightly with PAS and are diagnostically helpful in excluding other causes of paediatric microvesicular fatty liver such as Reye's syndrome (see below).

REYE'S SYNDROME

This is a serious and often fatal condition of encephalopathy and fatty change in the viscera of children under the age of 18. Viral infections (influenza B or A, varicella), salicylate ingestion and endotoxaemia have been implicated in the pathogenesis.[113–115] The incidence of Reye's syndrome declined throughout the 1980s, parallel with a decrease in the use of salicylates for childhood viral illnesses, but it is still seen in some parts of the world. Liver biopsy is an important part of the investigation. The specimen is abnormally pale or yellow on naked-eye examination and on light microscopy there is fine-droplet fatty change. This is panlobular in distribution and may be difficult to see without specific staining for fat because of the small size of the vacuoles. Droplets are smaller at the periphery of lobules than near portal tracts. Necrosis and inflammation are usually slight or absent, but in a few patients there is periportal ballooning or necrosis of hepatocytes.[116,117] Electron microscopy shows characteristic degenerative changes in liver-cell mitochondria; these are swollen and irregular in shape, with flocculent, electron-lucent matrix and reduced numbers of granules.[118] Succinic dehydrogenase activity is reduced. The differential diagnosis includes other conditions with microvesicular fat such as drug

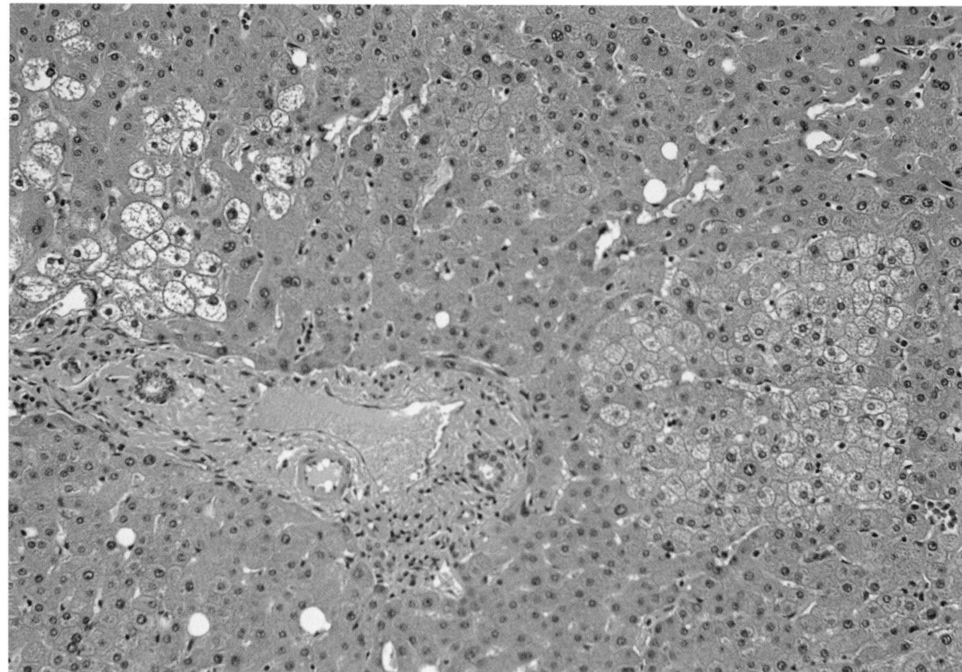

Figure 13.17 *Focal glycogenosis.* Two foci of glycogen-containing hepatocytes with clear cytoplasm are seen near the portal tract. The patient had undergone partial hepatectomy for metastatic adenocarcinoma. In individuals with deficiencies of urea cycle enzymes, this lesion is accompanied by microvesicular steatosis. (Partial hepatectomy, H&E).

hepatotoxicity, urea cycle defects (discussed above) and mitochondrial respiratory chain disorders.[119]

PARENTERAL NUTRITION

The effects of parenteral nutrition have been briefly mentioned in Chapter 8. It is pertinent to note here that in infants, **cholestasis** is the major lesion associated with parenteral nutrition;[120,121] this may occasion diagnostic difficulties when other causes of cholestasis such as sepsis or biliary obstruction are also under clinical consideration. These difficulties are compounded by the fact that with prolonged administration of parenteral nutrition the portal tracts show progressive changes which are very similar to those of bile-duct obstruction (Fig. 13.18). A ductular reaction may be present after 3 weeks of parenteral nutrition,[122] followed by portal fibrosis at 8 to 12 weeks and cirrhosis after 12 weeks.[123] Correlation of biopsy features with detailed clinical information regarding the duration of parenteral nutrition is clearly paramount in establishing the cause of jaundice in this population.

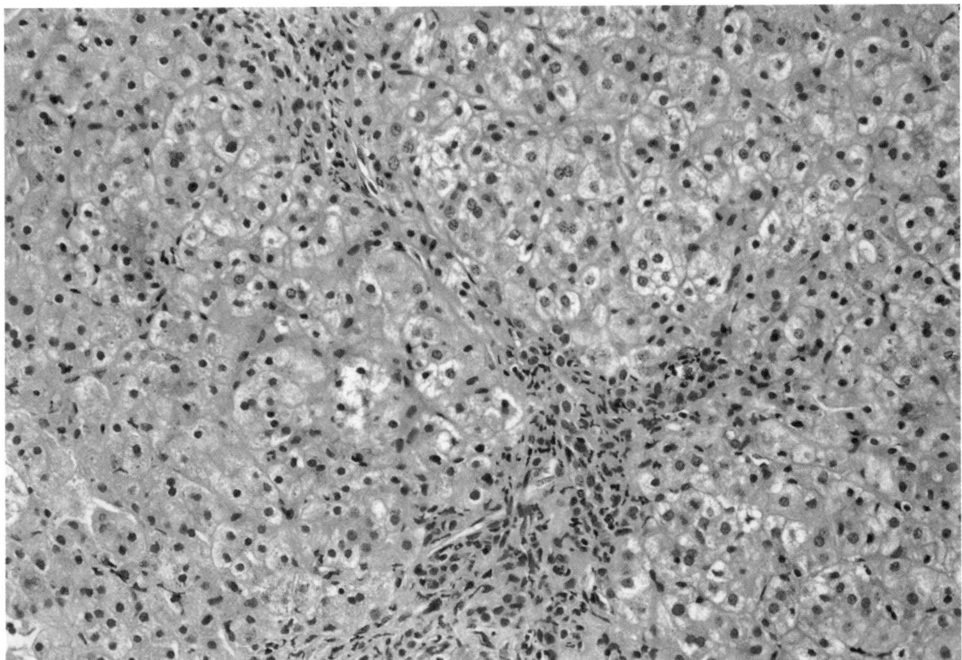

Figure 13.18 *Parenteral nutrition.* An irregular, fibrotic portal tract shows a ductular reaction and a mixed inflammatory cell infiltrate of neutrophilic leucocytes and lymphocytes. Parenchymal bile and cholestatic rosettes are present. (Needle biopsy, H&E).

CHRONIC GRANULOMATOUS DISEASE

Chronic granulomatous disease of childhood is an inherited disorder of leucocytes, which are unable to kill ingested organisms.[68] Patients are therefore susceptible to infections of different kinds. A variety of types of granulomas and microabscesses is found in the liver parenchyma. Pigmented and foamy PAS-positive macrophages are seen in portal tracts and lobular sinusoids.[124] Patients may die in childhood, but the disease is occasionally found in young adults.

HYPERBILIRUBINAEMIAS

In **Gilbert's syndrome,** a common form of familial unconjugated hyperbilirubinaemia,[125] the liver is histologically normal by light microscopy except that small amounts of stainable iron are often seen in hepatocytes. In the **Dubin-Johnson syndrome**, in which the serum bilirubin is mainly conjugated, canalicular excretion of bilirubin and some other organic substances is defective[126] because of a mutation in the gene for canalicular multi-specific-organic-anion transporter.[127] Other constituents of bile are excreted normally and there is no cholestasis. A complex dark brown pigment accumulates in hepatocytes, especially in perivenular areas, giving the liver a dark, speckled appearance to the naked eye. The pigment granules somewhat resemble normal lipofuscin pigment and occupy a similar pericanalicular site in hepatocytes, but are darker, more abundant, larger and more variable in size (Fig. 13.19). When the pigment is very abundant, its pericanalicular location is no longer evident. Simple histochemical characteristics such as PAS-positivity and acid-fastness do not reliably distinguish between Dubin-Johnson pigment and lipofuscin because both stain variably (see Table 3.1), but the distinction is usually clear on the basis of the above morphological features. When there is doubt, this may be resolved by electron microscopy which shows the Dubin-Johnson pigment granules to be composed of characteristic strands of electron-dense material in an electron-lucent background, together with scanty lipid droplets (see Fig. 17.2).

INHERITED CHOLESTATIC SYNDROMES

The cholestatic group of diseases termed **progressive familial intrahepatic cholestasis (PFIC)**, currently subdivided into three types (PFIC-1, -2 and -3), are autosomal recessive disorders in which gene mutations result in defective bile salt transporter proteins on the canalicular membrane.[127–129] Affected infants have jaundice, pruritus and intrahepatic cholestasis which progress to cirrhosis in childhood. The best known of these is **Byler disease** (PFIC-1) which affects kindred of the Amish settler Jacob Byler.[130,131] A clinically similar subgroup of PFIC-1 in non-Amish individuals is designated **Byler syndrome**. PFIC-1 is caused by mutations in *ATP8B1* on chromosome 18q21-22, which encodes FIC1 protein, which is expressed on bile

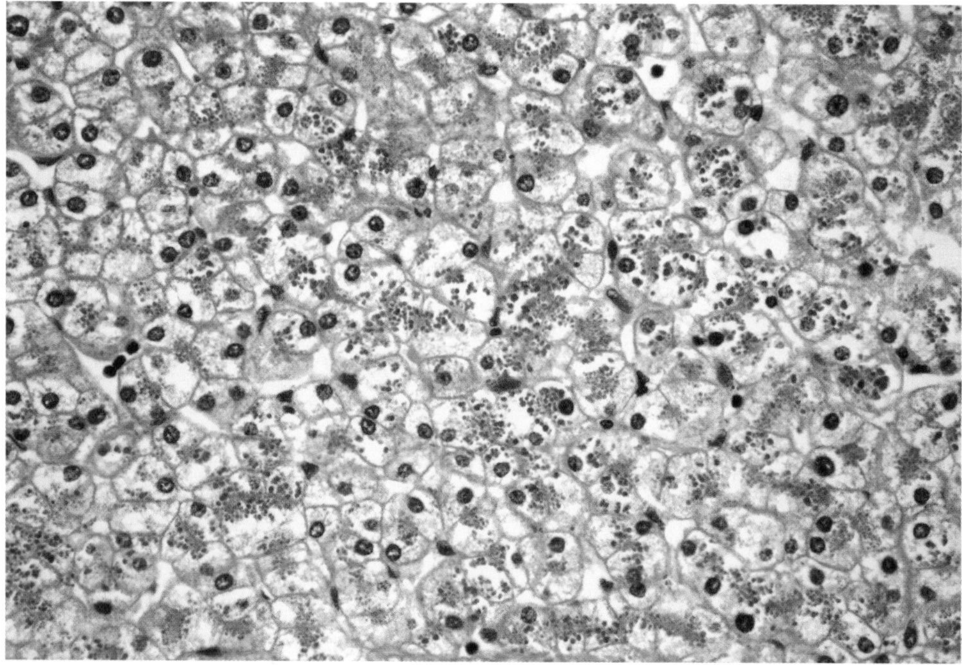

Figure 13.19 *Dubin-Johnson syndrome.* Hepatocytes contain abundant coarse, dark-brown pigment granules. (Needle biopsy, H&E).

canaliculi and intestinal epithelium. The presence of normal to low serum gamma glutamyl transferase (GGT) levels relative to the degree of cholestasis is an important diagnostic feature of Byler disease and syndrome. In both, the liver shows canalicular and sometimes hepatocellular bile plugs (Fig. 13.20). The bland cholestasis of Byler disease, however, contrasts with the features of 'neonatal hepatitis' (giant cells, chronic inflammation) and intrahepatic bile duct paucity seen in Byler syndrome and in PFIC-2 (caused by mutations in *ABCB11* which encodes the bile salt export pump-BSEP). Electron microscopy shows distinctive coarsely granular bile in Byler disease and filamentous or amorphous bile in Byler syndrome[130] (see Fig. 17.10). Portal fibrosis, ductular reaction and cirrhosis eventually develop and hepatocellular carcinoma has also been reported.[132] Many of these patients develop graft steatosis after liver transplantation, possibly because of the continued expression of dysfunctional FIC1 protein on intestinal epithelium.[133]

Two subtypes of **benign recurrent intrahepatic cholestasis (BRIC)** are recognised. Subtype 1 shows a gene mutation mapped to *ATP8B1* on chromosome 18 (as in PFIC-1) and in subtype 2 the *ABCB11* gene (also the target in PFIC-2) is mutated.[134] Affected patients have multiple attacks of jaundice and itching, often starting in childhood or early adult life.[127,128,135] Histologically, canalicular cholestasis is seen in attacks, usually unaccompanied by any substantial degree of inflammation (Fig. 13.21). Between attacks the liver returns to normal and there is no fibrosis or progression to cirrhosis. A clinical continuum between BRIC and PFIC is suggested in some cases.[136]

Additional congenital or familial cholestatic syndromes are described[137] including Norwegian cholestasis, North American Indian cholestasis,[29,131] Navajo neurohepatopathy[2] and recurrent cholestasis in the Faeroe Islands.[138]

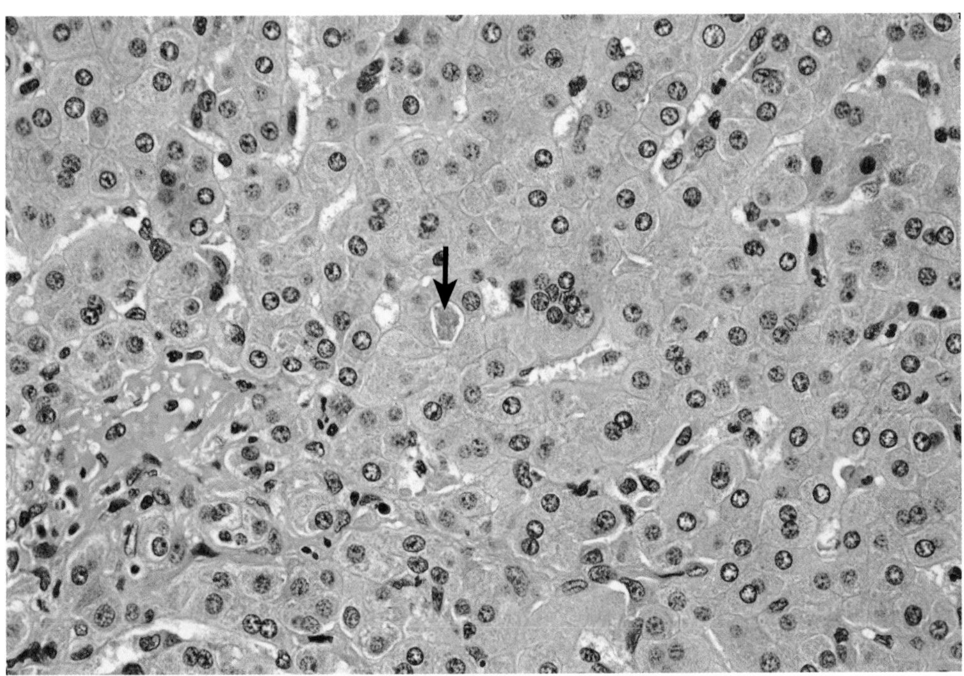

Figure 13.20 *Byler syndrome.* Canalicular bile (arrow) and multinucleated giant hepatocytes are present in this specimen from a non-Amish patient. (Explant liver, H&E).

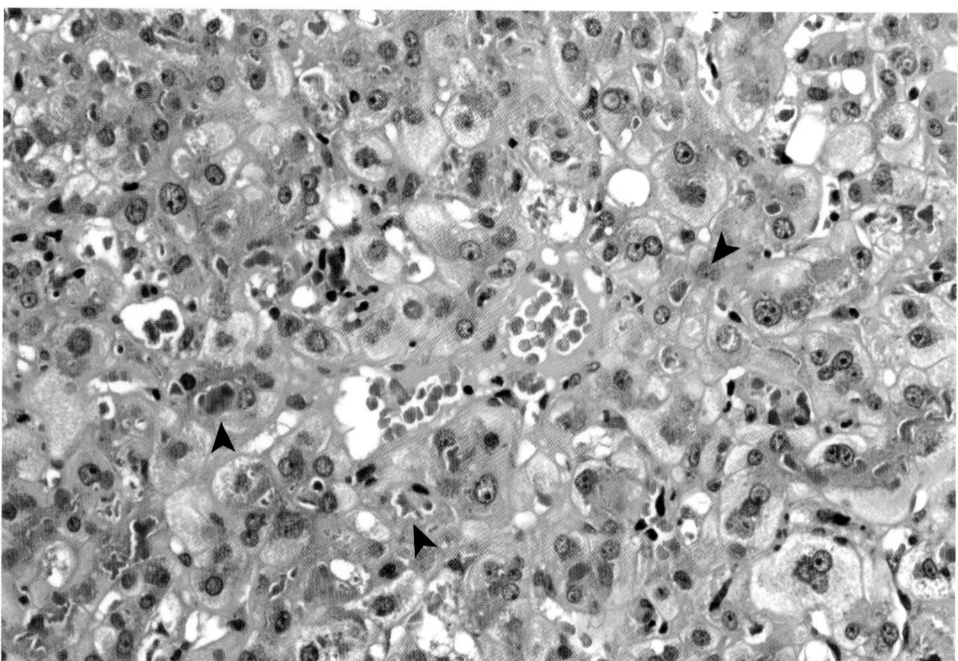

Figure 13.21 *Benign recurrent intrahepatic cholestasis* (*BRIC*). Bile canalicular cholestasis is diffusely prominent (arrowheads). (Needle biopsy, H&E).

CIRRHOSIS IN CHILDHOOD

Children are susceptible to many of the causal agents affecting adults, including hepatitis virus infections. As already noted, several inherited metabolic disorders lead to cirrhosis, and the possibility of Wilson's disease should always be considered in a child with chronic liver disease. Cirrhosis in young women should raise the question of autoimmune hepatitis, either type I (with anti-actin antibodies) or type II (anti-liver-kidney microsomal antibodies)[139] (see Ch. 9). Rare familial forms of cirrhosis have been described.[140] Not infrequently, the aetiology of some forms of childhood cirrhosis is obscure, as for example in the cerebral degenerative disorder Alper's disease[141] in which microvesicular fat is also present. Cryptogenic cirrhosis due to keratin mutations[142] is another consideration (see Ch. 10).

Indian childhood cirrhosis is a disease of young Indian children, with a high mortality and sometimes a familial incidence.[143] Scattered cases outside the Indian subcontinent have been reported.[144–150] Genetic factors and increased dietary copper ingestion through tap water or cooking utensils appear to play an important role in the pathogenesis.[147,151] Hepatocellular swelling in early stages is followed by ballooning, Mallory body formation and necrosis. Focal accumulations of neutrophils and pericellular fibrosis are seen as in alcoholic hepatitis, but there is little or no fatty change (Fig. 13.22). Large amounts of copper and copper-associated protein accumulate in affected hepatocytes.[152,153] In some patients tissue copper decreases after d-penicillamine therapy.[151] The small clusters of damaged hepatocytes surrounded by fibrosis eventually evolve to a cirrhosis characterised by very small nodules ('micro-micronodular cirrhosis').

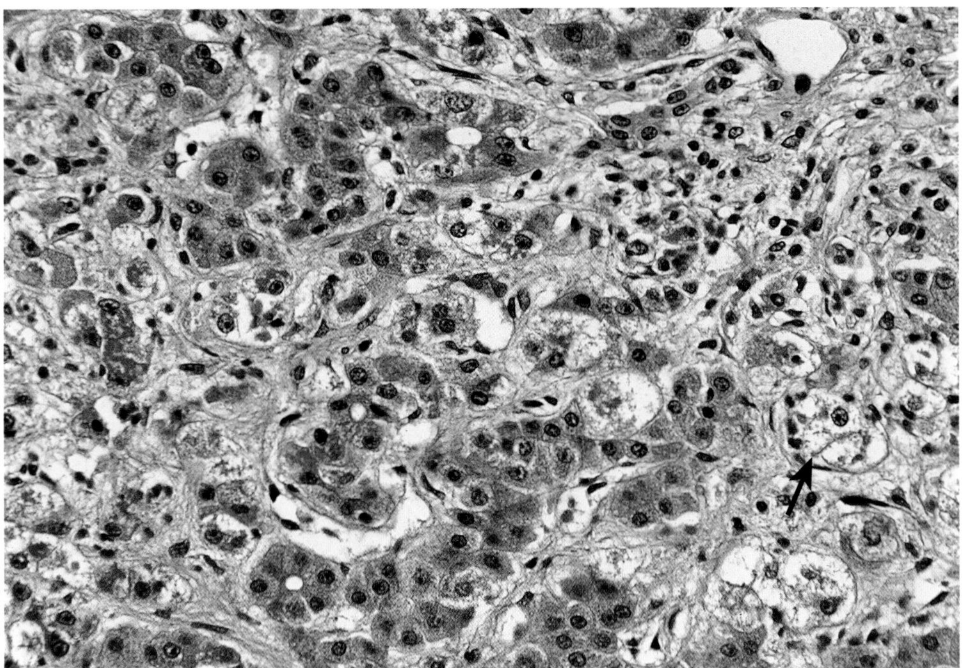

Figure 13.22 *Indian childhood cirrhosis.* Many liver cells are swollen (centre) and surrounded by fibrosis and mononuclear cells. Mallory bodies are present within some hepatocytes (arrow). Regenerating hepatocytes are organised into small clusters. (Post-mortem liver, H&E).

REFERENCES

1 Balistreri WF. Neonatal cholestasis. *J Pediatr* 1985; **106**: 171–184.
2 Vu TH, Tanji K, Holve SA, et al. Navajao neurohepatopathy: a mitochondrial DNA depletion syndrome? *Hepatology* 2001; **34**: 116–120.
3 Jansen PLM, Sturm E. Genetic cholestasis, causes and consequences for hepatobiliary transport. *Liver Int* 2003; **23**: 315–322.
4 Knisely AS, Mieli-Vergani G, Whitington PF. Neonatal hemochromatosis. *Gastroenterol Clin N Amer* 2003; **32**: 877–889.
5 Faa G, Liguori C, Columbano A, et al. Uneven copper distribution in the human newborn liver. *Hepatology* 1987; **7**: 838–842.
6 Faa G, Sciot R, Farci AMG, et al. Iron concentration and distribution in the newborn liver. *Liver* 1994; **14**: 193–199.
7 Bove KE, Daugherty CC, Tyson W, et al. Bile acid synthetic defects and liver disease. *Pediatr Dev Pathol* 2000; **3**: 1–16.
8 Müller-Höcker J, Muntau A, Schäfer S, et al. Depletion of mitochondrial DNA in the liver of an infant with neonatal giant cell hepatitis. *Hum Pathol* 2002; **33**: 247–253.
9 Ruchelli ED, Uri A, Dimmick JE, et al. Severe perinatal liver disease and Down syndrome: an apparent relationship. *Hum Pathol* 1991; **22**: 1274–1280.
10 Hadchouel M, Gautier M. Histopathologic study of the liver in the early cholestatic phase of alpha-1-antitrypsin deficiency. *J Pediatr* 1976; **89**: 211–215.
11 Perlmutter DH, Shepherd RW. Extrahepatic biliary atresia: a disease or a phenotype. *Hepatology* 2002; **35**: 1297–1304.
12 Gautier M, Eliot N. Extrahepatic biliary atresia. Morphological study of 98 biliary remnants. *Arch Pathol Lab Med* 1981; **105**: 397–402.
13 Chandra RS, Altman RP. Ductal remnants in extrahepatic biliary atresia:

a histopathologic study with clinical correlation. *J Pediatr* 1978; **93**: 196–200.

14 Gautier M, Jehan P, Odièvre M. Histologic study of biliary fibrous remnants in 48 cases of extrahepatic biliary atresia: correlation with postoperative bile flow restoration. *J Pediatr* 1976; **89**: 704–709.

15 Haas JE. Bile duct and liver pathology in biliary atresia. *World J Surg* 1978; **2**: 561–569.

16 Kasai M, Suzuki S. A new operation for 'non-correctable' biliary atresia. *Shujitsu* 1959; **13**: 173–179.

17 Logan S, Stanton A. Screening for biliary atresia. *Lancet* 1993; **342**: 256–256.

18 Lykaviens P, Chardot C, Sokhn M, Gauthier F, Valayer J, Bernard O. Outcome in adulthood of biliary atresia: a study of 63 patients who survived for over 20 years with their native liver. *Hepatology* 2005; **41**: 366–371.

19 Chen L, Goryachev A, Sun J, et al. Altered expression of genes involved in hepatic morphogenesis and fibrogenesis are identified by cDNA microarray analysis in biliary atresia. *Hepatology* 2003; **38**: 567–576.

20 Silveira TR, Salzano FM, Howard ER, et al. Congenital structural abnormalities in biliary atresia: evidence for etiopathogenic heterogeneity and therapeutic implications. *Acta Paediatr Scand* 1991; **80**: 1192–1199.

21 Fain JS, Lewin KJ. Intrahepatic biliary cysts in congenital biliary atresia. *Arch Pathol Lab Med* 1989; **113**: 1383–1386.

22 Zhang D-Y, Sabla G, Shivakumar P, et al. Coordinate expression of regulatory genes differentiates embryonic and perinatal forms of biliary atresia. *Hepatology* 2004; **39**: 954–962.

23 Raweily EA, Gibson AAM, Burt AD. Abnormalities of intrahepatic bile ducts in extrahepatic biliary atresia. *Histopathology* 1990; **17**: 521–527.

24 Nietgen GW, Vacanti JP, Perez-Atayde AR. Intrahepatic bile duct loss in biliary atresia despite portoenterostomy: a consequence of ongoing obstruction? *Gastroenterology* 1992; **102**: 2126–2133.

25 Alagille D. Extrahepatic biliary atresia. *Hepatology* 1984; **4**: 7S–10S.

26 Jørgensen MJ. The ductal plate malformation: a study of the intrahepatic bile-duct lesion in infantile polycystic disease and congenital hepatic fibrosis. *Acta Pathol Microbiol Scand* 1977; **257 (Suppl)**: 1–88.

27 Brough AJ, Bernstein J. Conjugated hyperbilirubinemia in early infancy. A reassessment of liver biopsy. *Hum Pathol* 1974; **5**: 507–516.

28 Ramm GA, Nair VG, Bridle KR, et al. Contribution of hepatic parenchymal and nonparenchymal cells to hepatic fibrogenesis in biliary atresia. *Am J Pathol* 1998; **153**: 527–535.

29 Riely CA. Familial intrahepatic cholestatic syndromes. *Semin Liver Dis* 1987; **7**: 119–133.

30 Dahms BB, Petrelli M, Wyllie R, et al. Arteriohepatic dysplasia in infancy and childhood: a longitudinal study of six patients. *Hepatology* 1982; **2**: 350–358.

31 Kahn EI, Daum F, Markowitz J, et al. Arteriohepatic dysplasia. II. Hepatobiliary morphology. *Hepatology* 1983; **3**: 77–84.

32 Nijjar SS, Crosby HA, Wallace L, et al. Notch receptor expression in adult human liver: a possible role in bile duct formation and hepatic neovascularization. *Hepatology* 2001; **34**: 1184–1192.

33 Emerick KM, Rand EB, Goldmuntz E, et al. Features of Alagille syndrome in 92 patients: frequency and relation to prognosis. *Hepatology* 1999; **29**: 822–829.

34 Finegold MJ, Carpenter RJ. Obliterative cholangitis due to cytomegalovirus: a possible precursor of paucity of intrahepatic bile ducts. *Hum Pathol* 1982; **13**: 662–665.

35 Bruguera M, Llach J, Rodés J. Nonsyndromic paucity of intrahepatic bile ducts in infancy and idiopathic ductopenia in adulthood: the same syndrome? *Hepatology* 1992; **15**: 830–834.

36 Ludwig J, Wiesner RH, Russo NF La. Idiopathic adulthood ductopenia: a cause of chronic cholestatic liver disease and biliary cirrhosis. *J Hepatol* 1988; **7**: 193–199.

37 Kahn E, Daum F, Markowitz J, et al. Nonsyndromatic paucity of interlobular bile ducts: light and electron microscopic evaluation of sequential liver biopsies in early childhood. *Hepatology* 1986; **6**: 890–901.

38 Heathcote J, Deodhar KP, Scheuer PJ, et al. Intrahepatic cholestasis in childhood. *N Engl J Med* 1976; **295**: 801–805.
39 Leblanc A, Hadchouel M, Jehan P, et al. Obstructive jaundice in children with histiocytosis X. *Gastroenterology* 1981; **80**: 134–139.
40 Kaplan KJ, Goodman ZD, Ishak KG. Liver involvement in Langerhans' cell histiocytosis: a study of nine cases. *Mod Pathol* 1999; **12**: 370–378.
41 Gregorio GV, Portmann B, Karani J, et al. Autoimmune hepatitis/sclerosing cholangitis overlap syndrome in childhood: a 16-year prospective study. *Hepatology* 2001; **33**: 544–553.
42 Summerfield JA, Nagafuchi Y, Sherlock S, et al. Hepatobiliary fibropolycystic diseases. A clinical and histological review of 51 patients. *J Hepatol* 1986; **2**: 141–156.
43 Desmet VJ. Congenital diseases of intrahepatic bile ducts: variations on the theme 'ductal plate malformation'. *Hepatology* 1992; **16**: 1069–1083.
44 Desmet VJ. What is congenital hepatic fibrosis? *Histopathology* 1992; **20**: 465–477.
45 Desmet VJ. Pathogenesis of ductal plate abnormalities. *Mayo Clin Proc* 1998; **73**: 80–89.
46 Scott J, Shousha S, Thomas HC, et al. Bile duct carcinoma: a late complication of congenital hepatic fibrosis. Case report and review of literature. *Am J Gastroenterol* 1980; **73**: 113–119.
47 Chaudhuri PK, Chaudhuri B, Schuler JJ, et al. Carcinoma associated with congenital cystic dilation of bile ducts. *Arch Surg* 1982; **117**: 1349–1351.
48 Honda N, Cobb C, Lechago J. Bile duct carcinoma associated with multiple von Meyenburg complexes in the liver. *Hum Pathol* 1986; **17**: 1287–1290.
49 Case records of the Massachusetts General Hospital. Case 48-1988. *N Engl J Med* 1988; **319**: 1465–1474.
50 Hodgson HJF, Davies DR, Thompson RPH. Congenital hepatic fibrosis. *J Clin Pathol* 1976; **29**: 11–16.
51 Koning TJ de, Nikkels PGJ, Dorland L, et al. Congenital hepatic fibrosis in 3 siblings with phosphomannose isomerase deficiency. *Virchow's Arch* 2000; **437**: 101–105.
52 Nakanuma Y, Terada T, Ohta G, et al. Caroli's disease in congenital hepatic fibrosis and infantile polycystic disease. *Liver* 1982; **2**: 346–354.
53 Ludwig J, MacCarty RL, LaRusso NF, et al. Intrahepatic cholangiectases and large-duct obliteration in primary sclerosing cholangitis. *Hepatology* 1986; **6**: 560–568.
54 Thommesen N. Biliary hamartomas (von Meyenburg complexes) in liver needle biopsies. *Acta Pathol Microbiol Scand A* 1978; **86**: 93–99.
55 Landing BH, Wells TR, Claireaux AE. Morphometric analysis of liver lesions in cystic diseases of childhood. *Hum Pathol* 1980; **11**: 549–560.
56 Chatelain D, Chailley-Heu B, Terris B, et al. The ciliated hepatic foregut cyst, an unusual bronchiolar foregut malformation: a histological, histochemical, and immunohistochemical study of 7 cases. *Hum Pathol* 2000; **31**: 241–246.
57 Forbes A, Murray-Lyon IM. Cystic disease of the liver and biliary tract. *Gut* 1991; **Suppl**: S116–S122.
58 Terada T, Nakanuma Y. Congenital biliary dilatation in autosomal dominant adult polycystic disease of the liver and kidneys. *Arch Pathol Lab Med* 1988; **112**: 1113–1116.
59 Ramos A, Torres VE, Holley KE, et al. The liver in autosomal dominant polycystic kidney disease. Implications for pathogenesis. *Arch Pathol Lab Med* 1990; **114**: 180–184.
59a Everson GT, Taylor MRG, Doctor RB. Polycystic disease of the liver. *Hepatology* 2004; **40**: 774–782.
60 Scott-Jupp R, Lama M, Tanner MS. Prevalence of liver disease in cystic fibrosis. *Arch Dis Child* 1991; **66**: 698–701.
61 Nagel RA, Westaby D, Javaid A, et al. Liver disease and bileduct abnormalities in adults with cystic fibrosis. *Lancet* 1989; **ii**: 1422–1425.
62 Marino CR, Gorelick FS. Scientific advances in cystic fibrosis. *Gastroenterology* 1992; **103**: 681–693.
63 Lindblad A, Hultcrantz R, Strandvik B. Bile-duct destruction and collagen deposition: a prominent ultrastructural feature of the liver in cystic fibrosis. *Hepatology* 1992; **16**: 372–381.
64 Furuya KN, Roberts EA, Canny GJ, et al. Neonatal hepatitis syndrome with

paucity of interlobular bile ducts in cystic fibrosis. *J Ped Gastroenterol Nutr* 1991; **12**: 127–130.
65 Isenberg JI. Cystic fibrosis: its influence on the liver, biliary tree, and bile salt metabolism. *Semin Liver Dis* 1982; **4**: 302–313.
66 Lewindon PJ, Pereira TN, Hoskins AC, et al. The role of hepatic stellate cells and transforming growth factor-beta-1 in cystic fibrosis liver disease. *Am J Pathol* 2002; **160**: 1705–1715.
67 Ishak KG. Hepatic morphology in the inherited metabolic diseases. *Semin Liver Dis* 1986; **6**: 246–258.
68 Ishak KG, Sharp HL. Metabolic errors and liver disease. In: MacSween RNM, Anthony PP, Scheuer PJ, et al., eds. Pathology of the Liver, 3 edn. Edinburgh: Churchill Livingstone, 1994: 123.
69 Portmann BC. Liver biopsy in the diagnosis of inherited metabolic disorders. In: Anthony PP, MacSween RNM, eds. Recent Advances in Histopathology, Vol 14. Edinburgh: Churchill Livingstone, 1989; 139–159.
70 Resnick JM, Whitley CB, Leonard AS, et al. Light and electron microscopic features of the liver in mucopolysaccharidosis. *Hum Pathol* 1994; **25**: 276–286.
71 Phillips MJ, Poucell S, Patterson J, et al. The liver. An Atlas and Text of Ultrastructural Pathology. New York, N.Y.: Raven Press, 1987.
72 Resnick JM, Krivit W, Snover DC, et al. Pathology of the liver in mucopolysaccharidosis: light and electron microscopic assessment before and after bone marrow transplantation. *Bone Marrow Transplant* 1992; **10**: 273–280.
73 Smanik EJ, Tavill AS, Jacobs GH, et al. Orthotopic liver transplantation in two adults with Niemann-Pick and Gaucher's diseases: implications for the treatment of inherited metabolic disease. *Hepatology* 1993; **17**: 42–49.
74 McAdams AJ, Hug G, Bove KE. Glycogen storage disease, types I to X: criteria for morphologic diagnosis. *Hum Pathol* 1974; **5**: 463–487.
75 Itoh S, Ishida Y, Matsuo S. Mallory bodies in a patient with type Ia glycogen storage disease. *Gastroenterology* 1987; **92**: 520–523.
76 Howell RR, Stevenson RE, Ben-Menachem Y, et al. Hepatic adenomata with type 1 glycogen storage disease. *JAMA* 1976; **236**: 1481–1484.
77 Coire CI, Qizilbash AH, Castelli MF. Hepatic adenomata in type Ia glycogen storage disease. *Arch Pathol Lab Med* 1987; **111**: 166–169.
78 Limmer J, Fleig WE, Leupold D, et al. Hepatocellular carcinoma in type I glycogen storage disease. *Hepatology* 1988; **8**: 531–537.
79 Markowitz AJ, Chen Y-T, Muenzer J, et al. A man with type III glycogenosis associated with cirrhosis and portal hypertension. *Gastroenterology* 1993; **105**: 1882–1885.
80 Bannayan GA, Dean WJ, Howell RR. Type IV glycogen-storage disease. Light-microscopic, electron-microscopic, and enzymatic study. *Am J Clin Pathol* 1976; **66**: 702–709.
81 Vázquez JJ. Ground glass hepatocytes: light and electron microscopy. Characterization of the different types. *Histol Histopathol* 1990; **5**: 379–386.
82 Jack CIA, Evans CC. Three cases of alpha-1-antitrypsin deficiency in the elderly. *Postgrad Med J* 1991; **67**: 840–842.
83 Rakela J, Goldschmiedt M, Ludwig J. Late manifestation of chronic liver disease in adults with alpha-1-antitrypsin deficiency. *Dig Dis Sci* 1987; **32**: 1358–1362.
84 Deutsch J, Becker H, Auböck L. Histopathological features of liver disease in alpha-1-antitrypsin deficiency. *Acta Paediatr* 1994; **393 (Suppl)**: 8–12.
85 Perlmutter DH. The cellular basis for liver injury in α_1-antitrypsin deficiency. *Hepatology* 1991; **13**: 172–185.
85a Aldonyte R, Jamsson L, Ljungberg O, Larsson S, Janciauskiene S. Polymerized α_1-antitrypsin is present on lung vascular endothelium. New insights into the biological significance of α_1-antitrypsin polymerization. *Histopathology* 2004; **45**: 587–592.
86 Carrell RW, Lomas DA. Alpha-1-antitrypsin deficiency – a model for conformational diseases. *N Engl J Med* 2002; **346**: 45–53.
87 Callea F, Fevery J, Groote J De, et al. Detection of Pi Z phenotype individuals by alpha-1-antitrypsin

(AAT) immunohistochemistry in paraffin-embedded liver tissue specimens. *J Hepatol* 1986; **2**: 389–401.
88 Theaker JM, Fleming KA. Alpha-1-antitrypsin and the liver: a routine immunohistological screen. *J Clin Pathol* 1986; **39**: 58–62.
89 Qizilbash A, Young-Pong O. Alpha 1 antitrypsin liver disease differential diagnosis of PAS-positive, diastase-resistant globules in liver cells. *Am J Clin Pathol* 1983; **79**: 697–702.
90 Hay CR, Preston FE, Triger DR, et al. Progressive liver disease in haemophilia: an understated problem? *Lancet* 1985; **1**: 1495–1498.
91 Geller SA, Nichols WS, Dycaico MJ, et al. Histopathology of α_1-antitrypsin liver disease in a transgenic mouse model. *Hepatology* 1990; **12**: 40–47.
92 Talbot IC, Mowat AP. Liver disease in infancy: histological features and relationship to alpha-antitrypsin phenotype. *J Clin Pathol* 1975; **28**: 559–563.
93 Odièvre M, Martin JP, Hadchouel M, et al. Alpha1-antitrypsin deficiency and liver disease in children: phenotypes, manifestations, and prognosis. *Pediatrics* 1976; **57**: 226–231.
94 Propst T, Propst A, Dietze O, et al. High prevalence of viral infection in adults with homozygous and heterozygous alpha-1-antitrypsin deficiency and chronic liver disease. *Ann Intern Med* 1992; **117**: 641–645.
95 Palmer PE, Wolfe HJ. Alpha-antitrypsin deposition in primary hepatic carcinomas. *Arch Pathol Lab Med* 1976; **100**: 232–236.
96 Reintoft I, Hagerstrand I. Demonstration of alpha 1-antitrypsin in hepatomas. *Arch Pathol Lab Med* 1979; **103**: 495–498.
97 Eriksson S, Carlson J, Velez R. Risk of cirrhosis and primary liver cancer in alpha 1- antitrypsin deficiency. *N Engl J Med* 1986; **314**: 736–739.
98 Graziadei IW, Joseph JJ, Wiesner RH, et al. Increased risk of chronic liver failure in adults with heterozygous α_1-antitrypsin deficiency. *Hepatology* 1998; **28**: 1058–1063.
99 Pittschieler K. Liver disease and heterozygous alpha-1-antitrypsin deficiency. *Acta Paediatr Scand* 1991; **80**: 323–327.
100 Marwick TH, Cooney PT, Kerlin P. Cirrhosis and hepatocellular carcinoma in a patient with heterozygous (MZ) alpha-1-antitrypsin deficiency. *Pathol* 1985; **17**: 649–652.
101 Reid CL, Wiener GJ, Cox DW, et al. Diffuse hepatocellular dysplasia and carcinoma associated with the Mmalton variant of α_1-antitrypsin. *Gastroenterology* 1987; **93**: 181–187.
102 Callea F, Brisigotti M, Fabbretti G, et al. Hepatic endoplasmic reticulum storage diseases. *Liver* 1992; **12**: 357–362.
103 Lindmark B, Eriksson S. Partial deficiency of α_1-antichymotrypsin is associated with chronic cryptogenic liver disease. *Scand J Gastroenterol* 1991; **26**: 508–512.
104 James SP, Stromeyer FW, Chang C, et al. Liver abnormalities in patients with Gaucher's disease. *Gastroenterology* 1981; **80**: 126–133.
105 Long RG, Lake BD, Pettit JE, et al. Adult Niemann-Pick disease: its relationship to the syndrome of the sea-blue histiocyte. *Am J Med* 1977; **62**: 627–635.
106 Tassoni JP, Fawaz KA, Johnston DE. Cirrhosis and portal hypertension in a patient with adult Niemann-Pick disease. *Gastroenterology* 1991; **100**: 567–569.
107 Lake BD, Patrick AD. Wolman's disease: deficiency of E600-resistant acid esterase activity with storage of lipids in lysosomes. *J Pediatr* 1970; **76**: 262–266.
108 Beaudet AL, Ferry GD, Nichols BL, Jr., et al. Cholesterol ester storage disease: clinical, biochemical, and pathological studies. *J Pediatr* 1977; **90**: 910–914.
109 Applebaum MN, Thaler MM. Reversibility of extensive liver damage in galactosemia. *Gastroenterology* 1975; **69**: 496–502.
110 Mieles LA, Esquivel COO, Thiel DH Van, et al. Liver transplantation for tyrosinemia: a review of 10 cases from the University of Pittsburgh. *Dig Dis Sci* 1990; **35**: 153–157.
111 Lichtenstein GR, Kaiser LR, Tuchman M, et al. Fatal hyperammonemia following orthotopic lung transplantation. *Gastroenterology* 1997; **112**: 236–240.
112 Badizadegan K, Perez-Atayde AR. Focal glycogenosis of the liver in

disorders of ureagenesis: its occurrence and diagnostic significance. *Hepatology* 1997; **26**: 365–373.
113 Kilpatrick-Smith L, Hale DE, Douglas SD. Progress in Reye syndrome: epidemiology, biochemical mechanisms and animal models. *Dig Dis* 1989; **7**: 135–146.
114 Lichtenstein PK, Heubi JE, Daugherty CC, et al. Grade I Reye's syndrome. A frequent cause of vomiting and liver dysfunction after varicella and upper-respiratory-tract infection. *N Engl J Med* 1983; **309**: 133–139.
115 Mowat AP. Reye's syndrome: 20 years on. *Br Med J Clin Res* 1983; **286**: 1999–2001.
116 Brown RE, Ishak KG. Hepatic zonal degeneration and necrosis in Reye's syndrome. *Arch Pathol Lab Med* 1976; **100**: 123–126.
117 Kimura S, Kobayashi T, Tanaka Y, et al. Liver histopathology in clinical Reye syndrome. *Brain Dev* 1991; **13**: 95–100.
118 Tonsgard JH. Effect of Reye's syndrome serum on the ultrastructure of isolated liver mitochondria. *Lab Invest* 1989; **60**: 568–573.
119 Mandel H, Hartman C, Berkowitz D, et al. The hepatic mitochondrial DNA depletion syndrome: ultrastructural changes in liver biopsies. *Hepatology* 2001; **34**: 776–784.
120 Balistreri WF, Bove KE. Hepatobiliary consequences of parenteral alimentation. In: Popper H, Schaffner F, eds. Progress in Liver Diseases, Vol IX, 1st edn. Philadelphia: WB Saunders, 1990: 567.
121 Quigley EMM, Marsh MN, Shaffer JL, et al. Hepatobiliary complications of total parenteral nutrition. *Gastroenterology* 1993; **104**: 286–301.
122 Cohen C, Olsen MM. Pediatric total parenteral nutrition. Liver histopathology. *Arch Pathol Lab Med* 1981; **105**: 152–156.
123 Mullick FG, Moran CA, Ishak KG. Total parenteral nutrition: a histopathologic analysis of the liver changes in 20 children. *Mod Pathol* 1994; **7**: 190–194.
124 Nakhleh RE, Glock M, Snover DC. Hepatic pathology of chronic granulomatous disease of childhood. *Arch Pathol Lab Med* 1992; **116**: 71–75.
125 Bosma PJ. Inherited disorders of bilirubin metabolism. *J Hepatol* 2003; **38**: 107–117.
126 Berthelot P, Dhumeaux D. New insights into the classification and mechanisms of hereditary, chronic, non-haemolytic hyperbilirubinaemias. *Gut* 1978; **19**: 474–480.
127 Traunder M, Meier PJ, Boyer JL. Molecular pathogenesis of cholestasis. *N Engl J Med* 1998; **339**: 1217–1227.
128 Oude Elferink RPJ, Berge Henegouwen GP Van. Cracking the genetic code for benign recurrent and progressive familial intrahepatic cholestasis. *J Hepatol* 1998; **29**: 317–320.
129 Müller M, Jansen PLM. The secretory function of the liver: new aspects of hepatobiliary transport. *J Hepatol* 1998; **28**: 344–354.
130 Bull LN, Carolton VEH, Stricker NL, et al. Genetic and morphological findings in progressive familial intrahepatic cholestasis (Byler Disease [PFIC-1] and Byler syndrome): evidence for heterogeneity. *Hepatology* 1997; **26**: 155–164.
131 Desmet VJ. Cholestasis: extrahepatic obstruction and secondary biliary cirrhosis. In: MacSween RNM, Anthony PP, Scheuer PJ, et al., eds. Pathology of the Liver, 3rd edn. Edinburgh: Churchill Livingstone, 1994: 425.
132 Ugarte N, Gonzalez-Crussi F. Hepatoma in siblings with progressive familial cholestatic cirrhosis of childhood. *Am J Clin Pathol* 1981; **76**: 172–177.
133 Lykavieris P, Mil S van, Cresteil D, et al. Progressive familial intrahepatic cholestasis type 1 and extrahepatic features: no catch-up of stature growth, exacerbation of diarrhea, and appearance of liver steatosis after liver transplantation. *J Hepatol* 2003; **39**: 447–452.
134 Mil SWC van, Woerd WL Van Der, Brugge G Van Der, et al. Benign recurrent intrahepatic cholestasis type 2 is caused by mutations in ABCB11. *Gastroenterology* 2004; **127**: 379–384.
135 Beaudoin M, Feldmann G, Erlinger S, et al. Benign recurrent cholestasis. *Digestion* 1973; **9**: 49–65.
136 Ooteghem NAM van, Klomp LWJ, Berge-Henegouwen GP van, et al. Benign recurrent intrahepatic

cholestasis progressing to progressive familial intrahepatic cholestasis: low GGT cholestasis is a clinical continuum. *J Hepatol* 2002; **36**: 439–443.
137 Jansen PLM, Müller M, Sturm E. Genes and cholestasis. *Hepatology* 2001; **34**: 1067–1074.
138 Tygstrup N, Steig BA, Juijn JA, et al. Recurrent familial intrahepatic cholestasis in the Faeroe Islands. Phenotypic heterogeneity but genetic homogeneity. *Hepatology* 1999; **29**: 506–508.
139 Johnson PJ, McFarlane IG, Eddleston ALWF. The natural course and heterogeneity of autoimmune-type chronic active hepatitis. *Semin Liver Dis* 1991; **11**: 187–196.
140 Barnett JL, Appelman HD, Moseley RH. A familial form of incomplete septal cirrhosis. *Gastroenterology* 1992; **102**: 674–678.
141 Narkewicz MR, Sokol RJ, Beckwith B, et al. Liver involvement in Alpers disease. *J Pediatr* 1991; **119**: 260–267.
142 Ku N-O, Gish R, Wright TL, et al. Keratin 8 mutations in patients with cryptogenic liver disease. *N Engl J Med* 2001; **344**: 1580–1587.
143 Millward-Sadler GH. Cirrhosis. In: MacSween RNM, Anthony PP, Scheuer PJ, et al., eds. Pathology of the Liver, 3rd edn. Edinburgh: Churchill Livingstone, 1994: Ch. 10.
144 Klass HJ, Kelly JK, Warnes TW. Indian childhood cirrhosis in the United Kingdom. *Gut* 1980; **21**: 344–350.
145 Lefkowitch JH, Honig CL, King ME, et al. Hepatic copper overload and features of Indian childhood cirrhosis in an American sibship. *N Engl J Med* 1982; **307**: 271–277.
146 Müller-Höcker J, Meyer U, Wiebecke B, et al. Copper storage disease of the liver and chronic dietary copper intoxication in two further German infants mimicking Indian childhood cirrhosis. *Path Res Pr* 1988; **183**: 39–45.
147 Adamson M, Reiner B, Olson JL, et al. Indian childhood cirrhosis in an American child. *Gastroenterology* 1992; **102**: 1771–1777.
148 Aljajeh IA, Mughal S, Al-Tahou B, et al. Indian childhood cirrhosis-like liver disease in an Arab child. A brief report. *Virchows Arch* 1994; **424**: 225–227.
149 Baker A, Gormally S, Saxena R, et al. Copper-associated liver disease in childhood. *J Hepatol* 1995; **23**: 538–543.
150 Müller T, Feichtinger H, Berger H, et al. Endemic Tyrolean infantile cirrhosis: an ecogenetic disorder. *Lancet* 1996; **347**: 877–880.
151 Bhusnurmath SR, Walia BNS, Singh S, et al. Sequential histopathologic alterations in Indian childhood cirrhosis treated with d-penicillamine. *Hum Pathol* 1991; **22**: 653–658.
152 Popper H, Goldfischer S, Sternlieb I, et al. Cytoplasmic copper and its toxic effects. Studies in Indian childhood cirrhosis. *Lancet* 1979; **1**: 1205–1208.
153 Tanner MS, Portmann B, Mowat AP, et al. Increased hepatic copper concentration in Indian childhood cirrhosis. *Lancet* 1979; **1**: 1203–1205.

GENERAL READING

Chandra RS, Stocker JT. The liver, gallbladder, and biliary tract. In: Stocker JT, Dehner LP, eds. Pediatric Pathology. Philadelphia: JB Lippincott, 1992: 703–790.

Ishak KG, Sharp HL. Developmental abnormalities and diseases in childhood. In: MacSween RNM, Anthony PP, Scheuer PJ, et al., eds. Pathology of the Liver, 4th edn. Edinburgh: Churchill Livingstone, 2002: 107–154.

Ishak KG, Sharp HL, Shwarzenberg SJ. Metabolic errors and liver disease. In: MacSween RNM, Anthony PP, Scheuer PJ, et al., eds. Pathology of the Liver, 4th edn. Edinburgh: Churchill Livingstone, 2002: 155–256.

Feingold MJ. Common diagnostic problems in pediatric liver pathology. *Clin Liver Dis* 2002; **6**: 421–454.

Ishak KG. Inherited metabolic diseases of the liver. *Clin Liver Dis* 2002; **6**: 455–480.

Jansen PLM, Müller M, Sturm E. Genes and cholestasis. *Hepatology* 2001; **34**: 1067–1074.

DISTURBANCES OF COPPER AND IRON METABOLISM

WILSON'S DISEASE (HEPATOLENTICULAR DEGENERATION)

Wilson's disease, an autosomal recessive disorder due to mutations in the gene *ATP7B* for copper-transporting ATPase located in the *trans*-Golgi network of the liver,[1] is an uncommon but important and treatable condition. Normal hepatic copper transport[2] is disrupted due to various *ATP7B* mutations[3] leading to the accumulation of copper in hepatocytes and liver disease. Liver biopsy is important for histological diagnosis and monitoring.

Chemical quantitation of copper concentration in the biopsy sample helps to establish the diagnosis and is sometimes used for determination of the genetic status of a patient's siblings.[4,5] Copper determination can be made from specimens obtained by routine liver biopsy or retrieved from paraffin blocks, without special copper-free solutions or instruments.[6] Homozygous subjects have increased liver copper levels from an early age, but do not develop symptoms of liver disease in the first few years of life. Increased liver copper levels precede the development of histological abnormalities. Hepatic copper is typically above 4 μmol/g dry weight (>250 μg/g dry weight).[6]

Histological lesions develop before the disease is clinically apparent. In the early, pre-cirrhotic phase, there is fatty change,[5] sometimes with the formation of fat granulomas.[4] Slender fibrous septa extend from portal tracts (Fig. 14.1). There may be unusually abundant lipofuscin pigment in hepatocytes and glycogen vacuolation of hepatocyte nuclei, but neither feature is easy to evaluate; both are found in normal subjects and nuclear vacuolation is particularly common in the young. Lipofuscin granules may be larger and less regular in outline than normal.[7] Inflammation is absent or mild in the early stages. Kupffer cells are sometimes enlarged and may stain for iron as a result of haemolysis. Electron microscopy helps in the diagnosis of both early and late disease because of characteristic changes in mitochondria and lysosomes.

In some patients, a phase of chronic hepatitis next develops and is difficult to distinguish histologically from chronic viral hepatitis. Stains for copper and copper-associated protein may be helpful, as discussed below. Cirrhosis develops in untreated patients, with or without a recognisable preceding phase of chronic hepatitis. A common though not invariable pattern is of an active cirrhosis with fatty change, ballooned hepatocytes, focally dense eosinophilic cytoplasm and glycogen vacuolation of nuclei (Fig. 14.2). Cholestasis may be present. Hepatocytes often contain Mallory bodies[7a] and these are sometimes very abundant. They are associated with an infiltrate rich in neutrophils, as in steatohepatitis (Fig. 14.3). Partial fibrous occlusion of efferent veins has been reported.[7] Hepatocellular carcinoma is a rare sequel of cirrhosis in Wilson's disease.[8,9]

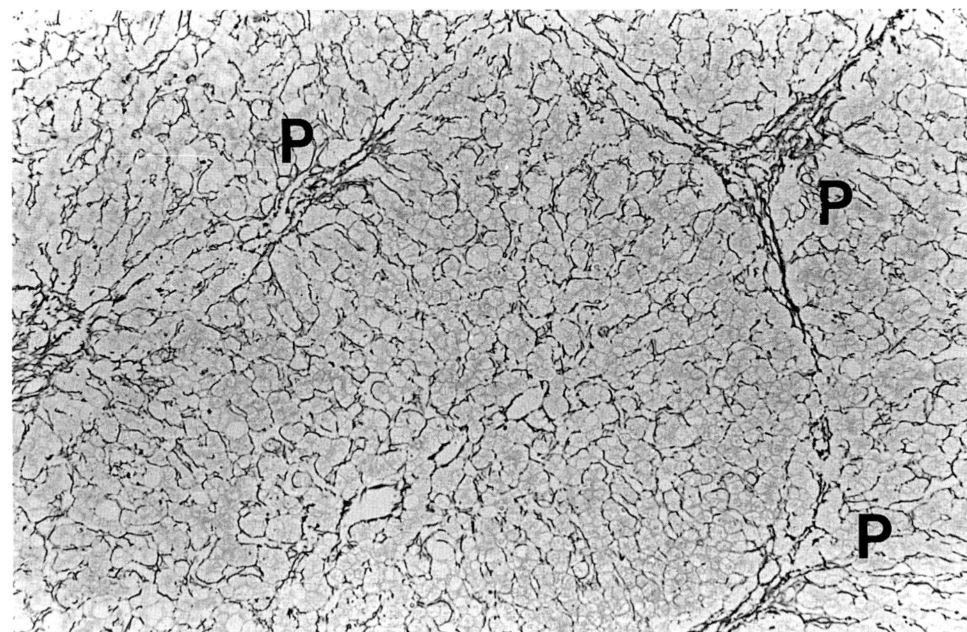

Figure 14.1 *Wilson's disease*. At this early stage slender septa extend from portal tracts (P) but lobular architecture is intact. There is steatosis, just visible in this reticulin preparation. (Wedge biopsy, reticulin).

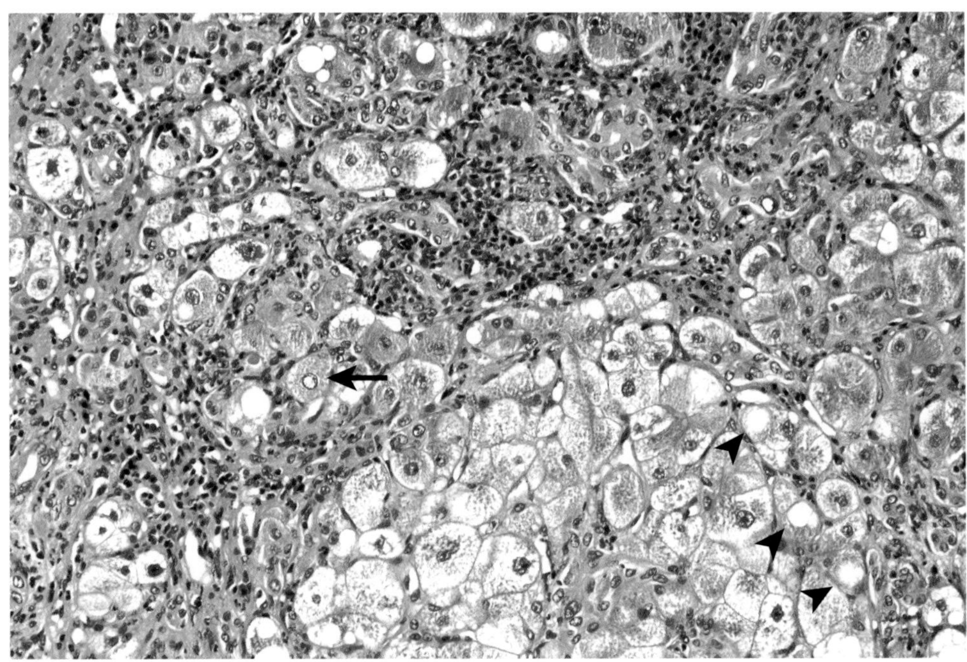

Figure 14.2 *Wilson's disease*. Active cirrhosis with liver-cell swelling, steatosis (arrowheads) and nuclear vacuolation (arrow). (Wedge biopsy, H&E).

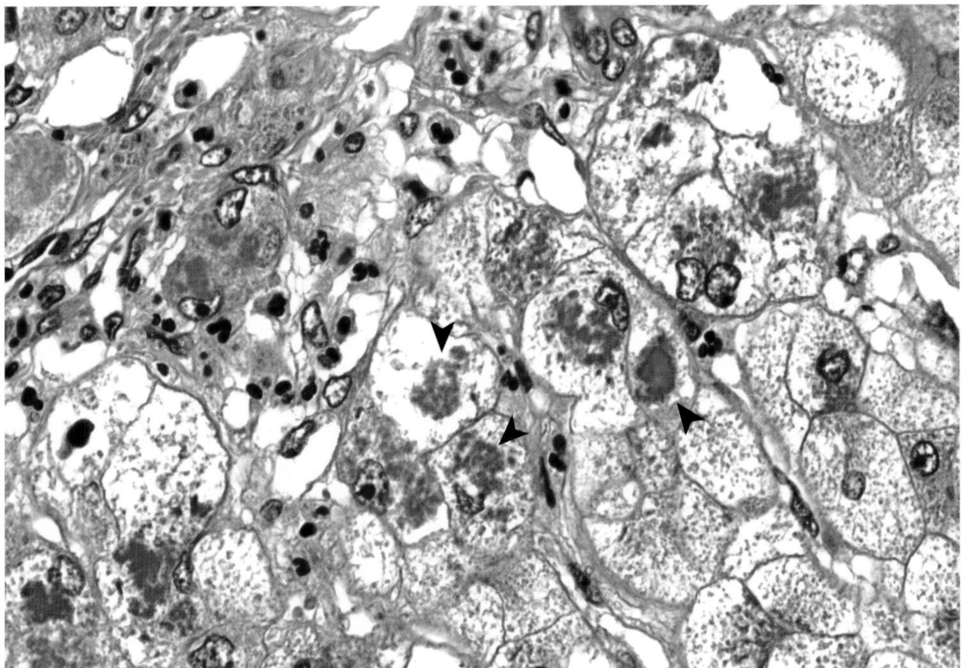

Figure 14.3 *Wilson's disease*. Numerous Mallory bodies (arrowheads) are seen within hepatocytes. (Post-mortem liver, H&E).

Fulminant hepatic failure may be the first manifestation of Wilson's disease and is a major indication for liver transplantation.[10] In one group of 11 patients studied, the livers were already cirrhotic and showed evidence of recent collapse. Nodules were mostly small and separated by septa in which there were abundant ductular structures, but relatively few inflammatory cells.[11] In an earlier study, all nine patients with fulminant hepatic failure were reported to have massive hepatic necrosis, eight of them with nodular regeneration.[12] The death of hepatocytes in the fulminant disease occurs by both apoptosis and necrosis.[13] The presence of much stainable copper and/or copper-associated protein distinguishes Wilson's disease from other causes of fulminant hepatic failure.

Staining for copper and copper-associated protein plays a part in the diagnosis of Wilson's disease, though staining results (as well as the copper concentration) can vary considerably throughout the liver.[14] Failure to stain either is common at some stages of the disease and does not therefore exclude the diagnosis. Conversely, both copper and copper-associated protein are found in other liver diseases, usually as a result of failure to secrete copper into the bile. Thus in a child with liver disease strong staining for copper might reflect loss of bile ducts rather than Wilson's disease. Other copper storage disorders have been described, including Indian childhood cirrhosis which is also occasionally seen elsewhere in the world.[15–17] Furthermore, neonatal liver is normally rich in copper.[18]

In the early phases of Wilson's disease, liver copper levels are high, but the copper is difficult to demonstrate histochemically. This is because it is diffusely distributed in hepatocytes and not concentrated in lysosomes. Sensitive histochemical methods (e.g. Timm's silver method or rhodanine) may show faint cytoplasmic staining. Later in the course of the disease copper begins to accumulate in liver-cell lysosomes and is then more easily stained. Once cirrhosis has developed, the distribution of copper is typically uneven, some nodules staining strongly, while others are negative (Fig. 14.4). Staining for copper and copper-protein may be dissociated, although in most cases, both are positive.[19,20] Timm's silver stain appears to be the most sensitive staining method for demonstrating copper in this disease.[21]

Because of the great variety of histological lesions in the liver, Wilson's disease can easily be mistaken for other liver disorders. Clinicians and pathologists should consider Wilson's disease in the differential diagnosis of hepatocellular disease at all ages and especially in the young. The disease can be arrested by treatment and its development prevented in siblings. The penalties for missing the diagnosis are therefore very great.

IRON OVERLOAD

Siderosis

Siderosis (or haemosiderosis) means the presence of demonstrable iron in tissues, irrespective of cause. The main forms of iron in hepatocytes are ferritin, haemosiderin and haem.[22] Stainable iron is mainly haemosiderin which is principally located in lysosomes and is seen as granules concentrated towards the biliary poles of the cells. Ferritin gives rise to more diffuse staining, imparting a bluish hue to the liver cell cytoplasm on iron stain. Hepatocellular siderosis almost always shows a diminishing gradient of intensity from the periphery of lobules

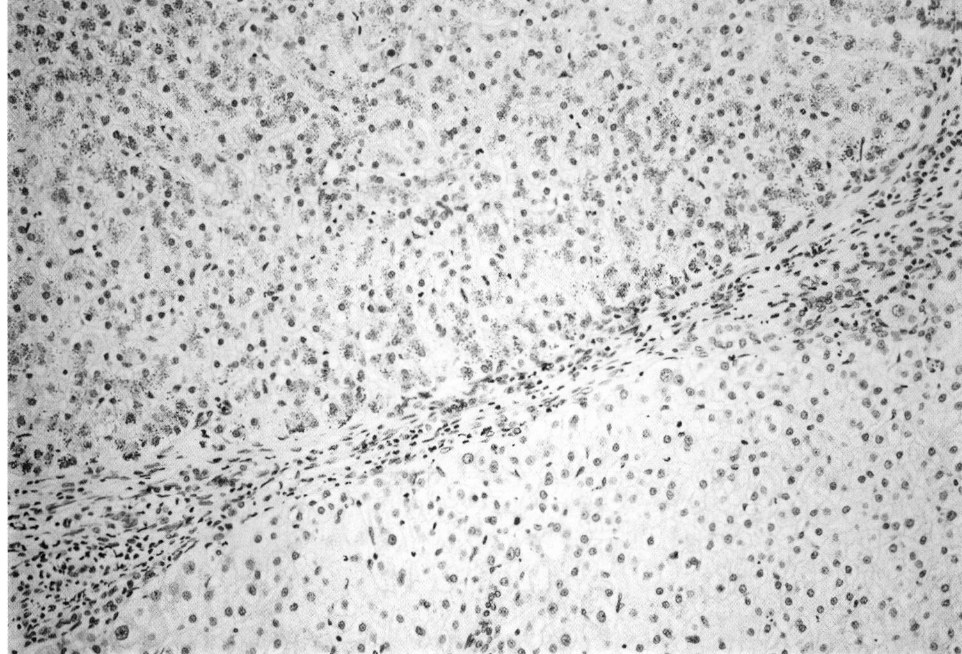

Figure 14.4 *Wilson's disease.* The upper nodule is strongly positive for copper, stained orange-red. The lower nodule is completely negative. (Wedge biopsy, rhodanine).

toward the central (efferent) veins. It is most severe in periportal regions (acinar zones 1), near small portal tracts, and least severe in centrilobular regions (acinar zones 3). The normal adult liver is usually negative on iron stain or at best shows minimal siderosis.[23] This is also true of the neonatal liver, although some cases may show mild periportal liver-cell siderosis (residual iron storage from the active period of hepatic haemopoiesis of the third trimester).[24]

Since iron stains of liver tissue are expected to be negative in most instances, a positive stain requires explanation. In this regard, two major categories of hepatic iron storage disease need to be considered, designated as **primary and secondary iron overload disorders**[25] (Table 14.1). The **primary disorders** are predominantly forms of hereditary haemochromatosis in which genetic mutations alter iron homeostasis in the gastrointestinal tract and liver. The **secondary disorders** are acquired conditions in which increased iron in the liver is due to exogenous sources of iron, abnormal erythrocyte destruction or changes in iron absorption and distribution related to underlying liver disease. The pathologist may be able to suggest the reason for the siderosis based on the distribution of the stainable iron. For example, in most of the primary iron overload disorders such as classic *HFE*-related haemochromatosis, the excess iron is mainly hepatocellular. In thalassaemia both hepatocytes and macrophages are positive, while exogenous iron overload leads to Kupffer cell storage in the first instance. Various types of underlying liver disease are also associated with siderosis. Cirrhotic livers of varied aetiology may contain much iron,[26,27] even within macroregenerative nodules.[28] In viral hepatitis and alcoholic liver disease small amounts of stainable iron are often found. Dense iron-positive granules are common in endothelial cells in a variety of conditions including acute hepatitis,[29] chronic hepatitis B and C,[30] and alcoholic liver disease, but their significance is not known.

The siderotic liver should be evaluated for the **distribution of stainable iron** among the various cell types, the **grade of siderosis**, the **presence of any related tissue damage** (fibrosis, cirrhosis, necrosis or even hepatocellular carcinoma) and

Table 14.1 Primary and secondary iron overload disorders

- Primary
  - Classic *HFE*-related hereditary haemochromatosis (Type 1[a])
  - Non-*HFE* hereditary haemochromatosis
    - Juvenile hereditary haemochromatosis
      - Haemojuvelin or *HJV* (*HFE2*)-related (Type 2A[a])
      - Hepcidin or *HAMP*-related (Type 2B[a])
    - Transferrin receptor 2-related haemochromatosis (Type 3[a])
    - Ferroportin-related iron overload (Type 4[a])
  - Aceruloplasminaemia
  - Others
- Secondary
  - Transfusion
  - Haemolysis
  - Haemodialysis
  - Dietary
  - Underlying liver disease (e.g. chronic hepatitis, fatty liver)

[a]Types 1–4 are classified as forms of hereditary haemochromatosis in the OMIM (Online Mendelian Inheritance in Man) database.[39]

coexisting liver disease of other aetiology. Various numerical methods of assessing the degree of siderosis (discussed below) are also helpful in evaluating causation and the effectiveness of therapeutic iron removal.

Numerical assessment of tissue iron

Many different systems have been devised for the quantification of iron in tissue sections.[31] **The histological grade of hepatocellular iron** can be simply scored on a scale from 1 to 4, grade 1 representing minimal deposition, grade 4 massive deposits with obliteration of the usual lobular gradient and grades 2 and 3 intermediate amounts. Examples are shown in various illustrations to this chapter. The alternative comprehensive grading system of Deugnier and colleagues[32] measures iron not only in hepatocytes but also in mesenchymal cells, bile duct epithelium, blood vessels and connective tissue, generating a score between 0 and 60. This has proved helpful in the assessment of patients with hereditary haemochromatosis.

Tissue for **measuring the iron concentration** can be taken separately at the time a specimen is obtained for histology or by fine needle aspiration biopsy,[33] or the actual paraffin block can be analyzed[34] after histological examination is complete. This has the advantage that the nature of the sample is known.[35] Once the hepatic iron concentration is determined, the hepatic iron index (HII) described by Bassett and colleagues[36] can be calculated: HII = tissue iron in μmol/g dry weight, divided by the age of the patient in years (or tissue iron in μg/g dry weight divided by (55.8 × age in years)).[35,36] Because of the progressive accumulation of iron in classic HFE-related hereditary haemochromatosis, this enables patients with the disease (who have an iron index of 1.9 or more) to be distinguished from heterozygous subjects and those with siderosis from other causes. However, in some patients with cirrhosis due to alcohol or other aetiologies unrelated to hereditary haemochromatosis, secondary accumulations of large amounts of iron in the liver may result in a calculated HII ≥1.9, thereby mimicking the hereditary disease.[26,27] Conversely, a small percentage of individuals with hereditary haemochromatosis may have an iron index of less than 1.9.[37] In recent years, genetic analysis has diminished the importance of these calculations.

The HII has been found to correlate well with a similar index derived from histological assessment and age, using the grading system of Deugnier and colleagues described above.[38] Use of this histological iron index avoids destruction of the tissue block and can be performed when the hepatic iron concentration is not available. Computerised image analysis is another approach to measuring iron deposition which correlates well with biochemical assay.[31]

PRIMARY IRON OVERLOAD DISORDERS

Molecular genetic studies have now defined a variety of heritable disorders affecting iron handling by the gastrointestinal tract and liver.[39] Several of these are listed in Table 14.1 and the reader is encouraged to consult the references in the section on 'General reading' at the end of this chapter for further details. The best understood of the primary iron overload disorders was first described in 1889 by von Recklinghausen[40] and is the disease referred to as 'hereditary haemochromatosis'. The majority of these cases are examples of what is currently known to be classic HFE-related hereditary haemochromatosis, which is discussed below. However, the identical picture of predominantly periportal hepatocellular iron overload can be found in patients with various combinations of the gene defects listed in Table 14.1. There is thus a pathological pattern of **classic haemochromatosis** with more than one possible cause.[39]

Classic *HFE*-related hereditary haemochromatosis

This autosomal recessive disorder is associated with progressive accumulation of iron in the liver, heart, pancreas and other organs. The frequency of homozygous disease is approximately one person in 300,[41] while heterozygotes are found in about one person in 8 to 10.[42] Overt disease may be found in as few as one in 5000[22] and even within families homozygous subjects may show different rates of iron accumulation.[43] The HFE gene, the gene for this type of haemochromatosis, is located on the short arm of chromosome 6 at some distance from the HLA-A locus.[42,44–47] A mis-sense mutation in HFE known as Cys282Tyr (C282Y) has been identified, which results in tyrosine substitution for cysteine at position 282 of the gene protein product.[47] The majority (80–100%) of individuals with the typical phenotype of hereditary haemochromatosis are homozygous for this mutation (designated C282Y/C282Y).[41,47] Genetic tests for C282Y can be performed on peripheral blood or on paraffin embedded tissue.[48] Expression of the mutated HFE protein on duodenal crypt epithelium is one of several factors that have been considered important in the pathogenesis of iron overload in haemochromatosis.[49] A second mutation, His63Asp (H63D) has been identified in fewer patients with haemochromatosis, either in homozygous form or as compound heterozygotes in conjunction with C282Y or the wild-type (normal) protein.[47] Other HFE mutations such as S65C (serine to cysteine) are also reported.[50] Non-HFE hereditary haemochromatosis[25] and other genetic disorders associated with iron overload are discussed later.

Until recently, a comprehensive panel of **diagnostic tests** combined with liver biopsy findings could be expected to provide a firm diagnosis of hereditary haemochromatosis (Table 14.2). However, the availability of genetic testing for HFE-related and other forms of haemochromatosis now sometimes obviates the need for liver biopsy, particularly if certain criteria indicate that the likelihood of hepatic fibrosis is low[51] (i.e. the patient is less than 40 years old, ferritin is less than 1000 ng/ml, serum liver tests are normal and hepatomegaly is absent). However, when there are coexisting liver diseases such as chronic hepatitis C or alcoholism that may accelerate hepatic fibrosis in the presence of a genetic iron overload disorder[52] or there are other reasons for direct morphologic assessment of liver tissue, liver biopsy continues to offer considerable information. Moreover, understanding the pathological progression of classic HFE-related hereditary haemochromatosis (discussed below) provides a useful comparative model of iron-related liver damage.

The first histological abnormality in homozygous HFE haemochromatosis is the appearance of stainable iron in periportal hepatocytes. This may be found incidentally in the course of investigation for other diseases. The unexplained presence of more than very small amounts of iron in hepatocytes should always raise the possibility of early hereditary haemochromatosis. The diagnosis can then be

Table 14.2 Characteristic diagnostic profile in *HFE* homozygous hereditary haemochromatosis

Diagnostic modality	Typical result(s)
Serum transferrin saturation	>62% (screening threshold is >45%[41])
Serum ferritin	≥300 μg/l (men); ≥200 μg/l (women)
Hepatic iron concentration	>2200 μg/g dry weight (men) >1600 μg/g dry weight (women)
Hepatic iron index	≥1.9
Genetic testing	C282Y/C282Y
Liver biopsy	Hepatocellular iron ≥grade 2 Minimal or no Kupffer cell iron

confirmed or refuted by means of genetic testing and/or calculating the hepatic iron index, as discussed previously. Early diagnosis is most important, because cirrhosis can be prevented by appropriate treatment both in patients and in their homozygous relatives, and life expectancy returned to normal.[53] In heterozygotes, stainable liver iron is either absent or very scanty.[38]

As iron stores increase, fibrosis begins to expand the portal tracts and slender septa extend from these to give a pattern of fibrosis resembling holly leaves (Fig. 14.5). The enlarged tracts contain iron-rich macrophages and a ductular reaction, but usually show little or no inflammatory infiltration. Iron may be seen in the ductular structures and in the epithelium of interlobular ducts in small amounts; larger quantities are not found until a later stage, when parenchymal siderosis is severe. It is a challenging paradox that in early haemochromatosis most of the iron is in hepatocytes but there is little or no evidence of liver-cell damage, liver-cell function remains virtually unimpaired, and the progressive lesion is portal in location. However, with increasing iron overload foci of sideronecrosis[32] are found, comprising eosinophilic or lytic necrosis of iron-laden hepatocytes, often in close association with clusters of macrophages (Fig. 14.6). The ratio of non-hepatocytic to hepatocytic iron, as assessed histologically, rises progressively. The ultrastructural progression of iron overload has also been examined.[54]

In fully developed hereditary haemochromatosis, the lobular gradient of iron staining is obliterated; iron in hepatocytes is now seen throughout the lobules whereas earlier, it is more abundant in periportal and mid-zonal regions.[32] Within individual hepatocytes, the iron is seen to be deposited in pericanalicular granules, outlining the bile canalicular system (Fig. 14.7). Cirrhosis slowly develops as fibrosis and hepatocellular hyperplasia alter the normal architectural relationships. True nodule formation is, however, a late event and for a long period there is fibrosis rather than cirrhosis, with irregular islands of parenchyma demarcated by fibrous septa (Fig. 14.8). The pattern is somewhat like that of chronic biliary tract disease. At this stage, some regression of fibrosis as a result of treatment remains possible. Once cirrhosis has developed, biopsy assessment of the effect of treatment on structural changes becomes more difficult because of a tendency for increasing nodule size and compression or remodelling of septa. The onset of cirrhosis marks a fall in life expectancy and an increased risk of hepatocellular carcinoma.[53] The presence of iron-free foci may represent an early stage of malignant transformation.[55,56] Carcinoma has been recorded in non-cirrhotic patients with hereditary haemochromatosis, but is very rare.[55,57]

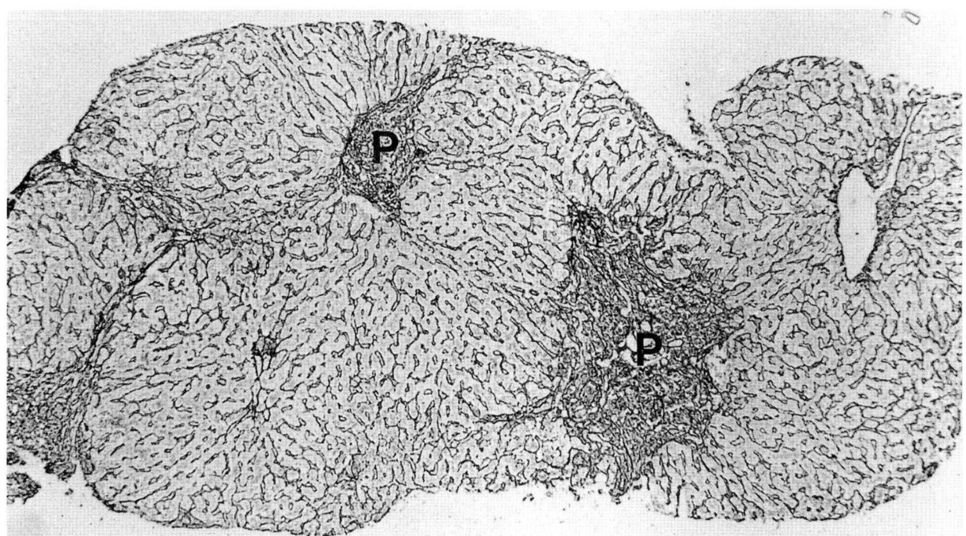

Figure 14.5 *Hereditary haemochromatosis*. At this early stage of fibrosis lobular architecture is still intact and vascular relationships are maintained. The portal tracts (P) are expanded by fibrous tissue. (Needle biopsy, reticulin).

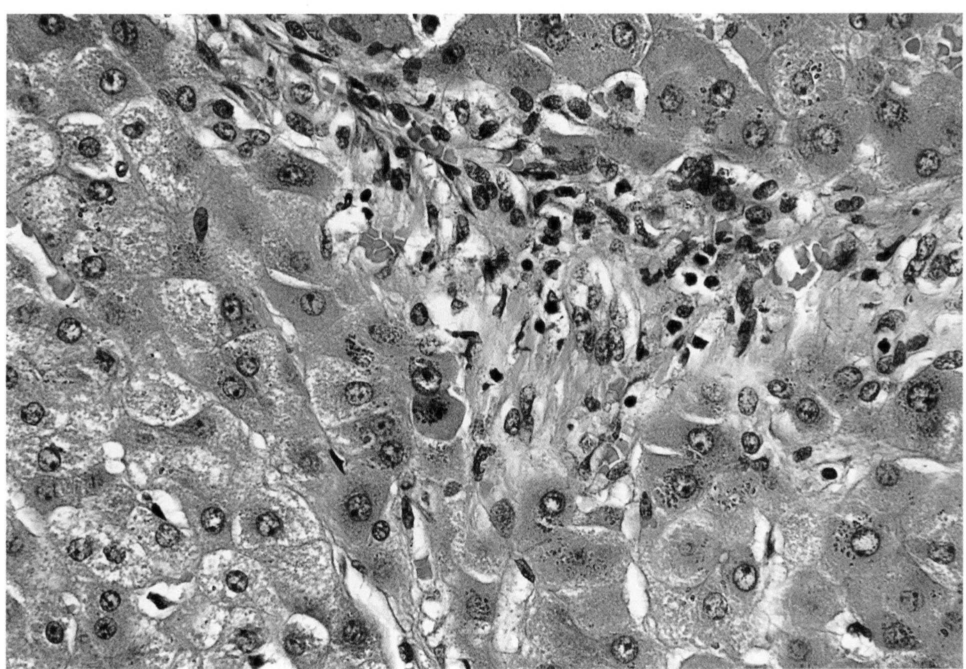

Figure 14.6 *Sideronecrosis*. Periportal hepatocytes contain haemosiderin granules and one siderotic hepatocyte near the centre of the field has undergone apoptosis. (Explant liver, H&E).

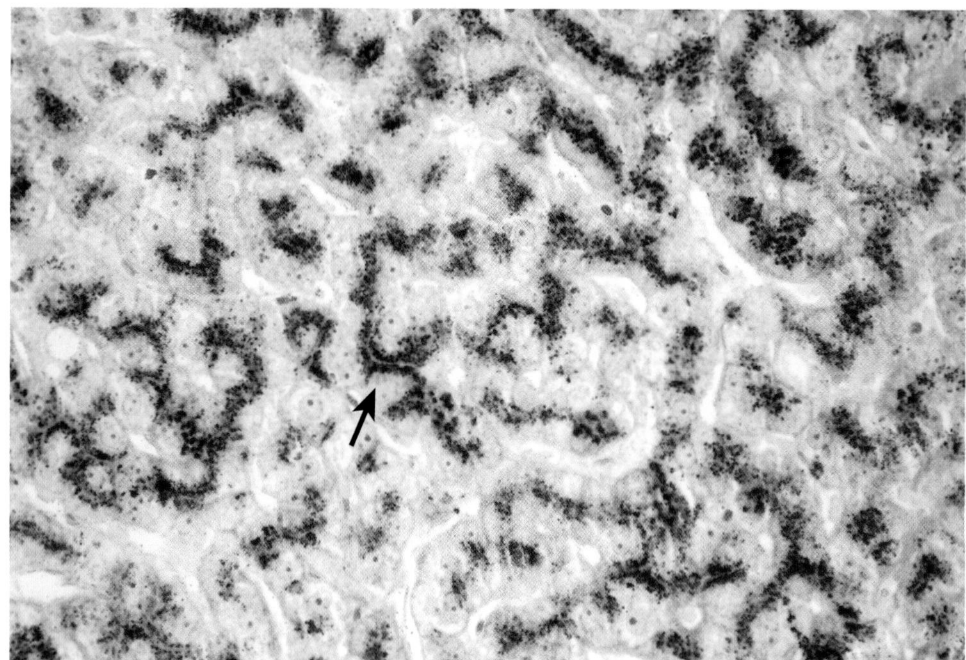

Figure 14.7 *Hereditary haemochromatosis*. Grade 4 (maximal) liver-cell siderosis. Iron-rich granules in a pericanalicular location outline bile canaliculi (arrow). (Needle biopsy, Perls' stain).

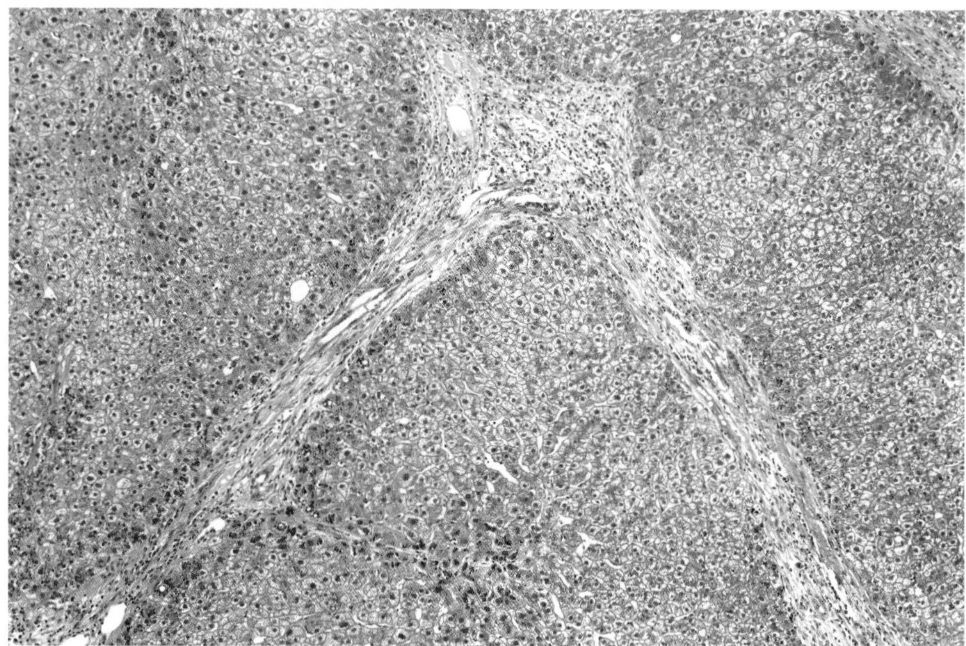

Figure 14.8 *Hereditary haemochromatosis*. Fibrous septa surround irregular islands of liver parenchyma. (Wedge biopsy, H&E).

Effective treatment leads to a steady reduction in stainable iron. Iron encrusted onto portal collagen is usually the most resistant to removal and may be the only stainable iron remaining in the liver. Removal of iron unmasks a brown lipofuscin-like pigment in hepatocytes and connective tissue. Following liver transplantation for haemochromatosis, there appears to be no significant re-accumulation of iron in the liver in most cases.[58]

Other primary iron overload disorders

Several types of **non-HFE haemochromatosis**[25] (Table 14.1) and other genetic diseases such as **aceruloplasminaemia**[59] result in hepatic iron overload, with marked hepatocellular siderosis present in the majority. However, some of these diseases show an atypical iron distribution. Both early and later stages of **ferroportin-related iron overload** feature abundant Kupffer cell siderosis (in contrast to *HFE*-related haemochromatosis). Liver-cell haemosiderin is absent or minimal in the early stage and as it progresses it is seen throughout the lobule, without the usual gradient from periportal to centrilobular regions.[25] The importance of ceruloplasmin in mediating egress of iron from cells is demonstrated in **aceruloplasminaemia**, where both hepatocytes and Kupffer cells accumulate haemosiderin.[59] Excessive Kupffer cell siderosis that cannot be accounted for by one of the causes of secondary iron overload (see below) should therefore also raise the suspicion of a genetic iron overload disorder.

SECONDARY IRON OVERLOAD DISORDERS

Neonatal iron overload (neonatal haemochromatosis)

This condition of severe iron overload in stillborn or premature infants is characterised by extensive hepatocellular necrosis, giant-cell formation, siderosis, fibrosis and nodule formation.[60–63] Whether the disease is a genetic or an acquired insult remains uncertain.[63] Intrauterine infection has been suggested as a possible cause,[64] but the condition is not related to hereditary haemochromatosis of adults. Periportal siderosis is a common finding in pathological livers of neonates[24] and may not itself be responsible for the liver damage in neonatal haemochromatosis.[65]

Iron overload in haematological disorders

Siderosis is found in patients with thalassaemia and, less commonly, other haematological disorders. The iron overload is partly the result of blood transfusion. In addition to the hepatocytic siderosis, portal fibrosis and septum formation seen in hereditary haemochromatosis, there is iron in macrophages from an early stage (Fig. 14.9) and haemopoietic cells may be present. There is often more infiltration of

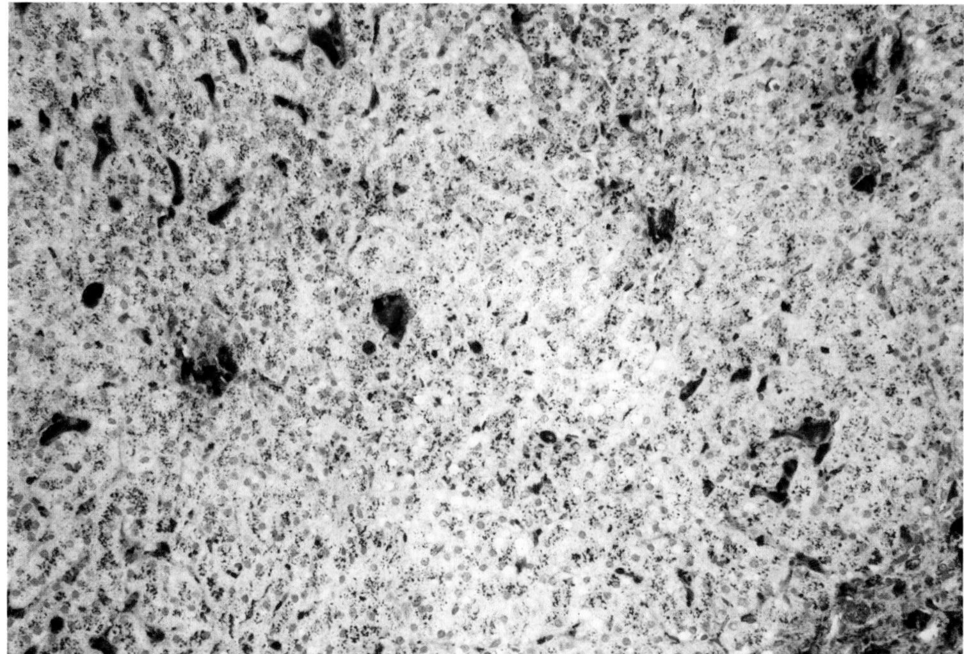

Figure 14.9 *Thalassaemia*. In this example of secondary iron overload hepatocytes show grade 3 siderosis. The darker clumps are iron-laden macrophages. (Needle biopsy, Perls' stain).

portal tracts, septa and sinusoids by lymphocytes than in hereditary haemochromatosis (Fig. 14.10). This, together with focal hepatocellular damage in some cases, is attributable to transfusion-related hepatitis, usually hepatitis C.[66,67] The pattern of fibrosis and degree of inflammation in a liver biopsy often help to determine the relative roles of iron overload and hepatitis C in the progression of the disease. Kupffer cell siderosis is a common finding in haemolysis, haemophagocytic syndrome,[68] haemodialysis and sickle cell disease.[69]

Liver disease of varied aetiology

Chronic viral hepatitis, alcoholic and non-alcoholic fatty liver disease and cirrhosis of diverse aetiologies unrelated to hereditary haemochromatosis[26,27] are often associated with variable degrees of siderosis (Fig. 14.11). In **chronic hepatitis**, serum iron and ferritin are sometimes increased as a result of release of iron from damaged hepatocytes and iron may be seen on liver biopsy. The iron may be located in periportal hepatocytes, in Kupffer cells or in the endothelium of portal vessels.[30,70] Patchy iron-rich foci of hepatocytes in an otherwise non-siderotic biopsy may occasionally be seen.[71] In chronic hepatitis C, iron overload adversely affects therapy with interferon.[72] The severe siderosis that can complicate **cirrhosis** due to viral hepatitis may sometimes mimic hereditary haemochromatosis,[26,27] with marked elevations in hepatic iron concentration and hepatic iron index. Such cases require a comprehensive correlation of the histopathologic features, biochemical test results, genetic analysis and other clinical data in order to clarify the aetiology of the iron

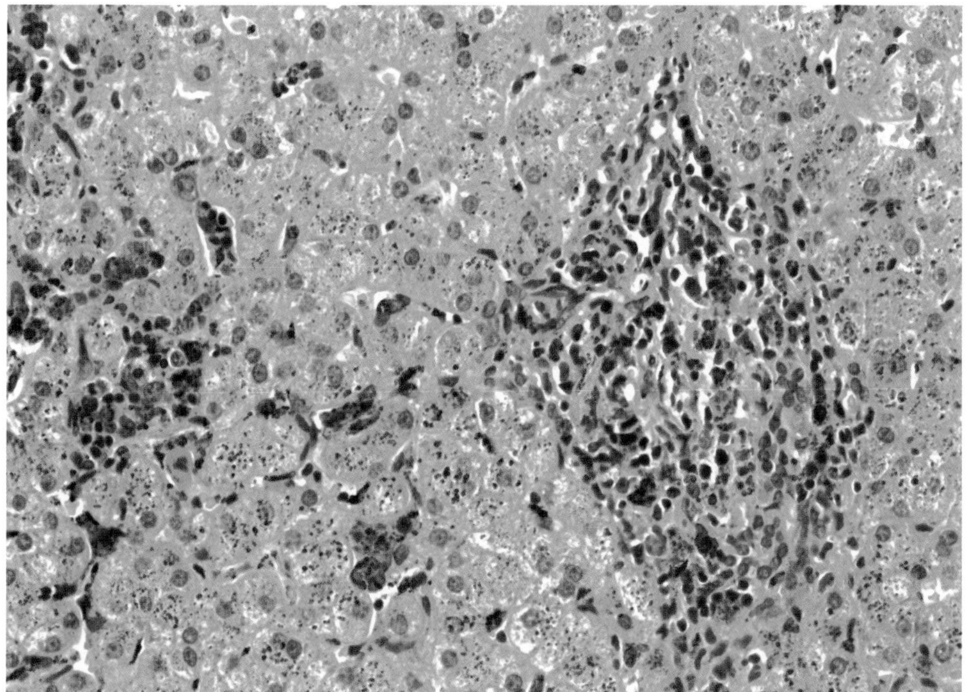

Figure 14.10 *Thalassaemia*. There are iron-laden macrophages in the portal tract and in sinusoids. Haemosiderin granules are also evident in hepatocytes. The portal inflammation is probably due to transfusion-transmitted hepatitis C. (Needle biopsy, H&E).

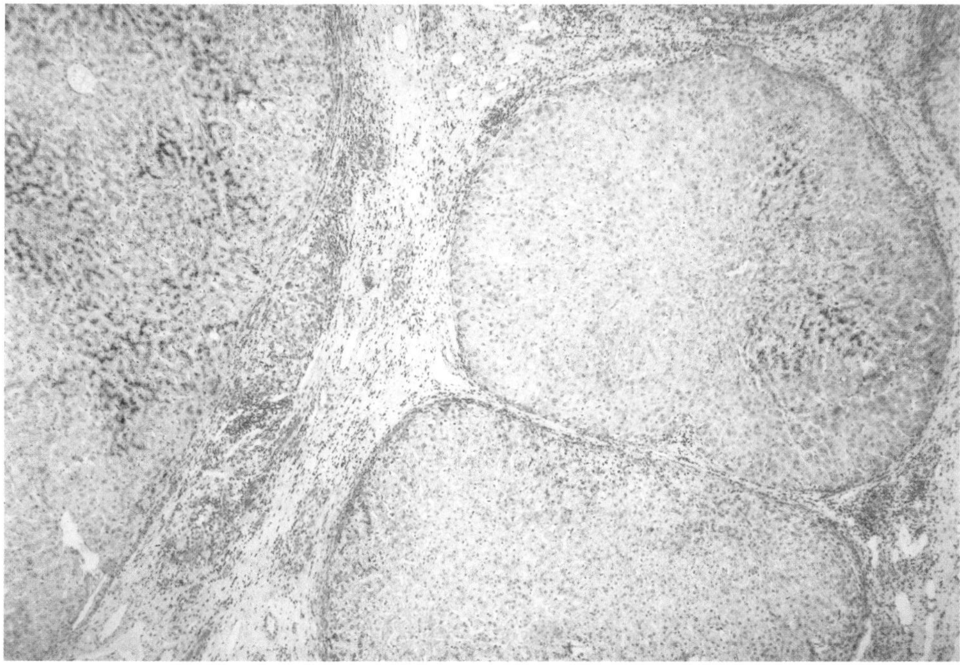

Figure 14.11 *Cirrhosis with siderosis*. This case of relatively inactive cirrhosis due to chronic hepatitis C demonstrates considerable variability in the degree of hepatocellular siderosis among the nodules. (Explant liver, Perls' stain).

overload. Biopsies from patients with **steatosis** sometimes show siderosis in periportal hepatocytes and in Kupffer cells, in which instance the possibility of **insulin resistance-iron overload/metabolic syndrome** (central obesity, hypertension, hyperlipidaemia, hyperglycaemia, insulin resistance) should be considered.[73]

The presence of underlying liver disease is not in itself necessarily sufficient to explain the presence of hepatocellular haemosiderosis nor does it preclude the diagnosis of a coexisting genetic iron overload disorder. An example of this is **porphyria cutanea tarda** in which siderosis is present and increased frequencies of both hepatitis C virus infection[74,75] and *HFE* gene mutations have been identified.[75] Histological siderosis in **alcoholic liver disease** (Fig. 14.12) may reflect underlying homozygous or heterozygous haemochromatosis or concomitant spur cell haemolytic anaemia.[76] Alcohol and chronic hepatitis C are known to accelerate the progression of liver disease in patients with *HFE*-related homozygous hereditary haemochromatosis.[52,77] However, no increased risk of fibrosis or cirrhosis appears to be present in alcoholics with mild hepatocellular siderosis who are C282Y heterozygotes.[78] Siderosis in certain individuals with **non-alcoholic steatohepatitis** (**NASH**) has also been linked to HFE C282Y mutations.[79]

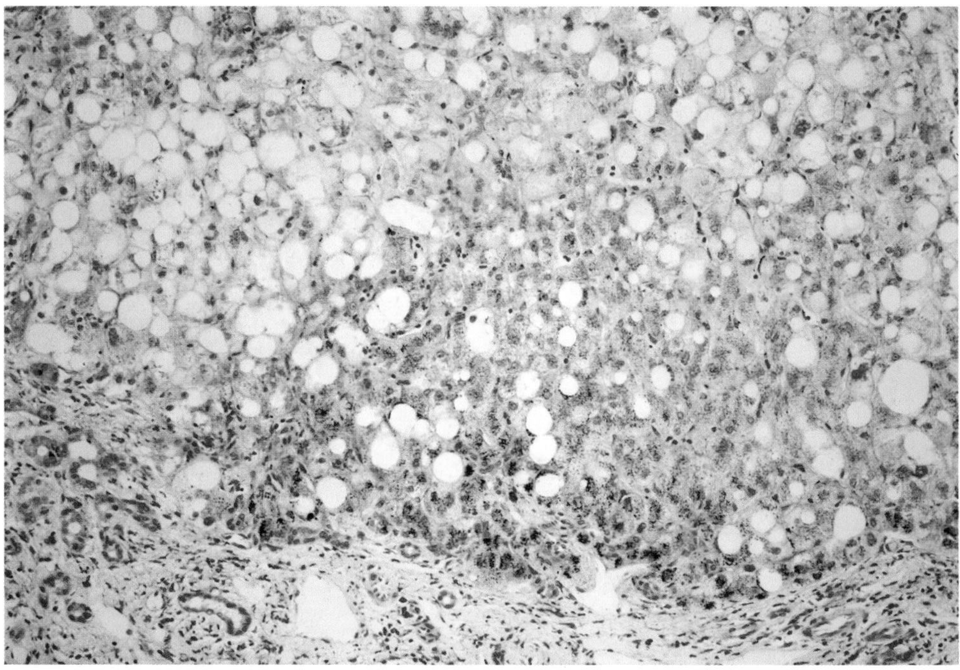

Figure 14.12 *Cirrhosis with siderosis.* In this fatty cirrhosis in an alcohol abuser there is grade 2 hepatocellular siderosis, the cause of which needs investigation. (Needle biopsy, Perls' stain).

REFERENCES

1 Riordan SM, Williams R. The Wilson's disease gene and phenotypic diversity. *J Hepatol* 2001; **34**: 165–171.

2 Tao TY, Gitlin JD. Hepatic copper metabolism: insights from genetic disease. *Hepatology* 2003; **37**: 1241–1247.

3 Huster D, Hoppert M, Lutsenko S, et al. Defective cellular localization of mutant ATP7B in Wilson's disease patients and hepatoma cell lines. *Gastroenterology* 2003; **124**: 335–345.

4 Scheinberg IH, Sternlieb I. Wilson's Disease. Major Problems in Internal Medicine, Vol. XXIII. Philadelphia: WB Saunders, 1984.

5 Walshe JM. Diagnosis and treatment of presymptomatic Wilson's disease. *Lancet* 1988; **ii**: 435–437.

6 Ludwig J, Moyer TP, Rakela J. The liver biopsy diagnosis of Wilson's disease. Methods in pathology. *Am J Clin Pathol* 1994; **102**: 443–446.

7 Stromeyer FW, Ishak KG. Histology of the liver in Wilson's disease: a study of 34 cases. *Am J Clin Pathol* 1980; **73**: 12–24.

7a Müller T, Langner C, Fuchsbichler A et al. Immunohistochemical analysis of Mallory bodies in Wilsonian and non-Wilsonian hepatic copper toxicosis. *Hepatology* 2004; **39**: 963–969.

8 Polio J, Enriquez RE, Chow A, et al. Hepatocellular carcinoma in Wilson's disease. Case report and review of the literature. *J Clin Gastroenterol* 1989; **11**: 220–224.

9 Cheng WSC, Govindarajan S, Redeker AG. Hepatocellular carcinoma in a case of Wilson's disease. *Liver* 1992; **12**: 42–45.

10 Schilsky ML, Scheinberg IH, Sternlieb I. Liver transplantation for Wilson's disease: indications and outcome. *Hepatology* 1994; **19**: 583–587.

11 Davies SE, Williams R, Portmann B. Hepatic morphology and histochemistry of Wilson's disease presenting as fulminant hepatic failure: a study of 11 cases. *Histopathology* 1989; **15**: 385–394.

12 McCullough AJ, Fleming CR, Thistle JL, et al. Diagnosis of Wilson's disease presenting as fulminant hepatic failure. *Gastroenterology* 1983; **84**: 161–167.

13 Strand S, Hofmann WJ, Grambihler A, et al. Hepatic failure and liver cell damage in acute Wilson's disease involve CD95 (APO-1/Fas) mediated apoptosis. *Nat Med* 1998; **4**: 588–593.

14 Faa G, Nurchi V, Demelia L, et al. Uneven hepatic copper distribution in Wilson's disease. *J Hepatol* 1995; **22**: 303–308.

15 Müller-Höcker J, Meyer U, Wiebecke B, et al. Copper storage disease of the liver and chronic dietary copper intoxication in two further German infants mimicking Indian childhood cirrhosis. *Path Res Pr* 1988; **183**: 39–45.

16 Baker A, Gormally S, Saxena R, et al. Copper-associated liver disease in childhood. *J Hepatol* 1995; **23**: 538–543.

17 Müller T, Feichtinger H, Berger H, et al. Endemic Tyrolean infantile cirrhosis: an ecogenetic disorder. *Lancet* 1996; **347**: 877–880.

18 Faa G, Liguori C, Columbano A, et al. Uneven copper distribution in the human newborn liver. *Hepatology* 1987; **7**: 838–842.

19 Elmes ME, Clarkson JP, Mahy NJ, et al. Metallothionein and copper in liver disease with copper retention – a histopathological study. *J Pathol* 1989; **158**: 131–137.

20 Mulder TPJ, Janssens AR, Verspaget HW, et al. Metallothionein concentration in the liver of patients with Wilson's disease, primary biliary cirrhosis, and liver metastasis of colorectal cancer. *J Hepatol* 1992; **16**: 346–350.

21 Pilloni L, Lecca S, Eyken P Van, et al. Value of histochemical stains for copper in the diagnosis of Wilson's disease. *Histopathology* 1998; **33**: 28–33.

22 Tavill AS, Sharma BK, Bacon BR. Iron and the liver: genetic hemochromatosis and other hepatic iron overload disorders. In: Popper H, Schaffner F, eds. Progress in Liver Diseases, Vol. IX. Philadelphia, PA: WB Saunders, 1990: 281.

23 Searle J, Leggett BA, Crawford DHG, et al. Iron storage diseases. In: MacSween RNM, Burt AD, Portmann BC, et al., eds. Pathology of the Liver, 4th edn. Edinburgh: Churchill Livingstone, 2002: 257.

24 Faa G, Sciot R, Farci AMG, et al. Iron concentration and distribution in the newborn liver. *Liver* 1994; **14**: 193–199.

25 Pietrangelo A. Non-HFE hemochromatosis. *Hepatology* 2004; **39**: 21–29.
26 Deugnier Y, Turlin B, Le Quilleuc D, et al. A reappraisal of hepatic siderosis in patients with end-stage cirrhosis: practical implications for the diagnosis of hemochromatosis. *Am J Surg Pathol* 1997; **21**: 669–675.
27 Ludwig J, Hashimoto E, Porayko MK, et al. Hemosiderosis in cirrhosis: a study of 447 native livers. *Gastroenterology* 1997; **112**: 882–888.
28 Terada T, Nakanuma Y. Survey of iron-accumulative macroregenerative nodules in cirrhotic livers. *Hepatology* 1989; **10**: 851–854.
29 Bardadin KA, Scheuer PJ. Endothelial cell changes in acute hepatitis. A light and electron microscopic study. *J Pathol* 1984; **144**: 213–220.
30 Kaji K, Nakanuma Y, Sasaki M, et al. Hemosiderin deposition in portal endothelial cells: a novel hepatic hemosiderosis frequent in chronic viral hepatitis B and C. *Hum Pathol* 1995; **26**: 1080–1085.
31 Olynyk J, Hall P, Sallie R, et al. Computerized measurement of iron in liver biopsies: a comparison with biochemical iron measurement. *Hepatology* 1990; **12**: 26–30.
32 Deugnier YM, Loréal O, Turlin B, et al. Liver pathology in genetic hemochromatosis: a review of 135 homozygous cases and their bioclinical correlations. *Gastroenterology* 1992; **102**: 2050–2059.
33 Olynyk J, Williams P, Fudge A, et al. Fine-needle aspiration biopsy for the measurement of hepatic iron concentration. *Hepatology* 1992; **15**: 502–506.
34 Olynyk JK, O'Neill R, Britton RS, et al. Determination of hepatic iron concentration in fresh and paraffin-embedded tissue: diagnostic implications. *Gastroenterology* 1994; **106**: 674–677.
35 Ludwig J, Batts KP, Moyer TP, et al. Liver biopsy diagnosis of homozygous hemochromatosis: a diagnostic algorithm. *Mayo Clin Proc* 1993; **68**: 263–267.
36 Bassett ML, Halliday JW, Powell LW. Value of hepatic iron measurements in early hemochromatosis and determination of the critical iron level associated with fibrosis. *Hepatology* 1986; **6**: 24–29.
37 Kowdley KV, Trainer TD, Saltzman JR, et al. Utility of hepatic iron index in American patients with hereditary hemochromatosis: a multicenter study. *Gastroenterology* 1997; **113**: 1270–1277.
38 Deugnier YM, Turlin B, Powell LW, et al. Differentiation between heterozygotes and homozygotes in genetic hemochromatosis by means of a histological hepatic iron index: a study of 192 cases. *Hepatology* 1993; **17**: 30–34.
39 Pietrangelo A. Hereditary hemochromatosis – a new look at an old disease. *N Engl J Med* 2004; **350**: 2383–2397.
40 von Recklinghausen FD. Hemochromatosis. Taggeblatt Versammlung Dtsch Naturforsch Arzte Heidelberg 1889; **62**: 324–325.
41 Powell LW, George K, McDonnell SM, et al. Diagnosis of hemochromatosis. *Ann Intern Med* 1998; **129**: 925–931.
42 Pietrangelo A. Hemochromatosis 1998: is one gene enough? *J Hepatol* 1998; **29**: 502–509.
43 Adams PC. Intrafamilial variation in hereditary hemochromatosis. *Dig Dis Sci* 1992; **37**: 361–363.
44 Riedel H-D, Stremmel W. The haemochromatosis gene. *J Hepatol* 1997; **26**: 941–944.
45 Ramrakhiani S, Bacon BR. Hemochromatosis. Advances in molecular genetics and clinical diagnosis. *J Clin Gastroenterol* 1998; **27**: 41–46.
46 Brissot P, Moirand R, Guyader D, et al. Hemochromatosis after the gene discovery: revisiting the diagnostic strategy. *J Hepatol* 1998; **28**: 14–18.
47 Bacon BR. Diagnosis and management of hemochromatosis. *Gastroenterology* 1997; **113**: 995–999.
48 Bartolo C, McAndrew PE, Sosolik RC, et al. Differential diagnosis of hereditary hemochromatosis from other liver disorders by genetic analysis. Gene mutation analysis of patients previously diagnosed with hemochromatosis by liver biopsy. *Arch Pathol Lab Med* 1998; **122**: 633–637.
49 Parkkila S, Niemelä O, Britton RS, et al.

Molecular aspects of iron absorption and HFE expression. *Gastroenterology* 2001; **121**: 1489–1496.
50 Wallace DF, Walker AP, Pietrangelo A, et al. Frequency of the S65C mutation of HFE and iron overload in 309 subjects heterozygous for C282Y. *J Hepatol* 2002; **36**: 474–479.
51 Harrison SA, Bacon BR. Hereditary hemochromatosis: update for 2003. *J Hepatol* 2003; **38**: S14–S23.
52 Diwarkaran HH, Befeler AS, Britton RS, et al. Accelerated hepatic fibrosis in patients with combined hereditary hemochromatosis and chronic hepatitis C infection. *J Hepatol* 2002; **36**: 687–691.
53 Niederau C, Fischer R, Sonnenberg A, et al. Survival and causes of death in cirrhotic and in noncirrhotic patients with primary hemochromatosis. *N Engl J Med* 1985; **313**: 1256–1262.
54 Iancu TC, Deugnier Y, Halliday JW, et al. Ultrastructural sequences during liver iron overload in genetic hemochromatosis. *J Hepatol* 1997; **27**: 628–638.
55 Deugnier YM, Guyuder D, Crantock I, et al. Primary liver cancer in genetic hemochromatosis: a clinical, pathological, and pathogenetic study of 54 cases. *Gastroenterology* 1993; **104**: 228–234.
56 Deugnier YM, Charalambous P, Le Quilleuc D, et al. Preneoplastic significance of hepatic iron-free foci in genetic hemochromatosis: a study of 185 patients. *Hepatology* 1993; **18**: 1363–1369.
57 Fellows IW, Stewart M, Jeffcoate WJ, et al. Hepatocellular carcinoma in primary haemochromatosis in the absence of cirrhosis. *Gut* 1988; **29**: 1603–1606.
58 Crawford DHG, Fletcher LM, Hubscher SG et al. Patient and graft survival after liver transplantation for hereditary hemochromatosis: implications for pathogenesis. *Hepatology* 2004; **39**: 1655–1662.
59 Loréal O, Turlin B, Pigeon C, et al. Aceruloplasminemia: new clinical, pathophysiological and therapeutic insights. *J Hepatol* 2002; **36**: 851–856.
60 Goldfischer S, Grotsky HW, Chang CH. Idiopathic neonatal iron storage involving the liver, pancreas, heart and endocrine and exocrine glands. *Hepatology* 1981; **1**: 58–64.
61 Blisard KS, Bartow SA. Neonatal hemochromatosis. *Hum Pathol* 1986; **17**: 376–383.
62 Moerman P, Pauwels P, Vandenberghe K, et al. Neonatal haemochromatosis. *Histopathology* 1990; **17**: 345–351.
63 Knisely AS, Mieli-Vergani G, Whitington PF. Neonatal hemochromatosis. *Gastroenterol Clin N Amer* 2003; **32**: 877–889.
64 Kershisnik MM, Knisely AS, Sun C-CJ, et al. Cytomegalovirus infection, fetal liver disease, and neonatal hemochromatosis. *Hum Pathol* 1992; **23**: 1075–1080.
65 Silver MM, Valberg LS, Cutz E, et al. Hepatic morphology and iron quantitation in perinatal hemochromatosis. Comparison with a large perinatal control population including cases with chronic liver disease. *Am J Pathol* 1993; **143**: 1312–1325.
66 Wonke B, Hoffbrand AV, Brown D, et al. Antibody to hepatitis C virus in multiply transfused patients with thalassaemia major. *J Clin Pathol* 1990; **43**: 638–640.
67 Donohue SM, Wonke B, Hoffbrand AV, et al. Alpha interferon in the treatment of chronic hepatitis C infection in thalassaemia major. *Br J Haematol* 1993; **83**: 491–497.
68 Kerguenec C de, Hillaire S, Molinié V, et al. Hepatic manifestations of hemophagocytic syndrome: a study of 30 cases. *Am J Gastroenterol* 2001; **96**: 852–857.
69 Banerjee S, Owen C, Chopra S. Sickle cell hepatopathy. *Hepatology* 2001; **33**: 1021–1028.
70 Haque S, Chandra B, Gerber MA, et al. Iron overload in patients with chronic hepatitis C: a clinicopathologic study. *Hum Pathol* 1996; **27**: 1277–1281.
71 Lefkowitch JH, Yee HT, Sweeting J, et al. Iron-rich foci in chronic hepatitis. *Hum Pathol* 1998; **29**: 116–118.
72 Bonkovsky HL, Banner BF, Rothman AL. Iron and chronic viral hepatitis. *Hepatology* 1997; **25**: 759–768.
73 Turlin B, Mendler MH, Moirand R, et al. Histologic features of the liver in insulin resistance-associated iron overload. A study of 139 patients. *Am J Clin Pathol* 2001; **116**: 263–270.
74 Nagy Z, Kászo F, Pár A, et al. Hemochromatosis (HFE) gene mutations and hepatitis C virus infection as risk

factors for porphyria cutanea tarda in Hungarian patients. *Liver Int* 2004; **24**: 16–20.

75 Bonkovsky HL, Poh-Fitzpatrick M, Pimstone N, et al. Porphyria cutanea tarda, hepatitis C and HFE gene mutations in North America. *Hepatology* 1998; **27**: 1661–1669.

76 Pascoe A, Kerlin P, Steadman C, et al. Spur cell anaemia and hepatic iron stores in patients with alcoholic liver disease undergoing orthotopic liver transplantation. *Gut* 1999; **45**: 301–305.

77 Fletcher LM, Dixon JL, Purdie DM, et al. Excess alcohol greatly increases the prevalence of cirrhosis in hereditary hemochromatosis. *Gastroenterology* 2002; **122**: 281–289.

78 Grove J, Daly AK, Burt AD, et al. Heterozygotes for HFE mutations have no increased risk of advanced alcoholic liver disease. *Gut* 1998; **43**: 262–266.

79 George DK, Goldwurm S, MacDonald GA, et al. Increased hepatic iron concentration in nonalcoholic steatohepatitis is associated with increased fibrosis. *Gastroenterology* 1998; **114**: 311–318.

GENERAL READING

Ishak KG, Sharp HL, Schwarzenberg SJ. Metabolic errors and liver disease. In: MacSween RNM, Burt AD, Portmann BC, et al., eds. Pathology of the Liver, 4th edn. Edinburgh: Churchill Livingstone, 2002: 155–256.

Ferenci P, Caca K, Loudianos G, et al. Diagnosis and phenotypic classification of Wilson disease. *Liver Int* 2003; **23**: 139–142.

Roberts EA, Schilsky ML. A practice guideline on Wilson disease. *Gastroenterology* 2003; **37**: 1475–1492.

Gitlin JD. Wilson disease. *Gastroenterology* 2003; **125**: 1868–1877.

Searle J, Leggett BA, Crawford DHG, Powell LW. Iron storage diseases. In: MacSween RNM, Burt AD, Portmann BC, et al., eds. Pathology of the Liver, 4th edn. Edinburgh: Churchill Livingstone, 2002: 257–272.

Harrison SA, Bacon BR. Hereditary hemochromatosis: update for 2003. *J Hepatol* 2003; **38**: S14–S23.

Pietrangelo A. Hereditary hemochromatosis – a new look at an old disease. *N Engl J Med* 2004; **350**: 2383–2397.

Pietrangelo A. Non-HFE hemochromatosis. *Hepatology* 2004; **39**: 21–29.

Sharma N, Butterworth J, Copper BT et al. The emerging role of the liver in iron metabolism. *Am J Gastroenterol* 2005; **100**: 201–206.

THE LIVER IN SYSTEMIC DISEASE AND PREGNANCY

INTRODUCTION

Liver biopsies are often obtained to evaluate abnormalities of liver function tests in patients with known or suspected systemic disease and in the investigation of pyrexia of unknown origin.[1] In the latter, liver biopsy provides diagnostic information in approximately 15–30% of cases.[2] The hepatic changes associated with systemic diseases vary from obvious granulomas or steatosis (discussed in Ch. 7) to more subtle findings such as an increase in liver-cell mitoses. The pathologist will want to know, whenever possible, whether or not the biopsy changes are specific for a systemic disease. For example, when granulomas are present, their aetiology usually has important therapeutic implications. Liver biopsy in patients with acquired immune deficiency syndrome may demonstrate suspected hepatotoxicity due to antiretroviral drugs or hepatic involvement by a micro-organism already identified elsewhere in the patient, or may disclose a new diagnosis such as lymphoma. Liver biopsy also provides tissue for culture and special stains. This chapter examines the pathology of hepatic granulomas, hepatic changes in a variety of infectious diseases and liver involvement in gastrointestinal and haemopoietic diseases and the porphyrias.

In the unusual situation where liver dysfunction is found in pregnancy, the histopathologist may be called upon to differentiate intercurrent conditions such as viral hepatitis from several varieties of liver disease unique to pregnancy. This differential diagnosis is discussed in the latter portion of this chapter.

GRANULOMAS

There are many causes of hepatic granulomas, including local irritants, infections, infestations and hypersensitivity to drugs. The constituents of these lesions, depending on the aetiology and inflammatory cytokines produced,[3] include large epithelioid cells, multinucleated giant cells, varied numbers of mononuclear cells and eosinophils. Hepatic granulomas can be further morphologically classified as **caseating (necrotising)**, **non-caseating**, **lipogranulomas** (see Ch. 7) and **fibrin-ring granulomas**.[4–6] The causes vary in frequency from one country to another. Although aetiology may be determined from the histological features, from special stains for micro-organisms, from culture of part of the biopsy specimen, or from clinical and serological data, the cause of hepatic granulomas may remain unknown in some 10–36% of cases.[7,8]

From a practical point of view, biopsies containing granulomas fall into one of four groups:

1. The cause of the granuloma is seen under the microscope. Examples are the granulomas around schistosome ova and the mineral oil lipogranulomas found in portal tracts or near terminal hepatic venules.
2. The cause is not seen, but other histological features and clinical circumstances make the diagnosis clear. For example, granulomas near damaged bile ducts in a patient with clinically and immunologically typical primary biliary cirrhosis are almost certainly due to this disease.
3. The cause is uncertain, but appearances favour one particular line of further investigation rather than another. For instance, sarcoidosis should be suspected when clusters of large granulomas with prominent epithelioid cells, large multinucleated giant cells and dense fibrosis are found in portal tracts.
4. The cause of the granulomas cannot be determined from the histological appearances. This is unfortunately common and the help that the pathologist can then give to the clinician is limited.

These four circumstances can be summarised as **see the cause**, **know the cause**, **suspect the cause** and **don't know the cause**. Some of the histological guidelines for evaluating granulomas are shown in Table 15.1.

Granulomas are found in up to 10% of liver biopsies.[9,10] They may be sparse and suspicion of granulomatous disease is an indication for examining step sections from different levels of a paraffin block, if no lesions are seen initially. Because identifiable granulomas are generally more than 50 μm in diameter, serial sections 5 μm thick are unnecessary, unless a single granuloma is to be further investigated.

Table 15.1 Histological features of hepatic granulomas

Aetiology	Favoured site(s)	Special features
Sarcoidosis	Portal/periportal	Clustering Hyalinisation Inclusions in giant cells May destroy bile ducts
Tuberculosis	None	Necrosis
PBC	Portal	Near damaged bile duct Lobular granulomas uncommon
Drug	None	Eosinophils Other lesions often present (hepatitis, fat, cholestasis)
Mineral oil	Portal, perivenous	Oil vacuoles
Q Fever, CMV, Allopurinol, etc.	None	Fibrin-ring granuloma
CGDC*	None	Brown pigment in macrophages May be necrotising
Cat scratch disease, tularaemia, yersinia	None	Purulent centre

*CGDC, chronic granulomatous disease of childhood.

Granulomas are commonly found in the liver in **sarcoidosis** and may even recur following liver transplantation.[11] The liver is usually one of several organs involved, but occasionally extrahepatic lesions are difficult to demonstrate and chest X-ray may be normal.[12] Liver biopsy is helpful for diagnosis, especially in patients with fever and arthralgia.[13] The lesions may be found both in portal tracts and in lobules and consist of well-defined rounded granulomas with variable infiltration by inflammatory cells including plasma cells and eosinophils (Fig. 15.1). The granulomas contain reticulin fibres (Fig. 15.2). Multinucleated giant cells may contain inclusions of different types.[14] Central necrosis may infrequently be present, but is never as extensive as in tuberculosis. The granulomas often cluster in portal and periportal regions[15] (Fig. 15.1) and older lesions show dense hyalinised collagen. The fibrosis may extend to interfere with normal acinar structure and in more severe cases, may progress to cirrhosis.[14,16] A surprising degree of reactive portal and lobular inflammation may occasionally be seen in association with sarcoid granulomas, raising the question of concomitant hepatitis.[16] The lobular component consists predominantly of hyperplastic Kupffer cells; acidophil bodies are rare. The portal tracts show considerable variability in the amount of lymphocytic inflammation and the most active portal inflammation is usually near granulomas. Serological tests for viral hepatitis should be obtained if there is serious diagnostic concern. In those few patient with sarcoidosis who develop portal hypertension,[17,18] it may be related to portal and periportal fibrosis or to broad areas of replacement fibrosis,[14] nodular regenerative hyperplasia[19] or cirrhosis.[14,16] Another rare complication of sarcoidosis is a primary biliary cirrhosis-like lesion, with destruction of bile ducts and a clinical picture of chronic cholestasis.[20] Portal features suggesting biliary obstruction may also be present.[14,16] It should be noted that a diagnosis of sarcoidosis cannot be proved by histological examination of the liver alone, because very similar lesions are found in other granulomatous diseases.

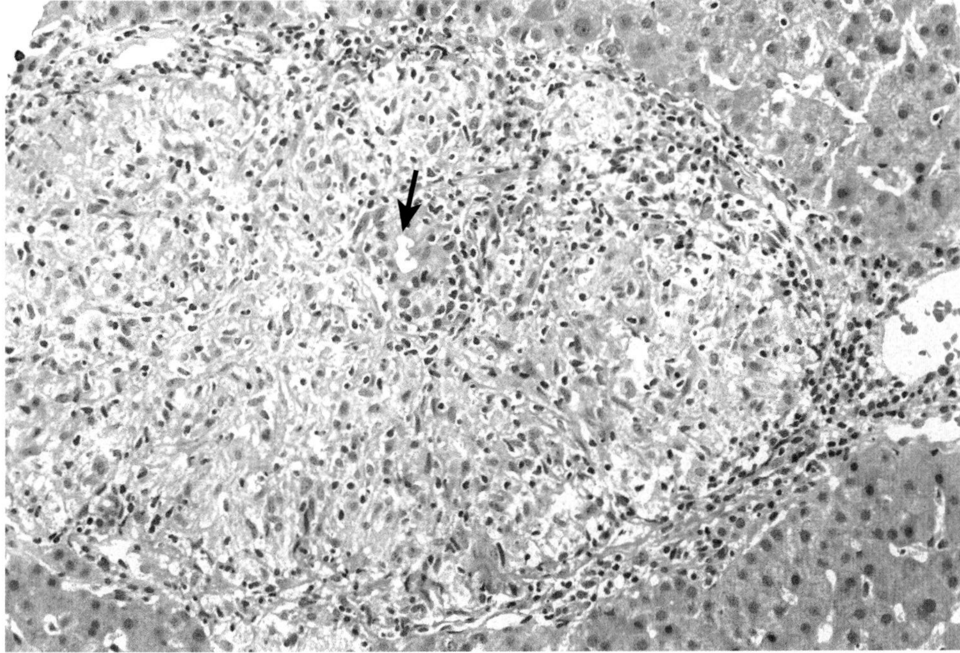

Figure 15.1 *Sarcoidosis*. A cluster of epithelioid-cell granulomas with giant cells has expanded a portal tract and surrounded a bile duct (arrow). (Needle biopsy, H&E).

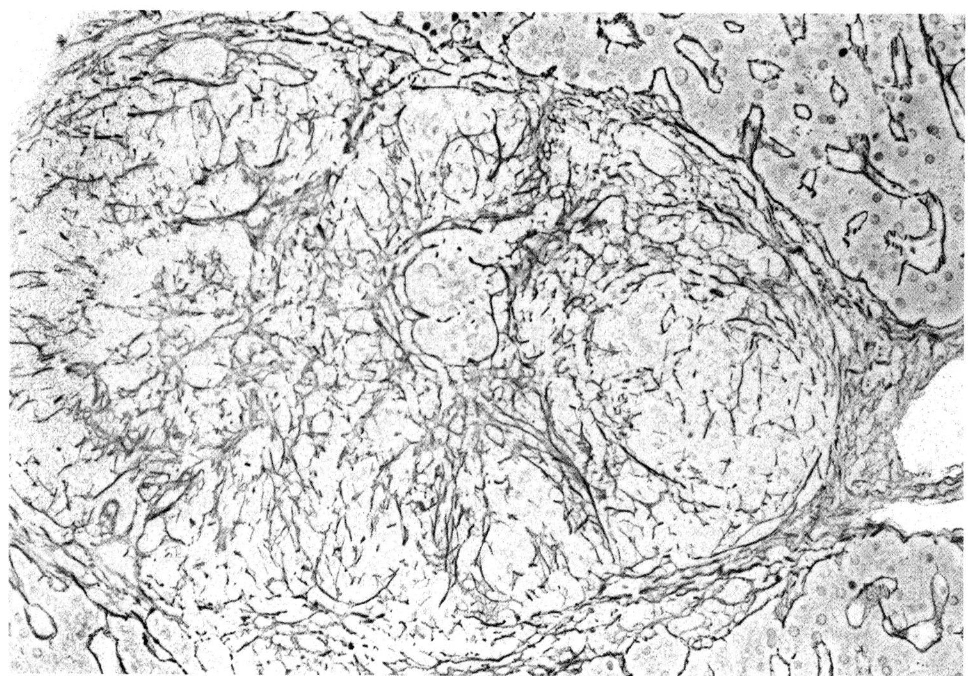

Figure 15.2 *Sarcoidosis*. The same field as in Figure 15.1. The granulomas are clustered and contain strands of reticulin. (Needle biopsy, reticulin).

In **chronic granulomatous disease of childhood**, defective neutrophil leucocyte function leads to the development of infective granulomas of different sizes, containing homogeneous eosinophilic material, necrotic debris or pus. Portal tracts are inflamed and there may be fibrosis. A brown pigment of ceroid type accumulates in portal macrophages and to a lesser extent in Kupffer cells.[21–23] The disease is sometimes first diagnosed in adult life.[24]

A small number of patients with **chronic hepatitis C** may show non-caseating granulomas in the liver, either portal or lobular in location.[25,26] In one series, nearly 10% of granulomas were ascribed to this infection.[8] Their pathogenesis is unknown. In some instances, other causes such as schistosomiasis may become apparent during a thorough evaluation.[27]

Drugs and toxins should be considered in the evaluation of hepatic granulomas (see Ch. 8), particularly if eosinophils are prominent.[28] A diverse array of particulate materials may cause granulomas, including aluminium,[29] feldspar[30] and silicone.[31] Biopsies with granulomas should therefore be examined under polarised light for evidence of particulate material. Dense reactive fibrosis may develop in the form of **sclerohyaline nodules** in individuals exposed in the workplace or by intravenous drug abuse to silica, chromium, cobalt and magnesium.[32]

The **fibrin-ring granuloma** is a distinctive, though non-specific,[33] form described in Q fever,[33–38] Hodgkin's disease,[39] allopurinol hypersensitivity,[40] cytomegalovirus[41] and Epstein-Barr virus infections,[42] leishmaniasis,[43] toxoplasmosis,[39] hepatitis A,[44,45] giant-cell arteritis[46] and systemic lupus erythematosus.[47] This granuloma is composed of a fat vacuole surrounded by a ring of fibrin, epithelioid cells, giant cells and neutrophils (Fig. 15.3). Serial sections may be needed to demonstrate the typical fibrin-ring or 'doughnut' lesion.[35]

Simon and Wolff[48] described a syndrome characterised by fever, constitutional symptoms and hepatic granulomas, not responding to antituberculous drugs but

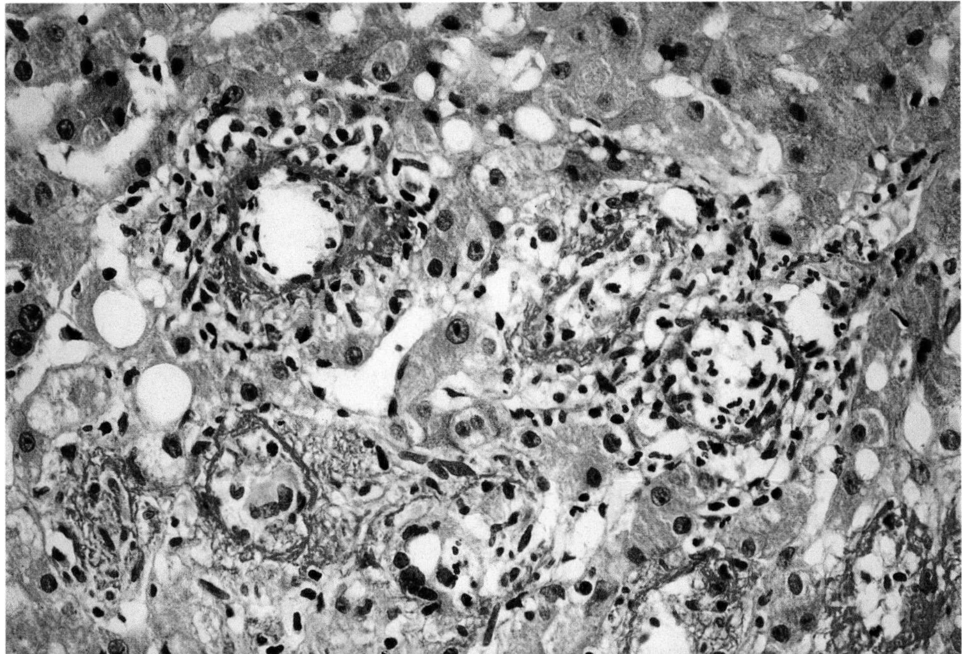

Figure 15.3 *Q fever*. Small granulomas containing giant cells, fat vacuoles and neutrophil leucocytes are surrounded by rings of fibrin, stained red. (Needle biopsy, MSB).

improving on corticosteroid therapy or sometimes with methotrexate.[49] In some patients the syndrome resolves spontaneously without treatment.[50] The cause has not been established.

VIRAL DISEASES

The pathological changes in the liver resulting from virus infections other than hepatitis viruses have been reviewed by Lucas.[51] The viral haemorrhagic fevers, such as mosquito-borne **Flavivirus** infection (**Dengue fever**[52]) and rodent-borne **Hantavirus** infections,[53] are characterised by mid-zonal or more extensive hepatic necrosis. In **yellow fever**, acidophil bodies are typically abundant; they were first described in this disease by Councilman over 100 years ago.[54,55]

Several viruses not normally associated with liver disease can occasionally cause liver damage. Examples include **herpes simplex virus** infection leading to irregular and randomly distributed areas of coagulative necrosis[56,57] (Fig. 15.4) and **adenovirus** infection.[58,59] In both infections, virus particles or antigens can be identified in hepatocytes. Paramyxovirus-like particles were described in adults with associated syncytial giant-cell hepatitis.[60] Multinucleated giant hepatocytes in liver biopsies from adults (**post-infantile giant cell hepatitis**) may also be seen in autoimmune hepatitis and other liver diseases.[61,62]

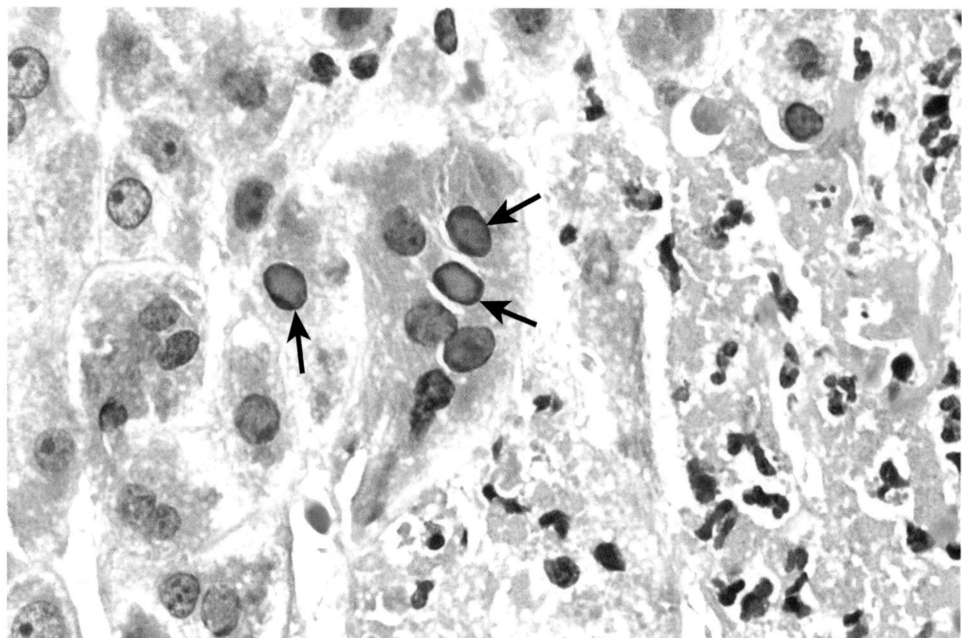

Figure 15.4 *Herpes simplex hepatitis.* Pale, ground-glass-like intranuclear inclusions are present in a multinucleated hepatocyte (near centre) and elsewhere (arrows). An adjacent focus of necrosis with neutrophils is seen at the right of the field. (Needle biopsy, H&E).

Cytomegalovirus infection

Cytomegalovirus (CMV) has been implicated in some children with neonatal hepatitis. Histological features include giant-cell formation as in other forms of neonatal liver damage, inflammation and cholestasis. Bile ducts are damaged and may be destroyed.[63] CMV genome can be identified by polymerase chain reaction in many cases.[64]

In later life, CMV infection can present as a mononucleosis-like illness, but also as a hepatitis. Asymptomatic infection is common in immunocompromised patients. In these, the histological changes are often mild, but typical CMV inclusions are found in hepatocytes, bile-duct epithelium and endothelial cells (Fig. 15.5). Specific immunocytochemical staining reveals CMV antigens even in cells without inclusions,[65] but sometimes with an abnormal granular basophilic cytoplasm.[66] Patients with CMV infection may also show aggregation of neutrophils in sinusoids, with or without evidence of CMV in neighbouring cells,[66] an important diagnostic consideration in immunocompromised patients or individuals who have received organ transplants. Larger accumulations of macrophages and lymphocytes can be seen and epithelioid-cell granulomas have been reported.[67] In immunocompetent patients, there are varying degrees of focal liver-cell and bile-duct damage, portal inflammation, infiltration of sinusoids with lymphoid cells and increased mitoses in hepatocytes.[68] In such patients, it may not be possible to demonstrate CMV inclusions or antigen, a situation possibly analogous to hepatitis B virus infection, where inclusions and antigen may be scanty or absent during the acute attack, while characteristic of the carrier state.[68]

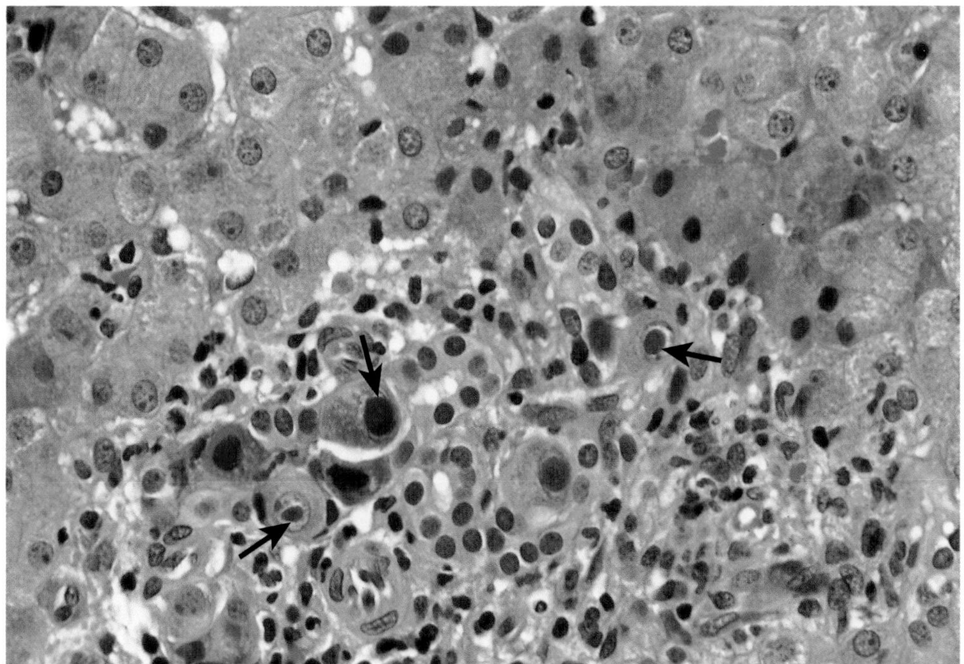

Figure 15.5 *Cytomegalovirus hepatitis in AIDS*. Numerous cytomegalovirus inclusions (arrows) are seen within bile duct epithelial cells. (Needle biopsy, H&E).

Infectious mononucleosis

The liver is histologically abnormal in infectious mononucleosis even when there is no clinical jaundice.[69] Dense accumulations of atypical lymphocytes are found in portal tracts and sinusoids (Fig. 15.6). Sinusoidal aggregates must be distinguished from the more heterogeneous collections of cells found in extramedullary haemopoiesis. The infiltration also mimics that of leukaemia. Kupffer cells are enlarged. Epithelioid-cell granulomas are occasionally present.[10] Small foci of hepatocellular necrosis and acidophil bodies may be seen, but the diffuse hepatocellular damage characteristic of viral hepatitis is usually absent and extensive necrosis[70] is rare. Cholestasis is absent or mild.

Acquired immune deficiency syndrome (AIDS)

A spectrum of hepatobiliary lesions has been associated with AIDS and HIV-1 infection since the onset of the epidemic[71–80] (Table 15.2). Liver biopsy continues to play an important diagnostic role in the evaluation of abnormal liver function tests in these patients,[73,74,81] particularly in managing the potential hepatotoxicity of highly active antiretroviral therapy (HAART)[82,83] and concurrent chronic hepatitis B and/or C which may be present. Although Kupffer cells and endothelial cells[84–88] are potential target cells for HIV-1 infection, there are no specific hepatic lesions due to HIV-1, a few cases of alleged 'HIV-1 hepatitis'[89,90] notwithstanding.

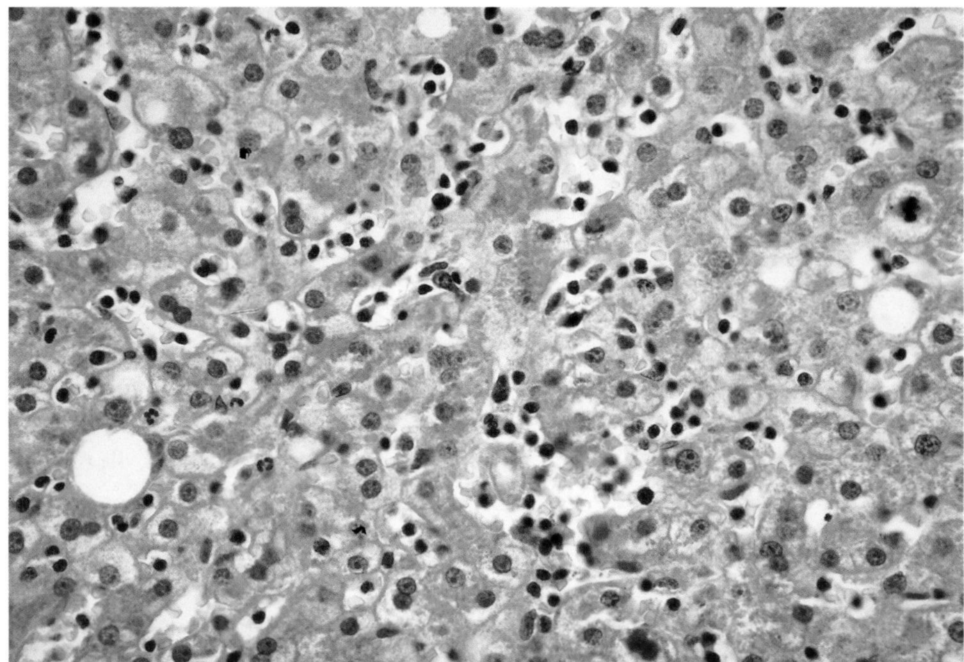

Figure 15.6 *Infectious mononucleosis*. A prominent sinusoidal 'beads-on-a-string' pattern is seen, consisting of atypical lymphocytes and hyperplastic Kupffer cells. (Needle biopsy, H&E).

Table 15.2 Hepatobiliary lesions in HIV-1 infection and AIDS

Lesion	Cause(s) or Type(s)
Granulomas	Mycobacteria, fungi, drugs
Abscesses	Staphylococci, streptococci, listeria
Bacillary peliosis	*Bartonella henselae*
Biliary tract disease (AIDS cholangiopathy)	CMV, cryptosporidia, microsporidia
Neoplasms	Kaposi's sarcoma, lymphoma, smooth muscle tumours
Chronic viral hepatitis	HBV, HCV, HDV
Other viral infections	CMV, herpes simplex, EBV, adenovirus
Vascular lesions	Peliosis hepatis, sinusoidal dilatation
Drug toxicity	Sulfa agents, antiretrovirals
Miscellaneous	Steatosis, haemosiderosis, stellate cell hypertrophy, amyloidosis

Despite the reduction in morbidity and mortality due to anti-retroviral therapy and prophylactic antibiotics,[91] opportunistic infections and neoplasms such as Kaposi's sarcoma and lymphoma must still be excluded on liver biopsy. Specimens should routinely be studied with acid-fast and silver stains for detection of high-incidence pathogens such as mycobacteria and fungi. Other methods such as Gram or Warthin-Starry stains can be applied, depending on the clinical and histological indications. A portion of the biopsy should be sent for culture.

Opportunistic infections and infestations

Opportunistic infections and infestations involving the liver and bile ducts in AIDS include *Mycobacterium avium-intracellulare* and *Mycobacterium tuberculosis* infection, cytomegalovirus infection, cryptococcosis, candidiasis, histoplasmosis, leishmaniasis,[92] malaria, cryptosporidiosis[93] and microsporidiosis.[94–96] Mycobacterial and fungal infections frequently produce **granulomas**. *Mycobacterium avium-intracellulare (MAI)* results in numerous granulomas and the organisms are readily demonstrated by staining with diastase-PAS or the Ziehl-Neelsen method[97–100] (Fig. 15.7). Each granuloma consists of foamy histiocytes with few lymphocytes. The histiocytes often show a striated appearance on haematoxylin and eosin staining due to the abundant packing of organisms in each cell. MAI organisms are also well stained with Gomori methenamine silver. For screening of liver biopsies, particularly for *Mycobacterium tuberculosis* which may be present in fewer numbers than MAI, the auramine-rhodamine fluorescent method[101,102] gives excellent results. Careful examination of special stains is of particular importance as some AIDS patients have mycobacterial infection without typical granuloma formation; scant, single mycobacteria may be present within sinusoids or portal tracts. *Pneumocystis carinii* may disseminate to the liver, producing acellular exudative masses, which closely resemble the pulmonary alveolar exudates.[103]

AIDS cholangiopathy

AIDS cholangiopathy resembles sclerosing cholangitis clinically and radiographically and is due to infections of the large bile ducts by several possible pathogens, including CMV, cryptosporidia and microsporidia.[94–96,104–106] Liver biopsy changes

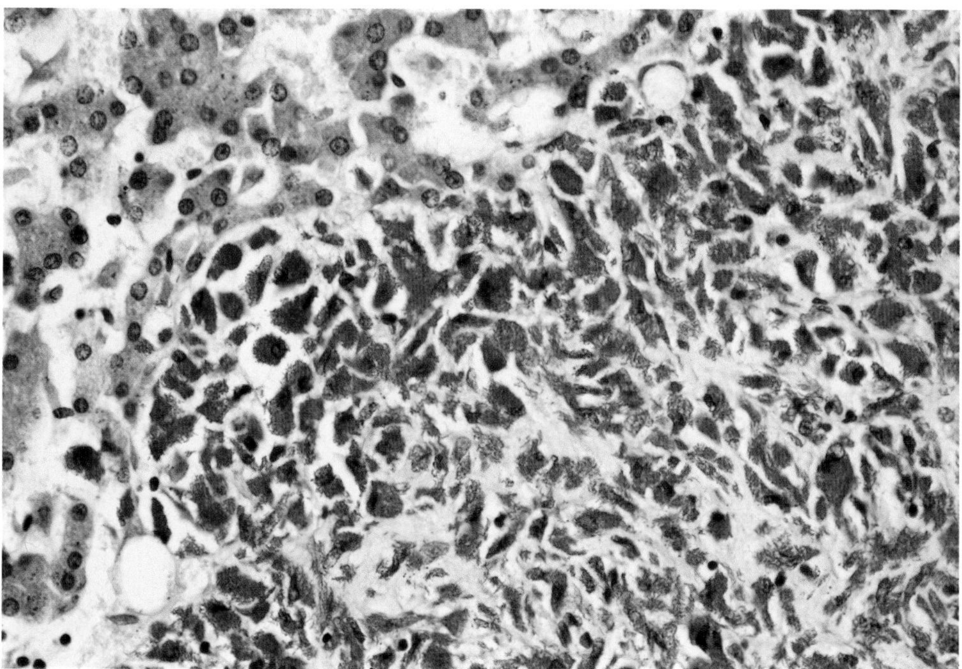

Figure 15.7 *Mycobacterium avium-intracellulare in AIDS.* Abundant macrophages with densely packed mycobacteria are present within a granuloma. Individual organisms are best seen in the centre of the field. Post mortem liver, Ziehl-Neelsen.

are those of large duct obstruction. Cryptosporidia and microsporidia are best identified in aspirates obtained at endoscopy, duodenal biopsies, or post mortem tissue samples of the major bile ducts.[94–96]

Peliosis hepatis

Peliosis hepatis[99,107,108] in AIDS has been postulated to be due to endothelial damage by HIV-1 infection.[88] Alternatively, **bacillary peliosis hepatis** may develop as a consequence of hepatic infection by the gram-negative bacillus *Bartonella henselae*.[109–112] Smudge-like or granular pink-to-purple material associated with a myxoid stroma is seen within dilated vascular spaces (Fig. 15.8) and the Warthin-Starry stain shows clumped bacilli in these areas.

Lymphomas

Lymphomas involve the liver as nodular masses or portal tract infiltrates (see Fig. 7.3) and are high-grade large cell, immunoblastic and Burkitt types.[113,114]

Chronic hepatitis

AIDS patients have many of the same risk factors for infection by hepatitis viruses and serum markers of prior infection or active viral hepatitis are often present. While the liver biopsy lesions of **chronic hepatitis B, C and delta** can vary considerably in persons infected with HIV,[115,116] it is now recognised that HIV infection may exert an adverse effect.[117–119] Fulminant hepatitis may occur[120] and in drug addicts, a

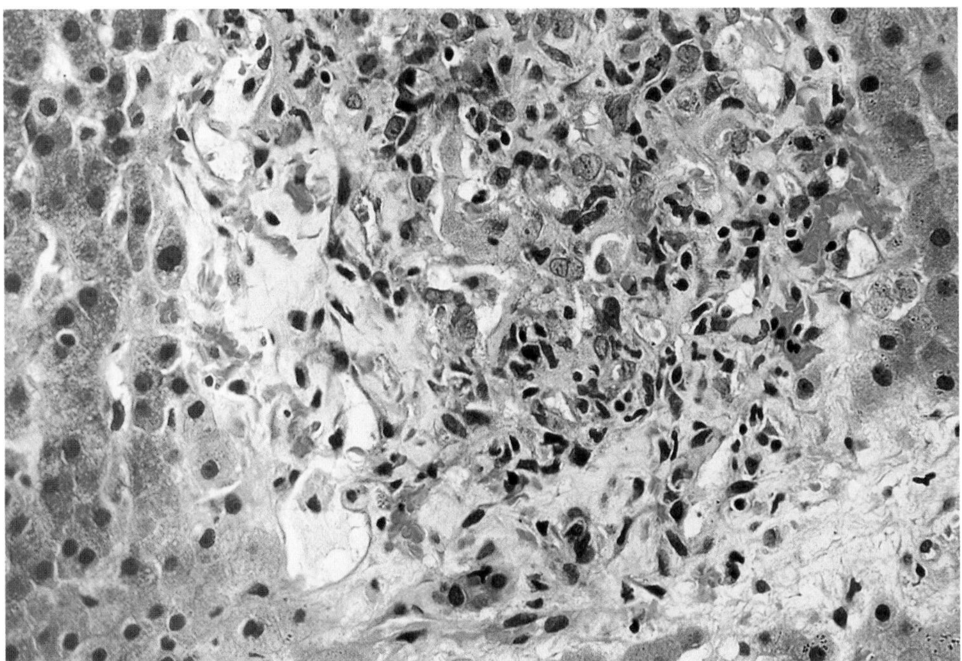

Figure 15.8 *Bacillary peliosis in AIDS*. The portal tract is expanded by dilated blood vessels (left and right), chronic inflammatory cells and pink-grey smudge-like material (arrow) which contains bacilli. (Needle biopsy, H&E).

propensity for more severe chronic hepatitis with progression to cirrhosis has been noted.[121]

Steatosis and other changes

Steatosis is common and may be periportal (see Fig. 7.3). Severe macrovesicular or microvesicular fat is cause for concern because this may reflect toxicity of anti-viral medications[82,83,122,123] and can be associated with liver failure.[124] **Siderosis** of Kupffer cells is related to transfusion or viraemia-associated erythrophagocytosis. In some cases, **non-specific changes** consisting of sparse portal or acinar lymphocytic inflammation with scattered acidophil bodies are seen, with no apparent aetiology.

Other lesions reported include **nodular regenerative hyperplasia**,[125] **amyloidosis**[126] and **hypertrophied perisinusoidal stellate (Ito) cells** containing numerous lipid droplets.[127] In children, **giant-cell hepatitis**,[89,128] **chronic hepatitis** of uncertain cause[129] and **primary leiomyosarcoma**[130] are described.

RICKETTSIAL, BACTERIAL AND FUNGAL INFECTIONS

Q fever

In Q fever, due to infection with *Coxiella burnetii*, liver involvement is common although only a few patients present clinically with liver disease. Histological changes include focal necrosis, non-specific inflammation and fatty change. The most characteristic lesion is the **fibrin-ring granuloma**[33–39] (Fig. 15.3), a granulomatous lesion also seen in several other infections and in some patients taking allopurinol.[40] Atypical lesions without annular arrangement or a central clear area but containing irregular fibrin strands are also found, as are non-specific granulomas without fibrin. In chronic Q fever, progressive fibrosis and cirrhosis have been reported.[131]

Brucellosis

In most patients with brucellosis, liver biopsy shows non-specific reactive changes comprising sinusoidal-cell hypertrophy, portal inflammation and focal necrosis. Non-necrotising granulomas, often small and located within the lobules, are more commonly found in the acute phase of the infection.[132]

Typhoid fever

Liver involvement is uncommon, but most patients with 'typhoid hepatitis' are jaundiced.[133] Liver biopsy shows a mild hepatitis with marked hyperplasia of mononuclear phagocytes and lymphocytoid cells in sinusoids.[134] Characteristic granuloma-like collections of mononuclear cells, the typhoid nodules, are described.[135] Other features include fatty change and portal inflammation.[133,136]

Cat scratch disease

Infection by a short gram-negative rod, *Bartonella henselae*, typically produces pyrexia and regional lymphadenopathy in children. Rarely, dissemination to the liver results in hepatic **granulomas with central stellate microabscesses** surrounded by palisaded macrophages, lymphocytes and an outer layer of fibroblasts.[137] The Warthin-Starry stain is used to identify the organisms.

Tuberculosis

Tuberculous lesions are present in the liver either as part of a generalised infection[138] or, less often, in the hepatobiliary form of the disease.[139] A normal chest X-ray does not exclude the diagnosis.[140] Granulomas are found randomly scattered in the parenchyma and also in the portal tracts. They range from small accumulations of macrophage-like cells to well-developed, large epithelioid-cell nodules with Langhans giant cells (Fig. 15.9). Central necrosis may or may not be present and its absence does not exclude the diagnosis. Extensive necrosis (Fig. 15.10) is more likely to be seen when there are widely disseminated granulomas in the liver. Mycobacteria are seen in a minority of biopsies. Acute lesions contain little reticulin, while chronic ones undergo scarring. Remaining liver tissue shows non-specific reactive features and fatty change. Patients with AIDS sometimes have mycobacterial infection without typical granulomas, or may form tuberculous abscesses.[141] In all patients in

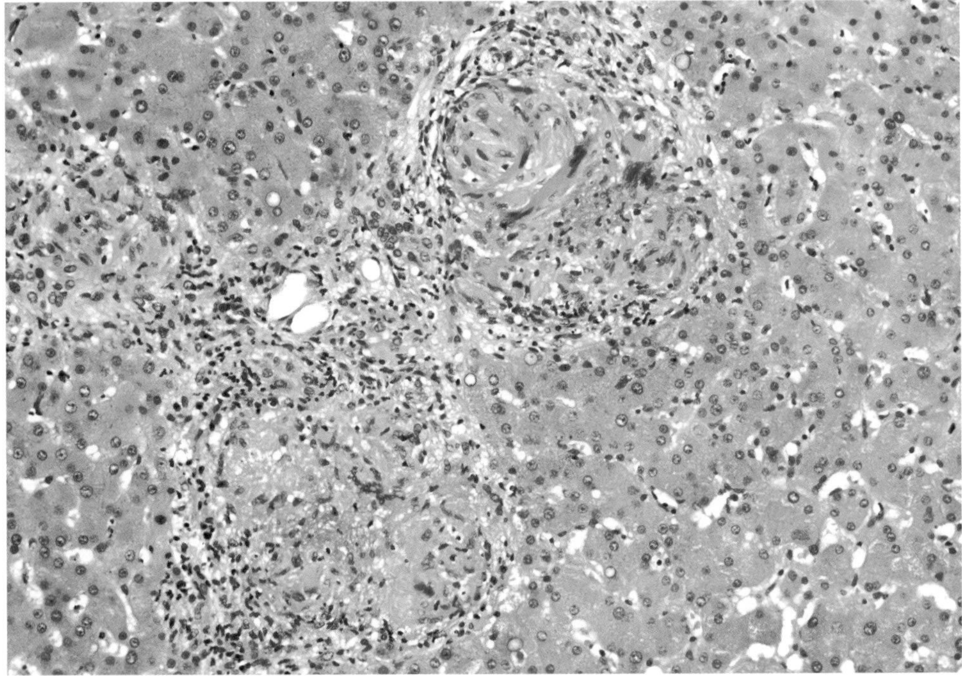

Figure 15.9 *Tuberculosis.* Three parenchymal granulomas abut a portal tract. Multinucleated giant cells are visible in two of the granulomas. (Needle biopsy, H&E).

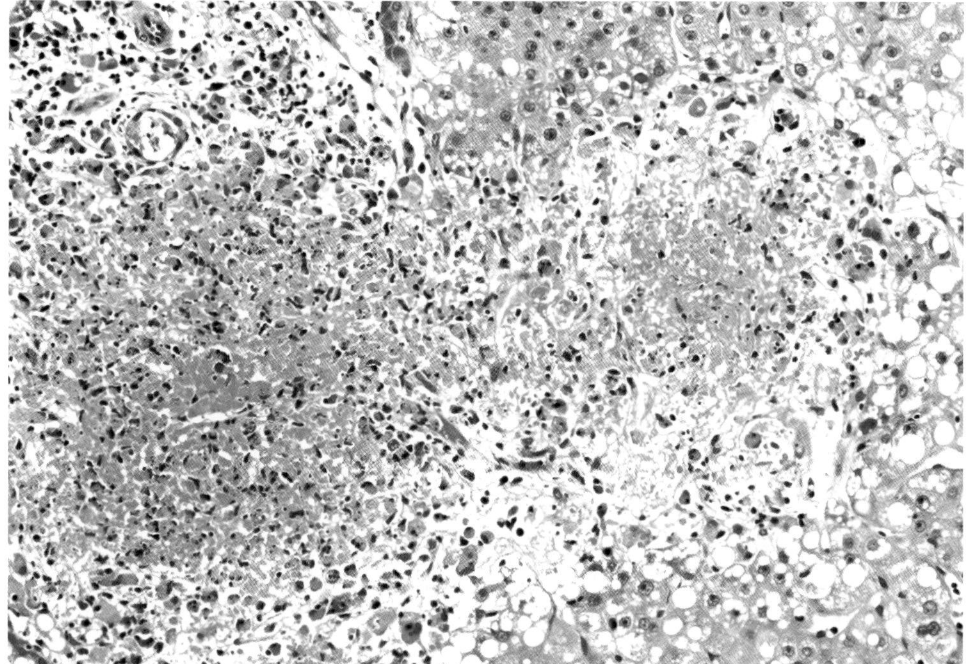

Figure 15.10 *Tuberculosis*. There is extensive necrosis with little residual evidence of granulomas. (Needle biopsy, H&E).

whom tuberculosis is suspected, part of the liver biopsy specimen should be cultured. Polymerase chain reaction studies may also be performed on biopsy samples.[142] Lesions similar to those of tuberculosis have been reported in patients given BCG immunotherapy.[143–146]

Leprosy

In lepromatous leprosy specific granuloma-like lesions composed of foam cells are found in the liver and often contain acid-fast bacilli.[147] Organisms are also seen in Kupffer cells. Epithelioid-cell granulomas of tuberculoid type, rare in lepromatous leprosy, are found in the livers of some patients with the tuberculoid form of the disease. Either type of granuloma is seen in borderline leprosy.[148]

Spirochaetal infection

Syphilis

In congenital syphilis, there is widespread fibrosis separating small groups of hepatocytes and spirochaetes are numerous. In early infections in adults, liver biopsies are normal or show non-specific changes.[149] Spirochaetes may be demonstrable histologically. In patients with secondary syphilis and jaundice or abnormal liver function tests, there is a variable degree of focal parenchymal inflammation, granuloma formation,[150] hepatocellular necrosis and portal inflammation. The portal reaction may mimic that of biliary obstruction,[151] and there may be inflammation of bile-duct epithelium as well as of the walls of small arteries and veins.[152,153] Because patients with syphilis often have other infections as well, lesions cannot always be confidently attributed to the syphilis itself.[154] The typical lesion of tertiary syphilis is the gumma, an area of necrosis surrounded by granulomatous tissue in which there is endarteritis. Healing is by fibrosis.

Leptospirosis

Most studies of the pathology of leptospirosis have dealt with autopsy material, in which disorganisation of liver-cell plates is a prominent feature. This is usually absent from liver biopsies.[155] Hepatocytes are swollen, especially in perivenular areas and there is an increase in mitotic figures. A few apoptotic bodies and fat vacuoles may be seen. Kupffer cells are prominent and there is a mild mononuclear-cell infiltrate in portal tracts. Cholestasis is common and may persist after resolution of the other changes.[156] The diagnosis can be confirmed by demonstrating leptospiral antigen in paraffin sections by immunocytochemistry.[157]

Lyme disease

Hepatomegaly, elevated serum aminotransferase activity and biopsy features resembling viral hepatitis may be seen in patients infected with the tick-borne spirochaete *Borrelia burgdorferi*.[158] Liver-cell ballooning and numerous mitoses are accompanied by sinusoidal inflammation (hyperplastic Kupffer cells, lymphocytes, plasma cells and neutrophilic leucocytes). The organism can be identified in liver tissue by Dieterle silver stain.

Candidiasis

The most common hepatic manifestations of candidiasis in immunocompromised hosts are **microabscesses** and **granulomas**.[159,160] The more acute lesions show microabscess formation with central necrosis, visible on gross examination as 1 to 2 mm yellow-white nodules. Yeasts and pseudohyphae can be seen in some, but not all, cases with diastase-PAS and Gomori methenamine silver stains. The predominantly neutrophilic infiltrates are replaced by epithelioid histiocytes and granulomas as the lesions evolve, sometimes surrounded by reactive fibrosis. Candidiasis is most often diagnosed post mortem, but should be suspected in the presence of fever, abdominal symptoms and elevated serum alkaline phosphatase activity. Systemic candidiasis has been noted as an important cause of mortality in patients with perivenular or multilobular hepatic necrosis due to **exertional heat-stroke**.[161]

Histoplasmosis

Hepatomegaly is common in disseminated histoplasmosis due to *Histoplasma capsulatum*. The disease is very occasionally seen in countries where it is not endemic.[162] The liver may rarely be the only organ clinically involved.[163] Liver biopsy shows non-specific inflammation as well as granulomas which may be mistaken for the lesions of tuberculosis.[164,165] The organisms may be scanty or abundant and are found in Kupffer cells and granulomas. They are round or oval, 1–5 μm across and have a capsule and central chromatin mass. Diastase-PAS and other stains for fungi can be used for their demonstration and differentiation from Leishman-Donovan bodies; the latter are PAS-negative in tissues.[166] Disseminated infection with *H. duboisii*, seen in Africa, also involves the liver. Nodular lesions contain the much larger and easily demonstrable organisms.[167]

Fibrous, calcified and even bony nodules are sometimes found in and deep to the liver capsule in long-standing histoplasmosis. The nodules, 1–3 mm in diameter, may have a necrotic core surrounded by granulomatous tissue and the organism is demonstrable in some instances.[168]

The liver in sepsis

Hepatic changes in sepsis are the result of infection of the liver itself, of circulating toxins, of ischaemia or of a combination of these factors. In many patients, the exact cause cannot be established.

Infective lesions include **liver abscess** and **bacterial cholangitis**. Less commonly, infection produces a diffuse bacterial hepatitis in which bacterial colonisation of the liver is associated with portal inflammation.[169] Infection in areas drained by the portal venous system can give rise to **pylephlebitis** (see Fig. 12.3). Rarely, cholangiographic and histologic features resembling primary sclerosing cholangitis develop in sepsis, possibly related to ischaemic damage to large ducts.[170] Post mortem liver sections from septic patients may show neutrophils aggregated within sinusoids and in sparse numbers dispersed throughout the connective tissue of portal tracts.

Patients with extrahepatic sepsis are often jaundiced, especially when the infection is due to gram-negative organisms.[171] Three histological patterns have been described in such patients. The commonest is **canalicular cholestasis**, most severe in perivenular areas. This is associated with various degrees of Kupffer-cell activation, fatty change and portal inflammation, but usually little or no hepatocellular necrosis.[172]

The second pattern is one of **ductular cholestasis and inflammation**.[171,173] Bile ductular structures and canals of Hering at the margins of portal tracts are dilated and filled with bile, often in the form of dense, highly pigmented deposits and neutrophils are seen within and around the affected ductules (Fig. 15.11). Perivenular cholestasis is usually present. Periportal canalicular bile is also sometimes present. These changes are not seen in uncomplicated bile-duct obstruction. They are common in the terminal stages of fatal acute or chronic liver disease complicated by sepsis. Damage to bile-duct epithelium has been reported,[174] but in most instances

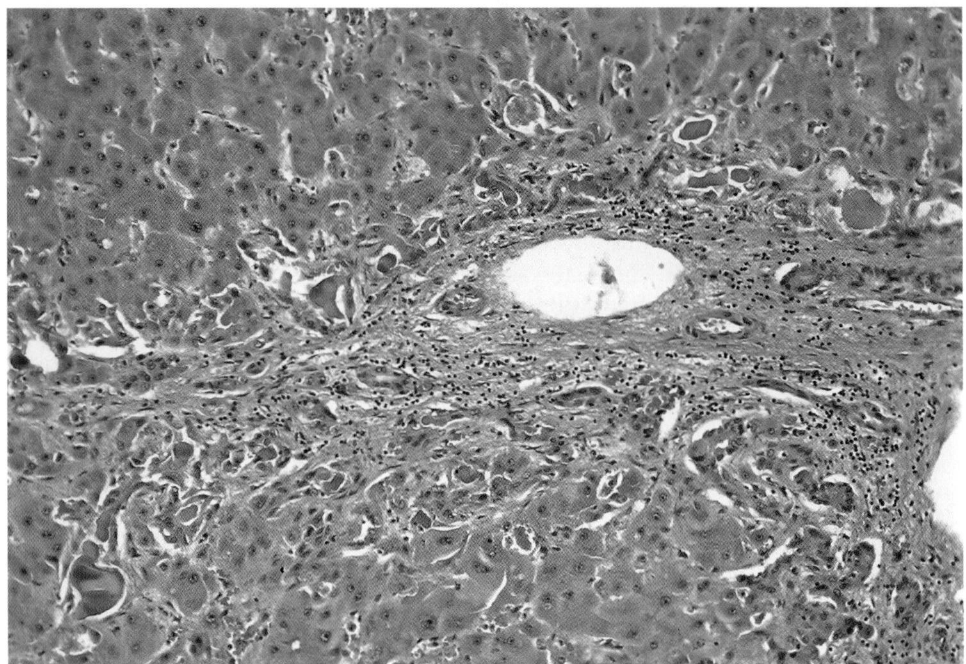

Figure 15.11 *Bile ductular cholestasis in sepsis.* Proliferated bile ductules at the edge of the portal tract contain inspissated bile. The patient died of septicaemia. (Post-mortem liver, H&E).

the interlobular bile ducts are not affected. Patients with the ductular cholestasis pattern have a disproportionately elevated serum bilirubin compared to alkaline phosphatase and aminotransferases.[175] Because of its dire implications, this biopsy finding should be communicated rapidly to the clinician and sepsis should be investigated.

The third pattern is **non-bacterial cholangitis**, seen in the **toxic shock syndrome**.[176] The histological features are similar to those of bacterial cholangitis, but the biliary tree is anatomically normal and the lesion is attributed to a circulating staphylococcal toxin rather than to bacteraemia. In many, but not all patients, the underlying lesion is a staphylococcal vaginitis associated with the use of tampons.

PARASITIC DISEASES

Toxoplasmosis

Toxoplasma gondii is occasionally responsible for neonatal liver injury. In adults, hepatic changes include extensive lymphocytic infiltration of sinusoids, evidence of mild liver-cell damage and granuloma formation.[10,177] Trophozoites may be seen within necrotic hepatocytes and can be identified by specific immunocytochemical methods.[178,179]

Malaria

In non-immune patients with malaria, there is hypertrophy of Kupffer cells and these contain malarial pigment (haemozoin) in the form of fine, dark-brown or black pigment granules (Fig. 15.12). In acute malaria due to *Plasmodium falciparum* they also contain erythrocytes, parasites and iron. Malarial pigment closely resembles schistosomal pigment. It often gives pin-point birefringence and, like formalin pigment, is soluble in alcoholic picric acid. This distinguishes it from carbon, with which it may be confused.[180] Following an attack of malaria the pigment clears from the lobules but can be found in portal macrophages.

The **tropical splenomegaly syndrome** (**hyper-reactive malarial splenomegaly**) probably represents an abnormal immune response of the patient to the malarial parasite.[181] Large numbers of small T-lymphocytes are seen in dilated hepatic sinusoids (Fig. 15.13). Kupffer cells are enlarged but hepatocytes remain normal. Malarial pigment is scanty or absent. The differential histological diagnosis is from leukaemia, hepatitis C virus infection, infectious mononucleosis, cytomegalovirus infection and toxoplasmosis.

Visceral leishmaniasis (kala-azar)

Infection by *Leishmania donovani* produces striking hypertrophy of Kupffer cells and portal macrophages. These cells contain variable, sometimes very large numbers of Leishman-Donovan bodies, easily visible in H&E-stained sections (Fig. 15.14). The

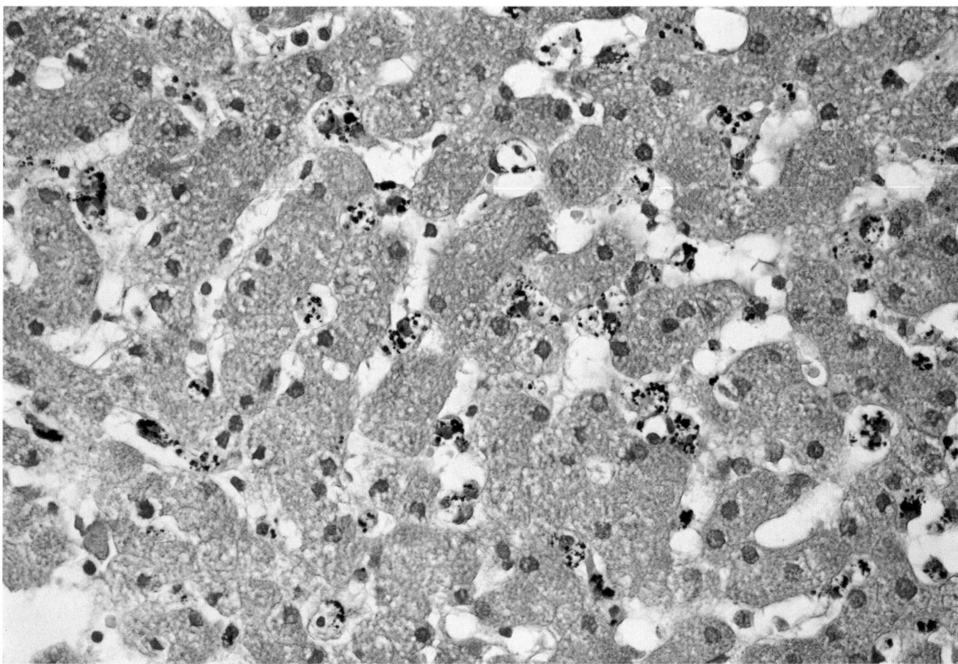

Figure 15.12 *Malaria*. Kupffer cells contain abundant dark granules of malarial pigment. (Needle biopsy, H&E).

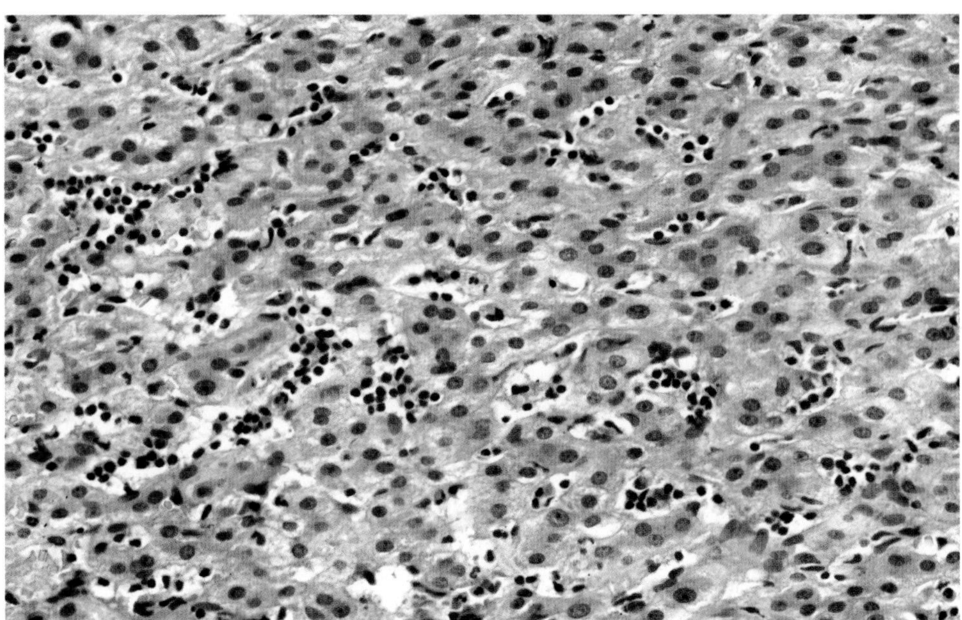

Figure 15.13 *Tropical splenomegaly syndrome (hyper-reactive malarial splenomegaly).* There are groups of lymphocytes in the sinusoids. Kupffer cells are enlarged. Hepatocytes appear normal. (Needle biopsy, H&E).

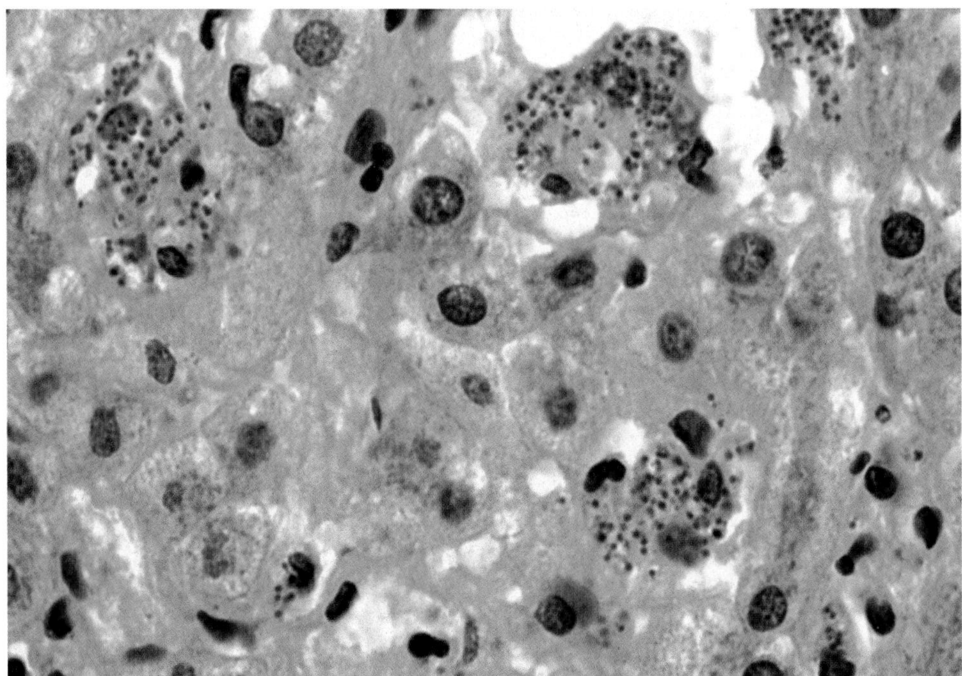

Figure 15.14 *Kala-azar*. There are many Leishman-Donovan bodies within several macrophages, just large enough to give the cells a stippled appearance at this magnification. (Post mortem liver, H&E).

PAS stain after diastase digestion is negative, in contrast to the positive staining obtained with *Histoplasma*. In some patients, the liver contains epithelioid-cell granulomas, which heal by fibrosis.[10,182]

Amoebiasis

In patients with liver abscesses due to *Entamoeba histolytica*,[183] the amoebae may be found at the margins of the lesion or, less often, within the necrotic debris. They may also be seen in the adjacent liver tissue. They are most easily demonstrated by the PAS or Giemsa methods. Organisms may be identified in fine needle aspiration biopsy specimens (Fig. 15.15).

Schistosomiasis

Liver lesions are usually caused by *Schistosoma mansoni* or *S. japonicum* and less commonly by other species.[184] In acute schistosomiasis due to *S. mansoni* the portal tracts are infiltrated by eosinophils, lymphocytes and macrophages. Kupffer cells are enlarged and there is focal hepatocellular necrosis. Granulomas around ova are rare.[185]

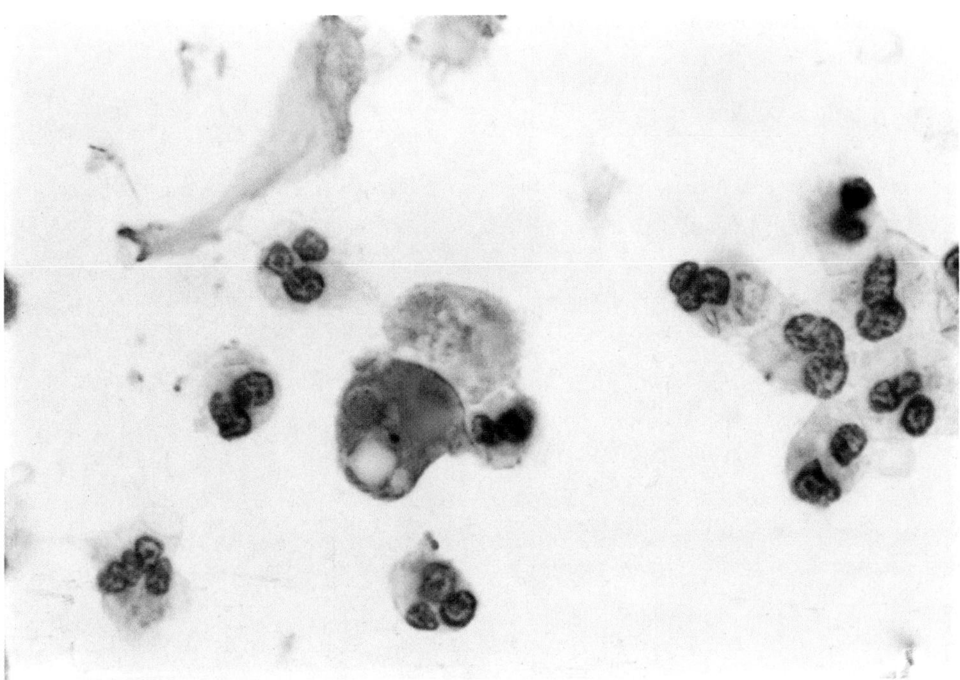

Figure 15.15 *Amoebic abscess.* A trophozoite of *Entamoeba* histolytica is present in this fine needle aspiration biopsy sample, with a round nucleus above several cytoplasmic glycogen vacuoles. Adjacent cells are neutrophilic leucocytes. Papanicolaou. (Figure kindly provided by Dr Alastair Deery, London).

More commonly schistosomiasis is chronic. Ova, initially containing live miracidia, are trapped in portal tracts where they excite a granulomatous reaction. This is composed of epithelioid cells, multinucleated giant cells, eosinophils and lymphocytes (Fig. 15.16). Healing is by fibrosis. When ova are scanty and granulomas are no longer seen, step sections may need to be searched. Ziehl-Neelsen staining is then helpful, because the ova of species other than *S. haematobium* are acid-fast.[186] Schistosomal pigment, found in portal tracts in some patients with chronic or past schistosomiasis, is a fine dark granular material closely resembling malarial pigment.

There are lesions in portal-vein branches of all sizes.[185] The smallest contain ova and granulomas. Angiomatoids, wide irregular thin-walled vascular channels, are characteristically found in fibrotic and enlarged portal tracts. Medium-sized veins show intimal thickening which may be eccentric and polypoid and in large veins there are thrombi and adult worms. In the course of portal scarring, isolated smooth muscle cells may become separated from the portal vein wall and entrapped in fibrous tissue, a helpful diagnostic feature.[187] Diffuse hyaline thickening and tortuosity of veins with surrounding fibrosis constitute 'clay pipestem fibrosis' in which hepatic artery branches and bile ducts are preserved[187] (Fig. 15.17).

Lobular changes are usually slight, but sinusoidal lining cells are prominent and there is an increase in fibre within the space of Disse.[188,189] Portal tract lymphocytic infiltrates and interface hepatitis are likely to reflect the presence of chronic hepatitis, as hepatitis B virus infection is increased in patients with hepatosplenic schistosomiasis,[190,191] as is hepatitis C.

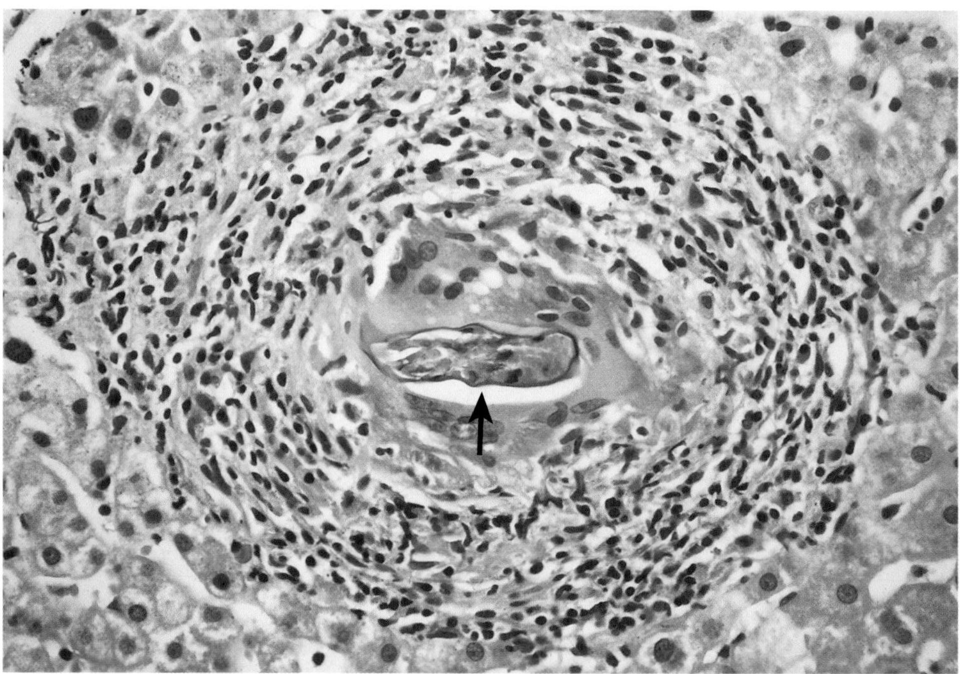

Figure 15.16 *Schistosomiasis*. An ovum (arrow) surrounded by giant cells is seen at the centre of a granuloma. The infiltrate is rich in eosinophil leucocytes. (Needle biopsy, H&E).

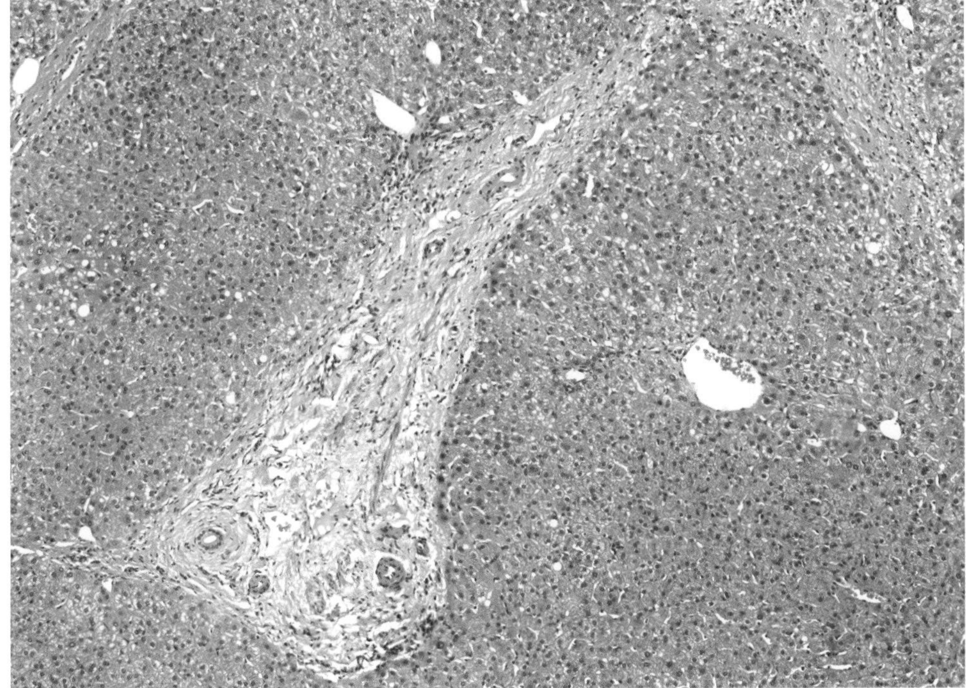

Figure 15.17 *Schistosomiasis*. Serpiginous septa contain many small blood vessels in this example of 'pipestem' fibrosis. (Wedge biopsy, H&E).

Liver flukes

Invasion of the biliary tree by the trematodes *Clonorchis sinensis* (the Chinese liver fluke), *Opisthorchis viverrini* and *O. felineus* is followed by proliferation of duct-like structures around the large bile ducts. The duct epithelium may undergo goblet-cell metaplasia.[192] Smaller ducts are surrounded by an eosinophil-rich infiltrate. Complications include bile-duct obstruction, infection, portal fibrosis and hypertension and bile-duct carcinoma.[193] Infestation may present several years after the patient has left an endemic area.[194]

The liver fluke *Fasciola hepatica* enters the liver from the peritoneal cavity and reaches the biliary tree some weeks later. White nodules are seen on the liver surface at the points of entry and may be mistaken for tumour. Migration tracks extend into the liver. Histologically capsular and subcapsular lesions are composed of serpiginous areas of necrosis containing eosinophils and Charcot-Leyden crystals and bordered by palisaded histiocytes (Fig. 15.18).[195] Elsewhere in the liver, portal tracts are infiltrated with eosinophils. The biliary phase of the infestation is marked by cholangitis with rather less bile-duct hyperplasia than in *Clonorchis* or *Opisthorchis* infections and both arterial and venous thrombosis. Features of bile-duct obstruction, periductal fibrosis and an ovum within a granuloma have also been reported.[196]

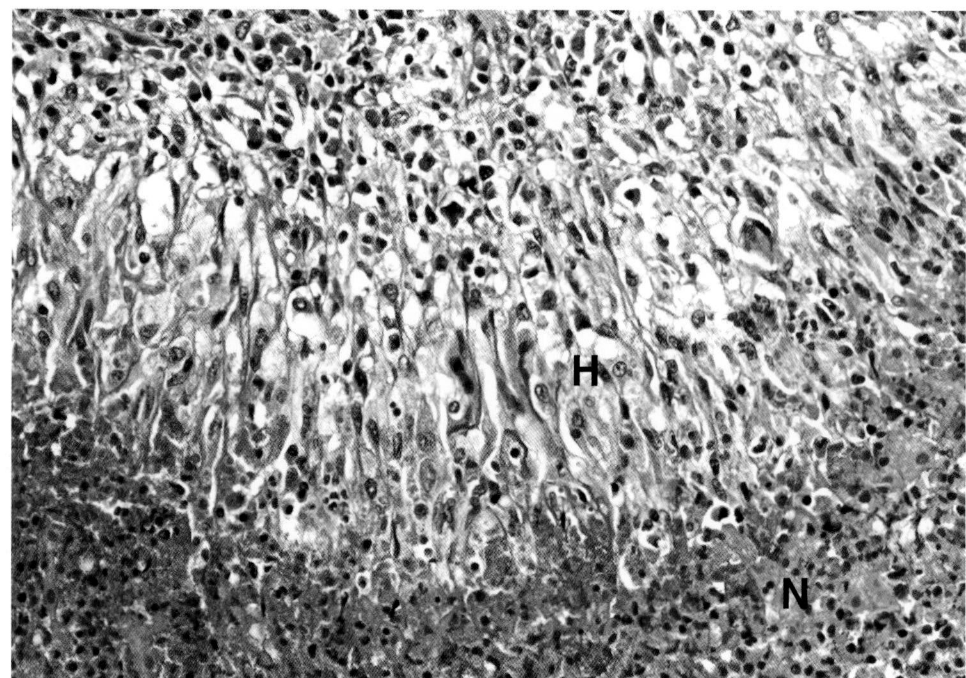

Figure 15.18 *Fascioliasis*. Part of a nodule near the surface of the liver. A central area of necrosis (N) filled with leucocytes is bordered by palisaded histiocytes (H). (Wedge biopsy, H&E).

Ascariasis

Focal areas of necrosis with infiltration by eosinophils and neutrophils are seen in the migratory phase, when larvae travel to the lungs via the liver. Adult worms may enter the biliary tree from the duodenum, giving rise to bile-duct obstruction, cholangitis and abscess formation.[186]

Larval diseases

In several parasitic diseases with larval stages, including infestation by *Toxocara*, the larvae may reach the liver and give rise to eosinophil-rich abscesses or granulomas. Larvae are sometimes seen within these lesions.[10] White capsular and subcapsular liver nodules composed of mature fibrous tissue with calcification and few infiltrating cells surround larval remnants in long-standing disease due to *Toxocara* or to arthropod larvae.[197]

Patients with **coeliac disease** sometimes have evidence of liver injury.[198] Lesions reported range from portal inflammation and fatty liver to chronic hepatitis, cirrhosis and hepatocellular carcinoma.[199] Isolated cases of coeliac disease associated with primary biliary cirrhosis,[200–202] primary sclerosing cholangitis[203] and autoimmune cholangitis[204] are also described. In **Whipple's disease** the characteristic foamy PAS-positive macrophages may be found in the liver[205] and epithelioid-cell granulomas have been reported.[206] Granulomas, associated with a heavy infiltration by eosinophils, have also been described in **eosinophilic gastroenteritis**.[207]

Chronic inflammatory bowel disease

The spectrum of liver lesions is generally similar in ulcerative colitis and Crohn's disease. In Crohn's disease, serious hepatic complications such as sclerosing cholangitis are much less common and there may be granulomas in the liver[208] or amyloid deposition.[209] Gallstones are more common in Crohn's disease than in the general population. In both Crohn's disease and ulcerative colitis, malnutrition, anaemia and toxaemia can lead to steatosis.[210]

A minority of patients with ulcerative colitis has persistent abnormalities of liver function tests.[211] Careful examination including cholangiography shows that most of these patients have primary sclerosing cholangitis, the pathology of which has already been described in detail earlier. Bile-duct carcinoma, sometimes accompanied by diffuse dysplasia of biliary epithelium[212,213] (see Fig. 5.18), is increased in patients with ulcerative colitis, probably reflecting underlying sclerosing cholangitis.[214,215] Portal inflammatory lesions with or without periductal fibrosis in ulcerative colitis have occasioned use of the term 'pericholangitis'. However, patients with such portal inflammation have largely been shown to have typical primary sclerosing cholangitis[216] or its small-duct variant.[217] Furthermore, some examples of so-called pericholangitis probably represent a non-specific inflammatory response to the colitis. The term pericholangitis should therefore be discarded.[217] While liver biopsies from patients with ulcerative colitis may show features of chronic hepatitis, this may be due to intercurrent viral hepatitis (for example, following blood transfusion). However, it should be noted that interface hepatitis is also common in primary sclerosing cholangitis. From a practical point of view, it therefore seems wise to consider the possibility of sclerosing cholangitis in all patients with ulcerative colitis and chronic liver disease.

HAEMATOLOGICAL DISORDERS AND THE LIVER

One of the most common findings in liver biopsies from patients with haematological disorders is diffuse **Kupffer cell siderosis**, usually reflecting prior transfusion (see Ch. 14). In **reactive haemophagocytic syndrome**,[218,219] diffuse

Kupffer cell hyperplasia with siderosis and phagocytosis of erythrocytes may be seen in patients with systemic infections, disseminated carcinoma, leukaemia and lymphoma. Phagocytosed red blood cells are well demonstrated on chromotrope aniline blue stain and the histiocytes stain much less intensely on diastase-PAS than those engaged in necrotizing processes such as viral hepatitis. Hepatic involvement by leukaemias and lymphomas is discussed in Chapter 11, the effects of thrombosis and sickle-cell disease in Chapter 12 and graft-versus-host disease following bone marrow transplantation in Chapter 16.

Haemophilia

Hepatitis viruses are readily transmitted in blood products and hepatitis is therefore common in patients with haemophilia.[220–223] Hepatitis C virus and possibly other putative non-A, non-E hepatitis viruses are the most important agents involved, but markers of infection with hepatitis B virus are also present in some patients. Liver histopathology is most often that of a mild chronic hepatitis;[223] cirrhosis is infrequent. The complications of infection by human immunodeficiency virus-1 (HIV-1) and AIDS have been seen in some haemophiliacs who received HIV-1-contaminated blood products prior to mandated screening for the virus which was initiated in the 1980s.

Extramedullary haemopoiesis

Haemopoiesis in the liver sinusoids is normal in fetal and neonatal life. In adults it is seen mainly in the myeloproliferative disorders and when bone marrow is invaded by tumours. Foci of haemopoiesis may also be seen in the congested liver of patients with cardiac failure,[224] in transplant livers with perivenular necrosis[225] or in the rare situation of graft-versus-host disease in liver transplant recipients.[226] The sinusoids and spaces of Disse of the enlarged liver contain discrete clumps of haemopoietic cells (Fig. 15.19) and there are similar cells in portal tracts. Features which distinguish haemopoiesis from the infiltrates of leukaemias, infectious mononucleosis, other infections and the tropical splenomegaly syndrome are the variety of cells in the aggregates and the presence of recognisable marrow cells such as normoblasts and eosinophil myelocytes. Megakaryocytes are commonly seen (Fig. 15.19) and are sometimes the only marrow elements found. Owing to the restraints of space, these cells are more elongated than in a section or smear of bone marrow. In the liver of neonates or stillborn infants with **Down syndrome**, megakaryocytes may be the predominant form of extramedullary haemopoiesis[227,228] and perisinusoidal fibrosis may also be present.[229]

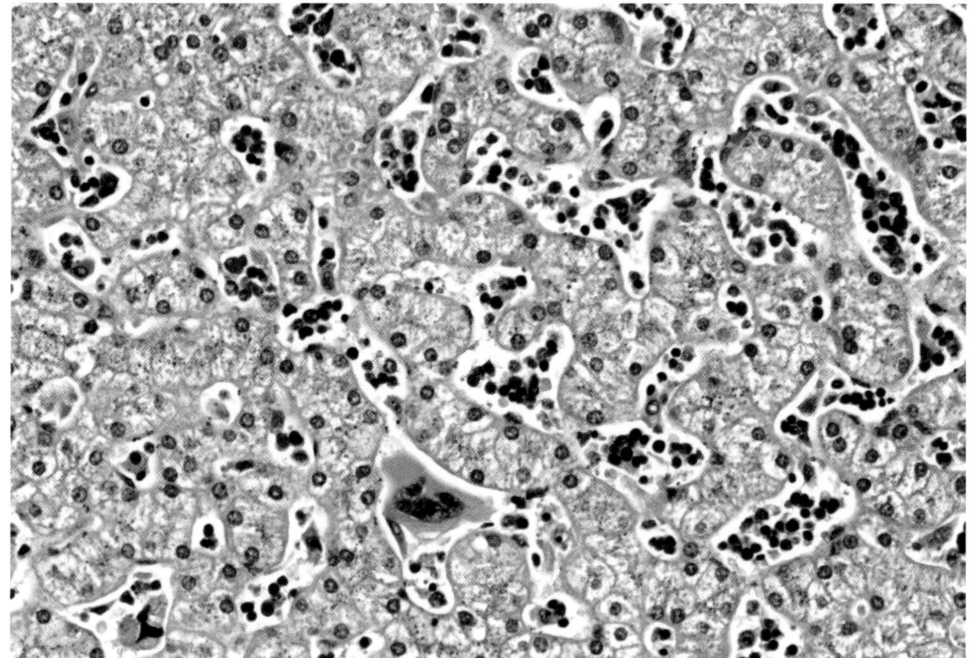

Figure 15.19 *Extramedullary haemopoiesis.* Clumps of haemopoietic cells are seen in the sinusoids, including a megakaryocyte at the bottom of the field. (Needle biopsy, H&E).

THE LIVER IN RHEUMATOID, IMMUNE-COMPLEX AND COLLAGEN DISEASES

Liver pathology is uncommon in this group of diseases, but when present is most often **steatosis**.[230] **Nodular regenerative hyperplasia** is also seen in many connective tissue diseases.[231,232] The presence of multisystem disordered immunity in these conditions may be reflected in some cases by associated immune damage to bile ducts (**primary biliary cirrhosis**) or in the form of hepatic vasculitis.[232]

Polyarteritis nodosa in small hepatic arteries can lead to infarction. Immune complexes containing hepatitis B surface antigen are sometimes demonstrable in vessel walls in this disease.[233] Both hepatitis B and C virus antigen-antibody complexes have been implicated in the pathogenesis of **essential (type II) mixed cryoglobulinaemia**.[234–237] In the **polymyalgia rheumatica-giant cell arteritis syndrome** the liver may contain granulomas.[238,239] Other findings reported include fatty change, venous congestion, non-specific hepatitis and prominent stellate cells.[240,241]

Patients with **rheumatoid arthritis** often have abnormal liver function tests, but liver biopsy more often shows non-specific changes or normal liver than definitive liver disease.[242–244] Amyloidosis or necrotising arteritis may be found and rheumatoid nodules in the liver like those typically found in subcutaneous tissue have been reported.[245] In **Felty's syndrome**[246] (rheumatoid arthritis, leukopenia and splenomegaly), the nodular lesions may be attributable to arteritis involving small intrahepatic vessels.[247]

Scleroderma and the **CRST syndrome** (calcinosis, Raynaud's phenomenon, sclerodactyly and telangiectasia) may be associated with primary biliary cirrhosis.[248,249] Giant, dense mitochondria on electron microscopy, with normal liver or non-specific changes on light microscopy, have been described in patients with **systemic sclerosis.**[250]

The majority of patients with **systemic lupus erythematosus (SLE)** do not have significant liver pathology. However, chronic hepatitis, cirrhosis and hepatic granulomas have been reported in several series.[251,252] Abnormal liver function tests may be present without serious lesions.[253,254] Steatosis, cholestasis, nodular regenerative hyperplasia and necrotizing arteritis involving arteries of 100–400 μm diameter have also been reported.[252] An unusual case of **malacoplakia** involving the liver in a steroid-treated patient with SLE and gram-negative bacterial infection showed aggregates of histiocytes with typical Michaelis-Gutmann bodies.[255] There appears to be no close relationship between systemic lupus and autoimmune (lupoid) hepatitis. A patient with chronic hepatitis and **mixed connective tissue disease** has been reported.[256]

AMYLOIDOSIS AND LIGHT CHAIN DEPOSITION

The liver is commonly involved in systemic amyloidosis. 'Primary' (AL) and reactive (AA) amyloidosis cannot definitively be distinguished by the pattern of liver involvement,[257,258] although sinusoidal deposition in AL and vascular involvement in AA are consistent patterns reported in several studies.[257,259] Histological distinction is made by the resistance of AL amyloid to potassium permanganate before Congo red staining[260] and by immunohistochemistry for immunoglobulin light chains, AA protein, transthyretin and other proteins.[258,261,262] In most patients the amyloid is deposited in portal arteries (Figs 15.20, 15.21) or diffusely in the perisinusoidal space of Disse (Fig. 15.22). The two patterns are often combined. The perisinusoidal deposits compress both the sinusoids and the liver-cell plates, occasionally leading to portal hypertension or to cholestasis.[263–265] Rarely, the amyloid is in the form of globular deposits[266–268] (Fig. 15.23), when it may be difficult to detect in haematoxylin and eosin-stained sections.

Amorphous perisinusoidal and portal deposits somewhat like amyloid are seen when the liver is involved in light chain deposit disease.[269] Immunoglobulin light chains, usually kappa, can be identified immunochemically. The characteristic green birefringence of amyloid after Congo red staining is absent. Occasionally amyloid and light chain deposits are found in the same patient.[270,271]

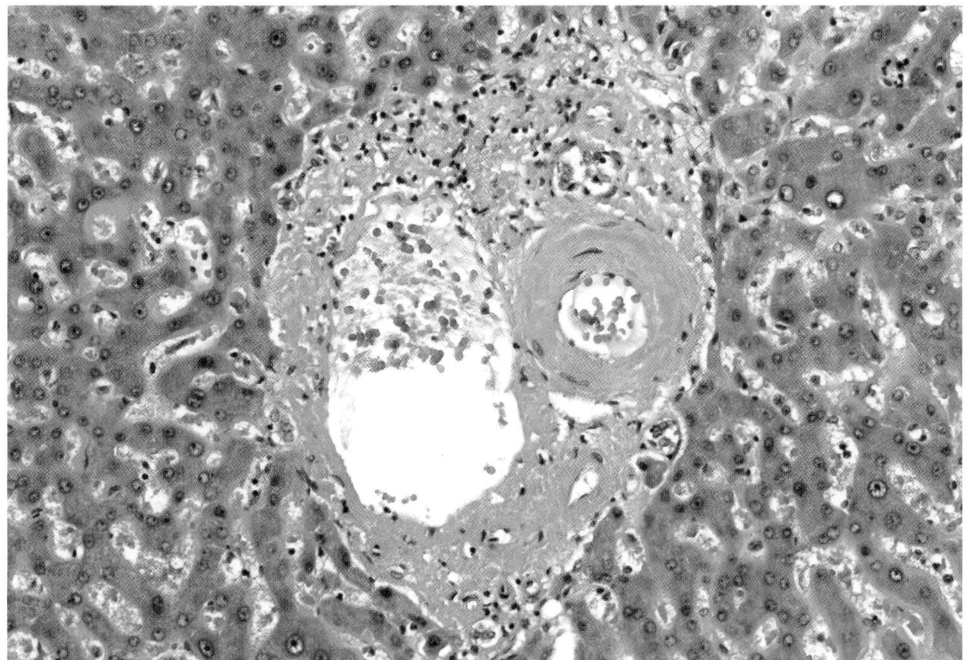

Figure 15.20 *Amyloidosis*. The artery at right within this portal tract is thickened by amyloid deposit. (Needle biopsy, H&E).

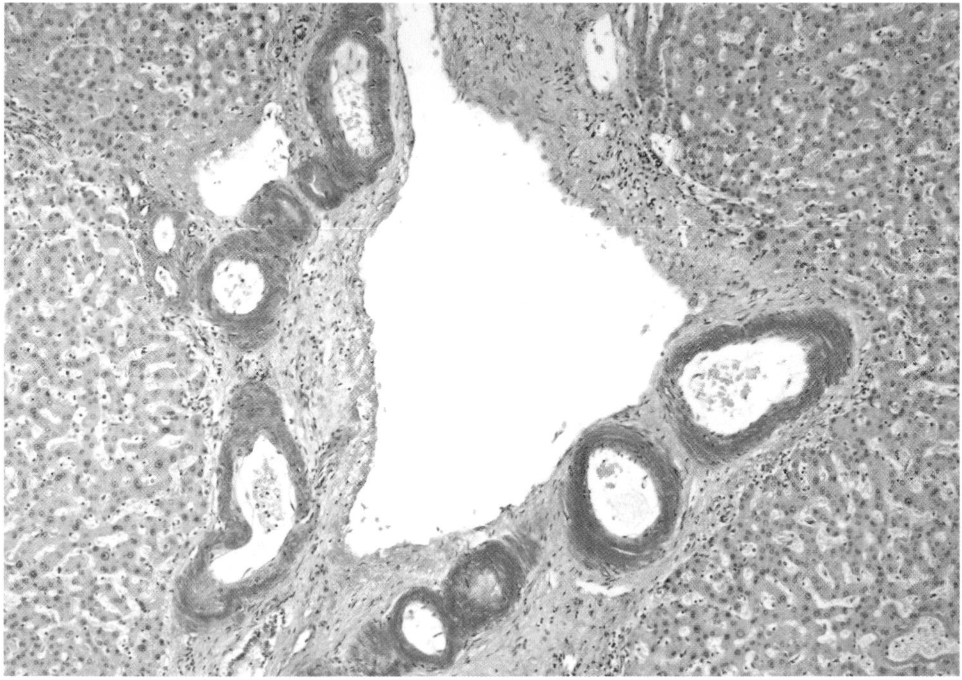

Figure 15.21 *Amyloidosis*. Arterial amyloid deposits in this large calibre portal tract are highlighted by Congo red staining. (Wedge biopsy, Congo red).

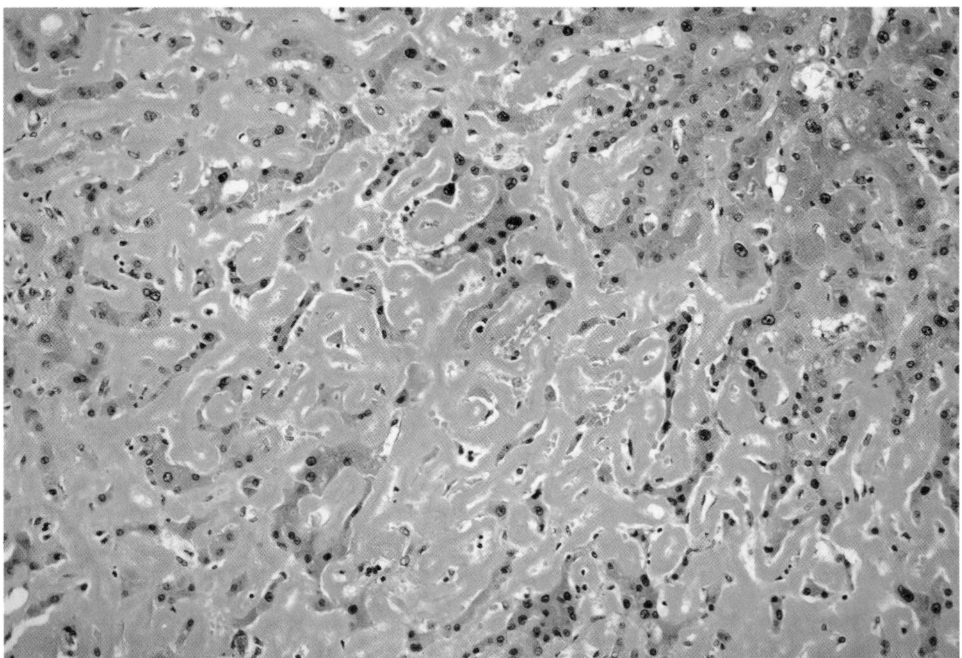

Figure 15.22 *Amyloidosis*. Amyloid has been laid down in the space of Disse. Liver-cell plates have undergone atrophy and sinusoids are narrowed. Cholestasis, an unusual complication of hepatic amyloidosis, is seen at upper right. (Explant liver, H&E).

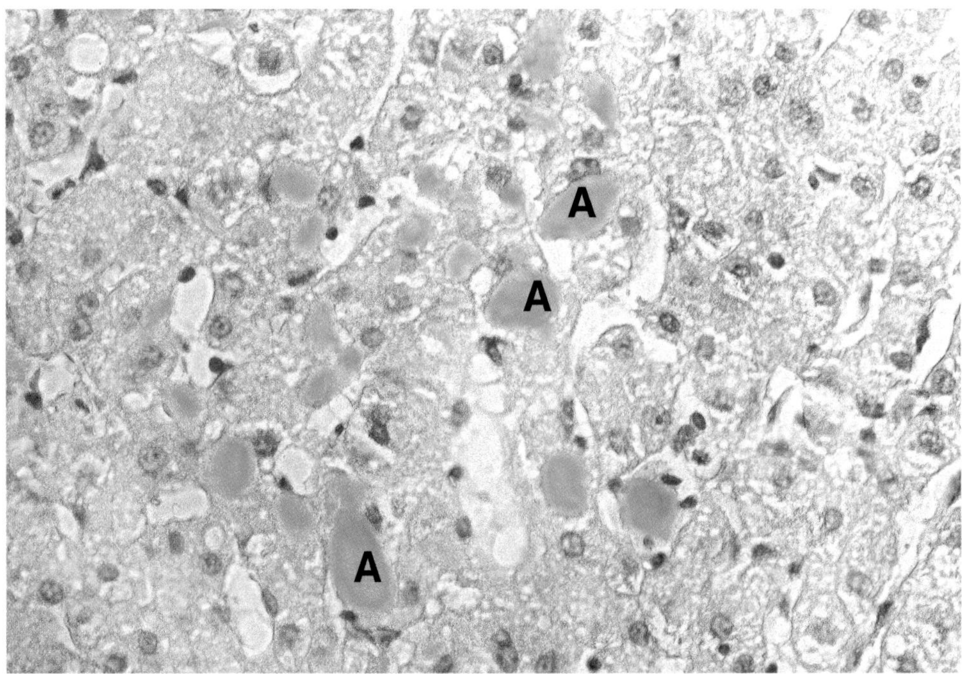

Figure 15.23 *Globular amyloid*. There are rounded deposits of amyloid (A) in the space of Disse. (Needle biopsy, Congo red).

Liver lesions are found in **porphyria cutanea tarda** and **protoporphyria**.[272] Red porphyrin fluorescence can be demonstrated in both diseases using unfixed liver tissue.

In **porphyria cutanea tarda (PCT)** hepatocytes contain needle-shaped birefringent porphyrin crystals, sufficiently water-soluble to make their demonstration difficult or impossible in routinely prepared paraffin sections. They can be seen in unstained paraffin sections, with a ferric ferricyanide reduction stain[273] and in haematoxylin and eosin-stained sections prepared with minimal exposure to water.[274] Fatty change and hepatocellular siderosis are common[275] and lobular clumps of iron- and ceroid-containing macrophages, fat droplets and inflammatory cells may also be present.[276] The role of *HFE* mutations in PCT varies geographically.[277–279] Alcohol contributes to the pathogenesis of PCT and biopsies should be critically examined for alcohol-related injury. More importantly, **chronic hepatitis** and **cirrhosis** are common in patients with PCT and the majority have hepatitis C virus infection.[280–283] The prevalence of chronic hepatitis C in this population is approximately 50%,[284,285] which may also explain the development of **hepatocellular carcinoma**.[272]

In **protoporphyria** (erythropoietic or erythrohepatic protoporphyria) dense, dark brown deposits of poorly soluble protoporphyrin accumulate in the liver (Fig. 15.24). These give a diagnostic red birefringence under polarised light, with a characteristic dark Maltese cross centrally.[286] There may be serious liver damage, with cholestasis, perisinusoidal and perivenular fibrosis and cirrhosis developing in some patients.[287,288]

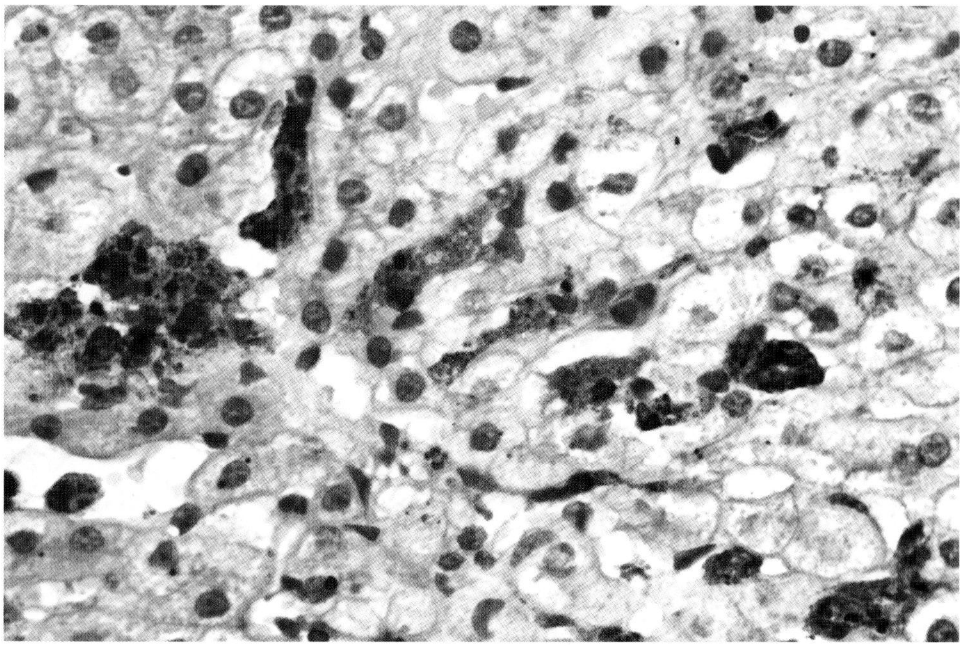

Figure 15.24 *Erythropoietic protoporphyria*. Dense brown protoporphyrin deposits are seen within sinusoids. (Needle biopsy, H&E).

NON-SPECIFIC REACTIVE CHANGES

A variety of changes including portal and lobular inflammation, fat accumulation and Kupffer-cell hypertrophy is seen in extrahepatic conditions, especially febrile, inflammatory or widespread neoplastic diseases. Focal hepatocellular necroses may be found in the parenchyma. The distinction of these reactive changes from a mild form of chronic hepatitis or from residual acute hepatitis requires clinical information. The latter may sometimes be suspected from a predominantly perivenular location of inflammation and liver-cell loss. Reactive changes near space-occupying lesions such as metastatic tumours are illustrated in Fig. 1.5.

THE LIVER IN PREGNANCY

In normal pregnancy there are no specific light microscopic findings in the liver. Electron microscopic changes reported in late pregnancy include giant mitochondria with paracrystalline inclusions, increase in the number of peroxisomes and proliferation of smooth endoplasmic reticulum.[289]

Liver disease in pregnancy is rare and falls into three categories:[290]

1 **Liver disease unique to pregnancy**. The four conditions included in this category[291] are **acute fatty liver of pregnancy (AFLP), pre-eclampsia/eclampsia**, the **HELLP syndrome (haemolysis, elevated liver enzymes and low platelets)** and **intrahepatic cholestasis of pregnancy (ICP)**.
2 **Intercurrent liver disease during pregnancy**. Viral hepatitis and cholelithiasis are examples. Hepatocellular carcinoma, including the fibrolamellar variety,[292] occurs rarely. **Viral hepatitis** is the most common form of liver disease encountered in pregnancy.
3 **Pre-existing liver disease in the pregnant patient**. Chronic hepatitis B viral infection and autoimmune hepatitis with or without cirrhosis are examples of this category.

Jaundice and elevated serum aminotransferases are important aspects of the clinical presentation of liver disease in pregnancy. The following discussion is limited to those diseases unique to pregnancy.

Acute fatty liver of pregnancy

This uncommon and serious complication of pregnancy develops in the last weeks of gestation.[290,293,294] Steatosis involves the greater part of each lobule, usually leaving a thin and incomplete rim of normal hepatocytes around the portal tracts.[295,296] The fat is mainly in the form of fine droplets, as in Reye's syndrome and other examples of microvesicular steatosis.[297] Large fat vacuoles of the kind seen in alcoholic liver disease are scanty and the cause of the hepatocellular swelling and pallor may not be readily apparent on examination of paraffin sections (Fig. 15.25). PAS and trichrome stains are sometimes more helpful than H&E for identifying the small fat vacuoles.

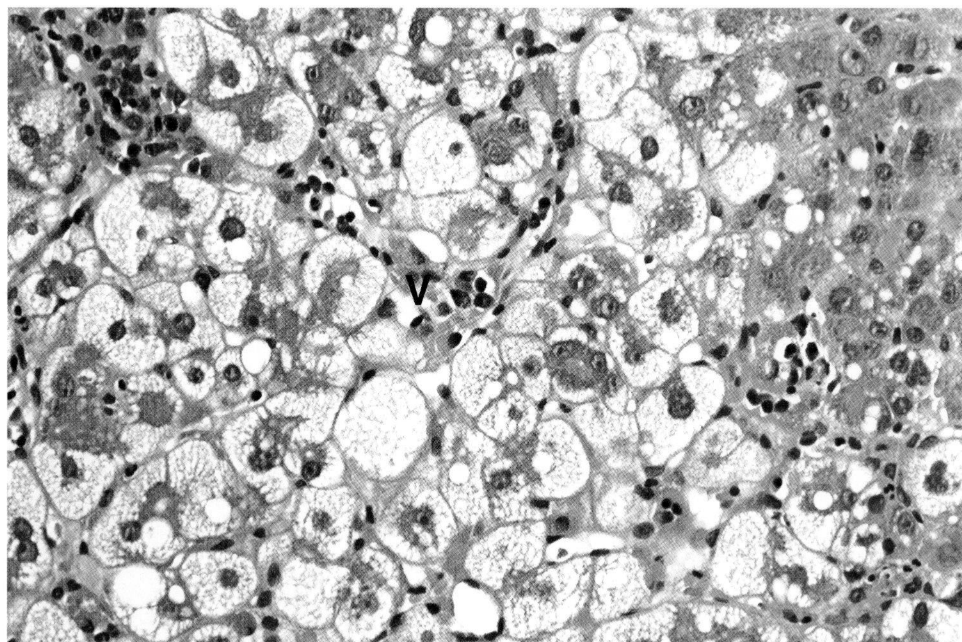

Figure 15.25 *Acute fatty liver of pregnancy.* Swollen pale-staining hepatocytes are seen around a terminal hepatic venule (V). The edge of a portal tract with a mild lymphocytic infiltrate is seen at the upper left corner. No large fat vacuoles are seen. (Post mortem liver, H&E).

Fat staining of frozen sections makes the diagnosis clear and a piece of the biopsy specimen should therefore be kept for frozen sectioning in patients with unexplained jaundice in late pregnancy. Inflammatory cells, mostly lymphocytes, are prominent in some examples and may lead to confusion with acute viral hepatitis,[298] in which microvesicular steatosis is not seen. In more severe examples of AFLP there is loss of hepatocytes leading to approximation of portal tracts. Fibrin deposits are occasionally demonstrable in hepatic sinusoids. One series showed cholestasis, extramedullary haemopoiesis and giant mitochondria[296] in some patients. With rare exception,[299] acute fatty liver does not recur in subsequent pregnancies.

Pre-eclampsia/eclampsia

Hypertension, proteinuria, peripheral oedema and occasional coagulation abnormalities in pregnancy constitute pre-eclampsia, or eclampsia if convulsions and hyperreflexia are also present. Liver involvement is unusual, but may be manifested by elevated serum aminotransferases and/or alkaline phosphatase. The incidence of preeclampsia is increased in patients with acute fatty liver.[298] The liver in pre-eclampsia shows fibrin thrombi in portal vessels and periportal sinusoids (Fig. 15.26) associated with necrosis and haemorrhage in more severe cases.[300,301] The identity of the fibrin can be established by phosphotungstic acid-haematoxylin (PTAH) staining or immunofluorescence.[302] These changes are not seen in all patients. Infarction, haematoma and rupture of the liver[303] are complications.

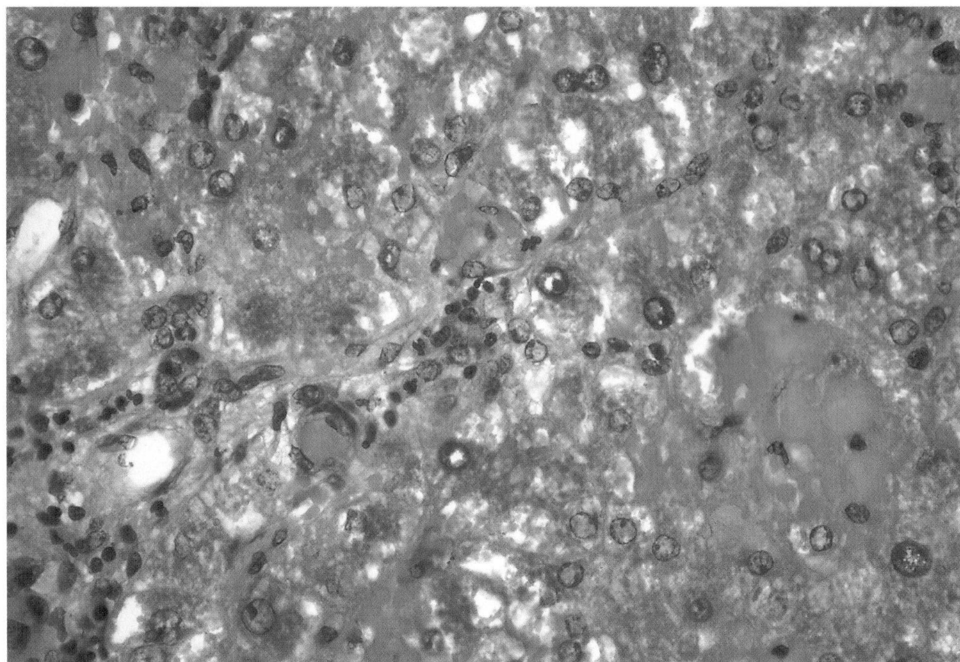

Figure 15.26 *Pre-eclampsia/eclampsia*. Fibrin is seen within the periportal sinusoids at lower right. (Needle biopsy, H&E).

HELLP syndrome

This syndrome is exceedingly uncommon in pregnancy[290,304] and is seen in 20% of patients with severe pre-eclampsia.[291] Liver biopsy changes range from non-specific portal inflammation and glycogenated hepatocyte nuclei[290,305–307] to the periportal fibrin and necrosis seen in pre-eclampsia.[291] One study demonstrated a relationship between maternal acute fatty liver of pregnancy and HELLP syndrome and a mitochondrial fatty acid beta-oxidation disorder with 3-hydroxyacyl-CoA dehydrogenase deficiency in their offspring.[308] Two of the children in the study had severe fatty change, necrosis and early nodules at autopsy.

Intrahepatic cholestasis of pregnancy (ICP)

Pruritus, with or without cholestatic jaundice, may develop in late pregnancy and recur in subsequent pregnancies. It regresses after delivery. Liver biopsy shows little apart from canalicular cholestasis, most severe in perivenular areas.[300] Minor hepatocellular changes and inflammation are attributable to the cholestasis itself. Portal inflammation is absent or mild. No histological abnormalities are detectable between pregnancies, but the jaundice has been shown to return on administration of oral contraceptives.[309] Concomitant intrahepatic cholestasis of pregnancy and acute fatty liver have been reported.[310] Mutations in the multidrug resistance 3 (*MDR3*) bile transport gene may have a pathogenetic role in ICP.[311]

REFERENCES

1 Bravo AA, Sheth SG, Chopra S. Liver biopsy. *N Engl J Med* 2001; **344**: 495–500.

2 Holtz T, Moseley RH, Scheiman JM. Liver biopsy in fever of unknown origin. A reappraisal. *J Clin Gastroenterol* 1993; **17**: 29–32.

3 Sandor M, Weinstock JV, Wynn TA. Granulomas in schistosome and mycobacterial infections: a model of local immune responses. *Trends Immunol* 2003; **24**: 44–52.

4 Lefkowitch JH. Hepatic granulomas. *J Hepatol* 1999; **30**: 40–45.

5 Ferrell LD. Hepatic granulomas: a morphologic approach to diagnosis. *Surg Pathol* 1990; **3**: 87–106.

6 Denk H, Scheuer PJ, Baptista A, et al. Guidelines for the diagnosis and interpretation of hepatic granulomas. *Histopathology* 1994; **25**: 209–218.

7 Fauci AS, Wolff SM. Granulomatous hepatitis. In: Popper H, Schaffner F, eds. Progress in Liver Diseases, Vol. V, 1st edn. New York, N.Y.: Grune & Stratton, 1976: 609.

8 Gaya DR, Thorburn KA, Oien KA, et al. Hepatic granulomas: a 10 year single centre experience. *J Clin Pathol* 2003; **56**: 850–853.

9 Guckian JC, Perry JE. Granulomatous hepatitis: an analysis of 63 cases and review of the literature. *Ann Intern Med* 1966; **65**: 1081–1100.

10 Ishak KG. Granulomas of the liver. In: Ioachim HL, ed. Pathology of Granulomas, 1st edn. New York, NY: Raven Press, 1983: 307.

11 Hunt J, Gordon FD, Jenkins RL, et al. Sarcoidosis with selective involvement of a second liver allograft: report of a case and review of the literature. *Mod Pathol* 1999; **12**: 325–328.

12 Israel HL, Margolis ML, Rose LJ. Hepatic granulomatosis and sarcoidosis. Further observations. *Dig Dis Sci* 1984; **29**: 353–356.

13 Hercules HD, Bethlem NM. Value of liver biopsy in sarcoidosis. *Arch Pathol Lab Med* 1984; **108**: 831–834.

14 Ishak KG. Sarcoidosis of the liver and bile ducts. *Mayo Clin Proc* 1998; **73**: 467–472.

15 Epstein MS, Devaney KO, Goodman ZD, et al. Liver disease in sarcoidosis. *Hepatology* 1990; **12**: 839A–839A.

16 Devaney K, Goodman ZD, Epstein MS, et al. Hepatic sarcoidosis. Clinicopathologic features in 100 patients. *Am J Surg Pathol* 1993; **17**: 1272–1280.

17 Maddrey WC, Johns CJ, Boitnott JK, et al. Sarcoidosis and chronic hepatic disease: a clinical and pathologic study of 20 patients. *Medicine* 1970; **49**: 375–395.

18 Tekeste H, Latour F, Levitt RE. Portal hypertension complicating sarcoid liver disease: case report and review of the literature. *Am J Gastroenterol* 1984; **79**: 389–396.

19 Moreno-Merlo F, Wanless IR, Shimamatsu K, et al. The role of granulomatous phlebitis and thrombosis in the pathogenesis of cirrhosis and portal hypertension in sarcoidosis. *Hepatology* 1997; **26**: 554–560.

20 Rudzki C, Ishak KG, Zimmerman HJ. Chronic intrahepatic cholestasis of sarcoidosis. *Am J Med* 1975; **59**: 373–387.

21 Bridges RA, Berendes H, Good RA. A fatal granulomatous disease of childhood. *Am J Dis Child* 1959; **97**: 387–408.

22 Ishak KG, Sharp HL. Metabolic errors and liver disease. In: MacSween RNM, Anthony PP, Scheuer PJ, et al., eds. Pathology of the Liver, 3rd edn. Edinburgh: Churchill Livingstone, 1994: 123.

23 Nakhleh RE, Glock M, Snover DC. Hepatic pathology of chronic granulomatous disease of childhood. *Arch Pathol Lab Med* 1992; **116**: 71–75.

24 Dilworth JA, Mandell GL. Adults with chronic granulomatous disease of 'childhood'. *Am J Med* 1977; **63**: 233–243.

25 Emile JF, Sebagh M, Ferray C, et al. The presence of epithelioid granulomas in hepatitis C virus-related cirrhosis. *Hum Pathol* 1993; **24**: 1095–1097.

26 Barceno R, Sanroman AL, Campo S Del, et al. Posttransplant liver granulomatosis associated with hepatitis C? *Transplantation* 1998; **65**: 1494–1495.

27 Goldin RD, Levine TS, Foster GR, et al. Granulomas and hepatitis C. *Histopathology* 1996; **28**: 265–267.

28 McMaster KR, Hennigar GR. Drug-induced granulomatous hepatitis. *Lab Invest* 1981; **44**: 61–73.

29 Kurumaya H, Kono N, Nakanuma Y, et al. Hepatic granulomata in long-term hemodialysis patients with hyperaluminumemia. *Arch Pathol Lab Med* 1989; **113**: 1132–1134.

30 Ballestri M, Baraldi A, Gatti AM, et al. Liver and kidney foreign bodies granulomatosis in a patient with malocclusion, bruxism and worn dental prostheses. *Gastroenterology* 2001; **121**: 1234–1238.

31 Leong ASY, Disney APS, Gove DW. Spallation and migration of silicone from blood-pump tubing in patients on hemodialysis. *N Engl J Med* 1982; **306**: 135–140.

32 Yao-Chang L, Tomashefski J, McMahon JT, et al. Mineral-associated hepatic injury: a report of seven cases with X-ray microanalysis. *Hum Pathol* 1991; **22**: 1120–1127.

33 Tjwa M, Hertogh G De, Neuville B, et al. Hepatic fibrin-ring granulomas in granulomatous hepatitis: report of four cases and review of the literature. *Acta Clin Belg* 2001; **56**: 341–348.

34 Bernstein M, Edmondson HA, Barbour BH. The liver lesion in Q-fever. Clinical and pathologic features. *Arch Intern Med* 1965; **116**: 491–498.

35 Pellegrin M, Delsol G, Auvergnat JC, et al. Granulomatous hepatitis in Q fever. *Hum Pathol* 1980; **11**: 51–57.

36 Hofmann CE, Heaton JW, Jr. Q fever hepatitis: clinical manifestations and pathological findings. *Gastroenterology* 1982; **83**: 474–479.

37 Qizilbash AH. The pathology of Q fever as seen on liver biopsy. *Arch Pathol Lab Med* 1983; **107**: 364–367.

38 Srigley JR, Vellend H, Palmer N, et al. Q-fever. The liver and bone marrow pathology. *Am J Surg Pathol* 1985; **9**: 752–758.

39 Marazuela M, Moreno A, Yebra M, et al. Hepatic fibrin-ring granulomas. A clinicopathologic study of 23 patients. *Hum Pathol* 1991; **22**: 607–613.

40 Vanderstigel M, Zafrani ES, Lejonc JL, et al. Allopurinol hypersensitivity syndrome as a cause of hepatic fibrin-ring granulomas. *Gastroenterology* 1986; **90**: 188–190.

41 Lobdell DH. 'Ring' granulomas in cytomegalovirus hepatitis. *Arch Pathol Lab Med* 1987; **111**: 881–882.

42 Nenert M, Mavier P, Dubuc N, et al. Epstein-Barr virus infection and hepatic fibrin-ring granulomas. *Hum Pathol* 1988; **19**: 608–610.

43 Moreno A, Marazuela M, Yebra M, et al. Hepatic fibrin-ring granulomas in visceral leishmaniasis. *Gastroenterology* 1988; **95**: 1123–1126.

44 Ponz E, García-Pagán JC, Bruguera M, et al. Hepatic fibrin-ring granulomas in a patient with hepatitis A. *Gastroenterology* 1991; **100**: 268–270.

45 Ruel M, Sevestre H, Henry-Biabaud E, et al. Fibrin ring granulomas in hepatitis A. *Dig Dis Sci* 1992; **37**: 1915–1917.

46 Bayser L De, Roblot P, Ramassamy A, et al. Hepatic fibrin-ring granulomas in giant cell arteritis. *Gastroenterology* 1993; **105**: 272–273.

47 Murphy E, Griffiths MR, Hunter JA, et al. Fibrin-ring granulomas: a non-specific reaction to liver injury? *Histopathology* 1991; **19**: 91–93.

48 Simon HB, Wolff SM. Granulomatous hepatitis and prolonged fever of unknown origin: a study of 13 patients. *Medicine* 1973; **52**: 1–21.

49 Knox TA, Kaplan MM, Gelfand JA, et al. Methotrexate treatment of idiopathic granulomatous hepatitis. *Ann Intern Med* 1995; **122**: 592–595.

50 Zoutman DE, Ralph ED, Frei JV. Granulomatous hepatitis and fever of unknown origin. An 11-year experience of 23 cases with three years' follow-up. *J Clin Gastroenterol* 1991; **13**: 69–75.

51 Lucas SB. Other viral and infectious diseases (including HIV-related liver disease). In: MacSween RNM, Burt AD, Portmann BC, et al., eds. Pathology of the Liver, 4th edn. Edinburgh: Churchill Livingstone, 2002: 363–414.

52 Huerre MR, Lan NT, Marianneau P, et al. Liver histopathology and biological correlates in five cases of fatal dengue fever in Vietnamese children. *Virchow's Arch* 2001; **438**: 107–115.

53 Elisaf M, Stefanaki S, Repanti M, et al. Liver involvement in hemorrhagic fever with renal syndrome. *J Clin Gastroenterol* 1993; **17**: 33–37.

54 Klotz O, Belt TH. The pathology of the liver in yellow fever. *Am J Pathol* 1930; **6**: 663–689.

55 Vieira WT, Gayotto LC, Lima CP de, et

al. Histopathology of the human liver in yellow fever with special emphasis on the diagnostic role of the Councilman body. *Histopathology* 1983; **7**: 195–208.
56 Goodman ZD, Ishak KG, Sesterhenn IA. Herpes simplex hepatitis in apparently immunocompetent adults. *Am J Clin Pathol* 1986; **85**: 694–699.
57 Jacques SM, Qureshi F. Herpes simplex virus hepatitis in pregnancy: a clinicopathologic study of three cases. *Hum Pathol* 1992; **23**: 183–187.
58 Carmichael GP, Jr., Zahradnik JM, Moyer GH et al. Adenovirus hepatitis in an immunosuppressed adult patient. *Am J Clin Pathol* 1979; **71**: 352–355.
59 Varki NM, Bhuta S, Drake T, et al. Adenovirus hepatitis in two successive liver transplants in a child. *Arch Pathol Lab Med* 1990; **114**: 106–109.
60 Phillips MJ, Glendis LM, Paucell S, et al. Syncytial giant-cell hepatitis. Sporadic hepatitis with distinctive pathologic features, a severe clinical course and paramyxoviral features. *N Engl J Med* 1991; **324**: 455–460.
61 Devaney K, Goodman ZD, Ishak KG. Postinfantile giant-cell transformation in hepatitis. *Hepatology* 1992; **16**: 327–333.
62 Lau J, Koukoulis G, Mieli-Vergani G, et al. Syncytial giant-cell hepatitis – a specific disease entity? *J Hepatol* 1992; **15**: 216–219.
63 Finegold MJ, Carpenter RJ. Obliterative cholangitis due to cytomegalovirus: a possible precursor of paucity of intrahepatic bile ducts. *Hum Pathol* 1982; **13**: 662–665.
64 Chang M-H, Huang H-H, Huang E-S, et al. Polymerase chain reaction to detect human cytomegalovirus in livers of infants with neonatal hepatitis. *Gastroenterology* 1992; **103**: 1022–1025.
65 Theise ND, Conn M, Thung SN. Localization of cytomegalovirus antigens in liver allografts over time. *Hum Pathol* 1993; **24**: 103–108.
66 Vanstapel MJ, Desmet VJ. Cytomegalovirus hepatitis: a histological and immunohistochemical study. *Appl Pathol* 1983; **1**: 41–49.
67 Clarke J, Craig RM, Saffro R, et al. Cytomegalovirus granulomatous hepatitis. *Am J Med* 1979; **66**: 264–269.
68 Snover DC, Horwitz CA. Liver disease in cytomegalovirus mononucleosis: a light microscopical and immunoperoxidase study of six cases. *Hepatology* 1984; **4**: 408–412.
69 Kilpatrick ZM. Structural and functional abnormalities of liver in infectious mononucleosis. *Arch Intern Med* 1966; **117**: 47–53.
70 Chang MY, Campbell WG, Jr. Fatal infectious mononucleosis. Association with liver necrosis and herpes-like virus particles. *Arch Pathol* 1975; **99**: 185–191.
71 Lebovics E, Thung SN, Schaffner F, et al. The liver in the acquired immunodeficiency syndrome: a clinical and histologic study. *Hepatology* 1985; **5**: 293–298.
72 Glasgow BJ, Anders K, Layfield LJ, et al. Clinical and pathologic findings of the liver in the acquired immune deficiency syndrome (AIDS). *Am J Clin Pathol* 1985; **83**: 582–588.
73 Dworkin BM, Stahl RE, Giardina MA, et al. The liver in acquired immune deficiency syndrome: emphasis on patients with intravenous drug abuse. *Am J Gastroenterol* 1987; **82**: 231–236.
74 Schneiderman DJ, Arenson DM, Cello JP, et al. Hepatic disease in patients with the acquired immune deficiency syndrome (AIDS). *Hepatology* 1987; **7**: 925–930.
75 Lebovics E, Dworkin BM, Heier SK, et al. The hepatobiliary manifestations of human immunodeficiency virus infection. *Am J Gastroenterol* 1988; **83**: 1–7.
76 Wilkins MJ, Lindley R, Dourakis SP, et al. Surgical pathology of the liver in HIV infection. *Histopathology* 1991; **18**: 459–464.
77 Comer GM. Hepatobiliary disease in AIDS. In: Kotler DP, ed. Gastrointestinal and nutritional manifestations of AIDS, 1st edn. New York, N.Y.: Raven Press, 1991: 119.
78 Bach N, Theise ND, Schaffner F. Hepatic histopathology in the acquired immunodeficiency syndrome. *Semin Liver Dis* 1992; **12**: 205–212.
79 Lefkowitch JH. The liver in AIDS. *Semin Liver Dis* 1997; **17**: 335–344.
80 Lefkowitch JH. Pathology of AIDS-related liver disease. *Dig Dis* 1994; **12**: 321–330.
81 Forsmark CE. AIDS and the gastrointestinal tract. *Postgrad Med* 1993; **93**: 143–152.
82 Clark SJ, Creighton S, Portmann B, et al. Acute liver failure associate with

antiretroviral treatment for HIV: a report of six cases. *J Hepatol* 2002; **36**: 295–301.
83 Spengler U, Lichterfeld M, Rockstroh JK. Antiretroviral drug toxicity – a challenge for the hepatologist? *J Hepatol* 2002; **36**: 283–294.
84 Scoazec JY, Feldmann G. Both macrophages and endothelial cells of the human hepatic sinusoid express the CD4 molecule, a receptor for the human immunodeficiency virus. *Hepatology* 1990; **12**: 505–510.
85 Housset C, Lamas E, Courgnaud V, et al. Presence of HIV-1 in human parenchymal and non-parenchymal liver cells in vivo. *J Hepatol* 1993; **19**: 252–258.
86 Steffan A-M, Lafon M-E, Gendrault J-L, et al. Primary cultures of endothelial cells from the human liver sinusoid are permissive for human immunodeficiency virus type 1. *Proc Natl Acad Sci* 1992; **89**: 1582–1586.
87 Housset C, Boucher O, Girard PM, et al. Immunohistochemical evidence for human immunodeficiency virus-1 infection of liver Kupffer cells. *Hum Pathol* 1990; **21**: 404–408.
88 Lafon M-E, Kirn A. Human immunodeficiency virus infection of the liver. *Semin Liver Dis* 1992; **12**: 197–204.
89 Witzleben CL, Marshall GS, Wenner W, et al. HIV as a cause of giant cell hepatitis. *Hum Pathol* 1988; **19**: 603–605.
90 Molina J-M, Welker Y, Ferchal F, et al. Hepatitis associated with primary HIV infection. *Gastroenterology* 1992; **102**: 739–746.
91 Palella FJ, Delaney KM, Moorman AC, et al. Declining morbidity and mortality among patients with advanced human immunodeficiency virus infection. *N Engl J Med* 1998; **338**: 853–860.
92 Hofman V, Marty P, Perrin C, et al. The histological spectrum of visceral leishmaniasis caused by *Leishmania infantum* MON-1 in acquired immune deficiency syndrome. *Hum Pathol* 2000; **31**: 75–84.
93 Kahn DG, Garfinkle JM, Klonoff DC, et al. Cryptosporidial and cytomegaloviral hepatitis and cholecystitis. *Arch Pathol Lab Med* 1987; **111**: 879–881.
94 Beaugerie L, Teilhac M-F, Deluol A-M, et al. Cholangiopathy associated with Microsporidia infection of the common bile duct mucosa in a patient with HIV infection. *Ann Intern Med* 1992; **117**: 401–402.
95 Pol S, Romana C, Richard S, et al. Enterocytozoon bieneusi infection in acquired-immunodeficiency syndrome-related sclerosing cholangitis. *Gastroenterology* 1992; **102**: 1778–1781.
96 Pol S, Romana CA, Richard S, et al. Microsporidia infection in patients with the human immunodeficiency virus and unexplained cholangitis. *N Engl J Med* 1993; **328**: 95–99.
97 Greene JB, Sidhu GS, Lewin S, et al. *Mycobacterium avium-intracellulare*: a cause of disseminated life-threatening infection in homosexuals and drug abusers. *Ann Intern Med* 1982; **97**: 539–546.
98 Orenstein MS, Tavitian A, Yonk B, et al. Granulomatous involvement of the liver in patients with AIDS. *Gut* 1985; **26**: 1220–1225.
99 Gordon SC, Reddy KR, Gould EE, et al. The spectrum of liver disease in the acquired immunodeficiency syndrome. *J Hepatol* 1986; **2**: 475–484.
100 Nakanuma Y, Liew CT, Peters RL, et al. Pathologic features of the liver in acquired immune deficiency syndrome (AIDS). *Liver* 1986; **6**: 158–166.
101 Stevens A. Micro-organisms. In: Bancroft JD, Stevens A, eds. Theory and Practice of Histological Techniques, 2nd edn. Edinburgh: Churchill Livingstone, 1982: 278.
102 Kuper SWA, May JR. Detection of acid-fast-organisms in tissue sections by fluorescence microscopy. *J Pathol Bacteriol* 1960; **79**: 59–68.
103 Poblete RB, Rodriguez K, Foust RT, et al. *Pneumocystis carinii* hepatitis in the acquired immunodeficiency syndrome (AIDS). *Ann Intern Med* 1989; **110**: 737–738.
104 Margulis SJ, Honig CL, Soave R, et al. Biliary tract obstruction in the acquired immunodeficiency syndrome [published erratum appears in *Ann Intern Med* 1986; **105**(4): 634]. *Ann Intern Med* 1986; **105**: 207–210.
105 Cello J. Human immunodeficiency virus-associated biliary tract disease. *Semin Liver Dis* 1992; **12**: 213–218.
106 Bouche H, Housset C, Dumont J-L, et al. AIDS-related cholangitis: diagnostic

features and course in 15 patients. *J Hepatol* 1993; **17**: 34–39.

107 Czapar CA, Weldon-Linne CM, Moore DM, et al. Peliosis hepatis in the acquired immunodeficiency syndrome. *Arch Pathol Lab Med* 1986; **110**: 611–613.

108 Boylston AW, Cook HT, Francis ND, et al. Biopsy pathology of acquired immune deficiency syndrome (AIDS). *J Clin Pathol* 1987; **40**: 1–8.

109 Perkocha LA, Geaghan SM, Yen TSB, et al. Clinical and pathological features of bacillary peliosis hepatis in association with human immunodeficiency virus infection. *N Engl J Med* 1990; **323**: 1581–1586.

110 Garcia-Tsao G, Panzini L, Yoselevitz M, et al. Bacillary peliosis hepatis as a cause of acute anemia in a patient with the acquired immunodeficiency syndrome. *Gastroenterology* 1992; **102**: 1065–1070.

111 Tappero JW, Koehler JE, Berger TG, et al. Bacillary angiomatosis and bacillary splenitis in immunocompetent adults. *Ann Intern Med* 1993; **118**: 363–365.

112 Koehler JE, Sanchez MA, Garrido CS, et al. Molecular epidemiology of bartonella infections in patients with bacillary angiomatosis-peliosis. *N Engl J Med* 1997; **337**: 1876–1883.

113 Caccamo D, Pervez NK, Marchevsky A. Primary lymphoma of the liver in the acquired immunodeficiency syndrome. *Arch Pathol Lab Med* 1986; **110**: 553–555.

114 Beral V, Peterman T, Berkelman R, et al. AIDS-associated non-Hodgkin lymphoma. *Lancet* 1991; **337**: 805–809.

115 Newell A, Francis N, Nelson M. Hepatitis and HIV: Interrelationship and interactions. *Br J Clin Pr* 1995; **49**: 247–251.

116 Horvath J, Raffanti SP. Clinical aspects of the interactions between human immunodeficiency virus and the hepatotropic viruses. *Clin Inf Dis* 1994; **18**: 339–347.

117 Colin J-F, Cazals-Hatem D, Loriot MA, et al. Influence of human immunodeficiency virus infection on chronic hepatitis B in homosexual men. *Hepatology* 1999; **29**: 1306–1310.

118 Collier J, Heathcote J. Hepatitis C viral infection in the immunosuppressed patient. *Hepatology* 1998; **27**: 1–6.

119 Di Martino V, Rufat P, Boyer N, et al. The influence of human immunodeficiency virus coinfection on chronic hepatitis C in injection drug users: a long-term retrospective cohort study. *Hepatology* 2001; **34**: 1193–1199.

120 Lichtenstein DR, Makadon HJ, Chopra S. Fulminant hepatitis B and delta virus coinfection in AIDS. *Am J Gastroenterol* 1992; **87**: 1643–1647.

121 Housset C, Pol S, Carnot F, et al. Interactions between human immunodeficiency virus-1, hepatitis delta virus and hepatitis B virus infections in 260 chronic carriers of hepatitis B virus. *Hepatology* 1992; **15**: 578–583.

122 Bissuel F, Bruneel F, Habersetzer F, et al. Fulminant hepatitis with severe lactate acidosis in HIV-infected patients on didanosine therapy. *J Int Med* 1994; **235**: 367–372.

123 Olano JP, Borucki MJ, Wen JW, et al. Massive hepatic steatosis and lactic acidosis in a patient with AIDS who was receiving zidovudine. *Clin Inf Dis* 1995; **21**: 973–976.

124 Freiman JP, Helfert KE, Hamrell MR, et al. Hepatomegaly with severe steatosis in HIV-seropositive patients. *AIDS* 1993; **7**: 379–385.

125 Fernandez-Miranda C, Colina F, Delgado JM, et al. Diffuse nodular regenerative hyperplasia of the liver associated with human immunodeficiency virus and visceral leishmaniasis. *Am J Gastroenterol* 1993; **88**: 433–435.

126 Osick LA, Lee T-P, Pedemonte MB, et al. Hepatic amyloidosis in intravenous drug abusers and AIDS patients. *J Hepatol* 1993; **19**: 79–84.

127 Kossaifi T, Dupon M, Le Bail B, et al. Perisinusoidal cell hypertrophy in a patient with acquired immunodeficiency syndrome. *Arch Pathol Lab Med* 1990; **114**: 876–879.

128 Kahn E, Greco A, Daum F, et al. Hepatic pathology in pediatric acquired immunodeficiency syndrome. *Hum Pathol* 1991; **22**: 1111–1119.

129 Duffy LF, Daum F, Kahn E, et al. Hepatitis in children with acquired immune deficiency syndrome. Histopathologic and immunocytologic features. *Gastroenterology* 1986; **90**: 173–181.

130 Ross JS, Rosario A Del, Bui HX, et al. Primary hepatic leiomyosarcoma in a child with the acquired immunodeficiency syndrome. *Hum Pathol* 1992; **23**: 69–72.

131 Turck WP, Howitt G, Turnberg LA, et al. Chronic Q fever. *Quart J Med* 1976; **45**: 193–217.

132 Cervantes F, Bruguera M, Carbonell J, et al. Liver disease in brucellosis. A clinical and pathological study of 40 cases. *Postgrad Med J* 1982; **58**: 346–350.

133 Khosla SN. Typhoid hepatitis. *Postgrad Med J* 1990; **66**: 923–925.

134 Brito T De, Trench Vieira W, D'Agostino Dias M. Jaundice in typhoid hepatitis: a light and electron microscopy study based on liver biopsies. *Acta Hepato Gastroenterol* 1977; **24**: 426–433.

135 Nasrallah SM, Nassar VH. Enteric fever: a clinicopathologic study of 104 cases. *Am J Gastroenterol* 1978; **69**: 63–69.

136 Pais P. A hepatitis like picture in typhoid fever. *Br Med J Clin Res* 1984; **289**: 225–226.

137 Lamps LW, Gray GF, Scott MA. The histologic spectrum of hepatic cat scratch disease. A series of six cases with confirmed *Bartonella henselae* infection. *Am J Surg Pathol* 1996; **20**: 1253–1259.

138 Asada Y, Hayashi T, Sumiyoshi A, et al. Miliary tuberculosis presenting as fever and jaundice with hepatic failure. *Hum Pathol* 1991; **22**: 92–94.

139 Alvarez SZ, Carpio R. Hepatobiliary tuberculosis. *Dig Dis Sci* 1983; **28**: 193–200.

140 Essop AR, Posen JA, Hodkinson JH, et al. Tuberculosis hepatitis: a clinical review of 96 cases. *Quart J Med* 1984; **53**: 465–477.

141 Pottipati AR, Dave PB, Gumaste V, et al. Tuberculous abscess of the liver in acquired immunodeficiency syndrome. *J Clin Gastroenterol* 1991; **13**: 549–553.

142 Alcantra-Payawal DE, Matsumura M, Shiratori Y, et al. Direct detection of Mycobacterium tuberculosis using polymerase chain reaction assay among patients with hepatic granuloma. *J Hepatol* 1997; **27**: 620–627.

143 Hunt JS, Silverstein MJ, Sparks FC, et al. Granulomatous hepatitis: a complication of B.C.G. immunotherapy. *Lancet* 1973; **2**: 820–821.

144 Bodurtha A, Kim YH, Laucius JF, et al. Hepatic granulomas and other hepatic lesions associated with BCG immunotherapy for cancer. *Am J Clin Pathol* 1974; **61**: 747–752.

145 Proctor DD, Chopra S, Rubenstein SC, et al. Mycobacteremia and granulomatous hepatitis following initial intravesical bacillus Calmette-Guerin instillation for bladder carcinoma. *Am J Gastroenterol* 1993; **88**: 1112–1115.

146 Case records of the Massachusetts General Hospital. Case 29-1998. *N Engl J Med* 1998; **339**: 831–837.

147 Karat AB, Job CK, Rao PS. Liver in leprosy: histological and biochemical findings. *BR MED J* 1971; **1**: 307–310.

148 Chen TS, Drutz DJ, Whelan GE. Hepatic granulomas in leprosy. Their relation to bacteremia. *Arch Pathol Lab Med* 1976; **100**: 182–185.

149 Terry SI, Hanchard B, Brooks SE, et al. Prevalence of liver abnormality in early syphilis. *Br J Vener Dis* 1984; **60**: 83–86.

150 Murray FE, O'Loughlin S, Dervan P, et al. Granulomatous hepatitis in secondary syphilis. *Ir J Med Sci* 1990; **159**: 53–54.

151 Sobel HJ, Wolf EH. Liver involvement in early syphilis. *Arch Pathol* 1972; **93**: 565–568.

152 Fehér J, Somogyi T, Timmer M, et al. Early syphilitic hepatitis. *Lancet* 1975; **2**: 896–899.

153 Romeu J, Rybak B, Dave P, et al. Spirochetal vasculitis and bile ductular damage in early hepatic syphilis. *Am J Gastroenterol* 1980; **74**: 352–354.

154 Veeravahu M. Diagnosis of liver involvement in early syphilis. A critical review. *Arch Intern Med* 1985; **145**: 132–134.

155 Brito T De, Machado MM, Montans SD, et al. Liver biopsy in human leptospirosis: a light and electron microscopy study. *Virchows Arch Pathol Anat Physiol* 1967; **342**: 61–69.

156 Brito T De, Penna DO, Hoshino S, et al. Cholestasis in human leptospirosis: a clinical, histochemical, biochemical and electron microscopy study based on liver biopsies. *Beiträge Pathol* 1970; **140**: 345–361.

157 Ferreira Alves VA, Vianna MR, Yasuda PH, et al. Detection of leptospiral

antigen in the human liver and kidney using an immunoperoxidase staining procedure. *J Pathol* 1987; **151**: 125–131.

158 Goellner MH, Agger WA, Burgess JH, et al. Hepatitis due to recurrent Lyme disease. *Ann Intern Med* 1988; **108**: 707–708.

159 Thaler M, Pastakia B, Shawker TH, et al. Hepatic candidiasis in cancer patients: the evolving picture of the syndrome. *Ann Intern Med* 1988; **108**: 88–100.

160 Lewis JH, Patel HR, Zimmerman HJ. The spectrum of hepatic candidiasis. *Hepatology* 1982; **2**: 479–487.

161 Hassanein T, Perper JA, Tepperman L, et al. Liver failure occurring as a component of exertional heatstroke. *Gastroenterology* 1991; **100**: 1442–1447.

162 Jariwalla A, Tulloch BR, Fox H, et al. Disseminated histoplasmosis in an English patient with diabetes mellitus. *Br Med J* 1977; **1**: 1002–1004.

163 Lanza FL, Nelson RS, Somayaji BN. Acute granulomatous hepatitis due to histoplasmosis. *Gastroenterology* 1970; **58**: 392–396.

164 Smith JW, Utz JP. Progressive disseminated histoplasmosis. A prospective study of 26 patients. *Ann Intern Med* 1972; **76**: 557–565.

165 Edmondson RP, Eykyn S, Davies DR, et al. Disseminated histoplasmosis successfully treated with amphotericin B. *J Clin Pathol* 1974; **27**: 308–310.

166 Ridley DS. The laboratory diagnosis of tropical diseases with special reference to Britain: a review. [Review]. *J Clin Pathol* 1974; **27**: 435–444.

167 Williams AO, Lawson EA, Lucas AO. African histoplasmosis due to *Histoplasma duboisii*. *Arch Pathol* 1971; **92**: 306–318.

168 Okudaira M, Straub M, Schwarz J. The etiology of discrete splenic and hepatic calcifications in an endemic area of histoplasmosis. *Am J Pathol* 1961; **39**: 599–611.

169 Weinstein L. Bacterial hepatitis: a case report on an unrecognized cause of fever of unknown origin. *N Engl J Med* 1978; **299**: 1052–1054.

170 Engler S, Elsing C, Flechtenmacher C, et al. Progressive sclerosing cholangitis after shock: a new variant of vanishing bile duct disorders. *Gut* 2003; **52**: 688–693.

171 Banks JG, Foulis AK, Ledingham IM, et al. Liver function in septic shock. *J Clin Pathol* 1982; **35**: 1249–1252.

172 Zimmerman HJ, Fang M, Utili R, et al. Jaundice due to bacterial infection. *Gastroenterology* 1979; **77**: 362–374.

173 Lefkowitch JH. Bile ductular cholestasis: an ominous histopathologic sign related to sepsis and 'cholangitis lenta'. *Hum Pathol* 1982; **13**: 19–24.

174 Vyberg M, Poulsen H. Abnormal bile duct epithelium accompanying septicaemia. *Virchows Arch A Pathol Anat Histopathol* 1984; **402**: 451–458.

175 Riely CA, Dean PJ, Park AL, et al. A distinct syndrome of liver disease with multisystem organ failure associated with bile ductular cholestasis. *Hepatology* 1989; **10**: 739A–739A.

176 Ishak KG, Rogers WA. Cryptogenic acute cholangitis – association with toxic shock syndrome. *Am J Clin Pathol* 1981; **76**: 619–626.

177 Weitberg AB, Alper JC, Diamond I, et al. Acute granulomatous hepatitis in the course of acquired toxoplasmosis. *N Engl J Med* 1979; **300**: 1093–1096.

178 Andres TL, Dorman SA, Winn W, Jr., et al. Immunohistochemical demonstration of *Toxoplasma gondii*. *Am J Clin Pathol* 1981; **75**: 431–434.

179 Conley FK, Jenkins KA, Remington JS. *Toxoplasma gondii* infection of the central nervous system. Use of the peroxidase-antiperoxidase method to demonstrate toxoplasma in formalin fixed, paraffin embedded tissue sections. *Hum Pathol* 1981; **12**: 690–698.

180 Pounder DJ. Malarial pigment and hepatic anthracosis [letter]. *Am J Surg Pathol* 1983; **7**: 501–502.

181 Anonymous. Annotation: Tropical splenomegaly syndrome. *Lancet* 1976; **i**: 1058–1059.

182 Daneshbod K. Visceral leishmaniasis (kala-azar) in Iran: a pathologic and electron microscopic study. *Am J Clin Pathol* 1972; **57**: 156–166.

183 Maltz G, Knauer CM. Amebic liver abscess: a 15-year experience. *Am J Gastroenterol* 1991; **86**: 704–710.

184 Dunn MA, Kamel R. Hepatic schistosomiasis. [Review]. *Hepatology* 1981; **1**: 653–661.

185 Andrade ZA. Hepatic schistosomiasis. Morphological aspects. In: Popper H,

Schaffner F, eds. Progress in Liver Diseases, Vol. II, 1st edn. New York, N.Y.: Grune & Stratton, 1965: 228.
186 Lucas SB. Other viral and infectious diseases. In: MacSween RNM, Anthony PP, Scheuer PJ, et al., eds. Pathology of the Liver, 3rd edn. Edinburgh: Churchill Livingstone, 1994: 269–316.
187 Andrade ZA, Peixoto E, Guerret S, et al. Hepatic connective tissue changes in hepatosplenic schistosomiasis. *Hum Pathol* 1992; **23**: 566–573.
188 Canto AL, Sesso A, Brito T De. Human chronic Mansonian schistosomiasis-cell proliferation and fibre formation in the hepatic sinusoidal wall: a morphometric, light and electron-microscopy study. *J Pathol* 1977; **123**: 35–44.
189 Grimaud JA, Borojevic R. Chronic human schistosomiasis mansoni. Pathology of the Disse's space. *Lab Invest* 1977; **36**: 268–273.
190 Lyra LG, Reboucas G, Andrade ZA. Hepatitis B surface antigen carrier state in hepatosplenic schistosomiasis. *Gastroenterology* 1976; **71**: 641–645.
191 Nash TE, Cheever AW, Ottesen EA, et al. Schistosome infections in humans: perspectives and recent findings. *Ann Intern Med* 1982; **97**: 740–754.
192 Sun T. Pathology and immunology of *Clonorchis sinensis* infection in the liver. *Ann Clin Lab Sci* 1984; **14**: 208–215.
193 Ona FV, Dytoc JNT. Clonorchis-associated cholangiocarcinoma: a report of two cases with unusual manifestations. *Gastroenterology* 1991; **101**: 831–839.
194 Hartley JP, Douglas AP. A case of clonorchiasis in England. *Br Med J* 1975; **3**: 575–575.
195 Acosta-Ferreira W, Vercelli-Retta J, Falconi LM. *Fasciola hepatica* human infection. Histopathological study of sixteen cases. *Virchows Arch A Pathol Anat Histol* 1979; **383**: 319–327.
196 Jones EA, Kay JM, Milligan HP, et al. Massive infection with *Fasciola hepatica* in man. *Am J Med* 1977; **63**: 836–842.
197 Drury RAB. Larval granulomata in the liver. *Gut* 1962; **3**: 289–294.
198 Hagander B, Berg NO, Brandt L, et al. Hepatic injury in adult coeliac disease. *Lancet* 1977; **2**: 270–272.
199 Pollock DJ. The liver in coeliac disease. *Histopathology* 1977; **1**: 421–430.
200 Gabrielsen TO, Hoel PS. Primary biliary cirrhosis associated with coeliac disease and dermatitis herpetiformis. *Dermatologica* 1985; **170**: 31–34.
201 Fouin-Fortunet H, Duprey F, Touchais O, et al. Coeliac disease associated with primary biliary cirrhosis. *Gastroenterol Clin Biol* 1985; **9**: 641–642.
202 Behr W, Barnert J. Adult coeliac disease and primary biliary cirrhosis. *Am J Gastroenterol* 1986; **81**: 796–799.
203 Hay JE, Wiesner RH, Shorter RG, et al. Primary sclerosing cholangitis and celiac disease. *Ann Intern Med* 1988; **109**: 713–717.
204 Gogos CA, Nikolopoulou V, Zolota V, et al. Autoimmune cholangitis in a patient with celiac disease: a case report and review of the literature. *J Hepatol* 1999; **30**: 321–324.
205 Burt AD, MacSween RNM. Liver pathology associated with diseases of other organs. In: MacSween RNM, Anthony PP, Scheuer PJ, et al., ed. Pathology of the Liver, 3rd edn. Edinburgh: Churchill Livingstone; 1994: 713–764.
206 Saint-Marc Girardin MF, Zafrani ES, Chaumette MT, et al. Hepatic granulomas in Whipple's disease. *Gastroenterology* 1984; **86**: 753–756.
207 Everett GD, Mitros FA. Eosinophilic gastroenteritis with hepatic eosinophilic granulomas. Report of a case with 30-year follow-up. *Am J Gastroenterol* 1980; **74**: 519–521.
208 Eade MN, Cooke WT, Brooke BN, et al. Liver disease in Crohn's colitis. A study of 21 consecutive patients having colectomy. *Ann Intern Med* 1971; **74**: 518–528.
209 Shorvon PJ. Amyloidosis and inflammatory bowel disease. *Am J Dig Dis* 1977; **22**: 209–213.
210 Quigley EMM, Zetterman RK. Hepatobiliary complications of malabsorption and malnutrition. *Semin Liver Dis* 1988; **8**: 218–228.
211 Shepherd HA, Selby WS, Chapman RW, et al. Ulcerative colitis and persistent liver dysfunction. *Quart J Med* 1983; **52**: 503–513.
212 Haworth AC, Manley PN, Groll A, et al. Bile duct carcinoma and biliary tract dysplasia in chronic ulcerative colitis. *Arch Pathol Lab Med* 1989; **113**: 434–436.

213 Fleming KA, Boberg KM, Glaumann H, et al. Biliary dysplasia as a marker of cholangiocarcinoma in primary sclerosing cholangitis. *J Hepatol* 2001; **34**: 360–365.
214 Wee A, Ludwig J, Coffey RJ, Jr., et al. Hepatobiliary carcinoma associated with primary sclerosing cholangitis and chronic ulcerative colitis. *Hum Pathol* 1985; **16**: 719–726.
215 Mir-Madjlessi SH, Farmer RG, Sivak MV, Jr. Bile duct carcinoma in patients with ulcerative colitis. Relationship to sclerosing cholangitis: report of six cases and review of the literature. [Review]. *Dig Dis Sci* 1987; **32**: 145–154.
216 Blackstone MO, Nemchausky BA. Cholangiographic abnormalities in ulcerative colitis associated pericholangitis which resemble sclerosing cholangitis. *Am J Dig Dis* 1978; **23**: 579–585.
217 Wee A, Ludwig J. Pericholangitis in chronic ulcerative colitis: primary sclerosing cholangitis of the small bile ducts? *Ann Intern Med* 1985; **102**: 581–587.
218 Tsui WMS, Wong KF, Tse CCH. Liver changes in reactive haemophagocytic syndrome. *Liver* 1992; **12**: 363–367.
219 Kerguenec C de, Hillaire S, Molinié V, et al. Hepatic manifestations of hemophagocytic syndrome: a study of 30 cases. *Am J Gastroenterol* 2001; **96**: 852–857.
220 Aledort LM, Levine PH, Hilgartner M, et al. A study of liver biopsies and liver disease among hemophiliacs. *Blood* 1985; **66**: 367–372.
221 Colombo M, Mannucci PM, Carnelli V, et al. Transmission of non-A, non-B hepatitis by heat-treated factor VIII concentrate. *Lancet* 1985; **ii**: 1–4.
222 Hay CR, Preston FE, Triger DR, et al. Progressive liver disease in haemophilia: an understated problem? *Lancet* 1985; **1**: 1495–1498.
223 Bianchi L, Desmet VJ, Popper H, et al. Histologic patterns of liver disease in hemophiliacs, with special reference to morphologic characteristics of non-A, non-B hepatitis. *Semin Liver Dis* 1987; **7**: 203–209.
224 Lefkowitch JH, Mendez L. Morphologic features of hepatic injury in cardiac disease and shock. *J Hepatol* 1986; **2**: 313–327.
225 Ludwig J, Gross JB, Perkins JD, et al. Persistent centrilobular necroses in hepatic allografts. *Hum Pathol* 1990; **21**: 656–661.
226 Collins RH, Anastasi J, Terstappen LWMM, et al. Brief report: donor-derived long-term multilineage hematopoiesis in a liver-transplant recipient. *N Engl J Med* 1993; **328**: 762–765.
227 Gilson TP, Bendon RW. Megakaryocytosis of the liver in a trisomy 21 stillbirth. *Arch Pathol Lab Med* 1993; **117**: 738–739.
228 Ruchelli ED, Uri A, Dimmick JE, et al. Severe perinatal liver disease and Down syndrome: an apparent relationship. *Hum Pathol* 1991; **22**: 1274–1280.
229 Arai H, Ishida A, Nakajima W, et al. Immunohistochemical study on transforming growth factor-beta 1 expression in liver fibrosis of Down's syndrome with transient abnormal myelopoiesis. *Hum Pathol* 1999; **30**: 474–476.
230 Youssef WI, Tavill AS. Connective tissue diseases and the liver. *J Clin Gastroenterol* 2002; **35**: 345–349.
231 Keshavarzian A, Rentsch R, Hodgson HJF. Clinical implications of liver biopsy findings in collagen-vascular disorders. *J Clin Gastroenterol* 1993; **17**: 219–226.
232 Matsumoto T, Kobayashi S, Shimizu H, et al. The liver in collagen diseases: pathologic study of 160 cases with particular reference to hepatic arteritis, primary biliary cirrhosis, autoimmune hepatitis and nodular regenerative hyperplasia of the liver. *Liver* 2000; **20**: 366–373.
233 Gocke DJ, Hsu K, Morgan C, et al. Association between polyarteritis and Australia antigen. *Lancet* 1970; **2**: 1149–1153.
234 Levo Y, Gorevic PD, Kassab HJ, et al. Liver involvement in the syndrome of mixed cryoglobulinemia. *Ann Intern Med* 1977; **87**: 287–292.
235 Misiani R, Bellavita P, Fenili D, et al. Hepatitis C virus infection in patients with essential mixed cryoglobulinemia. *Ann Intern Med* 1992; **117**: 573–577.
236 Agnello V, Chung RT, Kaplan LM. A role for hepatitis C virus infection in type II cryoglobulinemia. *N Engl J Med* 1992; **327**: 1490–1495.
237 Peña LR, Nand S, Maria N De, et al.

Hepatitis C virus infection and lymphoproliferative disorders. *Dig Dis Sci* 2000; **45**: 1854–1860.
238 Long R, James O. Polymyalgia rheumatica and liver disease. *Lancet* 1974; **1**: 77–79.
239 Litwack KD, Bohan A, Silverman L. Granulomatous liver disease and giant cell arteritis. Case report and literature review. *J Rheumatol* 1977; **4**: 307–312.
240 Gossmann HH, Dolle W, Korb G, et al. Liver changes in giant-cell arteritis: temporal arteritis and rheumatic polymyalgia (author's translation) [in German]. *Dtsch Med Wochenschr* 1979; **104**: 1199–1202.
241 Leong AS, Alp MH. Hepatocellular disease in the giant-cell arteritis/polymyalgia rheumatica syndrome. *Ann Rheum Dis* 1981; **40**: 92–95.
242 Rao R, Pfenniger K, Boni A. Liver function tests and liver biopsies in patients with rheumatoid arthritis. *Ann Rheum Dis* 1975; **34**: 198–199.
243 Mills PR, MacSween RN, Dick WC, et al. Liver disease in rheumatoid arthritis. *Scott Med J* 1980; **25**: 18–22.
244 Mills PR, Sturrock RD. Clinical associations between arthritis and liver disease. [Review]. *Ann Rheum Dis* 1982; **41**: 295–307.
245 Smits JG, Kooijman CD. Rheumatoid nodules in liver [letter]. *Histopathology* 1986; **10**: 1211–1213.
246 Thorne C, Urowitz MB, Wanless I, et al. Liver disease in Felty's syndrome. *Am J Med* 1982; **73**: 35–40.
247 Reynolds WJ, Wanless IR. Nodular regenerative hyperplasia of the liver in a patient with rheumatoid vasculitis: a morphometric study suggesting a role for hepatic arteritis in the pathogenesis. *J Rheumatol* 1984; **11**: 838–842.
248 Murray-Lyon IM, Thompson RP, Ansell ID, et al. Scleroderma and primary biliary cirrhosis. *Br Med J* 1970; **1**: 258–259.
249 Reynolds TB, Denison EK, Frankl HD, et al. Primary biliary cirrhosis with scleroderma, Raynaud's phenomenon and telangiectasia. New syndrome. *Am J Med* 1971; **50**: 302–312.
250 Feldmann G, Maurice M, Husson JM, et al. Hepatocyte giant mitochondria: an almost constant lesion in systemic scleroderma. *Virchows Arch A Pathol Anat Histol* 1977; **374**: 215–227.
251 Runyon BA, LaBrecque DR, Anuras S. The spectrum of liver disease in systemic lupus erythematosus. Report of 33 histologically-proved cases and review of the literature. *Am J Med* 1980; **69**: 187–194.
252 Matsumoto T, Yoshimine T, Shimouchi K, et al. The liver in systemic lupus erythematosus: pathologic analysis of 52 cases and review of Japanese autopsy registry data. *Hum Pathol* 1992; **23**: 1151–1158.
253 Gibson T, Myers AR. Subclinical liver disease in systemic lupus erythematosus. *J Rheumatol* 1981; **8**: 752–759.
254 Miller MH, Urowitz MB, Gladman DD, et al. The liver in systemic lupus erythematosus. *Quart J Med* 1984; **53**: 401–409.
255 Robertson SJ, Higgins RB, Powell C. Malacoplakia of liver: a case report. *Hum Pathol* 1991; **22**: 1294–1295.
256 Marshall JB, Ravendhran N, Sharp GC. Liver disease in mixed connective tissue disease. *Arch Intern Med* 1983; **143**: 1817–1818.
257 Chopra S, Rubinow A, Koff RS, et al. Hepatic amyloidosis. A histopathologic analysis of primary (AL) and secondary (AA) forms. *Am J Pathol* 1984; **115**: 186–193.
258 Buck FS, Koss MN. Hepatic amyloidosis: morphologic differences between systemic AL and AA types. *Hum Pathol* 1991; **22**: 904–907.
259 Looi L-M, Sumithran E. Morphologic differences in the pattern of liver infiltration between systemic AL and AA amyloidosis. *Hum Pathol* 1988; **19**: 732–735.
260 Wright JR, Calkins E, Humphrey RL. Potassium permanganate reaction in amyloidosis. A histologic method to assist in differentiating forms of this disease. *Lab Invest* 1977; **36**: 274–281.
261 Shirahama T, Skinner M, Cohen AS. Immunocytochemical identification of amyloid in formalin-fixed paraffin sections. *Histochemistry* 1981; **72**: 161–171.
262 Falk RH, Comenzo RL, Skinner M. The systemic amyloidoses. *N Engl J Med* 1997; **337**: 898–909.

263 Rubinow A, Koff RS, Cohen AS. Severe intrahepatic cholestasis in primary amyloidosis: a report of four cases and a review of the literature. *Am J Med* 1978; **64**: 937–946.
264 Finkelstein SD, Fornasier VL, Pruzanski W. Intrahepatic cholestasis with predominant pericentral deposition in systemic amyloidosis. *Hum Pathol* 1981; **12**: 470–472.
265 Case records of the Massachusetts General Hospital. Case 50-1987. *N Engl J Med* 1987; **317**: 1520–1531.
266 Livni N, Behar AJ, Lafair JS. Unusual amyloid bodies in human liver. Ultrastructural and freeze-etching studies. *Isr J Med Sci* 1977; **13**: 1163–1170.
267 French SW, Schloss GT, Stillman AE. Unusual amyloid bodies in human liver. *Am J Clin Pathol* 1981; **75**: 400–402.
268 Kanel GC, Uchida T, Peters RL. Globular hepatic amyloid – an unusual morphologic presentation. *Hepatology* 1981; **1**: 647–652.
269 Droz D, Noel LH, Carnot F, et al. Liver involvement in nonamyloid light chain deposits disease. *Lab Invest* 1984; **50**: 683–689.
270 Kirkpatrick CJ, Curry A, Galle J, et al. Systemic kappa light chain deposition and amyloidosis in multiple myeloma: novel morphological observations. *Histopathology* 1986; **10**: 1065–1076.
271 Smith NM, Malcolm AJ. Simultaneous AL-type amyloid and light chain deposit disease in a liver biopsy: a case report. *Histopathology* 1986; **10**: 1057–1064.
272 Bruguera M. Liver involvement in porphyria. *Sem Dermatol* 1986; **5**: 178–185.
273 Fakan F, Chlumská A. Demonstration of needle-shaped hepatic inclusions in porphyria cutanea tarda using the ferric ferricyanide reduction test. *Virchows Arch A* 1987; **411**: 365–368.
274 Cortés JM, Oliva H, Paradinas FJ, et al. The pathology of the liver in porphyria cutanea tarda. *Histopathology* 1980; **4**: 471–485.
275 Campo E, Bruguera M, Rodés J. Are there diagnostic histologic features of porphyria cutanea tarda in liver biopsy specimens? *Liver* 1990; **10**: 185–190.
276 Lefkowitch JH, Grossman ME. Hepatic pathology in porphyria cutanea tarda. *Liver* 1983; **3**: 19–29.
277 Nagy Z, Kószo F, Pár A, et al. Hemochromatosis (HFE) gene mutations and hepatitis C virus infection as risk factors for porphyria cutanea tarda in Hungarian patients. *Liver Int* 2004; **24**: 16–20.
278 Bonkovsky HL, Poh-Fitzpatrick M, Pimstone N, et al. Porphyria cutanea tarda, hepatitis C and HFE gene mutations in North America. *Hepatology* 1998; **27**: 1661–1669.
279 Bulaj ZJ, Phillips JD, Ajioka RS, et al. Hemochromatosis genes and other factors contributing to the pathogenesis of porphyria cutanea tarda. *Blood* 2000; **95**: 1565–1571.
280 Fargion S, Piperno A, Cappellini MD, et al. Hepatitis C virus and porphyria cutanea tarda: evidence of a strong association. *Hepatology* 1992; **16**: 1322–1326.
281 Herrero C, Vicente A, Bruguera M, et al. Is hepatitis C virus infection a trigger of porphyria cutanea tarda? *Lancet* 1993; **341**: 788–789.
282 DeCastro M, Sánchez J, Herrera JF, et al. Hepatitis C virus antibodies and liver disease in patients with porphyria cutanea tarda. *Hepatology* 1993; **17**: 551–557.
283 Bonkovsky H, Poh-Fitzpatrick M, Tattrie C, et al. Porphyria cutanea tarda and hepatitis C in the USA. *Hepatology* 1996; **24**: 486A.
284 Gisbert JP, García-Buey L, Pajares JM, et al. Prevalence of hepatitis C virus infection in porphyria cutanea tarda: systematic review and meta-analysis. *J Hepatol* 2003; **39**: 620–627.
285 Fargion S, Fracanzani AL. Prevalence of hepatitis C virus infection in porphyria cutanea tarda. *J Hepatol* 2003; **39**: 635–638.
286 Klatskin G, Bloomer JR. Birefringence of hepatic pigment deposits in erythropoietic protoporphyria. Specificity of polarization microscopy in the identification of hepatic protoporphyrin deposits. *Gastroenterology* 1974; **67**: 294–302.
287 Bloomer JR, Phillips MJ, Davidson DL, et al. Hepatic disease in erythropoietic protoporphyria. *Am J Med* 1975; **58**: 869–882.
288 Bonkovsky HL, Schned AR. Fatal liver failure in protoporphyria. Synergism

between ethanol excess and the genetic defect. *Gastroenterology* 1986; **90**: 191–201.
289 Pérez V, Gorodisch S, Casavilla F, et al. Ultrastructure of human liver at the end of normal pregnancy. *Am J Obs Gyn* 1971; **110**: 428–431.
290 Schorr-Lesnick B, Lebovics E, Dworkin B, et al. Liver diseases unique to pregnancy. *Am J Gastroenterol* 1991; **86**: 659–670.
291 Riely CA. Liver disease in the pregnant patient. *Am J Gastroenterol* 1999; **94**: 1728–1732.
292 Kroll D, Mazor M, Zirkin H, et al. Fibrolamellar carcinoma of the liver in pregnancy. A case report. *J Reprod Med* 1991; **36**: 823–827.
293 Samuels P, Cohen AW. Pregnancies complicated by liver disease and liver dysfunction. *Obstet Gynecol Clin N Amer* 1992; **19**: 745–763.
294 Kaplan MM. Acute fatty liver of pregnancy. *N Engl J Med* 1985; **313**: 367–370.
295 Burroughs AK, Seong NH, Dojcinov DM, et al. Idiopathic acute fatty liver of pregnancy in 12 patients. *Quart J Med* 1982; **51**: 481–497.
296 Rolfes DB, Ishak KG. Acute fatty liver of pregnancy: a clinicopathologic study of 35 cases. *Hepatology* 1985; **5**: 1149–1158.
297 Sherlock S. Acute fatty liver of pregnancy and the microvesicular fat diseases. *Gut* 1983; **24**: 265–269.
298 Riely CA. Acute fatty liver of pregnancy. *Semin Liver Dis* 1987; **7**: 47–54.
299 Schoeman MN, Batey RG, Wilcken B. Recurrent acute fatty liver of pregnancy associated with a fatty-acid oxidation defect in the offspring. *Gastroenterology* 1991; **100**: 544–548.
300 Rolfes DB, Ishak KG. Liver disease in toxemia of pregnancy. *Am J Gastroenterol* 1986; **81**: 1138–1144.
301 Rolfes DB, Ishak KG. Liver disease in pregnancy. [Review]. *Histopathology* 1986; **10**: 555–570.
302 Arias F, Mancilla-Jimenez R. Hepatic fibrinogen deposits in pre-eclampsia. Immunofluorescent evidence. *N Engl J Med* 1976; **295**: 578–582.
303 Cheung H, Hamzah H. Liver rupture in pregnancy: a typical case? *Singapore Med J* 1992; **33**: 89–91.
304 Schorr-Lesnick B, Dworkin B, Rosenthal WS. Hemolysis, elevated liver enzymes and low platelets in pregnancy (HELLP syndrome). A case report and literature review. *Dig Dis Sci* 1991; **36**: 1649–1652.
305 Weinstein L. Syndrome of hemolysis, elevated liver enzymes and low platelet count: a severe consequence of hypertension in pregnancy. *Am J Obstet Gynecol* 1982; **142**: 159–167.
306 Weinstein L. Preeclampsia/eclampsia with hemolysis, elevated liver enzymes and thrombocytopenia. *Obstet Gynecol* 1985; **66**: 657–660.
307 Baca L, Gibbons RB. The HELLP syndrome: a serious complication of pregnancy with hemolysis, elevated levels of liver enzymes and low platelet count. *Am J Med* 1988; **85**: 590–591.
308 Ibdah JA, Bennett MJ, Rinaldo P, et al. A fetal fatty-acid oxidation disorder as a cause of liver disease in pregnant women. *N Engl J Med* 1999; **340**: 1723–1731.
309 Adlercreutz H, Tenhunen R. Some aspects of the interaction between natural and synthetic female sex hormones and the liver. [Review]. *Am J Med* 1970; **49**: 630–648.
310 Vanjak D, Moreau R, Roche-Sicot J, et al. Intrahepatic cholestasis of pregnancy and acute fatty liver of pregnancy. An unusual but favorable association? *Gastroenterology* 1991; **100**: 1123–1125.
311 Dixon PH, Weerasekera N, Linton KJ, et al. Heterozygous MDR3 missense mutation associated with intrahepatic cholestasis of pregnancy: evidence for a defect in protein trafficking. *Hum Mol Genet* 2000; **9**: 1209–1217.

GENERAL READING

Ferrell LD. Hepatic granulomas: a morphologic approach to diagnosis. *Surg Pathol* 1990; **3**: 87–106.

Sartin JS, Walker RC. Granulomatous hepatitis: a retrospective review of 88 cases at the Mayo Clinic. *Mayo Clin Proc* 1991; **66**: 914–918.

Gaya DR, Thorburn KA, Oien KA, Morris AJ, Stanley AJ. Hepatic granulomas: a 10 year single centre experience. *J Clin Pathol* 2003; **56**: 850–853.

Sandor M, Weinstock JV, Wynn TA. Granulomas in schistosome and mycobacterial infections: a model of local immune responses. *Trends Immunol* 2003; **24**: 44–52.

Lucas SB. Other viral and infectious diseases (including HIV-related liver disease). In: MacSween RNM, Burt AD, Portmann BC, et al., eds. Pathology of the Liver, 4th edn. Edinburgh: Churchill Livingstone, 2002: 363–414.

Burt AD, Portmann BC, MacSween RNM. Liver pathology associated with diseases of other organs or systems. In: MacSween RNM, Burt AD, Portmann BC, et al., eds. Pathology of the Liver, 4th edn. Edinburgh: Churchill Livingstone, 2002: 827–884.

Benjaminov FS, Heathcote J. Liver disease in pregnancy. *Am J Gastroenterol* 2004; **99**: 2479–2488.

CHAPTER 16

THE LIVER IN ORGAN TRANSPLANTATION

INTRODUCTION

The pathologist is often asked to examine liver biopsies obtained to evaluate liver dysfunction in transplant patients, including recipients of liver, renal and bone marrow grafts. For liver transplantation, liver biopsy remains the diagnostic 'gold standard' when jaundice and allograft dysfunction develop, since biochemical tests do not adequately discriminate between rejection and other conditions that may develop in the allograft.[1] At the time of harvesting or engraftment, the donor liver may also require assessment, sometimes by frozen section, for lesions that may determine whether or not the graft can be used and that can affect the postoperative course and appearances of subsequent post-transplantation biopsies. This chapter reviews the histopathological features of liver transplant rejection and other conditions affecting the allograft. The concluding portions of the chapter discuss liver disease in recipients of renal and bone marrow transplants.

LIVER TRANSPLANTATION

General considerations

Percutaneous liver biopsies are obtained as part of a liver transplantation protocol or because of clinical deterioration.[2] In appropriate settings, fine needle aspiration biopsy of the liver may also provide diagnostic information.[3] Biopsy specimens taken at the time of transplantation provide a useful baseline and give an indication of the state of the donor liver. Specimens obtained intraoperatively, directly after revascularization of the graft, also allow evaluation of possible preservation (ischaemic/reperfusion) injury.[4] In anticipation of special investigations requiring snap-frozen tissue, a portion of the biopsy can be set aside for that purpose. Discussion with the clinical team and careful review of pertinent radiographic, biochemical and microbiological findings are critical to biopsy interpretation and institution of appropriate therapy. Serial biopsies may be necessary to resolve difficult diagnostic problems.

Frozen section of potential donor livers may be requested to exclude pre-existing disease. Pathologists providing frozen section coverage should be aware of three common reasons that frozen sections are requested: (1) to *determine if steatosis is present* and its degree; (2) *to exclude changes of chronic hepatitis* if the donor is known to be positive for antibodies to hepatitis B core antigen, but negative for surface antigen (i.e. possible occult hepatitis B) or is hepatitis C virus-positive and (3) to *evaluate a mass* found in the donor liver. Concern about a substantially **fatty liver** is based on the increased incidence of **primary graft dysfunction** or **nonfunction** when this is present.[5] The degree of macrovesicular (large droplet) fatty change should be categorised according to the percentage of parenchymal involvement as either absent, mild (<30%), moderate (30–60%) or marked (>60%).[6,7] Transplant surgeons have considered the last category unsuitable for use because of the high risk of primary dysfunction or non-function associated with severe steatosis.[5,7] Microvesicular (small droplet) fat is held not to be a contraindication, however,[8] but should also be graded and merits discussion with the transplant team if substantial. Diffuse portal mononuclear inflammatory cell infiltrates in donors with markers of hepatitis B or C viral infection support the presence of **chronic hepatitis**. The significance of this finding needs to be considered by the transplant team. With regard to **mass lesions** in the donor liver, demonstration of a malignant or metastatic tumour is an obvious contraindication to its use. However, the features of benign lesions such as focal nodular hyperplasia (Ch. 11) are important to recognise since they are often encountered in this setting.

There are many causes of allograft injury in addition to rejection (Table 16.1) and these should be considered in the context of the time elapsed since transplantation[9] (Fig. 16.1). For several weeks following transplantation, **functional cholestasis** may be present and must, if possible, be distinguished from the cholestasis of acute rejection, bile-duct obstruction, hepatitis, drug toxicity and sepsis. Bile is present within hepatocytes and canaliculi. This impairment of bile flow can be explained by exposure of the donor liver to cold ischaemia and reperfusion injury ('preservation injury') with resultant damage to liver-cell organelles.[10] Liver-cell death due to preservation injury actually shows features of both necrosis and apoptosis ('necrapoptosis').[11] Early postoperative cholestasis may also be due to a 'small-for-size' graft.[12] Cholestasis may be accompanied by **hepatocellular ballooning** in perivenular regions (Fig. 16.2) or in a diffuse distribution.[13,14] In the absence of frank perivenular necrosis, ballooning does not confer an unfavourable prognosis.[13] Hypoperfusion liver damage in the perioperative period may result in necrosis in periportal or perivenular regions and sometimes an irregular subcapsular band of

Table 16.1 Pathological considerations in the transplant liver

Graft rejection
Humoral (hyperacute)
Acute (cellular)
Chronic (ductopenic)
Functional cholestasis
Preservation injury
Bile duct obstruction
Thrombosis of hepatic artery or portal vein
Infections and sepsis
Drug toxicity
Recurrence of original disease
Neoplastic disease
Post-transplant lymphoproliferative disease
Hepatocellular carcinoma

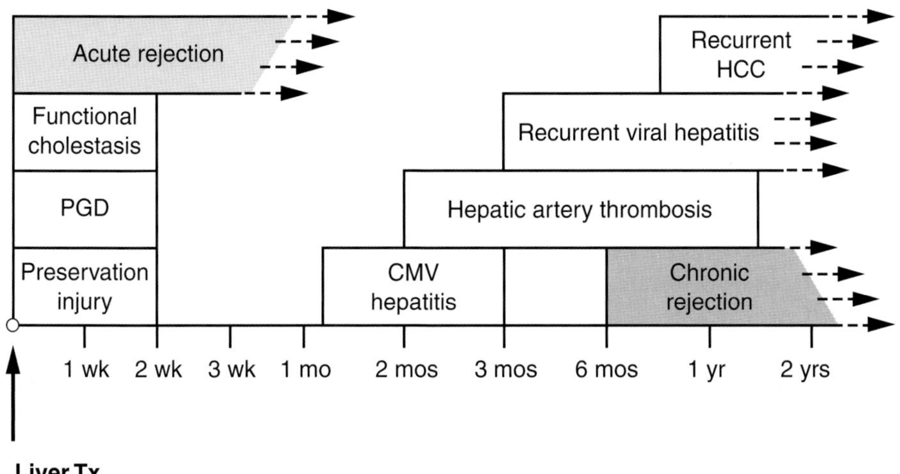

Figure 16.1 *Timeline of pathologic lesions after liver transplantation.* Common post-transplantation problems are shown correlated with the approximate time frame in which they develop. Dashed arrows indicate the potential for the condition to develop at a later time. CMV, cytomegalovirus; HCC, hepatocellular carcinoma; PGD, primary graft dysfunction.

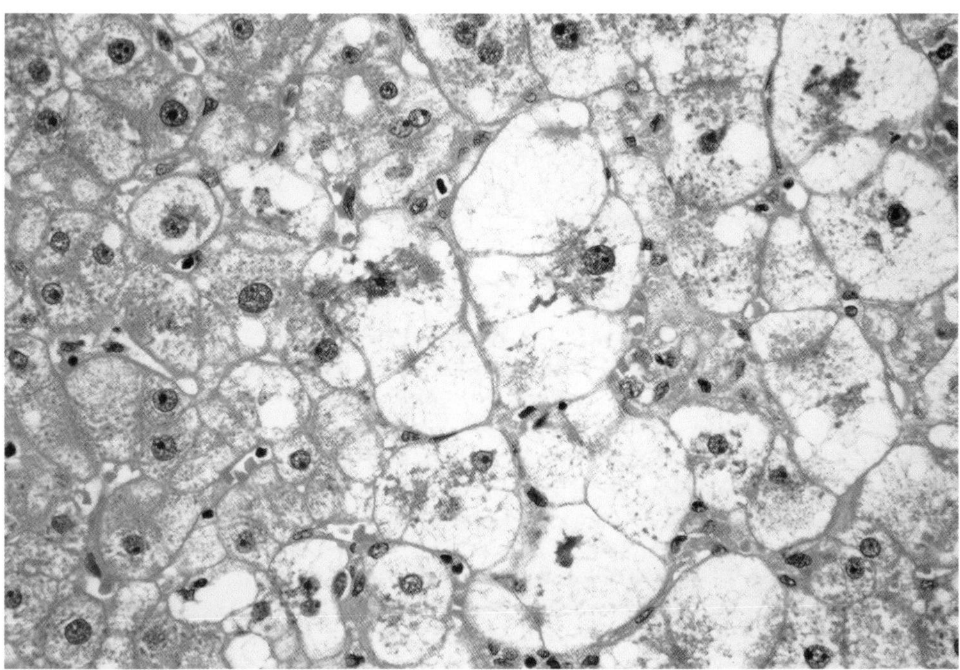

Figure 16.2 *Liver-cell ballooning after transplantation.* A liver biopsy obtained in week 2 following transplant shows ballooning of hepatocytes in a perivenular area. Intracellular cholestasis is visible. (Needle biopsy, H&E).

infarction.[15] If the donor liver is fatty, rupture of hepatocytes affected by preservation injury may rarely cause sinusoidal engorgement by lipid vacuoles (**lipopeliosis**)[16] (Fig. 16.3).

In evaluating post-transplant biopsies, special attention should be paid to the portal tracts, the major sites of rejection lesions. The type of cellular infiltrate, the bile ducts, portal vein branches and hepatic arterioles are examined to distinguish rejection from other conditions with portal tract pathology, particularly **bile duct obstruction, recurrent viral hepatitis, drug toxicity** and immunosuppression-related **lymphoproliferative disease** (see Differential diagnosis in transplant biopsies). The perivenular region also requires inspection for possible preservation injury, cholestasis or inflammation, and for necrosis which may accompany portal tract lesions in more severe cases of acute rejection[17] (see below). The lobular parenchyma shows few alterations in rejection apart from cholestasis, occasional acidophilic bodies and scattered liver-cell mitoses. As a result, in cases where confusion arises in the interpretation of portal changes, it is important to carefully evaluate the lobular parenchyma for evidence of intercurrent diseases such as viral or drug hepatitis. In the event that only a portion of the liver from a **living-related donor** is transplanted, enhancement of either apoptotic (acidophilic) bodies or hepatocellular mitosis is seen as the graft modulates to the appropriate size for the recipient. Postoperative portal tract biliary obstructive changes may also be present due to ischaemia or mechanical obstruction of the large bile ducts associated with this type of procedure.[18] *The pathologist should also bear in mind that a given biopsy may show superimposed features attributable to several different post-transplantation complications.*

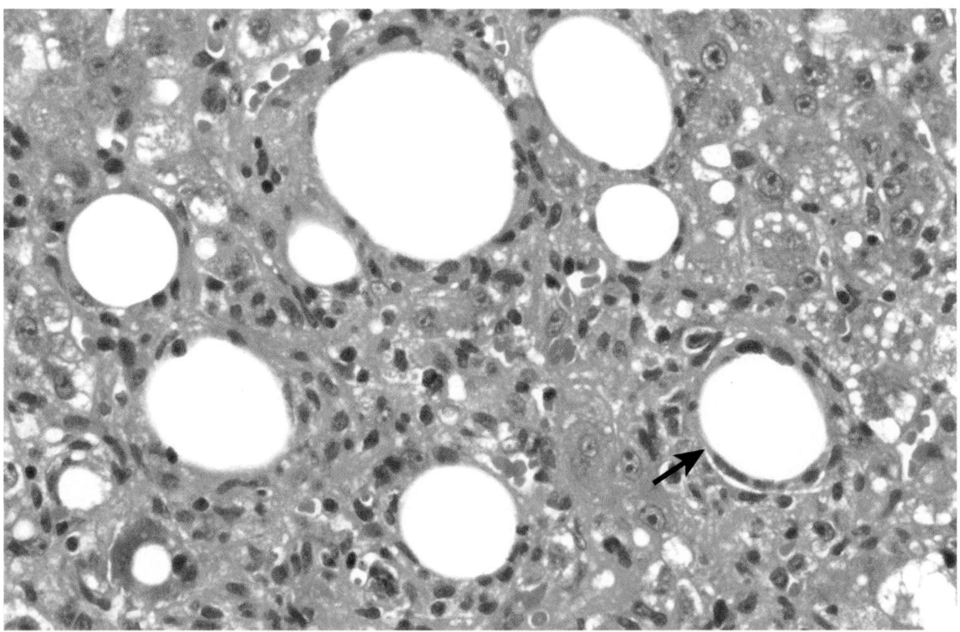

Figure 16.3 *Lipopeliosis.* The enlarged empty spaces in this perivenular region represent ruptured and coalescent lipid vacuoles within sinusoids. This developed due to necrosis and rupture of steatotic hepatocytes following allograft preservation injury. A Kupffer cell foreign body reaction engulfing the lipid is present (arrow). (Needle biopsy, H&E).

Graft rejection

The histopathological lesions of liver allograft rejection have been well characterised[19–23] and are classified as **humoral rejection, acute (cellular) rejection** and **chronic (ductopenic) rejection** as recommended by an international working party which met in 1994.[17] Acute and chronic rejection are the most common forms seen in clinical practice.

Humoral rejection

Humoral rejection (antibody-mediated or hyperacute rejection) is rare after liver transplantation, developing in patients with preformed antibodies or subsequently formed antibodies to an ABO blood group-incompatible donor liver. Microvascular damage evolves over the first few hours after transplantation, consisting of sinusoidal infiltrates of neutrophilic leucocytes, fibrin and red blood cells associated with focal haemorrhages. This progresses to portal and periportal edema with coagulative and haemorrhagic necrosis over the next few days[24] (Fig. 16.4). Immunofluorescent studies show linear deposits of IgG or IgM, complement fractions C1q, C3 and C4 and fibrinogen in arterial walls.[17,24] The graft may remain stable in some patients for the first few days, however, possibly because of Kupffer cell protection against the effects of circulating antibodies.[25] Graft failure within 2–4 weeks is associated with a progressive marked rise in serum aminotransferase activity. The liver appears mottled and cyanotic at gross examination. Recipients of ABO unmatched livers may also develop **graft-versus-host haemolysis**, associated with erythrophagocytosis and **Kupffer cell siderosis**.[26]

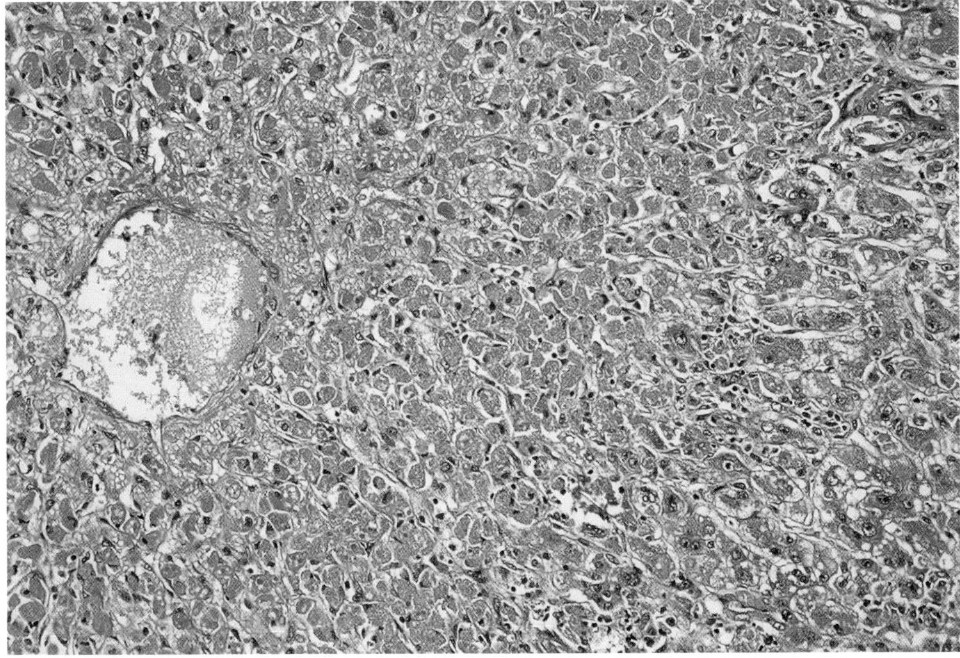

Figure 16.4 *Humoral (hyperacute) rejection*. Hepatocytes show extensive coagulative necrosis and apoptosis, and scattered neutrophils are present within sinusoids. Clumps of adherent platelets are seen in the terminal hepatic venule at left. The patient's serum contained antibodies to donor histocompatibility antigens. (Explant donor liver, H&E).

Acute (cellular) rejection

Acute (cellular) rejection, the most common form of rejection, is a cell-mediated immune injury directed at bile-duct epithelium and the endothelium of portal vein branches and terminal hepatic venules. This usually occurs within the first month to 6 weeks after transplantation,[27] but may be seen later if immunosuppression is lowered or discontinued. The characteristic histologic **triad** of cellular rejection includes **portal inflammation, bile duct damage,** and **endotheliitis (endothelialitis)**. Endotheliitis is not present in all cases. The portal inflammatory lesion is typically heterogeneous, with lymphocytes predominating among plasma cells, neutrophils and, occasionally, large lymphoid cells, some in mitosis (Fig. 16.5). Eosinophils are often abundant (Fig. 16.6) and are a very helpful diagnostic sign that acute rejection is present.[28,29] Bile ducts are surrounded and infiltrated by immune cells and damage to their epithelium takes the form of variation in nuclear size, vacuolation of cytoplasm, regions of cell stratification or cell loss and irregularity of duct outlines (Figs 16.5–16.7). Endotheliitis comprises attachment of lymphoid cells to the endothelium of portal-vein branches or terminal hepatic venules, variable degrees of endothelial damage, subendothelial inflammation (Figs 16.5, 16.6) and lifting off of endothelial cells from the underlying vein wall (Fig. 16.8). Sinusoidal endotheliitis is occasionally also present. Mild focal endotheliitis is sometimes found in association with hypoperfusion damage in baseline biopsies, but extensive endotheliitis in the postoperative period is very characteristic of rejection.[19] Necrosis of perivenular hepatocytes, accompanied by endotheliitis of terminal hepatic venules and expansive portal inflammatory lesions involving the periportal parenchyma, is indicative of severe acute rejection.[30] **Central venulitis** with nearby hepatocellular

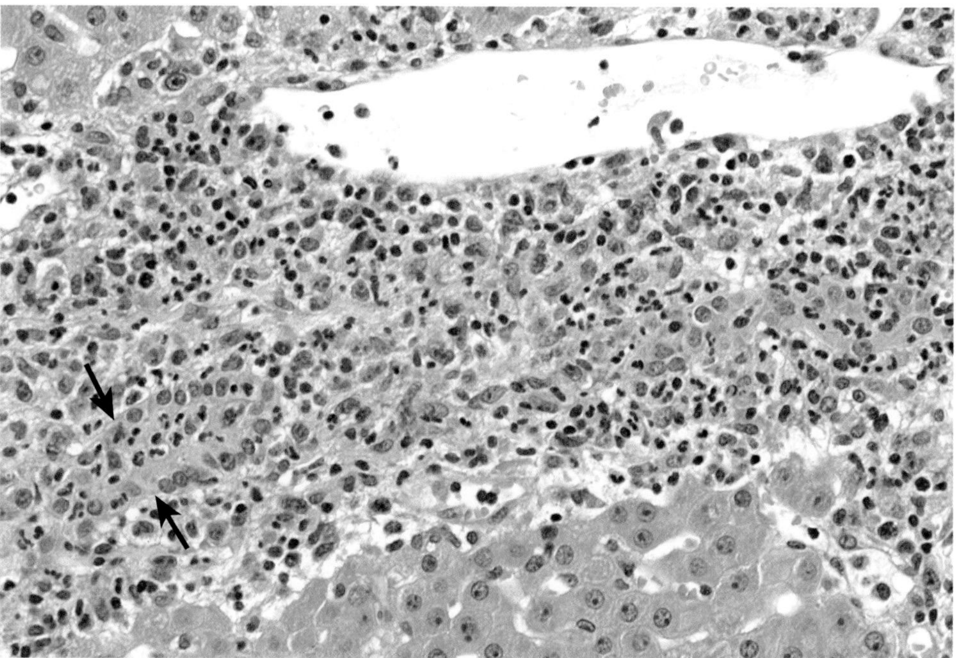

Figure 16.5 *Acute rejection.* Heterogeneous portal inflammation consisting of lymphocytes, plasma cells and scattered neutrophils infiltrates the bile duct (between arrows) and the portal vein branch at top. (Needle biopsy, H&E).

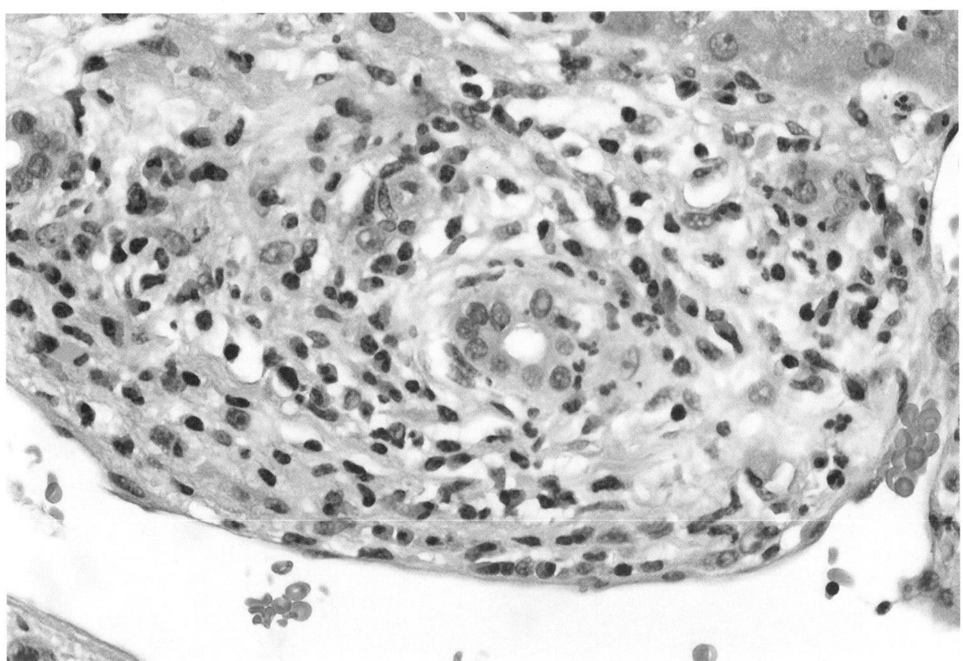

Figure 16.6 *Acute rejection*. The portal tract infiltrate is rich in eosinophils. The portal vein branch at bottom shows endotheliitis, with subendothelial lymphocytes and eosinophils. (Needle biopsy, H&E).

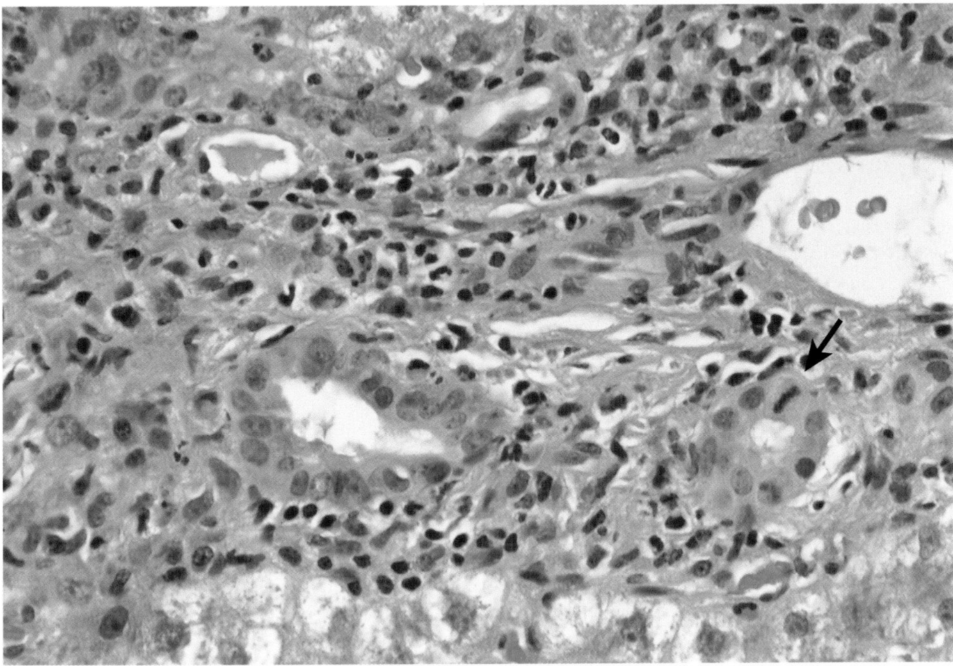

Figure 16.7 *Acute rejection*. A damaged bile duct, cut twice in this portal tract, shows irregular epithelium with mild nuclear pleomorphism. Neutrophils are admixed with lymphocytes around and above the duct at left. The duct profile at right shows a mitotic figure (arrow). (Needle biopsy, H&E). (Case kindly provided by Dr Jurgen Ludwig, Rochester, Minnesota).

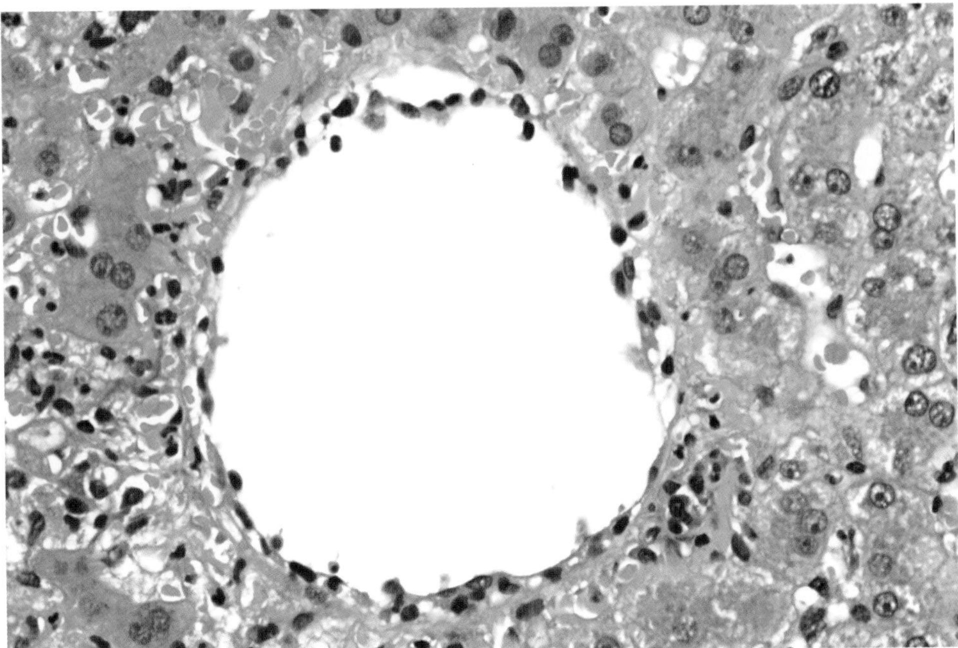

Figure 16.8 *Endotheliitis in acute rejection.* An efferent vein shows lymphocytic infiltration of its wall. The endothelium is focally lifted off the underlying vein wall and partially destroyed. (Needle biopsy, H&E).

dropout and apoptosis often presages later episodes of acute rejection and chronic ductopenic rejection.[31,31a]

Descriptive and semi-quantitative **grading of acute rejection** can effectively be accomplished using the scoring system presented in the Banff international consensus document[30] (Table 16.2). Using the semi-quantitative approach of assigning a numerical score to each component of the acute rejection triad, a total **Rejection Activity Index (RAI)** can be conveyed in the biopsy report. Alternatively, a simpler global assessment of the biopsy as showing indeterminate, mild, moderate or severe changes of acute rejection can be used (Table 16.3). The choice of grading system, as with grading and staging for chronic hepatitis, should be made after discussion with clinicians.

Chronic (ductopenic) rejection

Chronic (ductopenic) rejection ('vanishing bile duct syndrome') is defined as obliterative vasculopathy and loss of bile ducts occurring 60 days or longer after transplantation.[17,32] The incidence of chronic rejection in liver transplant patients has declined to less than 5% in some series[33–35] as immunosuppression regimens have improved. In most cases, vasculopathy and ductopenia occur together, but in a minority they can be present independently.[36] The diagnosis of chronic rejection can be problematic even for experienced hepatic pathologists,[37,38] particularly in the early stages.[17] Atrophy, nuclear pleomorphism and pyknosis of small ducts (bile-duct 'dystrophy') often precede frank ductopenia.[39] The presence of ductopenia is established when a formal count of small bile ducts and hepatic artery branches within portal tracts demonstrates loss of bile ducts from over 50% of portal tracts

Table 16.2 Banff grading scheme for acute rejection*

Category	Criteria	Score
Portal inflammation	Mostly lymphocytic inflammation involving, but not noticeably expanding, a minority of the triads	1
	Expansion of most or all of the triads, by a mixed infiltrate containing lymphocytes with occasional blasts, neutrophils and eosinophils	2
	Marked expansion of most or all of the triads by a mixed infiltrate containing numerous blasts and eosinophils with inflammatory spillover into the periportal parenchyma	3
Bile-duct inflammation damage	A minority of the ducts are cuffed and infiltrated by inflammatory cells and show only mild reactive changes such as increased nuclear:cytoplasmic ratio of the epithelial cells	1
	Most or all of the ducts infiltrated by inflammatory cells. More than an occasional duct shows degenerative changes such as nuclear pleomorphism, disordered polarity and cytoplasmic vacuolization of the epithelium	2
	As above for 2, with most or all of the ducts showing degenerative changes or focal luminal disruption	3
Venous endothelial inflammation	Subendothelial lymphocytic infiltration involving some, but not a majority of the portal and/or hepatic venules	1
	Subendothelial infiltration involving most or all of the portal and/or hepatic venules	2
	As above for 2, with moderate or severe perivenular inflammation that extends into the perivenular parenchyma and is associated with perivenular hepatocyte necrosis	3

Note: Total score = sum of components. Criteria that can be used to score liver allograft biopsies with acute rejection are as defined in the World Gastroenterology Consensus Document.
*The Rejection Activity Index (RAI) is the sum of the scores for each of the three components of acute rejection. RAI ≤ 4 (mild), RAI ≥ 6 (moderate or severe). (Table from Ref. 30, with permission.)

(Fig. 16.9). Progressive bile-duct loss results from a destructive cholangitis which in most cases stems from bouts of acute rejection that are not controlled by immunosuppression. Cytokeratin immunostaining may help identify remnants of bile duct epithelium.[22] Portal tract hepatic arterioles may also be lost.[32] Over time, portal inflammation becomes sparse and bile ducts disappear from the majority of portal tracts, usually without a ductular reaction[32] (Fig. 16.9). Episodes of acute rejection with increased inflammation and endotheliitis may develop superimposed on changes of chronic rejection. The pathology report in chronic rejection should therefore include consideration of the following points:[32] (1) whether acute rejection is present; (2) the degree of bile duct loss in portal tracts; (3) the presence of perivenular necrosis or fibrosis and (4) the degree of hepatic arteriole loss in relation to the total number of portal tracts.

Table 16.3 Descriptive terminology for acute rejection

Global Assessment*	Criteria
Indeterminate	Portal inflammatory infiltrate that fails to meet the criteria for the diagnosis of acute rejection (see text)
Mild	Rejection infiltrate in a minority of the triads, that is generally mild, and confined within the portal spaces
Moderate	Rejection infiltrate, expanding most or all the triads
Severe	As above for moderate, with spillover into periportal areas and moderate to severe perivenular inflammation that extends into the hepatic parenchyma and is associated with perivenular hepatocyte necrosis

Note: Global assessment of rejection grade is made on a review of the biopsy and after the diagnosis of rejection has been established.
*Verbal description of mild, moderate or severe acute rejection could also be labelled as grade I, II and III, respectively. (Table from Ref. 30, with permission.)

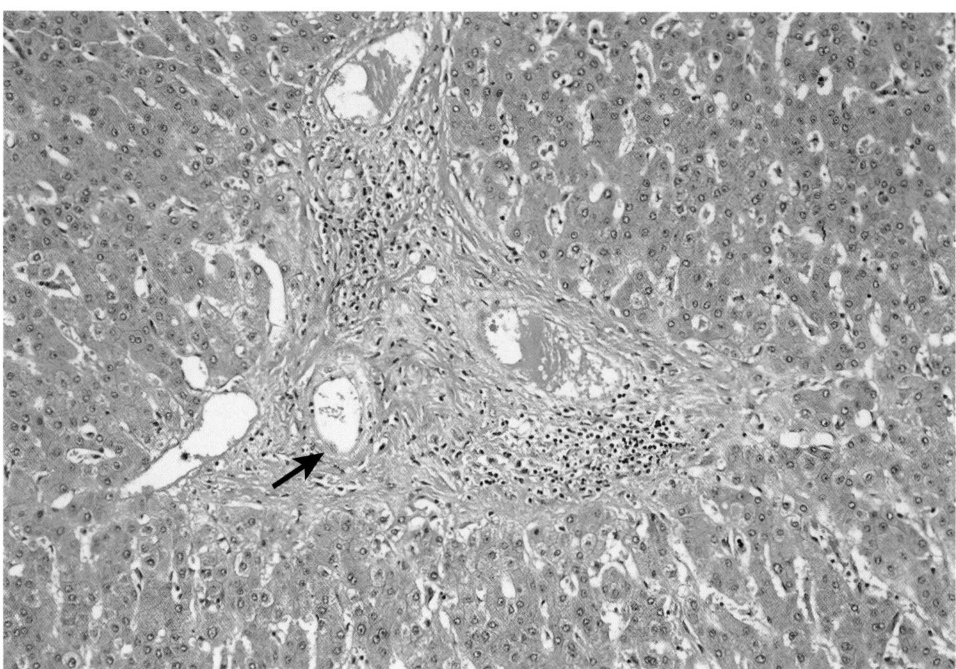

Figure 16.9 *Chronic (ductopenic) rejection.* An hepatic artery branch (arrow) is present in the portal tract but the corresponding interlobular bile duct has disappeared as a result of rejection. A sparse lymphocytic infiltrate remains. (Explanted donor liver, H&E). (Case kindly provided by Dr Jurgen Ludwig, Rochester, MN).

The presence of obliterative vasculopathy (rejection arteriopathy) may be more difficult to demonstrate on needle biopsies, since the characteristic subintimal accumulations of foamy histiocytes and myointimal cells predominantly affect the large-calibre arteries of the liver hilum[36,40] (Fig. 16.10). However, foam cell lesions can sometimes be demonstrated in medium-sized portal arterioles present in biopsies and occasionally in portal veins and sinusoids (Fig. 16.11). The presence of

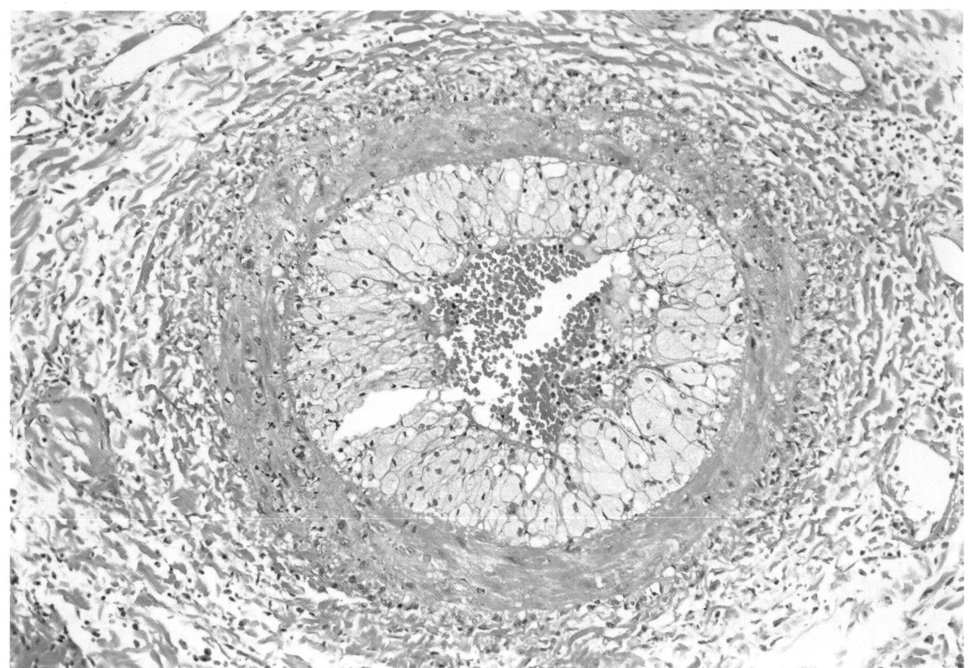

Figure 16.10 *Rejection arteriopathy*. A hilar artery from a transplant liver removed because of rejection shows an accumulation of subintimal foam cells. (Explanted donor liver, H&E). (Case kindly provided by Dr Jurgen Ludwig, Rochester, MN).

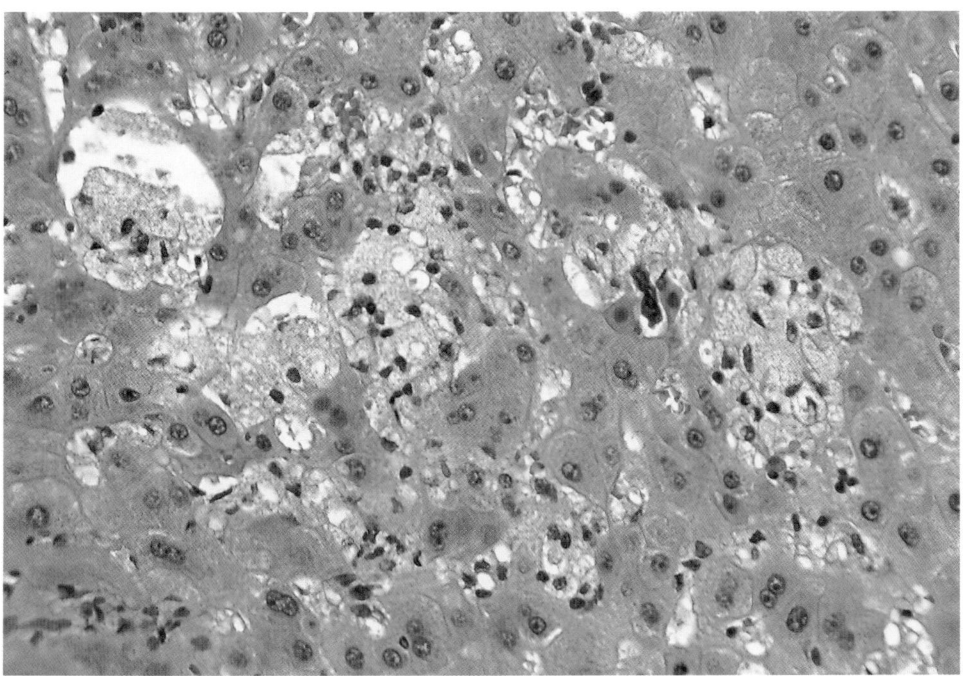

Figure 16.11 *Sinusoidal foam cells in transplant rejection*. Months after transplantation, foam cells may be deposited in large-calibre arteries and also within hepatic sinusoids. (Needle biopsy, H&E).

arteriopathy in most cases must be inferred when perivenular ischaemic necrosis and fibrosis are seen in liver biopsies obtained in the appropriate time frame of chronic rejection. Demonstration of perivenular necrosis in repeated biopsies indicates a poor prognosis.[41] Mismatch of recipient and donor histocompatibility antigens, activation of the complement membrane attack complex and persistent cytomegalovirus infection in the allograft have been invoked in the pathogenesis of bile duct loss and arteriopathy.[22,42–46]

Chronic rejection usually leads to irreversible graft failure, although some patients may recover.[22,47] The late stage characteristically shows marked cholestasis and bile duct loss, portal and periportal fibrosis, perivenular fibrosis and variable numbers of bridging fibrous septa linking portal tracts or central veins to portal tracts. Cirrhosis develops after liver transplantation in only a minority of patients and is typically due to recurrent or acquired viral hepatitis, rather than chronic rejection[48] (see Recurrent disease).

Other causes of graft dysfunction

Infection

Cytomegalovirus (CMV) is a common pathogen in liver allografts, most cases of CMV hepatitis occurring 4–8 weeks after transplant.[49] Typical intranuclear and cytoplasmic CMV inclusions (see Ch. 15) can be found in hepatocytes, bile duct epithelium (see Fig. 15.5) and endothelial cells. CMV infection should be suspected when small **microabscess**-like foci of necrosis with an infiltrate of neutrophils are present (Fig. 16.12). Smaller collections of parenchymal neutrophils (**'mini-microabscesses'**) are occasionally seen in patients without CMV infection, however, apparently without adverse effects on the graft.[50] CMV infection may also lead to formation of epithelioid granulomas. Immunohistochemical staining for CMV antigens is a sensitive method of demonstrating occult infection.[51] **Epstein-Barr Virus (EBV)** infection should be considered if portal tracts and sinusoids contain a preponderance of atypical lymphocytes and immunoblasts.[52–54] The possibility that as yet unidentified hepatitis viruses may cause post-transplantation liver dysfunction has been considered.[55]

Infection by **Gram-negative bacilli** may produce hepatocellular and canalicular cholestasis or, with sepsis, the more unusual picture of inspissated bile in periportal bile ductules ('bile ductular cholestasis') (see Ch. 15 and Fig. 15.11). Cholestasis due to infection and/or sepsis must be distinguished from that seen in bile duct obstruction and rejection. Assessment of portal tract changes as well as results of microbiological studies are important in making these distinctions. Culture and special stains of liver biopsy specimens which show microabscesses or granulomas are the best means of documenting **bacterial and fungal infections**.

Thrombosis

Thrombosis of the hepatic artery[56,57] or portal vein[58] (the latter, particularly in children) may develop within the first few weeks or months of transplantation, leading to infarction of the liver (see Ch. 12). Needle biopsy specimens may not be representative due to the irregular distribution of infarcted liver parenchyma.

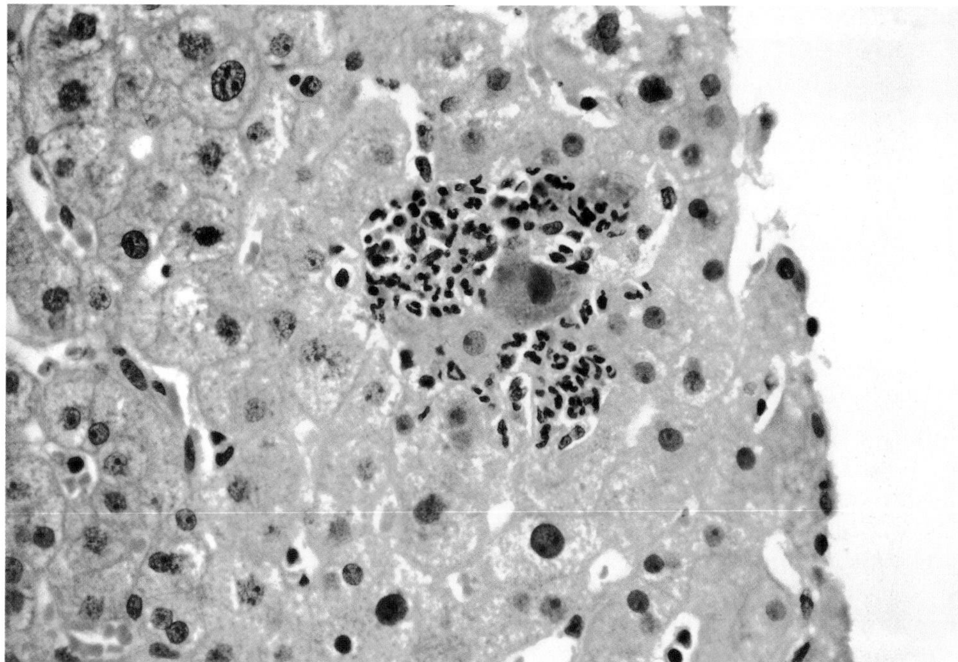

Figure 16.12 *Cytomegalovirus hepatitis*. A microabscess-like cluster of neutrophils surrounds a hepatocyte with a smudged intranuclear inclusion. (Needle biopsy, H&E).

Thrombosis, stricture or foam cell arteriopathy of perihilar arteries may cause necrosis, stricture, or cholangiectases of perihilar bile ducts due to impaired duct perfusion.[59] Liver biopsy in such cases may show features of biliary obstruction.[59]

Drug toxicity

The therapeutic regimen for immunosuppression in liver transplant patients includes several potentially hepatotoxic agents. **Azathioprine** hepatotoxicity has been reported primarily in renal transplant patients (see Renal transplantation). Elevated activities of serum aminotransferases with **sinusoidal congestion** and **perivenular necrosis** have been described in liver transplant patients treated with the drug[60] and veno-occlusive disease elsewhere in the graft should be suspected, even if not demonstrated in the biopsy sample. There may also be **fibrosis of terminal hepatic venules**, particularly in patients with cellular rejection and endotheliitis.[61] **Cyclosporine** may cause **cholestasis**[62] by inhibition of ATP-dependent bile salt transport.[63,64] Although a similar mechanism of cholestasis obtains for FK 506, hepatotoxicity is rare, probably due to the lower dose of FK 506 required for immunosuppression.[65,66]

Recurrent disease

Many of the diseases for which liver transplantation is performed have the potential to recur,[67] including viral hepatitis, malignant tumours, alcoholic and non-alcoholic steatohepatitis,[68–70] Budd-Chiari syndrome and variants of veno-occlusive disease,[71] autoimmune hepatitis, primary biliary cirrhosis and primary sclerosing cholangitis. The diagnosis of recurrent disease on liver biopsy can be controversial because some of these pre-transplant disorders have histopathological features which overlap with those seen in rejection or post-transplantation biliary obstruction.

Although the incidence of **recurrent viral hepatitis** in patients transplanted for severe liver disease due to hepatitis B, C and D varies at different transplantation centres, without prophylactic therapy it is an expected outcome in most cases. There are varied histopathological expressions of **recurrent hepatitis B**, including acute hepatitis, chronic hepatitis, cirrhosis, a carrier state with minimal histological disease, and fibrosing cholestatic hepatitis[72,73] (see below). Recurrent hepatitis B may evolve from chronic hepatitis to cirrhosis within a year after transplantation.[74] Hepatitis B and D (delta) antigens can be demonstrated by immunohistochemistry in allografts as early as 1 to 3 weeks after transplantation.[74] For patients with **co-infection by hepatitis B and hepatitis D** in the native liver, recurrence may follow a variable course. In some patients, delta virus recurs without demonstrable hepatitis B virus replication (absence of HBV core antigen on immunohistochemistry) or histological evidence of hepatitis.[75] Once HBV replication recurs and core antigen is present in the allograft, chronic hepatitis may then be seen on biopsy.[76] A minority of patients with recurrent hepatitis B infection may show a **fibrosing cholestatic hepatitis (FCH)** with large numbers of ground-glass inclusions, 'cytopathic' liver-cell ballooning, cholestasis and a network of periportal fibrosis[73,77–81] (Figs 16.13, 16.14). This pattern of disease recurrence is associated with a high rate of graft failure.

Recurrence of **hepatitis C** after transplantation results in a characteristic sequence of pathological changes.[82] Within the first several months, increased numbers of apoptotic bodies appear, an important histological marker of recurrence[83]

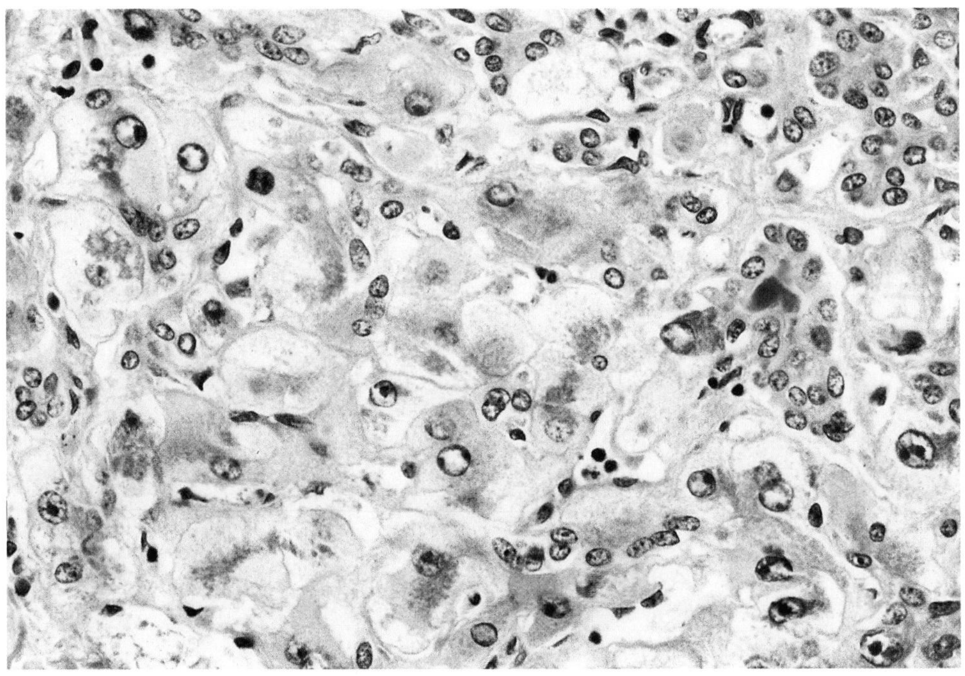

Figure 16.13 *Fibrosing cholestatic hepatitis.* Hepatocytes are swollen and many contain ground-glass inclusions. A bile thrombus is seen to the right of centre. (Explanted donor liver, H&E). (Case kindly provided by Dr Bernard Portmann, London).

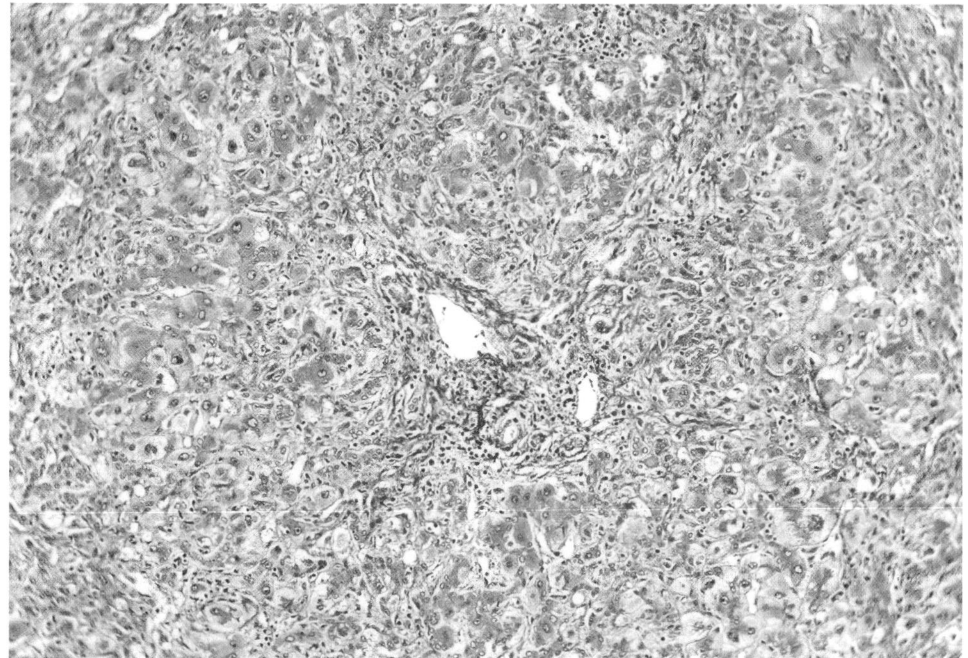

Figure 16.14 *Fibrosing cholestatic hepatitis.* Trichrome stain from the case depicted in Figure 16.12 shows an intricate network of fibrosis emanating from the portal tract (centre). (Explanted donor liver, trichrome). (Case kindly provided by Dr Bernard Portmann, London).

(Fig. 16.15). Their number and close proximity within the lobule far exceed that seen in acute rejection alone. Steatosis is often present and variable in degree, sometimes severe when genotype 3 infection recurs.[84] Increased lobular necroinflammation and liver-cell ballooning[85] follow and by 6 months to 1 year, the portal lesion of recurrent chronic hepatitis becomes established. This is manifested by the presence of lymphoid aggregates or follicles (sometimes an isolated finding in the first few months after transplant), lymphocytic or lymphoplasmacytic inflammation and variable degrees of interface hepatitis. The disease is frequently mild.[86,87] The inflammatory cell infiltrates are often polarised toward the edges of the portal tracts and periportal regions, in contrast to acute rejection where the infiltrates are more centrally localised around the bile ducts and portal vein branches. A ductular reaction is sometimes present in combination with the features of chronic hepatitis (Fig. 16.16) or may be the predominant portal lesion in the more serious **cholestatic recurrent hepatitis C**, which resembles fibrosing cholestatic hepatitis B.[88] These cases often show pronounced cholestasis and liver-cell ballooning (Fig. 16.16, *Inset*), features attributed to a direct cytopathic effects of the virus. Serum bilirubin and HCV titers are usually high.[89,90] The degree of fibrosis is more variable than in fibrosing cholestatic hepatitis B. Other forms of severe recurrent hepatitis C show confluent necrosis, liver cell ballooning, bridging fibrosis and cirrhosis.[89,90] Distinction of recurrent chronic hepatitis C from acute rejection is a common and challenging diagnostic problem,[82] often compounded when evidence of both processes are present in a given biopsy. Many histological parameters must therefore be evaluated (Table 16.4).

Following transplantation for **primary biliary cirrhosis (PBC)**, serum anti-mitochondrial antibodies may persist or recur, liver function tests (particularly

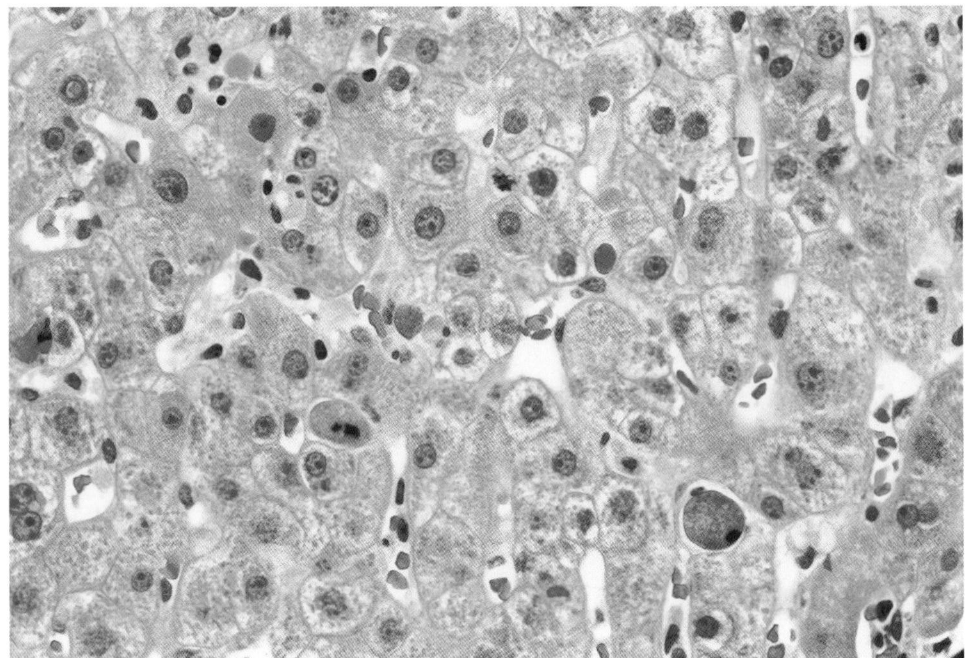

Figure 16.15 *Early recurrent hepatitis C after transplantation.* The numerous acidophilic (apoptotic) bodies shown here were the earliest histopathological evidence of recurrent hepatitis C in this case. (Needle biopsy, H&E).

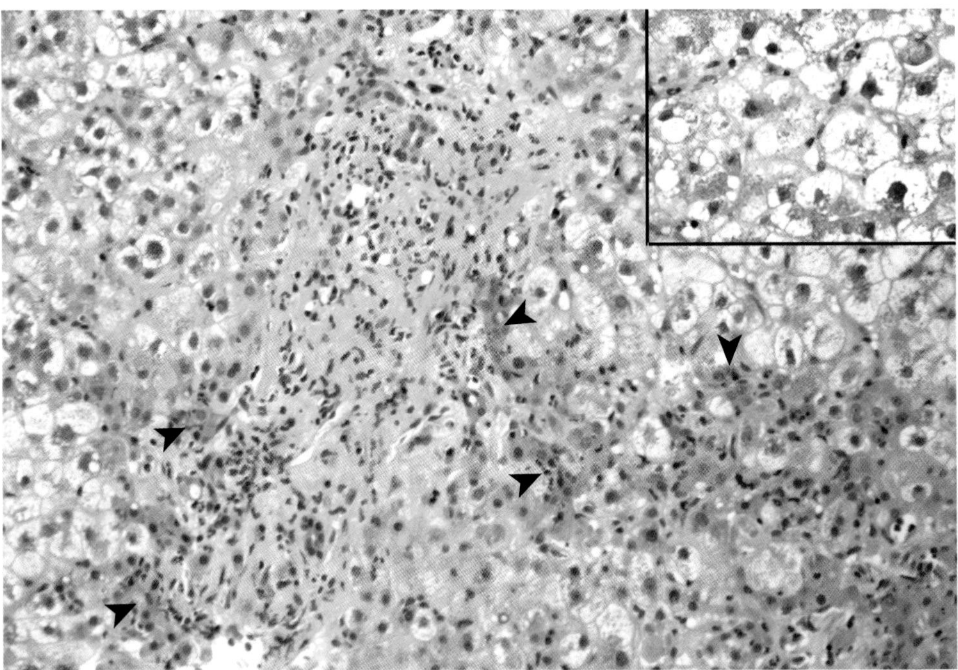

Figure 16.16 *Cholestatic recurrent chronic hepatitis C.* The portal tract shows mild chronic inflammation and fibrosis, with a prominent periportal ductular reaction (arrowheads). *Inset*: Hepatocytes show considerable ballooning cytopathic damage and cholestasis. (Needle biopsy, H&E).

Table 16.4 Comparative features of acute rejection *vs* recurrent chronic hepatitis C

Feature	Acute rejection	Recurrent hepatitis C
Lobular necroinflammation	No	Yes
Apoptotic bodies	Few	Many
Cholestasis	Mild	May be marked
Interface hepatitis	No (unless severe)	Often
Lymphoid aggregates/follicles	No	Yes
Portal inflammation	Heterogeneous	Lymphocytes, plasma cells
Fat	No (except with corticosteroid therapy)	Yes (genotype 3 especially)
Ductular reaction	No	Variable (common in cholestatic type)
Central venulitis	Often, diffuse	Uncommon, focal
Bile duct damage	Yes, diffuse	Focal or none
Portal/periportal fibrosis	No	Often

serum alkaline phosphatase activity) may worsen, and liver biopsy may demonstrate recurrent damage to bile ducts.[91] Florid bile-duct lesions and adjacent epithelioid granulomas are the most useful histological signs of recurrent disease. Ductular reaction and progressive copper deposition are other helpful features. There may also be portal lymphoid aggregates and mononuclear inflammation as well as ductopenia, but these can also be seen in hepatitis C virus infection and rejection. If there is uncertainty, hepatitis C virus infection should be serologically excluded. Recurrent PBC can progress to cirrhosis within several years.[92] **Autoimmune hepatitis** with high serum globulins and typical liver biopsy features has also been reported in patients transplanted for PBC.[93]

Recurrence of **primary sclerosing cholangitis (PSC)** after transplantation is reported,[94] but has been controversial because the radiological and histopathological features of PSC resemble those seen in biliary complications of the transplant procedure, such as biliary stricture due to hepatic artery thrombosis and bile duct or choledochojejunostomy anastomotic obstruction.[67] Biopsy features of cholestasis and portal obstructive changes therefore require cautious interpretation in the context of radiological and other data. Fibro-obliterative lesions (see Ch. 5) are more specific for recurrence.[94] Perihilar xanthogranulomatous cholangitis in the explanted PSC liver (see Ch. 5) has been associated with increased post-transplantation morbidity and mortality.

Studies of patients transplanted for **autoimmune hepatitis (AIH)** are at variance with regard to the incidence of recurrence.[67] An abrupt rise in serum aminotransferases, detectable autoantibodies, hypergammaglobulinaemia and portal inflammation with interface hepatitis on biopsy are consistent with recurrent disease. Lobular hepatitis may be the first sign of recurrence.[55] In children, recurrent AIH may be an aggressive disease resulting in cirrhosis and re-transplantation.[95]

De novo autoimmune hepatitis

Children and adults who have undergone liver transplantation for conditions other than autoimmune hepatitis infrequently develop *de novo* AIH, with elevated serum immunoglobulin levels and a variety of autoantibodies.[96] Lymphoplasmacytic interface hepatitis is the major histological criterion for this condition. The centrilobular necroinflammatory lesion of AIH (see Fig. 9.16) may also be present. A related, severe form of post-transplant liver disease, **graft dysfunction mimicking autoimmune hepatitis**,[97] can result in graft loss.

Neoplastic disease

Post-transplant lymphoproliferative disease (PTLD), chiefly B-cell lymphoma in lymph nodes and extranodal sites, is a complication of immunosuppression in patients with organ transplants. Special studies are important in determining whether the PTLD is polymorphic or monomorphic according to the current World Health Organization classification.[98] B-cell lymphoma in the liver has been reported as early as 2 months after liver transplantation,[99] but usually occurs one year or more after adult liver transplantation and within a year in children.[98] Lymphoma usually originates in recipient lymphoid tissue, but rarely it may be derived from donor lymphoid tissue present in the allograft.[100] Hepatic involvement consists of diffuse lymphoma nodules or portal tract infiltration by lymphoma cells (Fig. 16.17). Biopsy demonstration of Epstein-Barr virus, which is involved in the pathogenesis of most cases of PTLD,[98] is helpful in distinguishing this from rejection.[101] *De novo*[102,103] or recurrent[104] **hepatocellular carcinoma** has also developed in patients transplanted for chronic hepatitis B and C.

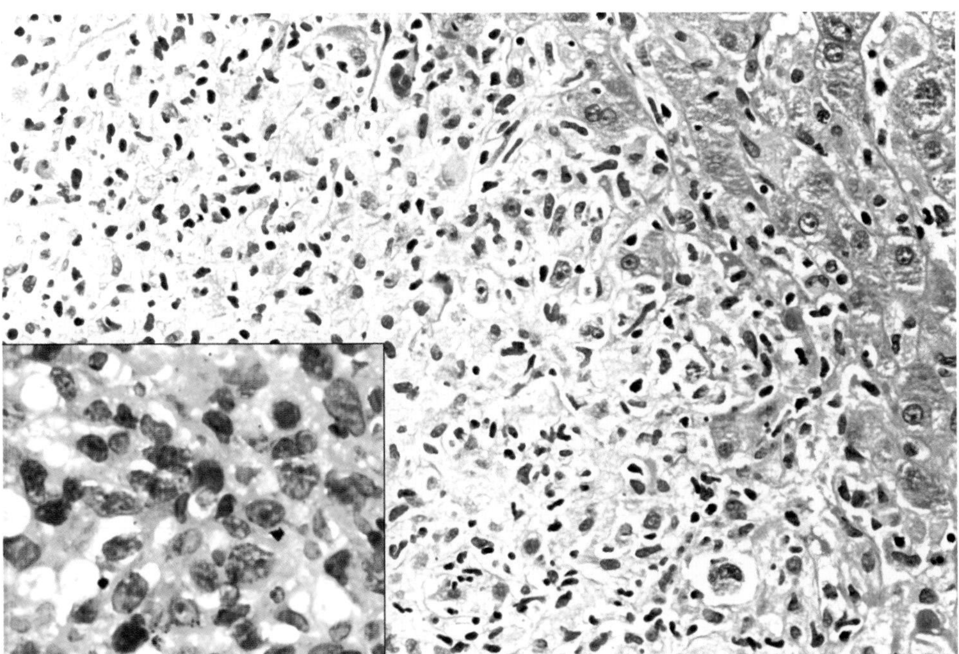

Figure 16.17 *Post-transplant lymphoproliferative disease*. The portal tract is infiltrated and overrun by a B-cell proliferation. *Inset*: The cytologic features are consistent with an immunoblastic lymphoma but immunotyping and other studies are necessary for definitive characterisation. (Needle biopsy, H&E).

Differential diagnosis in transplant biopsies

Most problems in biopsy interpretation after liver transplantation arise in distinguishing rejection from other conditions (Table 16.5). It should be kept in mind that rejection and other allograft disorders can coexist. Difficult pathological problems are usually resolved by discussion with clinicians, assessment of viral serologies and microbial culture results, and review of drug therapy. When necessary, patency of vascular or biliary anastomoses may need to be radiologically demonstrated.

While **endotheliitis** may be seen in several forms of liver disease,[105] when it is found in combination with bile duct damage and a mixed portal inflammatory infiltrate, the diagnosis of acute rejection is usually clear. Endotheliitis involving central veins (**central venulitis**) sometimes presents diagnostic difficulties.[106] Regular involvement of most central veins in a biopsy specimen favours rejection or the less common development of *de novo* autoimmune hepatitis. Central venulitis due to viral and drug hepatitis is more irregular in distribution. **Bile duct damage** represents a more difficult histological problem, because it is a feature seen in rejection, chronic hepatitis C and PBC. Portal tract lymphoid aggregates, numerous apoptotic bodies, interface hepatitis and prominent sinusoidal inflammation support the diagnosis of chronic hepatitis C. As noted earlier, the presence of a granulomatous, destructive cholangitis in a hepatitis C-seronegative patient transplanted for PBC is important evidence of recurrent PBC.

Neutrophils may be seen in the vicinity of damaged bile ducts in rejection (Fig. 16.5) and should not be mistaken for evidence of biliary obstruction. Obstruction can usually be excluded if portal tract oedema and ductular reaction are absent. **Eosinophils** are often prominent in rejection, but can be seen in fewer numbers in recurrent viral or autoimmune hepatitis. Subendothelial eosinophils in portal vein branches favours rejection. Drug hepatitis as a cause of eosinophil infiltrates may need consideration when there is antibiotic prophylaxis with sulfa agents such as trimethoprim-sulfamethoxazole, but the parenchymal changes of acute hepatitis usually help to distinguish this from rejection. **Cholestasis** may pose significant diagnostic problems because of several potential causes,[12] including biliary obstruction, rejection and sepsis. In biopsies obtained early (1–2 weeks) after transplantation, cholestasis is usually functional in nature. Small-for-size living donor grafts may also develop cholestasis. Cholestasis accompanied by portal oedema and a ductular reaction should prompt an assessment of the biliary anastomosis. The distinctive pattern of 'bile ductular cholestasis' is usually associated with sepsis. **Steatosis** of large droplet type in post-transplant biopsies may be due to several factors, including corticosteroid immunosuppression and recurrent hepatitis C virus infection. Genotype 3 re-infection particularly may result in severe fatty change.[84] Considerable fat also develops in allografts of children transplanted for progressive familial intrahepatic cholestasis type 1.[107] A few **apoptotic bodies** are common directly after transplantation, but months later their presence may be explained by episodes of acute rejection, recurrent hepatitis C, or occasionally in paediatric patients by intercurrent viral illnesses.

Table 16.5 Differential diagnostic features in transplant biopsies

	Condition				
Histological Feature	**Rejection**	**Recurrent HBV**	**Recurrent HCV**	**Biliary Obstruction**	**Ischaemia**
Cholestasis	+/–	Unusual (except in fibrosing cholestatic hepatitis)	Unusual	Yes	No
Portal inflammation					
Mixed (L,P,N,E)*	Yes	+/–	+/–	No	No
Lymphocytes, plasma cells	+/–	Yes	Yes	No	No
Neutrophils	+/–	No	No	Yes	No
Bile-duct damage	Yes	Unusual	Yes	No	No
Endotheliitis	Yes	Unusual	Unusual	No	Occasional
Zone 3 necrosis	Yes, if chronic	No	No	No	Yes
Sinusoidal inflammation	No	+/–	++	No	No
Apoptotic bodies	+/–	+	+++	No	No

+/– indicates a feature which is not characteristic, but which may sometimes be present.
*Mixed portal inflammation includes lymphocytes (L), plasma cells (P), neutrophils (N) and eosinophils (E).

RENAL TRANSPLANTATION

Patients who have undergone renal transplantation are exposed to many viruses capable of causing acute or chronic hepatitis, particularly hepatitis B[108] and hepatitis C.[109] Steatosis, chronic hepatitis and cirrhosis are often found on biopsy.[110] Fibrosing cholestatic hepatitis is infrequently seen in recipients with chronic hepatitis C.[111] There may be lesions related to administration of potentially hepatotoxic drugs such as azathioprine, which may cause cholestasis, veno-occlusive disease, nodular regenerative hyperplasia, and other lesions.[60,112–114] Cirrhosis develops in a small proportion of patients. Incrimination of a single aetiological agent is often difficult. Transfusions may cause substantial siderosis involving both hepatocytes and macrophages.[115,116] Vascular lesions following renal transplantation include narrowing or occlusion of efferent veins,[117] peliosis hepatis[118] and non-cirrhotic portal hypertension.[119] Portal hypertension associated with dilatation of sinusoids in acinar zones 2 and 3, with eventual development of fibrosis or cirrhosis, has also been reported.[120]

Patients who have been treated by **haemodialysis** may have birefringent material, probably derived from silicone tubing, in portal tracts. In some instances this material gives rise to a giant-cell or granulomatous reaction.[121–123] Haemodialysis patients also often have Kupffer cell siderosis.

BONE MARROW TRANSPLANTATION

Graft recipients are liable to liver damage from graft-versus-host disease, infection and idiosyncratic drug jaundice. **Graft-versus-host disease (GVHD)** involving the liver has varying histologic features depending on the stage of evolution.[124–126] The most characteristic features of acute (less than 90 days after transplant) GVHD are **bile duct damage** and **cholestasis.**[124,125] The ducts often appear attenuated, tapering and stretched lengthwise. The duct epithelium is irregular, with vacuolated or acidophilic cytoplasm, nuclear pleomorphism and multilayering, and increased nuclear-cytoplasmic ratio[124,127] (Fig. 16.18). Lymphocytes infiltrate the portal tracts and duct epithelium, but are sparse. In early GVHD (less than 35 days), duct changes are less apparent and numerous parenchymal acidophilic bodies may be present.[124] Histological features of GVHD resemble those seen in hepatitis C virus (HCV) infection and serological testing to exclude HCV may be required. More severe degrees of bile-duct atypia and duct destruction favour the diagnosis of GVHD over HCV infection. Endotheliitis is uncommon in comparison with acute liver allograft rejection. Siderosis is often present. Venous occlusion by loose or mature connective tissue is common.[128–132] In **chronic GVHD** (after 90 days) there is progressive bile-duct loss (ductopenia) with portal fibrosis.[124,126] The clinical and radiological picture may mimic intrahepatic primary sclerosing cholangitis.[133] Rarely, there are parenchymal changes of an acute hepatitis.[134] Cirrhosis of biliary type may finally develop.[135] Eosinophilic cytoplasmic inclusions in hepatocytes of patients dying after bone marrow transplantation have been described.[136]

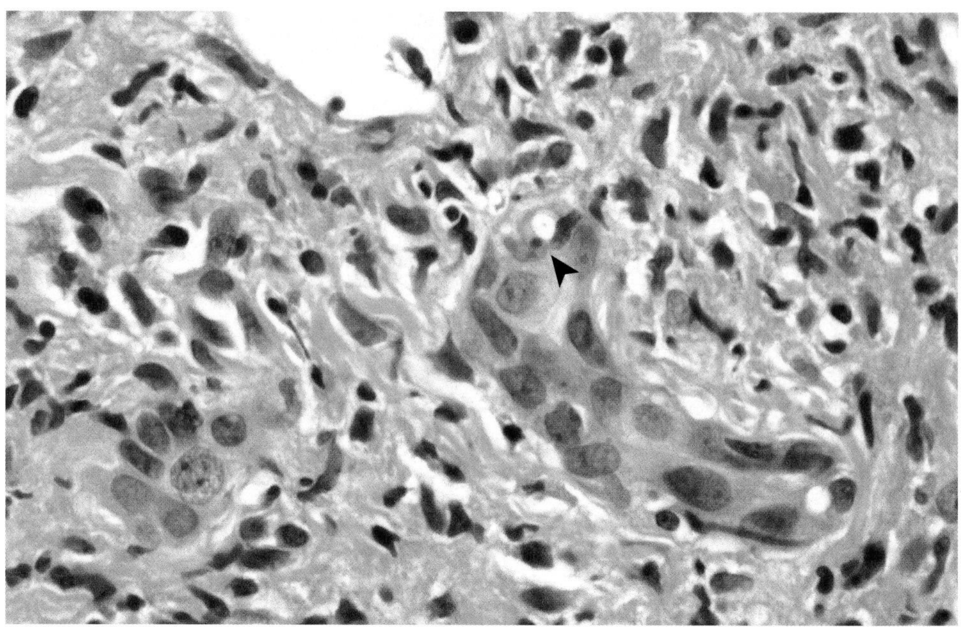

Figure 16.18 *Graft-versus-host disease.* The bile duct epithelium shows dyspolarity and attenuation. A small apoptotic nuclear fragment is seen at top (arrowhead) near an intracellular degenerative vacuole. The surrounding lymphocytic infiltrate is relatively mild. (Needle biopsy, H&E).

REFERENCES

1 Henley KS, Lucey MR, Appelman HD, et al. Biochemical and histopathological correlation in liver transplant: the first 180 days. *Hepatology* 1992; **16**: 688–693.

2 Eggink HF, Hofstee N, Gips CH, et al. Histopathology of serial graft biopsies from liver transplant recipients. *Am J Pathol* 1984; **114**: 18–31.

3 Kubota K, Ericzon B-G, Reinholt FP. Comparison of fine-needle aspiration biopsy and histology in human liver transplants. *Transplantation* 1991; **51**: 1010–1013.

4 Gaffey MJ, Boyd JC, Traweek ST, et al. Predictive value of intraoperative biopsies and liver function tests for preservation injury in orthotopic liver transplantation. *Hepatology* 1997; **25**: 184–189.

5 Verran D, Kusyk T, Painter D, et al. Clinical experience gained from the use of 120 steatotic donor livers for orthotopic liver transplantation. *Liver Transplant* 2003; **9**: 500–505.

6 Bzeizi KI, Jalan R, Plevris JN, et al. Primary graft dysfunction after liver transplantation: from pathogenesis to prevention. *Liver Transplant Surg* 1997; **3**: 137–148.

7 Trevisani F, Colantoni A, Caraceni P, et al. The use of donor fatty liver for liver transplantation: a challenge or a quagmire? *J Hepatol* 1996; **24**: 114–121.

8 Fishbein TM, Fiel MI, Emre S, et al. Use of livers with microvesicular fat safely expands the donor pool. *Transplantation* 1997; **64**: 248–251.

9 Ludwig J. Histopathology of the liver following transplantation. In: Maddrey WC, Sorrell MF, eds. Transplantation of the Liver, 2nd edn. Stamford, CT: Appleton and Lange, 1995: 267.

10 Williams JW, Vera S, Peters TG, et al. Cholestatic jaundice after hepatic transplantation. A nonimmunologically mediated event. *Am J Surg* 1986; **151**: 65–70.

11 Jaeschke H, LeMasters JJ. Apoptosis versus oncotic necrosis in hepatic ischemia/reperfusion injury. *Gastroenterology* 2003; **125**: 1246–1257.
12 Ben-Ari Z, Pappo O, Mor E. Intrahepatic cholestasis after liver transplantation. *Liver Transplant* 2003; **9**: 1005–1018.
13 Ng IOL, Burroughs AK, Rolles K, et al. Hepatocellular ballooning after liver transplantation: a light and electronmicroscopic study with clinicopathological correlation. *Histopathology* 1991; **18**: 323–330.
14 Goldstein NS, Hart J, Lewin KJ. Diffuse hepatocyte ballooning in liver biopsies from orthotopic liver transplant patients. *Histopathology* 1991; **18**: 331–338.
15 Russo PA, Yunis EJ. Subcapsular hepatic necrosis in orthotopic liver allografts. *Hepatology* 1986; **6**: 708–713.
16 Cha I, Bass N, Ferrell LD. Lipopeliosis. An immunohistochemical and clinicopathologic study of five cases. *Am J Surg Pathol* 1994; **18**: 789–795.
17 International Working Party. Terminology for hepatic allograft rejection. *Hepatology* 1995; **22**: 648–654.
18 Ayata G, Pomfret E, Pomposelli JJ, et al. Adult-to-adult live donor liver transplantation: a short-term clinicopathologic study. *Hum Pathol* 2001; **32**: 814–822.
19 Snover DC, Sibley RK, Freese DK, et al. Orthotopic liver transplantation: a pathological study of 63 serial liver biopsies from 17 patients with special reference to the diagnostic features and natural history of rejection. *Hepatology* 1984; **4**: 1212–1222.
20 Demetris AJ, Lasky S, Thiel DH Van, et al. Pathology of hepatic transplantation: A review of 62 adult allograft recipients immunosuppressed with a cyclosporine/steroid regimen. *Am J Pathol* 1985; **118**: 151–161.
21 Hubscher SG. Histological findings in liver allograft rejection – new insights into the pathogenesis of hepatocellular damage in liver allografts. *Histopathology* 1991; **18**: 377–383.
22 Freese DK, Snover DC, Sharp HL, et al. Chronic rejection after liver transplantation: a study of clinical, histopathological and immunological features. *Hepatology* 1991; **13**: 882–891.
23 Wiesner RH, Ludwig J, Krom RAF, et al. Hepatic allograft rejection: new developments in terminology, diagnosis, prevention, and treatment. *Mayo Clin Proc* 1993; **68**: 69–79.
24 Haga H, Egawa H, Shirase T et al. Periportal edema and necrosis as diagnostic histological features of early humoral rejection in ABO-incompatible liver transplantation. *Liver Transplant* 2004; **10**: 16–27.
25 Wardle EN. Kupffer cells and their function. *Liver* 1987; **7**: 63–75.
26 Clavien P-A, Camargo CA, Cameron R, et al. Kupffer cell erythrophagocytosis and graft-versus-host hemolysis in liver transplantation. *Gastroenterology* 1996; **110**: 1891–1896.
27 Wiesner RH, Demetris AJ, Belle SH, et al. Acute hepatic allograft rejection: incidence, risk factors and impact on outcome. *Hepatology* 1998; **28**: 638–645.
28 DeGroen PC, Kephart GM, Gleich GJ, et al. The eosinophil as an effector cell of the immune response during hepatic allograft rejection. *Hepatology* 1994; **20**: 654–662.
29 Nagral A, Ben-Ari Z, Dhillon AP, et al. Eosinophils in acute cellular rejection in liver allografts. *Liver Transplant Surg* 1998; **4**: 355–362.
30 International Panel. Banff schema for grading liver allograft rejection: an international consensus document. *Hepatology* 1997; **25**: 658–663.
31 Khettry U, Backer A, Ayata G, et al. Centrilobular histopathologic changes in liver transplant biopsies. *Hum Pathol* 2002; **33**: 270–276.
31a Lovell MO, Speeg KV, Halff GA et al. Acute hepatic allograft rejection: a comparison of patients with and without centrilobular alterations during first rejection episode. *Liver Transplant* 2004; **10**: 369–373.
32 International Panel. Update of the international Banff schema for liver allograft rejection: working recommendations for the histopathologic staging and reporting of chronic rejection. *Hepatology* 2000; **31**: 792–799.
33 Weisner RH, Batts KP, Krom RAF. Evolving concepts in the diagnosis, pathogenesis and treatment of chronic hepatic allograft rejection. *Liver Transplant Surg* 1999; **5**: 388–400.
34 Wiesner RH, Demetris AJ, Seaberg EC. Chronic hepatic allograft rejection:

defining clinical risk factors and assessing impact on graft outcome. *Hepatology* 1998; **28**: 314A.
35 Ludwig J, Hashimoto E, Porayko MK, et al. Failed allografts and causes of death after orthotopic liver transplantation from 1985 to 1995: decreasing prevalence of irreversible hepatic allograft rejection. *Liver Transplant Surg* 1996; **2**: 185–191.
36 McCaughan GW, Bishop GA. Atherosclerosis of the liver allograft. *J Hepatol* 1997; **27**: 592–598.
37 Demetris AJ, Belle SH, Hart J, et al. Intraobserver and interobserver variation in the histopathological assessment of liver allograft rejection. *Hepatology* 1991; **14**: 751–755.
38 Thung SN, Gerber MA. Histological features of liver allograft rejection: do you see what I see? *Hepatology* 1991; **14**: 949–951.
39 Sebagh M, Blakolmer K, Falissard B, et al. Accuracy of bile duct changes for the diagnosis of chronic liver allograft rejection: reliability of the 1999 Banff schema. *Hepatology* 2002; **35**: 117–125.
40 Liu G, Butany J, Wanless IR, et al. The vascular pathology of human hepatic allografts. *Hum Pathol* 1993; **24**: 182–188.
41 Ludwig J, Gross JB, Perkins JD, et al. Persistent centrilobular necroses in hepatic allografts. *Hum Pathol* 1990; **21**: 656–661.
42 Arnold JC, Portmann BC, O'Grady JG, et al. Cytomegalovirus infection persists in the liver graft in the vanishing bile duct syndrome. *Hepatology* 1992; **16**: 285–292.
43 Donaldson PT, Alexander GJM, O'Grady J, et al. Evidence for an immune response to HLA Class I antigens in the vanishing-bileduct syndrome after liver transplantation. *Lancet* 1987; **1**: 945–948.
44 O'Grady JG, Alexander GJM, Sutherland S, et al. Cytomegalovirus infection and donor/recipient HLA antigens: interdependent co-factors in pathogenesis of vanishing bileduct syndrome after liver transplantation. *Lancet* 1988; **2**: 302–305.
45 Lautenschlager I, Höckerstedt K, Jalanko H, et al. Persistent cytomegalovirus in liver allografts with chronic rejection. *Hepatology* 1997; **25**: 190–194.
46 Conti F, Grude P, Calmus Y, et al. Expression of the membrane attack complex of complement and its inhibitors during human liver allograft transplantation. *J Hepatol* 1997; **27**: 881–889.
47 Hubscher SG, Buckels JAC, Elias E, et al. Vanishing bile-duct syndrome following liver transplantation – is it reversible? *Transplantation* 1991; **51**: 1004–1010.
48 Tabatabai L, Lewis WD, Gordon F, et al. Fibrosis/cirrhosis after orthotopic liver transplantation. *Hum Pathol* 1999; **30**: 39–47.
49 Seehofer D, Rayes N, Tullius SG, et al. CMV hepatitis after liver transplantation: incidence, clinical course, and long-term follow-up. *Liver Transplant* 2002; **8**: 1138–1146.
50 MacDonald GA, Greenson JK, DelBuono EA, et al. Mini-microabscess syndrome in liver transplant patients. *Hepatology* 1997; **26**: 192–197.
51 Theise ND, Conn M, Thung SN. Localization of cytomegalovirus antigens in liver allografts over time. *Hum Pathol* 1993; **24**: 103–108.
52 Alshak NS, Jimenez AM, Gedebou M, et al. Epstein-Barr virus infection in liver transplantation patients: correlation of histopathology and semiquantitative Epstein-Barr virus-DNA recovery using polymerase chain reaction. *Hum Pathol* 1993; **24**: 1306–1312.
53 Markin RS. Manifestations of Epstein-Barr virus-associated disorders in liver. *Liver* 1994; **14**: 1–13.
54 Hubscher SG, Williams A, Davison SM, et al. Epstein-Barr virus in inflammatory diseases of the liver and liver allografts: an in situ hybridization study. *Hepatology* 1994; **20**: 899–907.
55 Pessoa MG, Terrault NA, Ferrell LD, et al. Hepatitis after liver transplantation: the role of the known and unknown viruses. *Liver Transplant Surg* 1998; **4**: 461–468.
56 Hertzler GL, Millikan WJ. The surgical pathologist's role in liver transplantation. *Arch Pathol Lab Med* 1991; **115**: 273–282.
57 Oh C-K, Pelletier SJ, Sawyer RG, et al. Uni- and multi-variate analysis of risk factors for early and late hepatic artery thrombosis after liver transplantation.

Transplantation 2001; **71**: 767–772.
58 Harper PL, Edgar PR, Luddington RJ, et al. Protein C deficiency and portal thrombosis in liver transplantation in children. *Lancet* 1988; **2**: 924–927.
59 Ludwig J, Batts KP, MacCarty RL. Ischemic cholangitis in hepatic allografts. *Mayo Clin Proc* 1992; **67**: 519–526.
60 Sterneck M, Wiesner R, Ascher N, et al. Azathioprine hepatotoxicity after liver transplantation. *Hepatology* 1991; **14**: 806–810.
61 Dhillon AP, Burroughs AK, Hudson M, et al. Hepatic venular stenosis after orthotopic liver transplantation. *Hepatology* 1994; **19**: 106–111.
62 Gulbis B, Adler M, Ooms HA, et al. Liver-function studies in heart-transplant recipients treated with cyclosporin A. *Clin Chem* 1988; **34**: 1772–1774.
63 Kadmon M, Klünemann C, Böhme M, et al. Inhibition by Cyclosporin A of adenosine triphosphate-dependent transport from the hepatocyte into bile. *Gastroenterology* 1993; **104**: 1507–1514.
64 Arias IM. Cyclosporin, the biology of the bile canaliculus, and cholestasis. *Gastroenterology* 1993; **104**: 1558–1560.
65 Thomson AW. FK-506 enters the clinic. *Immunol Today* 1990; **11**: 35–36.
66 Fung JJ, Todo S, Tzakis A, et al. Current status of FK 506 in liver transplantation. *Transplant Proc* 1991; **23**: 1902–1905.
67 Davern TJ, Lake JR. Recurrent disease after liver transplantation. *Semin Gastrointest Dis* 1998; **9**: 86–109.
68 Kim WR, Poterucha JJ, Porayko MK, et al. Recurrence of nonalcoholic steatohepatitis following liver transplantation. *Transplantation* 1996; **62**: 1802–1805.
69 Molloy RM, Komorowski R, Varma RR. Recurrent nonalcoholic steatohepatitis and cirrhosis after liver transplantation. *Liver Transplant Surg* 1997; **3**: 177–178.
70 Carson K, Washington MK, Treem WR, et al. Recurrence of nonalcoholic steatohepatitis in a liver transplant recipient. *Liver Transplant Surg* 1997; **3**: 174–176.
71 Fiel MI, Schiano TD, Klion FM, et al. Recurring fibro-obliterative venopathy in liver allografts. *Am J Surg Pathol* 1999; **23**: 734–737.
72 Walker N, Apel R, Kerlin P, et al. Hepatitis B virus infection in liver allografts. *Am J Surg Pathol* 1993; **17**: 666–677.
73 Lucey MR, Graham DM, Martin P, et al. Recurrence of hepatitis B and delta hepatitis after orthotopic liver transplantation. *Gut* 1992; **33**: 1390–1396.
74 Kate FJW ten, Schalm SW, Willemse PJA, et al. Course of hepatitis B and D virus infection in auxiliary liver grafts in hepatitis B-positive patients. A light-microscopic and immunohistochemical study. *J Hepatol* 1992; **14**: 168–175.
75 Ottobrelli A, Marzano A, Smedile A, et al. Patterns of hepatitis delta virus reinfection and disease in liver transplantation. *Gastroenterology* 1991; **101**: 1649–1655.
76 David E, Rahier J, Pucci A, et al. Recurrence of hepatitis D (delta) in liver transplants: histopathological aspects. *Gastroenterology* 1993; **104**: 1122–1128.
77 Davies SE, Portmann BC, O'Grady JG, et al. Hepatic histological findings after transplantation for chronic hepatitis B virus infection, including a unique pattern of fibrosing cholestatic hepatitis. *Hepatology* 1991; **13**: 150–157.
78 O'Grady JG, Smith HM, Davies SE, et al. Hepatitis B virus reinfection after orthotopic liver transplantation. Serological and clinical implications. *J Hepatol* 1992; **14**: 104–111.
79 Benner KG, Lee RG, Keeffe EB, et al. Fibrosing cytolytic liver failure secondary to recurrent hepatitis B after liver transplantation. *Gastroenterology* 1992; **103**: 1307–1312.
80 Lau JYN, Bain VG, Davies SE, et al. High-level expression of hepatitis B viral antigens in fibrosing cholestatic hepatitis. *Gastroenterology* 1992; **102**: 956–962.
81 Phillips MJ, Cameron R, Flowers MA, et al. Post-transplant recurrent hepatitis B viral liver disease. Viral-burden, steatoviral, and fibroviral hepatitis B. *Am J Pathol* 1992; **140**: 1295–1308.
82 Demetris AJ, Eghtesad B, Marcos A, et al. Recurrent hepatitis C in liver allografts. Prospective assessment of diagnostic accuracy, identification of pitfalls, and observations about pathogenesis. *Am J Surg Pathol* 2004; **28**: 658–669.

83 Saxena R, Crawford JM, Navarro VJ, et al. Utilization of acidophil bodies in the diagnosis of recurrent hepatitis C infection after orthotopic liver transplantation. *Mod Pathol* 2002; **15**: 897–903.
84 Gordon FD, Pomfret EA, Pomposelli JJ, et al. Severe steatosis as the initial histologic manifestation of recurrent hepatitis C genotype 3. *Hum Pathol* 2004; **35**: 636–638.
85 Guerrero RB, Batts KP, Burgart LJ, et al. Early detection of hepatitis C allograft reinfection after orthotopic liver transplantation: a molecular and histologic study. *Mod Pathol* 2000; **13**: 229–237.
86 Ferrell LD, Wright TL, Roberts J, et al. Hepatitis C viral infection in liver transplant recipients. *Hepatology* 1992; **16**: 865–876.
87 Böker KHW, Dalley G, Bahr MJ, et al. Long-term outcome of hepatitis C virus infection after liver transplantation. *Hepatology* 1997; **25**: 203–210.
88 Dickson RC, Caldwell SH, Ishitani MB, et al. Clinical and histologic patterns of early graft failure due to recurrent hepatitis C in four patients after liver transplantation. *Transplantation* 1996; **61**: 701–705.
89 Taga SA, Washington MK, Terrault N, et al. Cholestatic hepatitis C in liver allografts. *Liver Transplant Surg* 1998; **4**: 304–310.
90 Schluger LK, Sheiner PA, Thung SN, et al. Severe recurrent cholestatic hepatitis C following orthotopic liver transplantation. *Hepatology* 1996; **23**: 971–976.
91 Sylvestre PB, Batts KP, Burgart LJ, et al. Recurrence of primary biliary cirrhosis after liver transplantation: histologic estimate of incidence and natural history. *Liver Transplant* 2003; **9**: 1086–1093.
92 Hubscher SG, Elias E, Buckels JAC, et al. Primary biliary cirrhosis. Histological evidence of disease recurrence after liver transplantation. *J Hepatol* 1993; **18**: 173–184.
93 Khettry U, Anand N, Faul PN, et al. Liver transplantation for primary biliary cirrhosis: a long-term pathologic study. *Liver Transplant* 2003; **9**: 87–96.
94 Graziadei IW, Wiesner RH, Batts KP, et al. Recurrence of primary sclerosing cholangitis following liver transplantation. *Hepatology* 1999; **29**: 1050–1056.
95 Birnbaum AH, Benkov KJ, Pittman NS, et al. Recurrence of autoimmune hepatitis in children after liver transplantation. *J Ped Gastroenterol Nutr* 1997; **25**: 20–25.
96 Mieli-Vergani G, Vergani D. De novo autoimmune hepatitis after liver transplantation. *J Hepatol* 2004; **40**: 3–7.
97 Heneghan MA, Portmann BC, Norris SM, et al. Graft dysfunction mimicking autoimmune hepatitis following liver transplantation in adults. *Hepatology* 2001; **34**: 464–470.
98 Leblond V, Choquet S. Lymphoproliferative disorders after liver transplantation. *J Hepatol* 2004; **40**: 728–735.
99 Palazzo JP, Lundquist K, Mitchell D, et al. Rapid development of lymphoma following liver transplantation in a recipient with hepatitis B and primary hemochromatosis. *Am J Gastroenterol* 1991; **88**: 102–104.
100 Spiro IJ, Yandell DW, Li C, et al. Brief report: lymphoma of donor origin occurring in the porta hepatis of a transplanted liver. *N Engl J Med* 1993; **329**: 27–29.
101 Lones MA, Shintaku IP, Weiss LM, et al. Posttransplant lymphoproliferative disorder in liver allograft biopsies: a comparison of three methods for the demonstration of Epstein-Barr virus. *Hum Pathol* 1997; **28**: 533–539.
102 Luketic VA, Shiffman ML, McCall JB, et al. Primary hepatocellular carcinoma after orthotopic liver transplantation for chronic hepatitis B infection. *Ann Intern Med* 1991; **114**: 212–213.
103 Saxena R, Ye MQ, Emre S, et al. De novo hepatocellular carcinoma in a hepatic allograft with recurrent hepatitis C cirrhosis. *Liver Transplant Surg* 1999; **5**: 81–82.
104 McPeake JR, O'Grady JG, Zaman S, et al. Liver transplantation for primary hepatocellular carcinoma: tumor size and number determine outcome. *J Hepatol* 1993; **18**: 226–234.
105 Nonomura A, Mizukami Y, Matsubara F, et al. Clinicopathological study of lymphocyte attachment to endothelial cells (endothelialitis) in various liver diseases. *Liver* 1991; **11**: 78–88.

106 Demetris AJ. Central venulitis in liver allografts: considerations of differential diagnosis. *Hepatology* 2001; **33**: 1329–1330.
107 Lykavieris P, Mil S van, Cresteil D, et al. Progressive familial intrahepatic cholestasis type 1 and extrahepatic features: no catch-up of stature growth, exacerbation of diarrhea, and appearance of liver steatosis after liver transplantation. *J Hepatol* 2003; **39**: 447–452.
108 Degos F, Degott C. Hepatitis in renal transplant recipients. *J Hepatol* 1989; **9**: 114–123.
109 Chan T-M, Lok ASF, Cheng IKP, et al. A prospective study of hepatitis C virus infection among renal transplant recipients. *Gastroenterology* 1993; **104**: 862–868.
110 Rao KV, Anderson WR, Kasiske BL, et al. Value of liver biopsy in the evaluation and management of chronic liver disease in renal transplant recipients. *Am J Med* 1993; **94**: 241–250.
111 Delladetsima JK, Boletis JN, Makris F, et al. Fibrosing cholestatic hepatitis in renal transplant recipients with hepatitis C virus infection. *Liver Transplant Surg* 1999; **5**: 294–300.
112 Sopko J, Anuras S. Liver disease in renal transplant recipients. [Review]. *Am J Med* 1978; **64**: 139–146.
113 Ware AJ, Luby JP, Hollinger B, et al. Etiology of liver disease in renal-transplant patients. *Ann Intern Med* 1979; **91**: 364–371.
114 Weir MR, Kirkman RL, Strom TB, et al. Liver disease in recipients of long-functioning renal allografts. *Kidney Int* 1985; **28**: 839–844.
115 Rao KV, Anderson WR. Hemosiderosis: an unrecognized complication in renal allograft recipients. *Transplantation* 1982; **33**: 115–117.
116 Rao KV, Anderson WR. Hemosiderosis and hemochromatosis in renal transplant recipients. Clinical and pathological features, diagnostic correlations, predisposing factors, and treatment. *Am J Nephrol* 1985; **5**: 419–430.
117 Marubbio AT, Danielson B. Hepatic veno-occlusive disease in a renal transplant patient receiving azathioprine. *Gastroenterology* 1975; **69**: 739–743.
118 Degott C, Rueff B, Kreis H, et al. Peliosis hepatis in recipients of renal transplants. *Gut* 1978; **19**: 748–753.
119 Nataf C, Feldmann G, Lebrec D, et al. Idiopathic portal hypertension (perisinusoidal fibrosis) after renal transplantation. *Gut* 1979; **20**: 531–537.
120 Gerlag PG, Lobatto S, Driessen WM, et al. Hepatic sinusoidal dilatation with portal hypertension during azathioprine treatment after kidney transplantation. *J Hepatol* 1985; **1**: 339–348.
121 Krempien B, Bommer J, Ritz E. Foreign body giant cell reaction in lungs, liver and spleen. A complication of long term haemodialysis. *Virchows Arch A Pathol Anat Histol* 1981; **392**: 73–80.
122 Leong AS, Disney AP, Gove DW. Refractile particles in liver of haemodialysis patients [letter]. *Lancet* 1981; **1**: 889–890.
123 Parfrey PS, O'Driscoll JB, Paradinas FJ. Refractile material in the liver of haemodialysis patients [letter]. *Lancet* 1981; **1**: 1101–1102.
124 Shulman HM, Sharma P, Amos D, et al. A coded histologic study of hepatic graft-versus-host disease after human bone marrow transplantation. *Hepatology* 1988; **8**: 463–470.
125 McDonald GB, Shulman HM, Sullivan KM, et al. Intestinal and hepatic complications of human bone marrow transplantation, Part I. *Gastroenterol* 1986; **90**: 460–477.
126 McDonald GB, Shulman HM, Sullivan KM, et al. Intestinal and hepatic complications of human bone marrow transplantation, Part II. *Gastroenterol* 1986; **90**: 770–784.
127 Snover DC, Weisdorf SA, Ramsay NK, et al. Hepatic graft versus host disease: a study of the predictive value of liver biopsy in diagnosis. *Hepatology* 1984; **4**: 123–130.
128 Berk PD, Popper H, Krueger GR, et al. Veno-occlusive disease of the liver after allogeneic bone marrow transplantation: possible association with graft-versus-host disease. *Ann Intern Med* 1979; **90**: 158–164.
129 Sloane JP, Farthing MJ, Powles RL. Histopathological changes in the liver after allogeneic bone marrow transplantation. *J Clin Pathol* 1980; **33**: 344–350.
130 Farthing MJ, Clark ML, Sloane JP, et al. Liver disease after bone marrow transplantation. *Gut* 1982; **23**: 465–474.

131 McDonald GB, Sharma P, Matthews DE, et al. Venocclusive disease of the liver after bone marrow transplantation: diagnosis, incidence, and predisposing factors. *Hepatology* 1984; **4**: 116–122.
132 Shulman HM, Fisher LB, Schoch HG et al. Venoocclusive disease of the liver after marrow transplantation: histological correlates of clinical signs and symptoms. *Hepatology* 1994; **19**: 1171–1180.
133 Geubel AP, Cnudde A, Ferrant A, et al. Diffuse biliary tract involvement mimicking primary sclerosing cholangitis after bone marrow transplantation. *J Hepatol* 1990; **10**: 23–28.
134 Strasser SI, Shulman HM, Flowers ME, et al. Chronic graft-versus-host disease of the liver: presentation as an acute hepatitis. *Hepatology* 2000; **32**: 1265–1271.
135 Knapp AB, Crawford JM, Rappeport JM, et al. Cirrhosis as a consequence of graft-versus-host disease. *Gastroenterology* 1987; **92**: 513–519.
136 Zubair I, Herrera GA, Pretlow TG, et al. Cytoplasmic inclusions in hepatocytes of bone marrow transplant patients: light and electron microscopic characterization. *Am J Clin Pathol* 1985; **83**: 65–68.

GENERAL READING

Hübscher S, Portmann BC. Transplantation pathology. In: MacSween RNM, Burt AD, Portmann B, et al., eds. Pathology of the Liver, 4th edn. Edinburgh: Churchill Livingstone, 2002: 885–943.

Demetris AJ, Crawford JM, Nalesnik M, et al. Transplantation pathology of the liver. In: Odze RD, Goldblum JR, Crawford JM, eds. Surgical Pathology of the GI Tract, Liver, Biliary Tract, Liver, Biliary Tract, and Pancreas. Philadelphia, PA: WB Saunders, 2004: 909–966.

Ludwig J, Lefkowitch JH. Histopathology of the liver following transplantation. In: Maddrey WC, Schiff ER, Sorrell MF, eds. Transplantation of the Liver, 3rd edn. Philadelphia, PA: Lippincott Williams & Wilkins, 2001: 229–250.

International panel. Banff schema for grading liver allograft rejection: an international consensus document. *Hepatology* 1997; **25**: 658–663.

International panel. Update of the international Banff schema for liver allograft rejection: working recommendations for the histopathologic staging and reporting of chronic rejection. *Hepatology* 2000; **31**: 792–799.

Lefkowitch JH. Diagnostic issues in liver transplantation pathology. *Clin Liver Dis* 2002; **6**: 555–570.

Regev A, Molina R et al. Reliability of histopathologic assessment for the differentiation of recurrent hepatitis C from acute rejection after liver transplantation. *Liver Transplant* 2004; **10**: 1233–1239.

CHAPTER 17

ELECTRON MICROSCOPY AND OTHER TECHNIQUES

INTRODUCTION

This chapter will focus primarily on the role of transmission electron microscopy in the assessment of liver ultrastructure and disease. It also describes, in brief, the principles and uses of other methodologies. The special conditions required for tissue processing in each of these techniques (Table 17.1) should be carefully planned for in advance of obtaining specimens. While some of these methods are not universally available in pathology departments, other departments at one's institution or at other centres of investigation may be consulted in cases of particular diagnostic or research interest. Procedures for fixation and processing for transmission electron microscopy are available in several of the 'General reading' references at the end of the chapter.

ELECTRON MICROSCOPY OF LIVER BIOPSIES

Transmission electron microscopy (TEM) continues to provide important information about the normal cellular and extracellular constituents of the liver and their alterations in disease. Recent interest in the relationships between the various sinusoidal cells of the liver has benefited from TEM studies[1,2] as have investigations of hepatic progenitor cells.[3] Data from standard TEM studies can be enhanced by the application of immunohistochemical stains (see Immunoelectron microscopy), digitised three-dimensional computer reconstructions[4–6] and morphometry. Transmission electron microscopy is sometimes limited by the lack of specificity of certain ultrastructural changes and the problem of sampling error in lesions that may not be uniformly distributed. The first of these limitations is well illustrated in cholestasis; various features of cholestasis such as loss of canalicular microvilli are easily recognised under the electron microscope, but many causes produce these changes. Sampling error can sometimes be reduced by the combination of light and electron microscopy in a single instrument.[7]

In diagnostic work, transmission electron microscopy should be seriously considered under five circumstances:

1 **To establish the nature of an inborn error of metabolism**. In a number of storage diseases, the ultrastructural changes are diagnostic or give an indication of the type of disease to be considered.[8,9] Specific features are seen, for example,

Table 17.1 Liver tissue processing for various techniques

Technique	Tissue preparation
Transmission electron microscopy	Glutaraldehyde fixation
Scanning electron microscopy	Perfusion-fixation; critical point drying; coating with gold or platinum
Immunoelectron microscopy	Glutaraldehyde/paraformaldehyde fixation
Immunoperoxidase of tissue sections	Fixation in 10% neutral formalin or alternative fixative
Immunoperoxidase and immunofluorescence of frozen sections	Snap freeze after embedding in OCT compound
In situ hybridisation	Snap freeze after embedding in OCT compound
Flow cytometry	Fresh tissue
Confocal laser scanning microscopy	Snap freeze after embedding in OCT compound
Laser capture microdissection	Conventional tissue sections for light microscopy
Gene array analysis	Snap freeze in liquid nitrogen; store at −80°C

in type II glycogenosis, in Gaucher's disease and in Niemann-Pick disease (Fig. 17.1). Storage diseases can and should often be diagnosed by other, usually biochemical methods, but even then electron microscopy can reduce the period of investigation by drawing attention to a likely diagnosis. Electron microscopy may show whether a liver-cell pigment is lipofuscin or the pigment of the Dubin-Johnson syndrome (Fig. 17.2) and can therefore be helpful when this syndrome is suspected but not fully proved by light microscopy.[10] In some patients with Wilson's disease, characteristic changes may be seen in liver-cell mitochondria (see below).

2 **To establish the presence of viral infection**. Electron microscopy of liver biopsies may prove to be important when serological test results or cultures for suspected viral infection are unavailable or incomplete. Both intranuclear and intracytoplasmic virions may be identified by the appearances of their spherical or hexagonal capsids, dense core material, surface envelopes and paracrystalline and lattice-like arrays. These features can be compared with published micrographs for identification of the candidate virion.[11,12] For example, some adult patients with the unusual finding of giant-cell hepatitis on routine light microscopy have been shown to have paramyxovirus-like particles in the liver as a result of electron microscopic studies of biopsy material.[13,14] Glutaraldehyde fixation of biopsy specimens is preferred, but viral particles can also be identified in formalin-fixed tissues which are washed and then processed for electron microscopy.

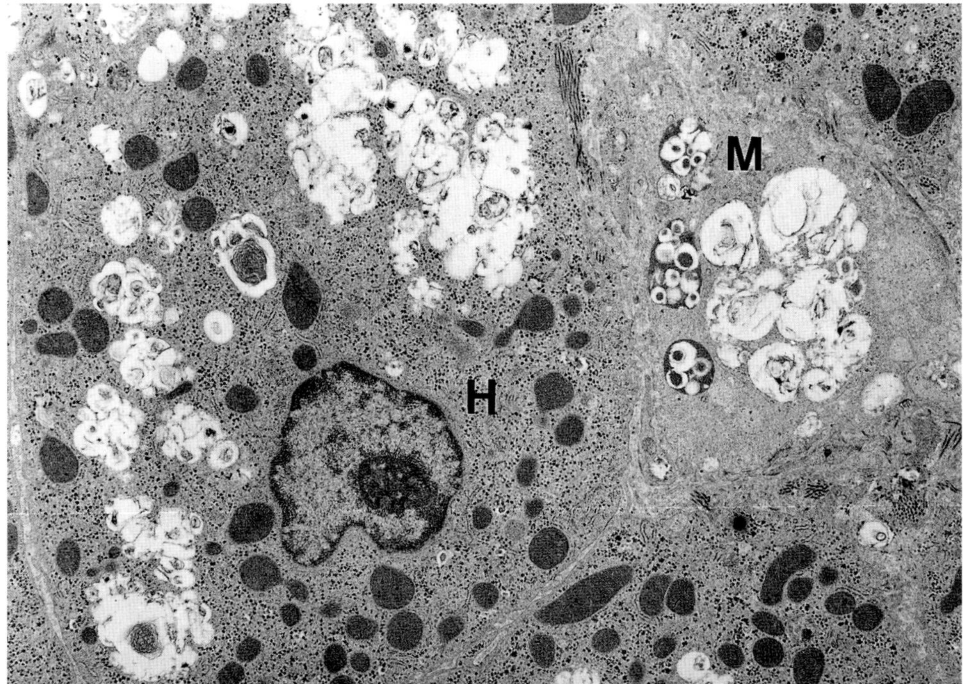

Figure 17.1 *Liver tissue from a patient with Niemann-Pick disease.* Macrophages (M) and hepatocytes (H) contain abundant vacuoles in which there are lamellar lipid inclusions. (Needle biopsy, lead citrate; ×4600).

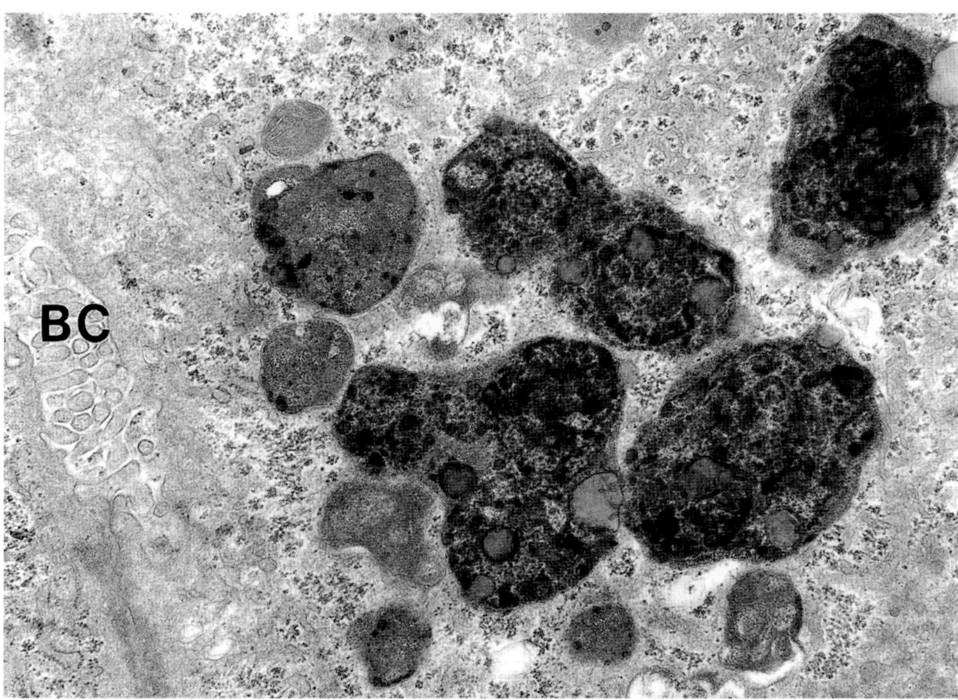

Figure 17.2 *Dubin-Johnson syndrome.* Large, characteristically complex dense bodies are seen near a bile canaliculus (BC). (Needle biopsy, lead citrate; ×18 900).

3 **To establish the nature of a tumour of doubtful histogenesis**. The ultrastructural features of many tumours, including neuroendocrine tumours and malignant melanomas, help in making a firm diagnosis.[15] The more obvious features such as neurosecretory granules in neuroendocrine tumours survive paraffin embedding; re-embedding of paraffin material for electron microscopy should therefore be considered.
4 **To establish the presence of specific drug-related changes**. In liver damage due to a small number of drugs, including perhexiline maleate[16] and amiodarone,[17–20] hepatocytes contain lysosomes filled with lamellar phospholipid material (Fig. 17.3).
5 **To provide material for research**. Electron microscopy offers wide potential for research into human liver disease and it may be that future research will increase the diagnostic value of electron microscopy in this field. If liver biopsy is performed in a patient having a disease with potentially helpful or interesting ultrastructural features, small pieces of the specimen can be embedded for electron microscopy and stored indefinitely in block form. The extent to which this is done clearly depends on the resources of the particular laboratory.

Whenever electron microscopy of a liver biopsy specimen is considered, the laboratory should be contacted beforehand and arrangements made for collection and fixation of the specimen at the bedside. Proper processing of the tissue, including optimal fixation, provides the basis for accurate analysis of ultrastructural changes.

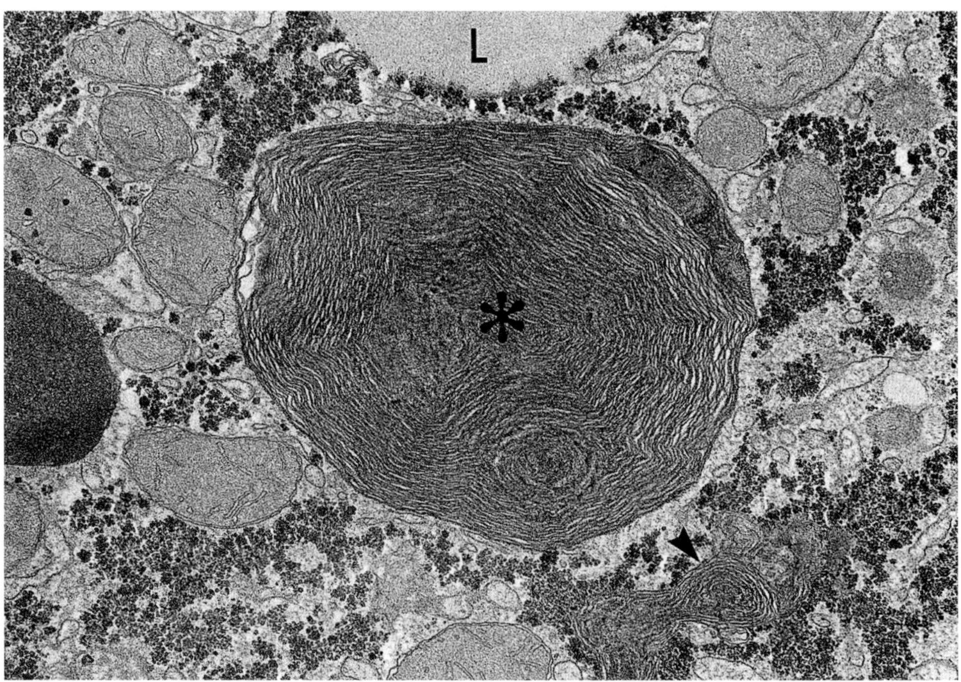

Figure 17.3 *Amiodarone-induced phospholipidosis*. An enlarged lysosome (asterisk), resembling a myelin figure, contains densely packed, concentrically arranged osmiophilic lipids, thought to represent drug–lipid complexes. A smaller membranous whorl (arrowhead) is seen in the cytoplasm. L, lipid. (Figure kindly provided by Dr S. Poucell and Professor MJ Phillips, Toronto). (Ferrocyanide; ×38 000).

THE NORMAL LIVER AND EXAMPLES OF ULTRASTRUCTURAL CHANGES IN DISEASE

The following description of the liver under the transmission electron microscope is a general one. It should be noted that the quality of fixation will influence the appearance of cells and organelles. The letters in the description of normal liver refer to Figures 17.4 and 17.5.

Several cell types are found in the hepatic lobules. The hepatocytes or parenchymal cells (PC) are separated from the sinusoidal endothelial cells (EC) by the space of Disse (SD), in which there are collagen fibres and stellate cells (SC), formerly known as perisinusoidal cells, Ito cells or fat-storing cells. Within the sinusoidal lumen are Kupffer cells (KC), the hepatic macrophages and large granular lymphocytes (also called pit cells), with natural killer activity.

Hepatocyte (liver cell, parenchymal cell)

Hepatocytes have similar features in different lobular regions, but vary in detailed structure. For example, there are more lysosomes and mitochondria in periportal than in perivenular hepatocytes, while the converse is true for the smooth-surfaced endoplasmic reticulum. The hepatocyte is a highly polarised cell with surfaces facing the space of Disse, other hepatocytes and the bile canaliculus. The plasma membrane is specialised in these three areas. Many microvilli project into the space of Disse and into the bile canaliculus. This is a potential space formed by two or three hepatocytes in normal liver and sometimes more in disease. The intercellular membrane of the hepatocyte is relatively smooth and forms several types of intercellular junctions.

The nucleus

The nucleus (N) is normally limited by a double membrane, the nuclear envelope, which is continuous with the rough-surfaced endoplasmic reticulum. The nuclear envelope has small pores which are thought to serve as a route of communication between the nucleoplasm and the cytoplasm. Within the nucleus there is irregularly distributed chromatin and a nucleolus is often visible.

Structural changes

Large amounts of monoparticulate glycogen are seen in some hepatocyte nuclei in diabetes mellitus, in children and also in normal subjects. In type B hepatitis, core virus particles are seen (Fig. 17.6). Intranuclear virions are also seen in infections due to cytomegalovirus, herpesvirus, echovirus and adenovirus.

Mitochondria

Mitochondria (M) are the sites of oxidative enzyme activity and are involved in the metabolism of amino acids, lipids and carbohydrates. There are approximately 2000 mitochondria within the hepatocyte.[21] A smooth outer limiting membrane and an inner membrane with deep infoldings, the cristae, give the mitochondria a

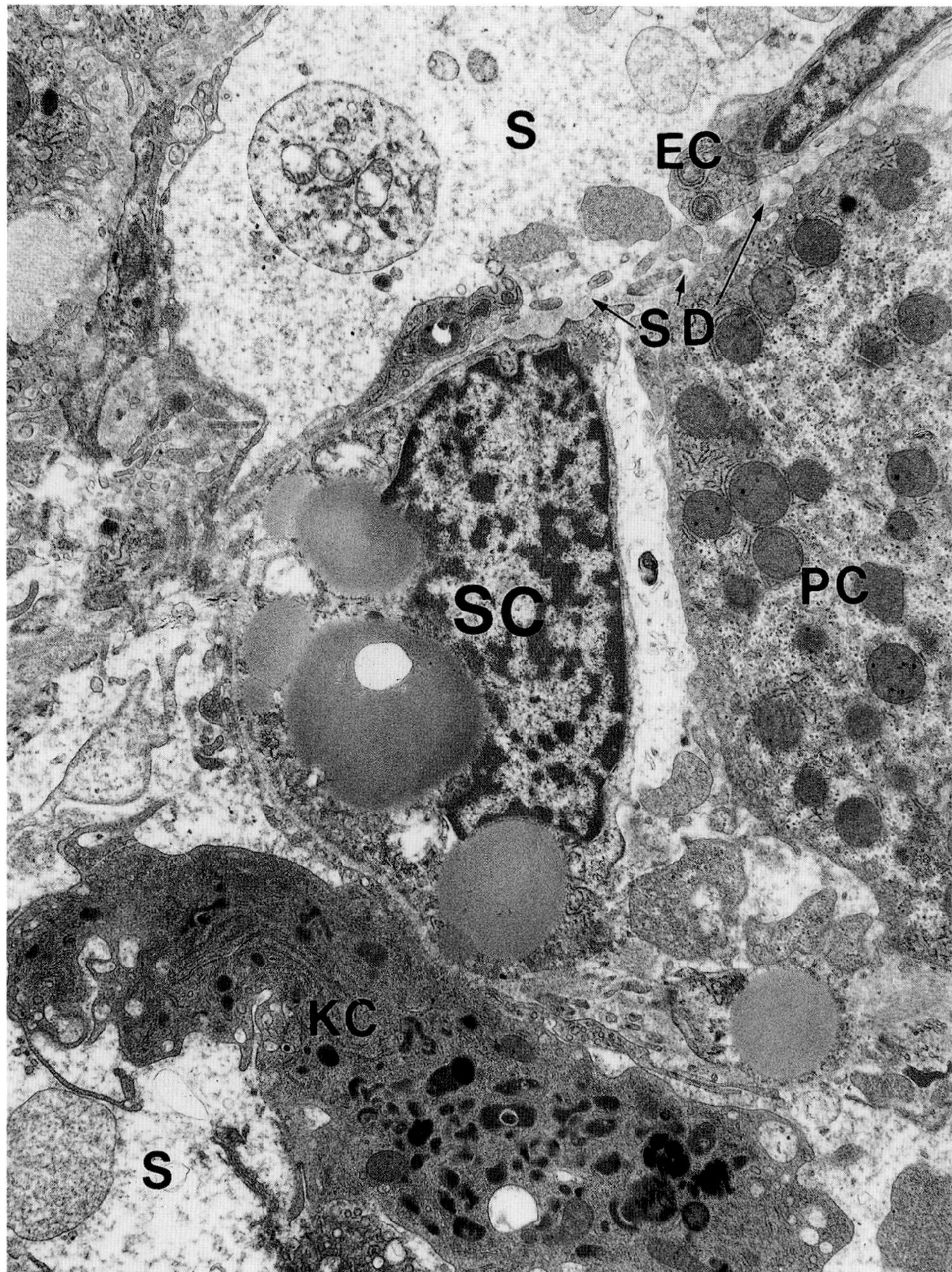

Figure 17.4 *Normal human liver*. At the edge of a liver-cell plate the parenchymal cell (PC) is separated from the sinusoidal lumen (S) by an endothelial cell (EC) and Kupffer cell (KC). SC, stellate cell; SD, space of Disse. (Needle biopsy, lead citrate; ×10 000).

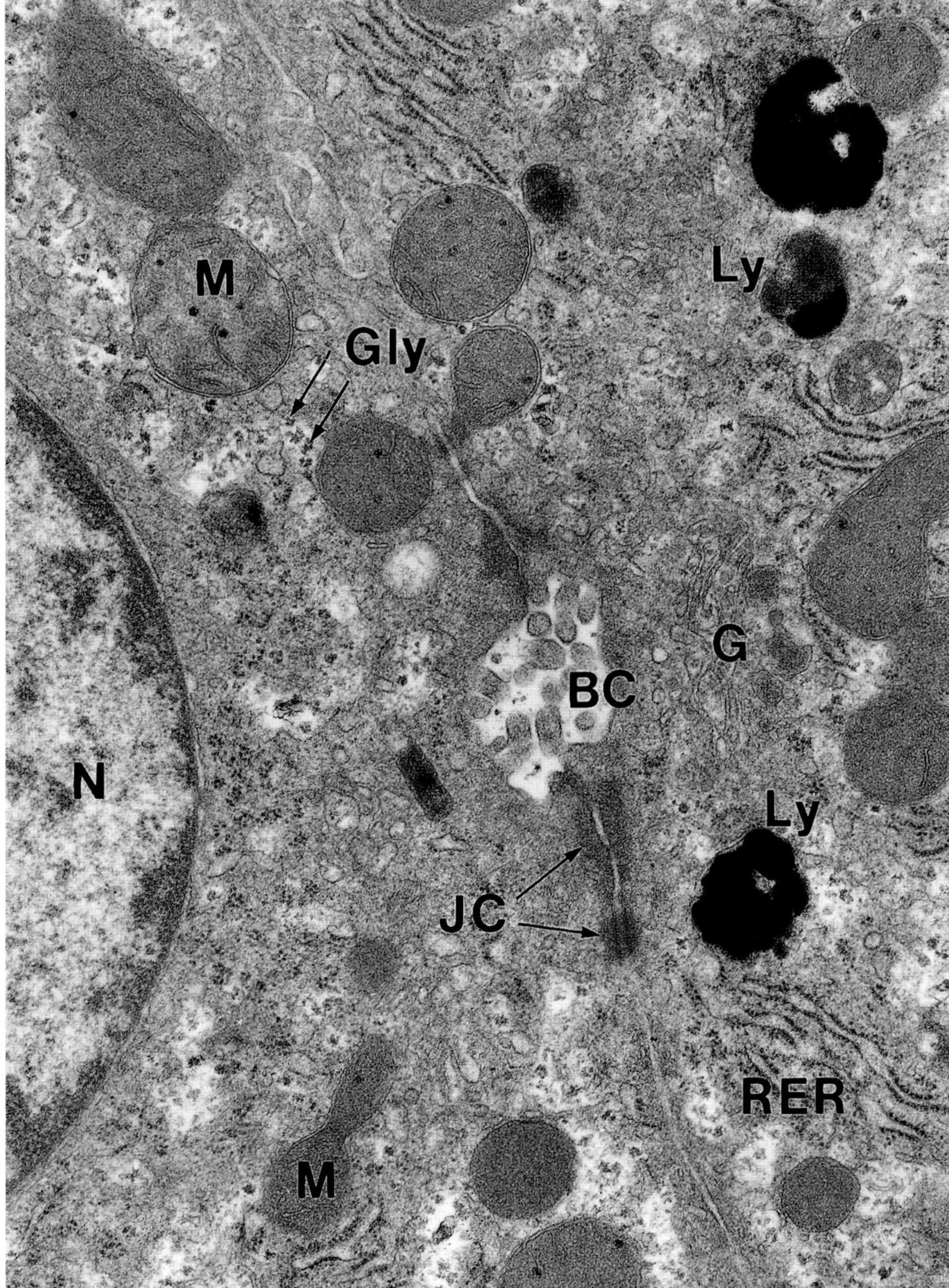

Figure 17.5 *Normal human liver*. Two parenchymal cells have formed a bile canaliculus (BC) delimited by junctional complexes (JC). Lysosomes (Ly) have varying density, the darker ones corresponding to lipofuscin as seen under the light microscope. N, nucleus; M, mitochondria; Gly, glycogen; RER, rough-surfaced endoplasmic reticulum; G, Golgi apparatus. (Needle biopsy, lead citrate; ×24 000).

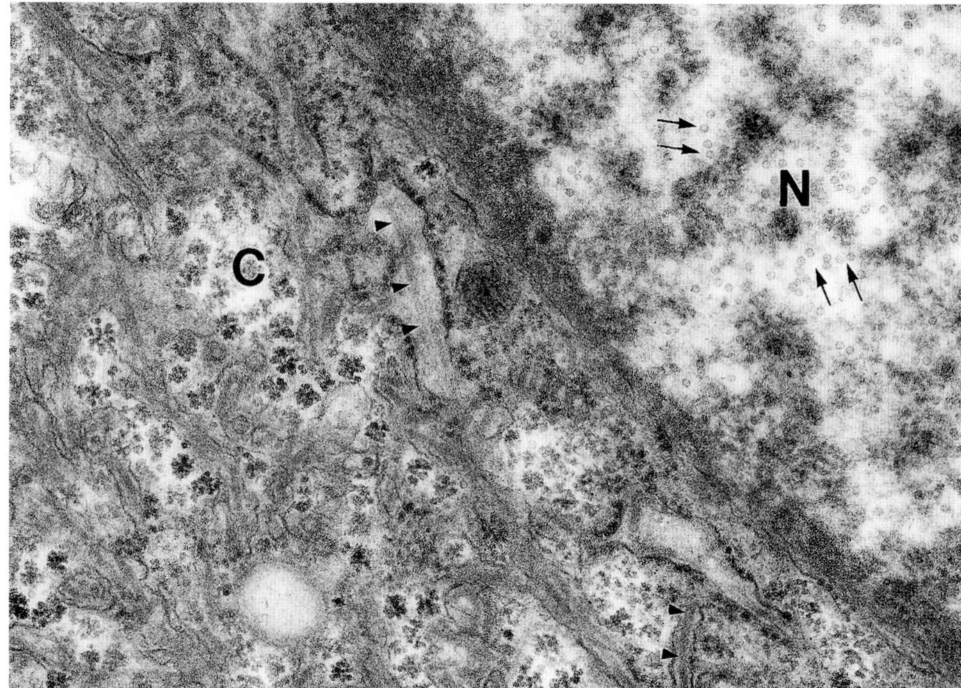

Figure 17.6 *Hepatocyte in HBsAg-positive chronic hepatitis.* In the nucleus (N) there are numerous core particles (arrows). The cytoplasm (C) contains irregularly shaped cisternae of the endoplasmic reticulum in which there are tubules (arrowheads), the morphological *in situ* counterpart of surface antigen. (Needle biopsy, lead citrate; ×45 000).

characteristic appearance. The inner membrane surrounds the mitochondrial matrix, which contains many dense granules.

Structural changes

Cristae of atypical shape, crystalline inclusions and enlarged or unusually scanty granules are found in a wide variety of conditions and sometimes also in the normal liver. Giant mitochondria are seen most often in alcoholic liver disease[22] but are also found in non-alcoholic fatty liver disease[22a] and other conditions.[23] Immunohistochemistry and immunoelectron microscopy can assist in their detection.[24] They are frequently found in patients with systemic sclerosis.[25] In early stages of Wilson's disease mitochondria show variation in shape, increased electron density, widening of the spaces between membranes, vacuolation, enlargement of matrix granules and deposition of crystalline material[26,27] (Fig. 17.7). Three types of Wilsonian mitochondria are described which show intrafamilial concordance.[28] Abnormal, swollen and irregular mitochondria are found in hepatocytes in Reye's syndrome[29] and other microvesicular fat syndromes.[30]

Endoplasmic reticulum

This is an important site of protein synthesis and transport. It also contains enzymes involved in drug and steroid metabolism. Morphologically the endoplasmic reticulum is a cisternal membrane-bound system continuous with the nuclear envelope. It is the morphological counterpart of the microsomes. Two main types of

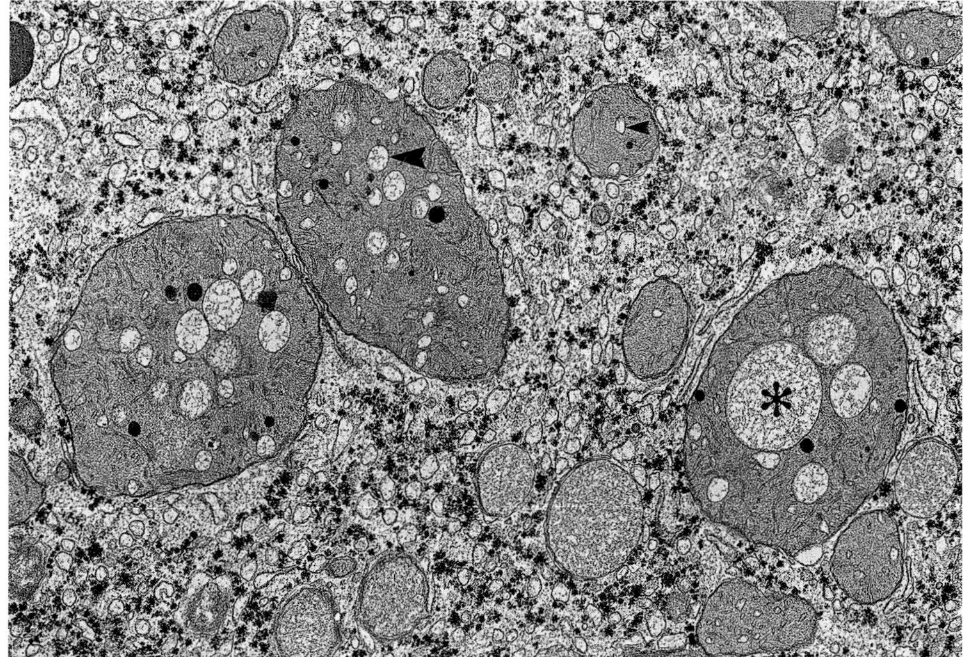

Figure 17.7 *Wilson's disease*. Hepatocyte cytoplasm with mitochondria showing dilatation of intracristal spaces (arrowheads). Some are microcystic and their contents finely granular (asterisk). Dense granules are prominent. (Figure kindly supplied by Professor MJ Phillips and Ms JS Patterson, Toronto). (Ferrocyanide; ×11 400).

endoplasmic reticulum can be recognised. The **rough-surfaced endoplasmic reticulum (RER)** is studded with ribosomes and is often arranged in a lamellar pattern. The **smooth-surfaced endoplasmic reticulum (SER)** lacks ribosomes and has a tubular or vesicular appearance.

Structural changes

Dilatation, degranulation, vesiculation and proliferation of the endoplasmic reticulum can be seen in many conditions. Some of these 'changes' are also influenced by the fixation procedure, making them difficult to evaluate. Their accurate quantitation requires carefully controlled processing conditions and morphometric analysis. However, in α_1-antitrypsin deficiency, the dilatation of endoplasmic reticulum is striking, and finely granular material accumulates in the cisternae (Fig. 17.8). In chronic type B hepatitis the cisternae are also dilated and contain tubular structures representing the surface material of the hepatitis B virus (Fig. 17.6) and sometimes complete Dane particles.

Lysosomes (Ly)

These organelles carry many different lytic enzymes and are involved in the breakdown of proteins, carbohydrates and lipids. **Primary lysosomes** are small vesicles containing enzymes, but not yet involved in catabolic processes. **Secondary lysosomes** are membrane-bound, often irregularly shaped electron-dense bodies in which the breakdown processes take place. When undigested residues accumulate and enzyme activity is diminished, the secondary lysosomes are called residual

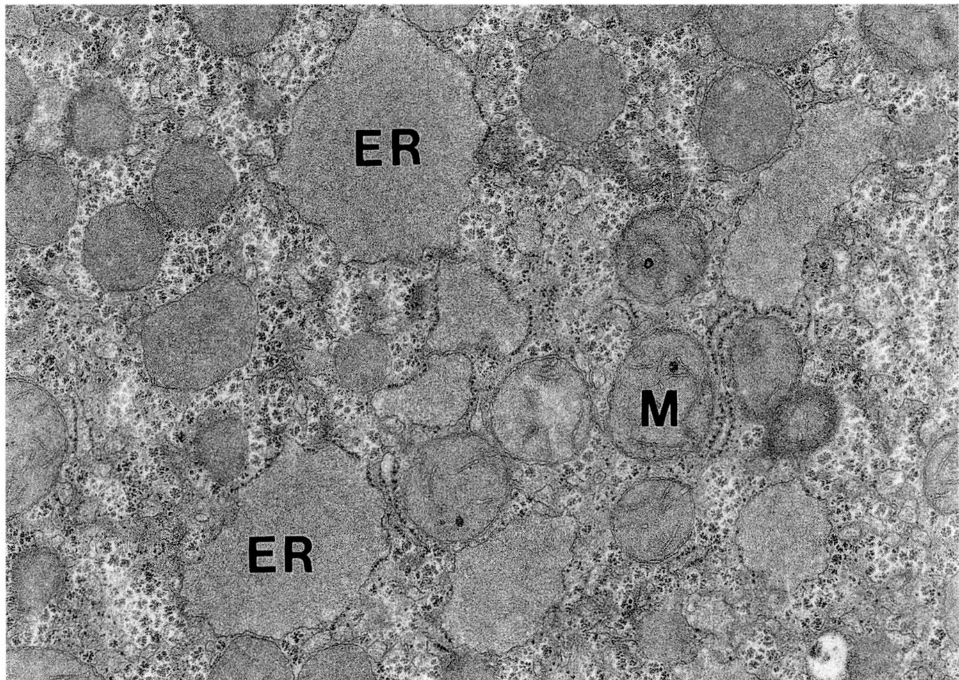

Figure 17.8 α_1-*Antitrypsin deficiency*. In this parenchymal cell the cisternae of the endoplasmic reticulum (ER) are dilated and filled with finely granular material. M, mitochondrion. (Needle biopsy, lead citrate; ×16 000).

bodies. These are the lipofuscin granules. All types of secondary lysosomes tend to be concentrated around the bile canaliculi.

Structural changes

Lysosomes accumulate iron pigment in various forms of iron overload, including hereditary haemochromatosis.[31] They can be strikingly enlarged in inborn errors of metabolism, such as Niemann-Pick disease (Fig. 17.1) and type II glycogenosis, or show characteristic changes as in the Dubin-Johnson syndrome (Fig. 17.2). Lamellar and reticular inclusions are seen within them in acquired, drug-related phospholipidosis.[16–20]

Peroxisomes

These are round or oval bodies with an even, granular matrix bounded by a single membrane. Human peroxisomes infrequently have a nucleoid, whereas this is seen in other species. They are most numerous in perivenular hepatocytes. They contain numerous oxidative enzymes and are involved in β-oxidation of long-chain fatty acids and synthesis of bile acids and prostaglandins. Their catalase enzyme mediates conversion of peroxidase to water.

Structural changes

Peroxisomes are absent in Zellweger's syndrome (cerebro-hepato-renal syndrome).[32] In alcoholic and drug hepatitis, catalase content of peroxisomes is decreased[33] and they show irregular shapes.[33,34] Increased numbers of peroxisomes are seen in alcoholic and drug hepatitis as well as in cirrhosis.[35]

Golgi system

The Golgi system (G) is a membranous system involved in excretory functions of the cell. It contains enzymes such as glycosyl transferases and is involved in glycoprotein metabolism. Morphologically it is composed of small groups of flattened sacs with associated vesicles.

Structural changes
The appearance of the Golgi system is influenced by fixation and changes are therefore difficult to quantify, but dilatation is evident in regenerating liver and in hepatocellular carcinoma. Electron-dense liposomes accumulate in the system during the development of fatty liver.

Cell sap (cytosol)

The soluble portion of the cytoplasm (cell sap) contains variable amounts of glycogen, free ribosomes, microtubules, intermediate filaments and microfilaments. A few lipid droplets and scanty iron-containing granules are also seen.

Structural changes
Ferritin particles accumulate in iron storage disorders.[31] Fat droplets are numerous in fatty liver, but the amount of fat varies greatly with the patient's state of nutrition. Core particles of hepatitis B virus can be identified in the cytoplasm in many cases of chronic type B hepatitis. Cytoplasmic crystalline inclusions are seen both in normal and in diseased livers. In alcoholic hepatitis, the Mallory bodies found in ballooned hepatocytes are composed of accumulations of cytokeratin and other proteins in the form of filaments (Fig. 17.9).

Bile canaliculus

The bile canaliculus (BC) measures approximately 0.75 μm and is formed by membranes of several contiguous hepatocytes, which are joined by tight junctions.[36] Surface microvilli covered with a thin glycoprotein coat project into the canalicular lumen. Actin filaments are present within the microvilli and extend downward into a pericanalicular web also composed of actin, functioning in canalicular contraction.

Structural changes
Alterations in the bile canaliculus are similar in many forms of cholestasis. Loss of microvilli, formation of surface membrane blebs and disorganisation of the pericanalicular actin filament web are common features. In the cholestasis related to preservation injury after liver transplantation, for example, ischaemia and reperfusion injury result in canalicular dilatation, loss of microvilli and compaction of actin filaments.[37] Intracanalicular bile appears as electron-dense filamentous material. Coarsely granular canalicular bile ('Byler bile') is a characteristic of progressive familial intrahepatic cholestasis type 1 (Byler disease) seen in Amish children and others with this disorder[38] (Fig. 17.10).

Kupffer cell

The Kupffer cell (KC) has an irregular outline, with many finger-like protrusions of the cell surface by which it is anchored to endothelial cells. It is rich in phagocytic

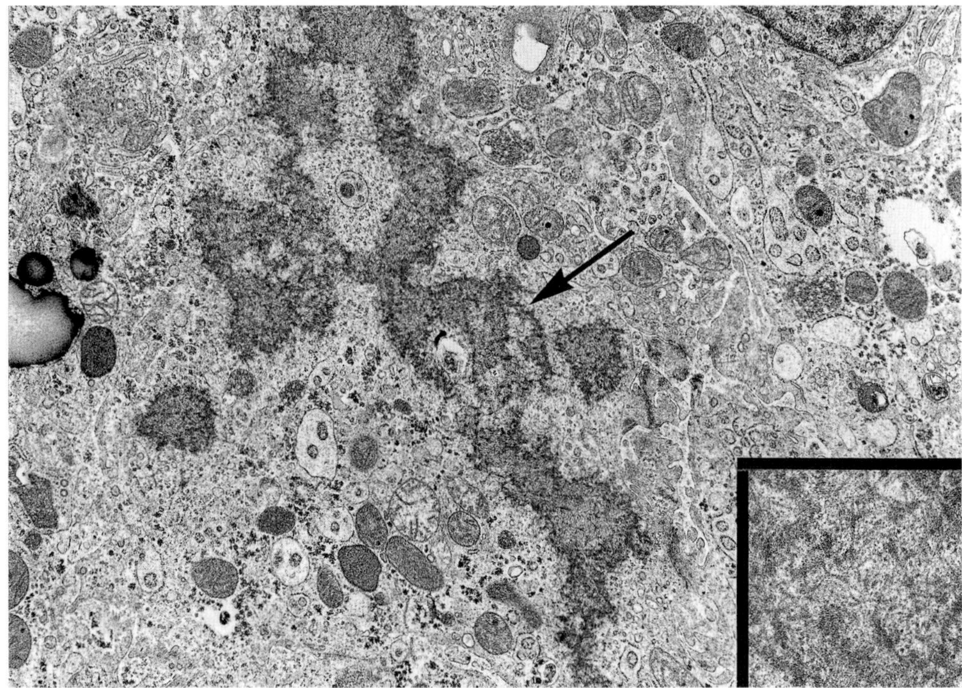

Figure 17.9 *Mallory bodies.* Irregular electron-dense material (arrow) is seen in the cytoplasm of a hepatocyte. The fibrillar nature of the material is evident at the higher magnification shown in the inset. (Needle biopsy, uranyl acetate and lead citrate; ×8600; *inset* ×27 000).

vacuoles (phagosomes), lysosomes and mitochondria, while the endoplasmic reticulum is only moderately well developed. The nucleus is irregular in shape, with a tendency for the chromatin to be concentrated at the nuclear periphery.

Structural changes

Hypertrophied Kupffer cells can be seen in all conditions of parenchymal cell destruction (e.g. hepatitis) and in pigment overload (e.g. cholestasis, siderosis). Many storage disorders affect the Kupffer cells; in Niemann-Pick disease, for example, both Kupffer cells and hepatocytes are enlarged and filled with vacuoles containing accumulated sphingomyelin (Fig. 17.1).

Endothelial cell

The endothelial cell (EC) is a flattened cell with a smooth surface, showing small fenestrations, which are thought to provide direct communication between the sinusoidal lumen and the space of Disse.[39] The cytoplasmic volume is relatively small. Many micropinocytotic vesicles can be seen beneath the plasma membrane.

Structural changes

In hepatitis and other conditions, endothelial cells undergo several changes, including the accumulation of iron-rich siderosomes and the formation of basement membrane material on the aspect of the cells facing the space of Disse.[40] In patients with chronic viral hepatitis and acquired immune deficiency syndrome,

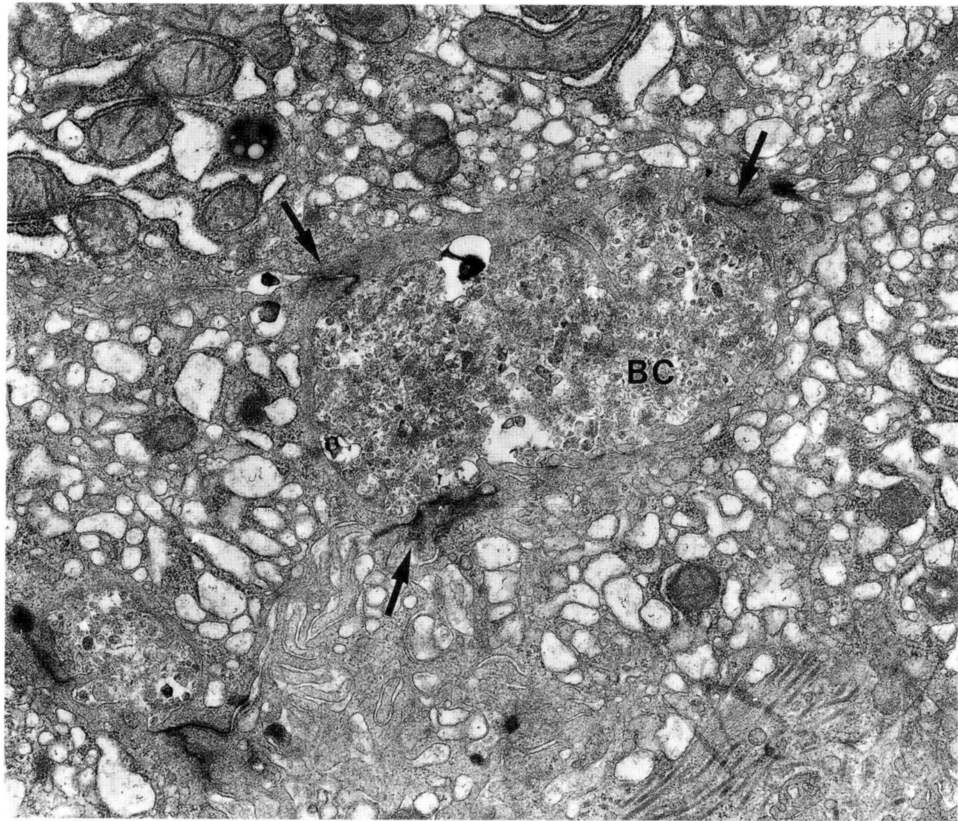

Figure 17.10 *Progressive familial intrahepatic cholestasis, type 1 (PFIC-1).* The dilated bile canaliculus (BC) contains coarsely granular bile ('Byler bile'), a feature associated with cholestasis in Amish children. The canaliculus is delimited by several junctional complexes (arrows) and has a reduced number of microvilli. (Figure kindly provided by Dr AS Knisely, Galveston, Texas). (Needle biopsy, lead citrate; ×24 475).

tubuloreticular structures and **cylindrical confronting cisternae** develop within the rough endoplasmic reticulum of endothelial cells and sometimes within Kupffer cells, stellate cells (see below) and lymphocytes.[41,42] Tubuloreticular structures are reticular aggregates of branching tubules within the cisternae of the endoplasmic reticulum and sometimes the perinuclear envelope. Cylindrical confronting cisternae are cylinders of fused membranous lamellae derived from two or more cisternae of endoplasmic reticulum, one inside the other. They appear to be a result of increased endogenous levels of α- and β-interferon. Membrane-bound dense bodies, seen on light microscopy as PAS-diastase-positive cytoplasmic granules, are sometimes present in chronic hepatitis B and C and autoimmune hepatitis[43] (see Fig. 9.10).

Stellate cell

The stellate cell (SC), previously known as the Ito cell, fat-storing cell, perisinusoidal cell or lipocyte, is a major storage site for vitamin A. In liver injury, it becomes a transitional cell or myofibroblast-like cell capable of synthesising collagen type I, III and IV, as well as laminin.[44] Stellate cells are located within the space of Disse and have conspicuous rough endoplasmic reticulum, a large Golgi apparatus and large lipid droplets containing vitamin A. In alcoholic liver disease, hypervitaminosis A and methotrexate toxicity stellate cells undergo hyperplasia and are associated with increased collagen fibres within the space of Disse. Multivesicular stellate cells with numerous lipid droplets have been reported in primary biliary cirrhosis.[45]

Pit cell (large granular lymphocyte)

This cell is located within the sinusoidal lumen, preferentially in the periportal region compared with the acinar zone 3.[46] Its surface uropodia and pseudopodia are often in close contact with endothelial cells or Kupffer cells. The nucleus is dense, eccentrically located in the cell and indented. The cell's name derives from its characteristic electron-dense, membrane-bound granules of cytotoxic enzymes, which resemble 'pits' or 'pips' in fruit. The cytoplasm contains profiles of rough endoplasmic reticulum, a well-developed Golgi apparatus, centrioles and occasional rod-cored vesicles. Pit cells function as natural killer cells and have been identified in autoimmune hepatitis and in increased numbers in livers with malignant tumours.[47]

Immunoelectron microscopy

The principles employed in immunohistochemical staining of liver biopsy sections for light microscopy (see Immunohistochemistry) can be adapted for use in electron microscopy.[48] Following fixation of the specimen in a mixture of glutaraldehyde and paraformaldehyde, the tissue is treated with borohydride, cryoprotected and frozen for storage. Thick sections of 20–40 μm are later cut from the thawed samples and stained by either a direct or indirect immunoperoxidase method.[49] The stained sections are then post-fixed in osmium tetroxide, dehydrated and embedded in Epon. Under the electron microscope, electron-dense immunoreactive material is seen at the site of the target antigen.

Availability of a wide variety of monoclonal and polyclonal antibodies to tissue antigens and receptors has greatly expanded investigations of interactions of hepatocytes with immune cells and with the extracellular matrix. Intercellular adhesion molecules, histocompatibility antigens and interferon receptors are among the potential list of antigens that can be studied by immunoelectron microscopy.[50–52] An example of this technique is shown in Figure 17.11 which demonstrates the up-regulation of the type A receptor for tumour necrosis factor on hepatocyte membranes in a patient with chronic hepatitis B.[53]

Scanning electron microscopy

The three-dimensional structure of the liver can be assessed by scanning electron microscopy (SEM) of specially prepared tissues,[54] or even of sections from paraffin blocks.[55] X-ray microanalysis may be combined with the scanning technique and is

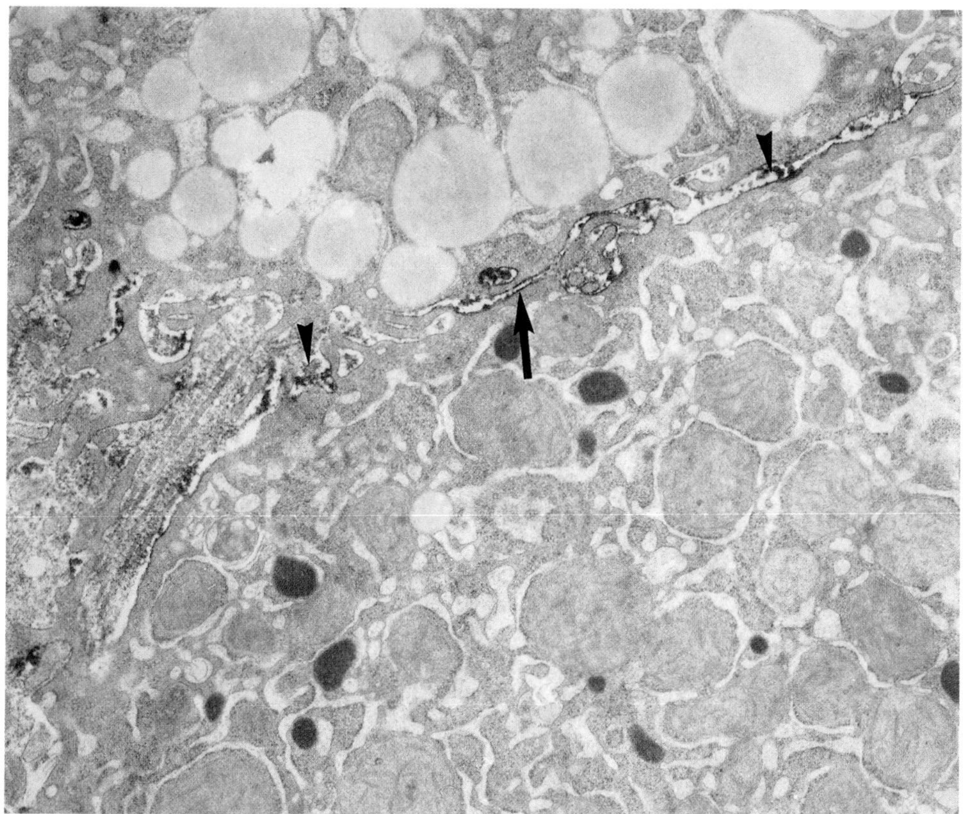

Figure 17.11 *Type A receptor for tumour necrosis factor (TNF).* A case of hepatitis B virus-positive chronic hepatitis stained with monoclonal antibody utr-1 (directed against type A receptor of TNF) shows positive staining on the membranes of two adjacent hepatocytes in a discontinuous pattern (arrow) and in the intercellular space (arrowheads). (Figure kindly provided by Drs VJ Desmet, R Volpes, J Van den Oord and R De Vos, Leuven). (Immunoelectron microscopy, ×18 400).

useful in elemental analysis. Laboratories with scanning electron microscopes are best equipped to provide details on appropriate tissue fixation, critical point drying and coating of specimens with gold or platinum. SEM is useful in examining bile ducts[56] and resin casts of hepatic vasculature.[57–60]

IMMUNOHISTOCHEMISTRY

Immunohistochemical techniques are now widely available in pathology laboratories and the methods for both immunoperoxidase stains and immunofluorescence microscopy are covered in standard textbooks.[61] Both direct and indirect labelling methods are used to detect antigens in liver biopsy tissue; the indirect method is the more popular and more sensitive. Important variables that may affect results include the type and duration of fixation, the vendor or other source used to obtain the antibodies and the type of label attached to the antibody for detection of the antigen. Microwave treatment of tissue sections in certain cases may improve antigen exposure for staining. While fixation in 10% neutral formalin is acceptable for many immunohistochemical stains, some will require alternative fixatives or cryostat sections and these factors should be considered when the biopsy specimen is initially processed.

In routine diagnostic work immunohistochemistry is helpful in four major areas:

1. *To ascertain the histogenesis of malignant tumours in the liver.* In distinguishing metastatic carcinoma from primary hepatocellular carcinoma, the former usually stain positively for epithelial membrane antigen and with the pooled monoclonal anti-keratin antibody AE1/AE3. Hepatocellular carcinomas show negative staining for cytokeratin 7 and 20.[62] α-Fetoprotein staining gives disappointing results in many hepatocellular carcinomas but is usually positive in hepatoblastomas. (This is discussed further in Ch. 11.)
2. *Staining for α_1-antitrypsin* (Fig. 13.14) is important in confirming the identity of diastase-resistant, PAS-positive periportal granules in chronic hepatitis, cirrhosis and in neonatal hepatitis.
3. *Identification of bile-duct epithelium.* Biopsy specimens which show an apparent paucity of interlobular bile ducts may benefit from specific staining for biliary cytokeratins 7 and 19 of the catalogue of Moll.[63] Biliary epithelium that may be obscured by inflammatory cell infiltrates in chronic biliary disease, drug-related hepatitis or liver transplant rejection can thereby be identified (see Figs 5.24, 5.25. Residual duct epithelium in segments of atretic ducts resected at the time of Kasai surgery for extrahepatic biliary atresia can also be demonstrated. Unusual patterns of the ductular reaction or remnants of the bile-duct plate (Fig. 13.5) can be studied with cytokeratin stains. AE1/AE3 pooled antibody generally gives good staining results.
4. *Localisation of viral antigens.* For patients with hepatitis B virus infection, immunohistochemical demonstration of surface antigen is more sensitive than non-immunohistochemical methods such as orcein or Victoria blue. In addition, assessment of the distribution of core and surface antigens when correlated with serum markers of viral replication and biopsy features on light microscopy usually provides a more comprehensive perspective regarding viral liver disease in any given patient. In some patients, demonstration of hepatitis D antigen by immunohistochemistry is the first evidence of delta virus infection or recurrence. Attempts at immunohistochemical staining of hepatitis C virus antigens using commercially available reagents have met with mixed results and other techniques such as *in situ* hybridisation[64] or polymerase chain reaction[65,66] may be more sensitive (also discussed in Chapter 9). Immunohistochemical staining for cytomegalovirus in post-transplantation liver biopsies is frequently required.[67]

Scientific questions of a more basic nature concerning the interaction of the immune system with the liver in various forms of injury, the composition of the extracellular matrix and factors involved in hepatocellular proliferation can be addressed with immunohistochemistry. For example, expression of intercellular adhesion molecules on the surfaces of hepatocytes for binding lymphocytes is of fundamental importance in interface hepatitis associated with chronic viral hepatitis[50] (Fig. 17.12). A histological index of liver-cell proliferation in acute and chronic liver disease can be obtained by staining for proliferating cell nuclear antigen (PCNA), an intranuclear auxiliary protein of DNA polymerase-δ,[68–71] and other markers.

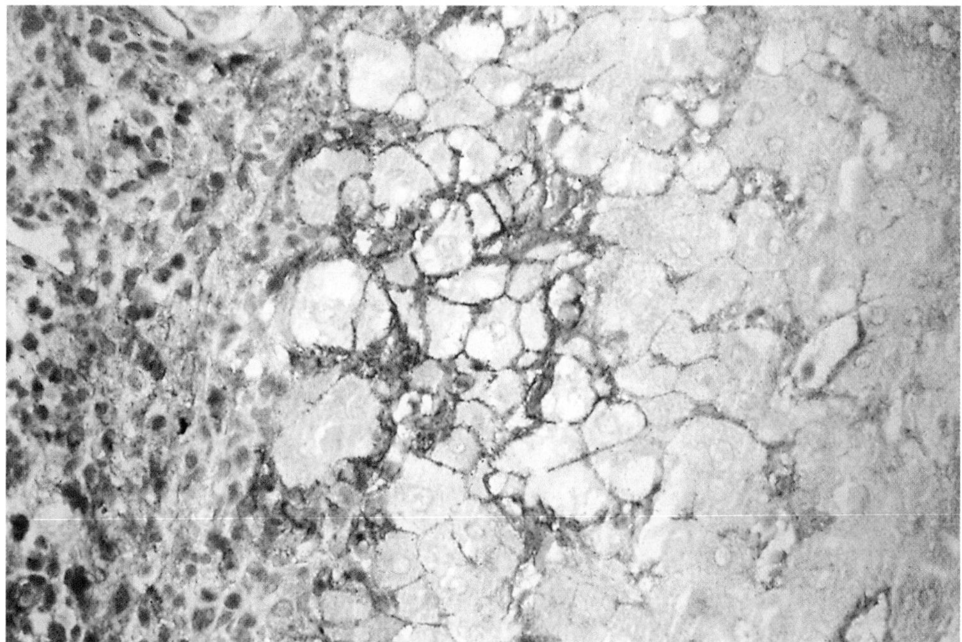

Figure 17.12 *Intercellular adhesion molecule-1 (ICAM-1) expression on hepatocytes.* Brown immunoreaction product to ICAM-1 is seen on periportal hepatocyte membranes in a case of chronic hepatitis. An inflamed portal tract is seen at left. The section was stained with monoclonal antibody 84H10 directed against ICAM-1. (Figure kindly provided by Drs VJ Desmet, R Volpes, J Van den Oord and R De Vos, Leuven).

IN SITU HYBRIDISATION

In this technique, radioactively labelled probes for specific RNA or DNA sequences are applied to cryostat tissue sections. Biotinylated probes can also be used on formalin-fixed, paraffin embedded sections.[72] Probes are prepared by cloning of genetic material and subcloning into plasmids. After preparation of the tissue sections, the probe is applied directly and hybridised. Slides treated with radiolabelled probes are then exposed to photographic emulsion for 1–2 weeks, resulting in a distribution of silver grains over cells containing the target RNA or DNA sequences. *In situ* hybridisation is widely used in research laboratories to localise gene sequences encoding hepatic secretory proteins such as albumin and extracellular matrix proteins. One of its major applications is in the identification of viral sequences, including cytomegalovirus[72] (see Fig. 1.10), hepatitis B virus and hepatitis C virus.[64] The sensitivity of *in situ* hybridisation can be improved by combination with **polymerase chain reaction**[73,74] (see below).

FLOW CYTOMETRY OF LYMPHOCYTES FROM LIVER BIOPSIES

In order to immunotype lymphocytes present in liver biopsy specimens, fresh samples of liver tissue are treated with enzymatic digestion and gradient centrifugation.[75] This technique has been used to analyse lymphocyte subpopulations in various forms of liver disease, including chronic hepatitis, primary biliary cirrhosis and alcoholic liver disease.[76,77]

CONFOCAL LASER SCANNING MICROSCOPY

The confocal laser scanning microscope has been referred to as an 'opto-digital microtome'[78] because of its capacity to obtain two-dimensional images from very thin optical sections of tissues or cells and to process them into three-dimensional data with digitised computer software. The primary advantages of this form of microscopy are its high resolution and enhanced contrast. These two advantages are obtained by using a very thin plane of focus provided by a laser light source (usually argon ion) filtered through several dichroic mirrors. The light emanating from a focal point in the specimen is imaged by back projection onto a detector pinhole aperture; the emanating light and the imaged light are in common focus, hence the name 'confocal'.

Following specimen fixation (usually by an aldehyde agent), one or more fluorescent reagents are used to label the specific antigen(s) under investigation. A series of two-dimensional images in a thin focal plane of approximately 0.6 to 1.5 μm are obtained through the confocal laser scanning microscope. These images are then aligned pixel by pixel using specific software image processing in order to generate three-dimensional data. Elements to be considered in planning confocal microscopy include the wavelength of light which the laser source can provide for excitation of the fluorochrome, appropriate stability of the antigen in tissue after fixation, mounting medium used and type(s) of fluorochrome to be utilised.[78] Dyes with widely separated excitation and emission wavelengths are optimal, such as fluorescein (FITC) or acridine orange for simultaneous DNA and RNA staining.

This technique is versatile; one can examine protein traffic in cells, localisation of matrix proteins,[79] metabolites produced in chemical hepatotoxicity,[80] DNA of individual chromosomes and ploidy status of tumours. *In situ* hybridisation can also be performed.

POLYMERASE CHAIN REACTION (PCR)

This is an *in vitro* method of nucleic acid synthesis by which small targeted segments of DNA (or RNA) can be amplified from biological samples. The ingredients for this method include two oligonucleotide primers that complement opposite ends of each strand in the target sequence, thermostable *Taq* DNA polymerase (or reverse transcriptase, in detecting RNA) and four deoxynucleotide triphosphates (dNTPs) in a buffered solution. The DNA strands are first separated by boiling. The oligonucleotide primers are then annealed to the target DNA, after which the primers are extended by *Taq* DNA polymerase. These extension products or daughter strands are complementary to and can bind the two primers, thereby allowing repeated cycles of denaturation and amplification and an exponential (2(n)) production of the target segment.[81–84]

Liver samples for polymerase chain reaction must be frozen in most instances.[85] However, extraction of nucleic acids from formalin-fixed, paraffin-embedded sections is also feasible and can be used in the diagnosis of genetic mutations, for example in the *HFE* gene in hereditary haemochromatosis.[86]

LASER CAPTURE MICRODISSECTION (LCM)

This technique obtains well-defined target cell populations (including immunostained cells) from formalin-fixed, paraffin-embedded tissue sections for molecular analysis using PCR. A thermoplastic polymer coating attached to a rigid support is placed in contact with a tissue section and is bonded to microscopically selected cell clusters by a near-infrared laser pulse.[87] The selected cells are then subjected to PCR. LCM improves the sensitivity of detecting genetic alterations in archival tissue samples[88] and can be applied to diagnostic and research problems in hepatic pathology, such as detection of hepatitis C virus RNA sequences in liver biopsies.[89]

GENE ARRAY ANALYSIS

The recent elucidation of the human genome has resulted in a number of functional genomics techniques by which gene profiling in normal and disease states can be undertaken. The liver transcriptosome expresses some 25–40% of the 39 000 genes in the human genome.[90] Snap frozen liver tissue can be used for comparative studies utilising oligonucleotide gene chip arrays and other methods and preliminary data have become available for a wide range of liver diseases. The relevance of this technique to liver disease has recently been reviewed.[90] As yet in its infancy, its potential applications provide the opportunity to directly correlate gene expression with cellular function, phenotype and alterations in disease.

REFERENCES

1 Burt AD, Le Bail B, Balabaud C, et al. Morphologic investigation of sinusoidal cells. *Semin Liver Dis* 1993; **13**: 21–38.

2 Rieder H. Meyer zum Büschenfelde K-H, Ramadori G. Functional spectrum of sinusoidal endothelial liver cells. Filtration, endocytosis, synthetic capacities and intercellular communication. *J Hepatol* 1992; **15**: 237–250.

3 Xiao J-C, Ruck P, Adam A, et al. Small epithelial cells in human liver cirrhosis exhibit features of hepatic stem-like cells: immunohistochemical, electron

microscopic and immunoelectron microscopic findings. *Histopathology* 2003; **42**: 141–149.
4 Nagore N, Howe S, Boxer L, et al. Liver cell rosettes: structural differences in cholestasis and hepatitis. *Liver* 1989; **9**: 43–51.
5 Nagore N, Howe S, Scheuer PJ. The three-dimensional liver. In: Popper H, Schaffner F, eds. Progress in Liver Diseases, Vol. IX, 1st edn. Philadelphia, PA: WB Saunders, 1989: 1.
6 Ludwig J, Ritman EL, LaRusso NF, et al. Anatomy of the human biliary system studied by quantitative computer-aided three-dimensional imaging techniques. *Hepatology* 1998; **27**: 893–899.
7 Jones S, Chapman SK, Crocker PR, et al. Combined light and electron microscope in routine histopathology. *J Clin Pathol* 1982; **35**: 425–429.
8 Spycher MA. Electron microscopy: a method for the diagnosis of inherited metabolic storage diseases. Electron microscopy in diagnosis. Pathology. *Res Pract* 1980; **167**: 118–135.
9 Ishak KG, Sharp HL. Metabolic errors and liver disease. In: MacSween RNM, Anthony PP, Scheuer PJ, et al., eds. Pathology of the Liver, 3rd edn. Edinburgh: Churchill Livingstone, 1994: 123.
10 Toker C, Trevino N. Hepatic ultrastructure in chronic idiopathic jaundice. *Arch Pathol* 1965; **80**: 453–460.
11 Miller SE. Detection and identification of viruses by electron microscopy. *J Electron Micro Tech* 1986; **4**: 265–301.
12 Phillips MJ, Poucell S, Patterson J, et al. The liver. An Atlas and Text of Ultrastructural Pathology. New York, N.Y.: Raven Press, 1987.
13 Phillips MJ, Glendis LM, Paucell S, et al. Syncytial giant-cell hepatitis. Sporadic hepatitis with distinctive pathologic features, a severe clinical course, and paramyxoviral features. *N Engl J Med* 1991; **324**: 455–460.
14 Fimmel CJ, Guo L, Compans RW, et al. A case of syncytial giant cell hepatitis with features of a paramyxoviral infection. *Am J Gastroenterol* 1998; **93**: 1931–1937.
15 Lloreta-Trull J, Serrano S. The current role of electron microscopy in the diagnosis of epithelial and epithelioid tumors. *Sem Diagn Pathol* 2003; **20**: 46–59.
16 Pessayre D, Bichara M, Degott C, et al. Perhexiline maleate-induced cirrhosis. *Gastroenterology* 1979; **76**: 170–177.
17 Poucell S, Ireton J, Valencia-Mayoral P, et al. Amiodarone-associated phospholipidosis and fibrosis of the liver. Light, immunohistochemical, and electron microscopic studies. *Gastroenterology* 1984; **86**: 926–936.
18 Simon JB, Manley PN, Brien JF, et al. Amiodarone hepatotoxicity simulating alcoholic liver disease. *N Engl J Med* 1984; **311**: 167–172.
19 Pirovino M, Müller O, Zysset T, et al. Amiodarone-induced hepatic phospholipidosis: correlation of morphological and biochemical findings in an animal model. *Hepatology* 1988; **8**: 591–598.
20 Lewis JH, Ranard RC, Caruso A, et al. Amiodarone hepatotoxicity: prevalence and clinicopathologic correlations among 104 patients. *Hepatology* 1989; **9**: 679–685.
21 Rohr HP, Lüthy J, Gudat F, et al. Stereology: a new supplement to the study of human liver biopsy specimens. In: Popper H, Schaffner F, eds. Progress in Liver Diseases, Vol. V, 1st edn. New York, N.Y.: Grune & Stratton, 1976: 24.
22 Uchida T, Kronborg I, Peters RL. Alcoholic hyalin-containing hepatocytes – a characteristic morphologic appearance. *Liver* 1984; **4**: 233–243.
22a Le TH, Caldwell SH, Redick JA et al. The zonal distribution of megamitochondria with crystalline inclusions in nonalcoholic steatohepatitis. *Hepatology* 2004; **39**: 1423–1429.
23 Chedid A, Jao W, Port J. Megamitochondria in hepatic and renal disease. *Am J Gastroenterol* 1980; **73**: 319–324.
24 Foschini MP, Macchia S, Losi L, et al. Identification of mitochondria in liver biopsies. A study by immunohistochemistry, immunogold and Western blot analysis. *Virchows Arch* 1998; **433**: 267–273.
25 Feldmann G, Maurice M, Husson JM, et al. Hepatocyte giant mitochondria: an almost constant lesion in systemic scleroderma. *Virchows Arch A Pathol Anat Histol* 1977; **374**: 215–227.

26 Sternlieb I. Evolution of the hepatic lesion in Wilson's disease (hepatolenticular degeneration). In: Popper H, Schaffner F, eds. Progress in Liver Diseases, Vol. IV, 1st edn. New York, N.Y.: Grune & Stratton, 1972: 511.
27 Scheinberg IH, Sternlieb I. Wilson's disease. Major Problems in Internal Medicine, Vol. XXIII. Philadelphia: WB Saunders, 1984.
28 Sternlieb I. Fraternal concordance of types of abnormal hepatocellular mitochondria in Wilson's disease. *Hepatology* 1992; **16**: 728–732.
29 Tonsgard JH. Effect of Reye's syndrome serum on the ultrastructure of isolated liver mitochondria. *Lab Invest* 1989; **60**: 568–573.
30 Lichtenstein GR, Kaiser LR, Tuchman M, et al. Fatal hyperammonemia following orthotopic lung transplantation. *Gastroenterology* 1997; **112**: 236–240.
31 Iancu TC, Deugnier Y, Halliday JW, et al. Ultrastructural sequences during liver iron overload in genetic hemochromatosis. *J Hepatol* 1997; **27**: 628–638.
32 Mooi WJ, Dingemans KP, Bergh Weerman MA Van Den, et al. Ultrastructure of the liver in cerebrohepatorenal syndrome of Zellweger. *Ultrastruct Pathol* 1983; **5**: 135–144.
33 Craemer D De, Kerckaert I, Roels F. Hepatocellular peroxisomes in human alcoholic and drug-induced hepatitis: a quantitative study. *Hepatology* 1991; **14**: 811–817.
34 Sternlieb I, Quintana N. The peroxisomes of human hepatocytes. *Lab Invest* 1977; **36**: 140–149.
35 Craemer D De, Pauwels M, Roels F. Peroxisomes in cirrhosis of the human liver: a cytochemical, ultrastructural and quantitative study. *Hepatology* 1993; **17**: 404–410.
36 Arias IM, Che M, Gatmaitan Z, et al. The biology of the bile canaliculus. *Hepatology* 1993; **17**: 318–329.
37 Cutrin JC, Cantino D, Biasi F, et al. Reperfusion damage to the bile canaliculi in transplanted human liver. *Hepatology* 1996; **24**: 1053–1057.
38 Bull LN, Carolton VEH, Stricker NL, et al. Genetic and morphological findings in progressive familial intrahepatic cholestasis (Byler Disease [PFIC-1] and Byler syndrome): evidence for heterogeneity. *Hepatology* 1997; **26**: 155–164.
39 Horn T, Lyon H, Christoffersen P. The blood hepatocytic barrier: a light microscopical, transmission- and scanning electron microscopic study. *Liver* 1986; **6**: 233–245.
40 Bardadin KA, Scheuer PJ. Endothelial cell changes in acute hepatitis. A light and electron microscopic study. *J Pathol* 1984; **144**: 213–220.
41 Schaff Z, Hoofnagle JH, Grimley PM. Hepatic inclusions during interferon therapy in chronic viral hepatitis. *Hepatology* 1986; **6**: 966–970.
42 Luu J, Bockus D, Remington F, et al. Tubuloreticular structures and cylindrical confronting cisternae: a review. *Hum Pathol* 1989; **20**: 617–627.
43 Iwamura S, Enzan H, Saibara T, et al. Appearance of sinusoidal inclusion-containing endothelial cells in liver disease. *Hepatology* 1994; **20**: 604–610.
44 Friedman SL. The cellular basis of hepatic fibrosis. *N Engl J Med* 1993; **328**: 1828–1835.
45 Cameron RG, Neuman MG, Shear N, et al. Multivesicular stellate cells in primary biliary cirrhosis. *Hepatology* 1997; **26**: 819–822.
46 Luo D, Vanderkerken K, Bouwens L, et al. The number and distribution of hepatic natural killer cells (pit cells) in normal rat liver: an immunohistochemical study. *Hepatology* 1995; **21**: 1690–1694.
47 Nakatani K, Kaneda K, Seki S et al. Pit cells as liver-associated natural killer cells: morphology and function. *Med Electron Microsc* 2004; **37**: 29–36.
48 Vos R De, Wolf-Peeters C De, Oord JJ van den, et al. A recommended procedure for ultrastructural immunohistochemistry on small human tissue samples. *J Histochem Cytochem* 1985; **33**: 959–964.
49 Elias JM. Immunohistopathology. A Practical Approach to Diagnosis. Chicago: ASCP Press, 1990.
50 Volpes R, Oord JJ van den, Desmet VJ. Can hepatocytes serve as 'activated' immunomodulating cells in the immune response? *J Hepatol* 1992; **16**: 228–240.

51 Horiike N, Onji M, Kumon I, et al. Intercellular adhesion molecule-1 expression on the hepatocyte membrane of patients with chronic hepatitis B and C. *Liver* 1993; **13**: 10–14.

52 Volpes R, Oord JJ van den, Vos R De, et al. Expression of interferon-gamma receptor in normal and pathological human liver tissue. *J Hepatol* 1991; **12**: 195–202.

53 Volpes R, Oord JJ van den, Vos R De, et al. Hepatic expression of type A and type B receptors for tumor necrosis factor. *J Hepatol* 1992; **14**: 361–369.

54 Vonnahme F-J. The Human Liver. A Scanning Electron Microscopic Atlas. Basel and Freiburg: Karger, 1993.

55 Ishak KG. Applications of scanning electron microscopy to the study of liver disease. In: Popper H, Schaffner F, eds. Progress in Liver Diseases, Vol. VIII, 1st edn. New York, N.Y.: Grune & Stratton, 1986: 1.

56 Petersen C, Grasshoff S, Luciano L. Diverse morphology of biliary atresia in an animal model. *J Hepatol* 1998; **28**: 603–607.

57 Haratake J, Hisaoka M, Furuta A, et al. A scanning electron microscopic study of postnatal development of rat peribiliary plexus. *Hepatology* 1991; **14**: 1196–1200.

58 Haratake J, Hisaoka M, Yamamoto O, et al. Morphological changes of hepatic microcirculation in experimental rat cirrhosis: a scanning electron microscopic study. *Hepatology* 1991; **13**: 952–956.

59 Gaudio E, Pannarale L, Onori P, et al. A scanning electron microscopic study of liver microcirculation disarrangement in experimental rat cirrhosis. *Hepatology* 1993; **17**: 477–485.

60 Terada T, Ishida F, Nakanuma Y. Vascular plexus around intrahepatic bile ducts in normal livers and portal hypertension. *J Hepatol* 1989; **8**: 139–149.

61 Taylor CR, Cote RJ. Immunomicroscopy: A Diagnostic Tool for the Surgical Pathologist (Major Problems in Pathology, Vol. 19). Philadelphia, PA: WB Saunders, 1994.

62 Wang NP, Zee S, Zarbo RJ, et al. Coordinate expression of cytokeratins 7 and 20 defines unique subsets of carcinomas. *Appl Immunohistochem* 1995; **3**: 99–107.

63 Moll R, Franke WW, Schiller D, et al. The catalog of human cytokeratins: pattern of expression in normal epithelia, tumors and cultured cells. *Cell* 1982; **31**: 11–24.

64 Felger RE, Montone KT, Furth EE. A rapid method for the detection of hepatitis C virus RNA by in situ hybridization. *Mod Pathol* 1996; **9**: 696–702.

65 Park YN, Abe K, Li H, et al. Detection of hepatitis C virus RNA using ligation-dependent polymerase chain reaction in formalin-fixed, paraffin-embedded liver tissues. *Am J Pathol* 1996; **149**: 1485–1491.

66 Lau GKK, Davis GL, Wu SPC, et al. Hepatic expression of hepatitis C virus RNA in chronic hepatitis C: a study by in situ reverse-transcription polymerase chain reaction. *Hepatology* 1996; **23**: 1318–1323.

67 Theise ND, Conn M, Thung SN. Localization of cytomegalovirus antigens in liver allografts over time. *Hum Pathol* 1993; **24**: 103–108.

68 Wolf HK, Michalopoulos GK. Hepatocyte regeneration in acute fulminant and nonfulminant hepatitis: a study of proliferating cell nuclear antigen expression. *Hepatology* 1992; **15**: 707–713.

69 Kayano K, Yasunaga M, Kubota M, et al. Detection of proliferating hepatocytes by immunohistochemical staining for proliferating cell nuclear antigen (PCNA) in patients with acute hepatic failure. *Liver* 1992; **12**: 132–136.

70 Kawakita N, Seki S, Sakaguchi H, et al. Analysis of proliferating hepatocytes using a monoclonal antibody against proliferating cell nuclear antigen/cyclin in embedded tissues from various liver diseases fixed in formaldehyde. *Am J Pathol* 1992; **140**: 513–520.

71 Siitonen SM, Kallioniemi O-P, Isola JJ. Proliferating cell nuclear antigen immunohistochemistry using monoclonal antibody 19A2 and a new antigen retrieval technique has prognostic impact in archival paraffin-embedded node-negative breast cancer. *Am J Pathol* 1993; **142**: 1081–1089.

72 Naoumov NV, Alexander GJM, O'Grady JG, et al. Rapid diagnosis of cytomegalovirus infection by in-situ

hybridisation in liver grafts. *Lancet* 1988; **1**: 1361–1364.

73 Nuovo GJ, Lidonnici K, MacConnell P, et al. Intracellular localization of polymerase chain reaction (PCR)-amplified hepatitis C cDNA. *Am J Surg Pathol* 1993; **17**: 683–690.

74 Komminoth P, Long AA, Ray R, et al. In situ polymerase chain reaction detection of viral DNA, single-copy genes, and gene rearrangements in cell suspensions and cytospins. *Diagn Mol Pathol* 1992; **1**: 85–97.

75 Hata K, Zhang XR, Iwatsuki S, et al. Isolation, phenotyping and functional analysis of lymphocytes from human liver. *Clin Immunol Immunopathol* 1990; **56**: 401–419.

76 Hata K, Thiel DH Van, Herberman RB, et al. Phenotypic and functional characteristics of lymphocytes isolated from liver biopsy specimens from patients with active liver disease. *Hepatology* 1992; **15**: 816–823.

77 Li X, Jeffers LJ, Reddy KR, et al. Immunophenotyping of lymphocytes in liver tissue of patients with chronic liver diseases by flow cytometry. *Hepatology* 1991; **14**: 121–127.

78 Neri LM, Martelli AM, Previati M, et al. From two dimensional (2D) to three dimensional (3D) analysis by confocal microscopy. *Liver* 1992; **12**: 268–279.

79 Vassy J, Rigaut JP, Briane D, et al. Confocal microscopy immuno-fluorescence localization of desmin and other intermediate filament proteins in fetal rat livers. *Hepatology* 1993; **17**: 293–300.

80 Pompella A, Comporti M. Imaging of oxidative stress at subcellular level by confocal laser scanning microscopy after fluorescent derivatization of cellular carbonyls. *Am J Pathol* 1993; **142**: 1353–1357.

81 Berk PD, Worman HJ. An introduction to molecular biology and recombinant DNA technology for the hepatologist. *Semin Liver Dis* 1992; **12**: 227–245.

82 Rose EA. Applications of the polymerase chain reaction to genome analysis. *FASEB J* 1991; **5**: 46–54.

83 Mullis KB. The unusual origin of the polymerase chain reaction. *Sci Am* 1990; **262**: 56–65.

84 Eisenstein BI. The polymerase chain reaction. A new method of using molecular genetics for medical diagnosis. *N Engl J Med* 1990; **322**: 178–183.

85 Shieh YSC, Shim K-S, Lampertico P, et al. Detection of hepatitis C virus sequences in liver tissue by the polymerase chain reaction. *Lab Invest* 1991; **65**: 408–411.

86 Press RD, Flora K, Gross C, et al. Hepatic iron overload. Direct HFE (HLA-H) mutation analysis vs. quantitative iron assays for the diagnosis of hereditary hemochromatosis. *Am J Clin Pathol* 1998; **109**: 577–584.

87 Suarez-Quian CA, Goldstein SR, Pohida T, et al. Laser capture microdissection of single cells from complex tissues. *Biotechniques* 1999; **26**: 328–335.

88 Giercksky HE, Thorstensen L, Qvist H, et al. Comparison of genetic changes in frozen biopsies and microdissected archival material from the same colorectal liver metastases. *Diagn Mol Pathol* 1997; **6**: 318–325.

89 Saito K, Sullivan D, Haruna Y, et al. Detection of hepatitis C virus RNA sequences in hepatocellular carcinoma and its precursors by microdissection polymerase chain reaction. *Arch Pathol Lab Med* 1997; **121**: 400–403.

90 Shackel NA, Gorrell MD, McCaughan GW. Gene array analysis and the liver. *Hepatology* 2002; **36**: 1313–1325.

GENERAL READING

Taylor CR, Cote RJ. Immunomicroscopy: A Diagnostic Tool for the Surgical Pathologist (Major Problems in Pathology, Vol. 19), 2nd edn. Philadelphia, PA: WB Saunders, 1994.

Berk PD, Worman HJ. An introduction to molecular biology and recombinant DNA technology for the hepatologist. *Sem Liv Dis* 1992; **12**: 227–245.

Watson JD, Gilman M, Witkowski J, Zoller M. Recombinant DNA, 2nd edn. New York, N.Y.: Scientific American Books, 1992.

Vonnahme F-J. The Human Liver. A Scanning Electron Microscopic Atlas. Basel and Freiburg: Karger, 1993.
Phillips MJ, Poucell S, Patterson J, Valencia P. The Liver. An Atlas and Text of Ultrastructural Pathology. New York, N.Y.: Raven Press, 1987.
Ghadially FN. Ultrastructural Pathology of the Cell and Matrix, 3rd edn. London: Butterworths, 1988.
Shackel NA, Gorrell MD, McCaughan GW. Gene array analysis and the liver. *Hepatology* 2002; **36**: 1313–1325.

Glossary

Note: Words in *italics* are defined elsewhere in the glossary.

Acidophil body (Fig. 6.2) A *hepatocyte* which has undergone *apoptosis*; now often referred to as an apoptotic body. See also *Councilman bodies*.

Acinus (Fig. 3.1) An anatomical unit based on blood supply, its three parenchymal zones containing successively less oxygenated blood. Zone 1 is nearest to the terminal portal vessels in a small portal tract.

Activity (Figs 9.7 and 9.8) In histological terms, an expression of the degree of hepatocellular damage and associated inflammation. Especially used in chronic hepatitis and cirrhosis, in which it forms the basis of *grading*.

Apoptosis (Fig. 6.2) Shrinkage and fragmentation of cells, seen in the liver mainly in the form of densely-stained rounded structures derived from hepatocytes but lying free outside the liver-cell plates.

Autoimmune hepatitis A form of hepatitis associated with high titres of autoantibodies in serum. Usually responds to immunosuppressive therapy.

Ballooning degeneration Swelling and rounding of hepatocytes, with loss of their normal polygonal shape. Different forms of ballooning are seen in viral hepatitis (Fig. 6.2) and steatohepatitis (Fig. 7.16).

Bile canaliculus (Fig. 5.2) The tubular space formed between the biliary poles of two or three *hepatocytes*, or more in diseased liver. The canaliculus has no separate epithelial lining of its own.

Bile duct (Fig. 3.2) The smallest ducts, the interlobular bile ducts, are centrally located in small portal tracts and are usually accompanied by blood vessels. In practice they are sometimes difficult to distinguish from *bile ductules*, the transition being gradual.

Bile ductule and canal of Hering (Fig. 3.3) At the portal–parenchymal interface the canalicular system drains into the *canals of Hering* which are partly lined by hepatocytes and partly by biliary epithelial cells (*cholangiocytes*). These in turn connect with bile ductules, fully lined by biliary epithelium.

Bile extravasate (Fig. 5.9) Leakage of bile from a duct into the connective tissue of the portal tract, occasionally seen in large bile-duct obstruction.

Bile infarct (Fig. 5.4) An area of liver-cell death in a cholestatic liver; often periportal whereas canalicular cholestasis is mainly perivenular. Bile staining is variable and may be absent. Bile infarcts are easily mistaken for accumulations of foamy macrophages.

Bile lake An accumulation of bile outside a liver-cell plate.

Bile thrombus (Fig. 5.2) Synonymous with bile plug: the accumulation of visible bile in a *bile canaliculus*.

Bilirubinostasis A term sometimes used for histological *cholestasis*.

Bridging fibrosis (Fig. 7.13) Linking of portal tracts and/or efferent venules by fibrous tissue.

Bridging necrosis (Fig. 6.8) Confluent hepatocellular necrosis and *collapse* linking vascular structures; usually and preferably confined to linking of portal tracts to efferent venules

Canals of Hering (Fig. 3.3) Structures lined partly by *hepatocytes* and partly by bile ductular epithelium. They are a probable site of *progenitor cells*.

Ceroid pigment (Fig. 6.4) Brown pigment

in macrophages, found after hepatocellular injury; rich in oxidised lipids and PAS-positive after diastase digestion. Distinct from *lipofuscin*.

Cholangiocyte Epithelial cell of the biliary tract.

Cholate stasis (Fig. 5.10) A term sometimes used for chronic cholestasis, on the assumption that the hepatocellular changes result from the accumulation of toxic bile salts. Also known as *precholestasis* or *pseudoxanthomatous change*.

Cholestasis (Fig. 5.2) In morphological terms, *bilirubinostasis* or visible bile in a section of liver. Also defined as failure of bile to reach the duodenum and biochemically as a type of jaundice with dark urine, pale stools, conjugated hyperbilirubinaemia and raised serum alkaline phosphatase.

Cirrhosis The transformation of the normal hepatic architecture into nodules separated by *fibrosis*.

Collapse (Fig. 4.2) Condensation of pre-existing reticulin framework as a result of necrosis. May be followed by *fibrosis*.

Confluent necrosis (Fig. 8.4) Death of groups of adjacent *hepatocytes*.

Councilman bodies *Hepatocytes* which have undergone *apoptosis*. The term is best restricted to yellow fever, the disease in which they were described by Dr Councilman.

Disse space (Fig.17.4) The space between the sinusoidal endothelium and *hepatocytes*; contents include extracellular matrix and *hepatic stellate cells*.

Ductopenia (Fig. 16.9) Loss of significant numbers of interlobular *bile ducts*. Causes include rejection of liver grafts, graft-versus-host disease, primary biliary cirrhosis, primary sclerosing cholangitis and drug injury. Diseases characterised by ductopenia are known as *vanishing bile duct syndromes*.

Ductular proliferation Use of this term is discouraged for the reason given in the next definition.

Ductular reaction (Fig. 4.6) A reaction of ductular phenotype, seen as an increase in ductular structures. This may be the result of proliferation of pre-existing ductules, but the new structures could also arise from biliary metaplasia of *hepatocytes* or from transformation of *progenitor cells*.

Dysplasia (Figs 10.8 and 10.9) A change in the size, nuclear-cytoplasmic ratio and/or nuclear appearances of hepatocytes, usually in chronic hepatitis and cirrhosis. Large-cell and small-cell types are described. Also known as large- and small-cell change.

Fat-storing cells *Hepatic stellate cells*.

Fatty liver disease Includes both steatosis and steatohepatitis, as in alcoholic fatty liver disease (AFLD) and nonalcoholic fatty liver disease (NAFLD).

Feathery degeneration (Fig. 5.3) A type of liver-cell injury in *cholestasis*, attributed to toxic effects of bile salts. Affected *hepatocytes*, often single cells lying within normal parenchyma, are swollen and have pale-staining feathery cytoplasm.

Fibrosis Formation of new collagen fibres. It may follow *collapse* of pre-existing connective tissue framework or arise *de novo*.

Focal necrosis (Fig. 9.7) Death of *hepatocytes*, singly or in small groups. Because of the rapid disappearance of the dead cells, focal necrosis is usually recognised by the presence of inflammatory cells and by a break in continuity of a liver-cell plate rather than by the presence of necrotic tissue.

Follicle See *lymphoid follicle*.

Glycogen vacuolation See *nuclear vacuolation*.

Grading Semi-quantitative scoring of the various processes comprising hepatocellular damage and inflammation, usually in chronic hepatitis. Numerical assessment of histological activity.

Granuloma (Fig. 15.1) A focal accumulation of epithelioid cells, which are modified macrophages with abundant cytoplasm and often curved, elongated nuclei. To be distinguished from simple accumulations of macrophages.

Ground-glass hepatocytes (Fig. 9.11) *Hepatocytes* with a well-defined, lightly eosinophilic homogeneous area occupying much of the cytoplasm. The commonest form is seen in the livers of patients infected with the hepatitis B virus.

Haemochromatosis (See also *siderosis*) A condition in which hepatic fibrosis and cirrhosis ultimately develop as a result of iron overload. The common form, hereditary haemochromatosis, is usually the result of mutations of the *HFE* gene on chromosome 6.

Hepatic stellate cells (Figs 8.9 and 17.4) Cells containing vacuoles rich in vitamin A, lying within the *Disse space*. In pathological conditions, they are able to transform into myofibroblasts and produce extracellular matrix components. Previously used synonyms include *fat-storing cells, Ito cells, lipocytes, parasinusoidal cells* and *perisinusoidal cells.*

Hepatocytes Liver cells.

Interface hepatitis (Figs 9.3 and 9.4) Death of hepatocytes at the interface of connective tissue and parenchyma in chronic liver disease, accompanied by inflammatory-cell infiltration. Characteristic of chronic hepatitis and synonymous with the older term *piecemeal necrosis.*

Ito cells *Hepatic stellate cells.*

Kupffer cells The resident macrophages of the liver, straddling the sinusoidal lumens.

Limiting plate The layer of *hepatocytes* next to a portal tract.

Lipocytes *Hepatic stellate cells.*

Lipofuscin (Fig 3.6) Pigmented granular material in *hepatocytes*, of lysosomal origin and most abundant at the biliary poles of the cells. Found in normal liver in greatly varying amounts.

Liver-cell plates (Fig. 3.5) Interconnecting walls of *hepatocytes*, one cell thick in adults. Thicker plates are found in children and in regenerating liver.

Lobular activity (Fig. 9.7) Inflammation and hepatocellular damage deep within the lobules, in contrast to *interface hepatitis.*

Lobule (Fig. 3.1) An anatomical unit with an efferent (centrilobular) vein at its centre and portal tracts peripherally.

Lupoid hepatitis An old term for *autoimmune hepatitis*, no longer in use.

Lymphoid follicle (Fig. 9.12) A structured accumulation of lymphocytes resembling the follicles of normal lymph nodes.

Mallory bodies (Fig. 7.11) Irregular, dense cytoplasmic inclusions with a cytokeratin component, often in the form of strands or garlands. Electron microscopy reveals a filamentous structure.

Massive necrosis (Fig. 6.11) *Multilobular necrosis* involving a substantial part of the whole liver. This usually leads to severe liver insufficiency.

Multilobular necrosis (Fig. 6.11) *Confluent necrosis* involving the whole of several adjacent *lobules*. The clinical effects are variable, depending on the extent of the lesion.

Non-alcoholic steatohepatitis (NASH) (Fig. 7.16) A form of hepatitis resembling alcoholic steatohepatitis but associated with other causes such as obesity, diabetes or drugs.

Nuclear vacuolation (Fig. 7.4) Empty *hepatocyte* nuclei in paraffin sections. May be due to glycogen accumulation, lipid, or invagination of cytoplasm. Glycogen nuclei, common in the young, the obese and the diabetic, are typically enlarged and have prominent nuclear membranes. The glycogen may be demonstrable histochemically but is often lost during processing.

Panacinar necrosis (Fig. 6.11) Necrosis of an entire *acinus.*

Panlobular necrosis (Fig. 6.11) Necrosis of an entire *lobule.*

Parasinusoidal cells *Hepatic stellate cells.*

Parenchyma The specialised tissue of the liver, as opposed to the connective tissue. Often used loosely to describe the contents of the *lobules* as opposed to the portal tracts.

Periportal The part of the hepatic *lobule* or *acinus* next to a small portal tract.

Perisinusoidal cells *Hepatic stellate cells.*

Piecemeal necrosis *Interface hepatitis* is now often used for this process, because it almost certainly involves *apoptosis* rather than, or as well as, necrosis.

Polyploidy (Fig. 3.9) The coexistence of different classes of nuclei containing multiple sets of chromosomes (e.g. quadriploid, octaploid); a normal state in adult human liver.

Portal triad (Fig. 3.2) The triad of artery, vein and *bile duct* present in most portal tracts.

Precholestasis (Fig. 5.10) See *cholate stasis.*

Progenitor cell A partly committed cell capable of producing a range of specialised cell types. In the liver, progenitor cells are probably located in *bile ductules* or *canals of Hering*. See also *stem cell.*

Pseudoacini *Rosettes.*

Pseudoxanthomatous change (Fig. 5.10) See *cholate stasis.*

Regeneration (Fig. 10.6) Loosely used to describe hepatocellular hyperplasia following injury or loss. Not easily recognised in conventional sections because of low mitotic rate; characterised by increase in the thickness of the cell plates.

Rosettes (Figs 4.4, 9.8 and 9.14) In liver pathology this term refers to a change of the normal plate pattern of *hepatocytes* to glandular structures formed by several *hepatocytes*. Different types of rosette formation are seen in *cholestasis* and in chronic hepatitis.

Septa (Fig. 10.16) Walls of fibrous tissue, seen in two-dimensional sections as lines or bands. Septa may be formed by *collapse* ('passive septa'), by new fibre formation ('active septa') or by both.

Siderosis The presence of stainable iron in any component of liver tissue. The many causes of siderosis include several diseases under the heading of *haemochromatosis*, in which progressive iron accumulation leads to *fibrosis* and *cirrhosis*. However, at an early stage of hereditary *haemochromatosis* there is iron deposition without *fibrosis*.

Spotty necrosis Widespread, but patchy hepatocellular necrosis, typical of acute hepatitis.

Staging The semi-quantitative assessment of structural changes including *fibrosis* and *cirrhosis*.

Steatohepatitis (Fig. 7.8) A form of hepatitis characterised by *steatosis*, hepatocellular *ballooning*, *Mallory bodies* and pericellular fibrosis.

Steatosis (Figs 7.1 and 7.2) The accumulation of excess lipid in *hepatocytes*

Stellate cells The same as *hepatic stellate cells*.

Stem cell A self-renewing cell with the potential to give rise to a variety of cells including *progenitor cells*.

Vanishing bile duct syndromes Disorders characterised by loss of bile ducts leading to *ductopenia* (paucity of ducts) with consequent *cholestasis*.

Index

Bold numbers denote **main entries**

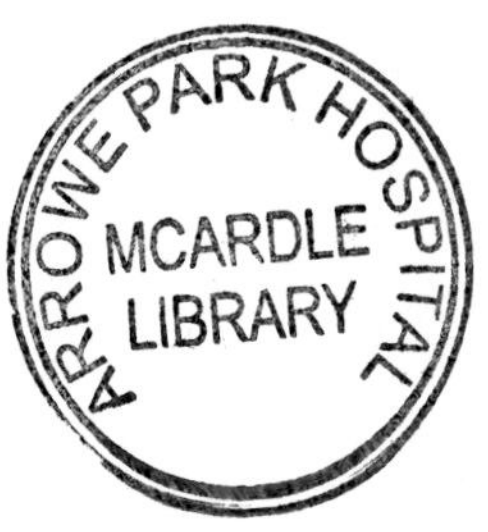